Different **types of images**:
- Realistic and detailed anatomical illustrations for in-depth views
- Schematic illustrations to see functional relationships
- Photos of surface anatomy
- Orientation sketches
- Photographs of imaging processes

The figures

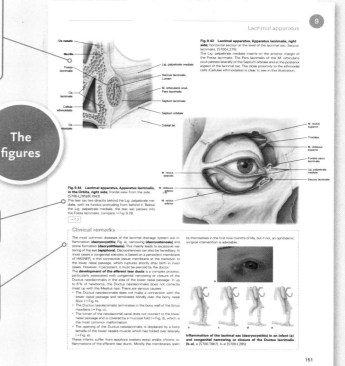

Detailed figure captions clarify the most important structures and topographical relationships.

The **illustrated Clinical remarks** feature shows a picture of the affected body area, which helps you to remember what you have learnt.

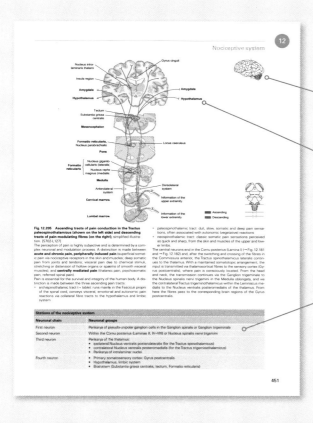

Orientation sketches give you the anatomical section depicted at a glance.

Learning tip: important structures are shown in **bold**.

Tables help to identify the relevant relationships.

Sample questions from the exam

Sample questions from an **oral anatomy exam** are given at the end of each chapter to test your knowledge.

You will find these topics in the 17th edition

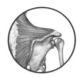
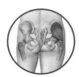
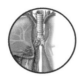
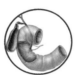

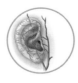

General Anatomy and Musculoskeletal System

Volume 1 General Anatomy and Musculoskeletal System

Inner Organs

Volume 2 Inner Organs

Head, Neck and Neuroanatomy

Volume 3 Head, Neck and Neuroanatomy

Learning Tables

F. Paulsen, J. Waschke

Sobotta

Atlas of Anatomy

Translated by
T. Klonisch and S. Hombach-Klonisch

Friedrich Paulsen, Jens Waschke (eds.)

Sobotta

Atlas of Anatomy

Head, Neck and Neuroanatomy

17th Edition

English version with Latin nomenclature

Translated by
T. Klonisch and S. Hombach-Klonisch,
Winnipeg, Canada

ELSEVIER

Original Publication
Sobotta Atlas der Anatomie, 25. Auflage
© Elsevier GmbH, 2022.
All rights reserved.
ISBN 978-3-437-44150-9

This translation of Sobotta Atlas der Anatomie, 25th edition by Friedrich Paulsen and Jens Waschke was undertaken by Elsevier GmbH.

Elsevier GmbH, Bernhard-Wicki-Str. 5, 80636 Munich, Germany
We are grateful for any feedback and suggestions sent to:
kundendienst@elsevier.com

ISBN 978-0-7020-6767-9

Notice
Practitioners and researchers must always rely on their own experience and knowledge in evaluating and using any information, methods, compounds or experiments described herein. Because of rapid advances in the medical sciences, in particular, independent verification of diagnoses and drug dosages should be made. To the fullest extent of the law, no responsibility is assumed by Elsevier, authors, editors or contributors for any injury and/or damage to persons or property as a matter of products liability, negligence or otherwise, or from any use or operation of any methods, products, instructions, or ideas contained in the material herein.

Bibliographical information published by the Deutsche Nationalbibliothek
The Deutsche Nationalbibliothek lists this publication in the Deutsche Nationalbibliografie: detailed bibliographic data are available on the internet at https://www.dnb.de

23 24 25 26 27   5 4 3 2 1

For copyright details for illustrations, see the credits for respective images.

Content strategist: Sonja Frankl
Project management: Dr. Andrea Beilmann, Sibylle Hartl
Editing and translating: Marieke O'Connor, Oxford, U.K.
Media rights management: Sophia Höver, Munich, Germany
Production management: Dr. Andrea Beilmann, Sibylle Hartl
Design: Nicola Kerber, Olching, Germany
Typesetting: abavo GmbH, Buchloe, Germany
Printing and binding: Drukarnia Dimograf Sp. z o. o., Bielsko-Biała, Poland
Cover design: Stefan Hilden, hilden_design, Munich; SpieszDesign, Neu-Ulm, Germany

Updated information is available on the internet at **www.elsevier.de**

This atlas was founded by Johannes Sobotta †, former Professor of Anatomy and Director of the Anatomical Institute of the University in Bonn, Germany.

German editions:
1st Edition: 1904–1907 J. F. Lehmanns Verlag, Munich, Germany
2nd–11th Edition: 1913–1944 J. F. Lehmanns Verlag, Munich, Germany
12th Edition: 1948 and following editions Urban & Schwarzenberg, Munich, Germany
13th Edition: 1953, ed. H. Becher
14th Edition: 1956, ed. H. Becher
15th Edition: 1957, ed. H. Becher
16th Edition: 1967, ed. H. Becher
17th Edition: 1972, eds. H. Ferner and J. Staubesand
18th Edition: 1982, eds. H. Ferner and J. Staubesand
19th Edition: 1988, ed. J. Staubesand
20th Edition: 1993, eds. R. Putz and R. Pabst, Urban & Schwarzenberg, Munich, Germany
21st Edition: 2000, eds. R. Putz and R. Pabst, Urban & Fischer, Munich, Germany
22nd Edition: 2006, eds. R. Putz and R. Pabst, Urban & Fischer, Munich, Germany
23rd Edition: 2010, eds. F. Paulsen and J. Waschke, Urban & Fischer, Elsevier, Munich, Germany
24th Edition: 2017, eds. F. Paulsen and J. Waschke, Elsevier, Munich, Germany
25th Edition: 2022, eds. F. Paulsen and J. Waschke, Elsevier, Munich, Germany

Foreign Editions:
Arabic
Chinese
Croatian
Czech
English (nomenclature in English or Latin)
French
Greek
Hungarian
Indonesian
Italian
Japanese
Korean
Polish
Portuguese
Russian
Spanish
Turkish
Ukrainian

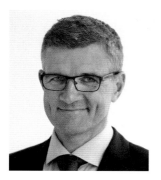

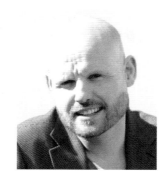

Prof. Dr. Friedrich Paulsen
Dissecting courses for students

In his teaching, Friedrich Paulsen puts great emphasis on students actually being able to dissect the cadavers of body donors. *'The hands-on experience in dissection is extremely important not only for the three-dimensional understanding of anatomy and as the basis for virtually every medical profession, but for many students also clearly addresses the issue of death and dying for the first time. The members of the dissection team not only study anatomy but also learn to deal with a particular situation. Medical students will never again come into such close contact with their classmates and teachers.'*

Friedrich Paulsen was born in Kiel in 1965. After completing his school education in Brunswick he first trained as a nurse. He then studied human medicine at the Christian-Albrecht University of Kiel (CAU). After acting as an AiP (Doctor in Practice) at the university clinic for Oral and Maxillofacial Surgery, and after acting as a doctor's assistant at the University ENT Clinic, he took on the position of assistant at the Anatomical Institute of the CAU in 1998, during an *'Ärzteschwemme'*, obtaining a qualification in the subject of anatomy under Prof Dr Bernhard Tillmann, MD. In 2003 he was appointed to the posts of C3-Professor for Anatomy at the Ludwig-Maximilians-University in Munich and the Martin Luther University, Halle-Wittenberg. In Halle he founded a further Education Centre for Clinical Anatomy. Further posts followed at the ordinariat at the Universities of Saarland, Tübingen and Vienna, as well as at the Friedrich Alexander University (FAU), Erlangen-Nuremberg, where he has been the Professor for Anatomy and the Institute Director since 2010. From 2016 to 2018 he was Vice President for Education and from 2018 until 2022 Vice President for the People, and thereby a part of the FAU university leadership. Since 2006 he has been the publisher of the magazine 'Annals of Anatomy' and since 2014 he has belonged to the Commission of Experts of the IMPP (Institute for medical and pharmaceutical examination issues). Friedrich Paulsen is honorary member of the Anatomical Society (Great Britain and Ireland) as well as of the Societatea Anatomistilor (Rumania). Since 2006 he has been the secretary of the Anatomical Society, from 2009 to 2019 he was the Secretary-General of the International Federation of Associations of Anatomy (IFAA), the international governing body of the anatomists and since 2021 he has been the president of the European Federation of Experimental Morphology (EFEM), the governing body of European anatomists. In addition, he is the Visiting Professor at the Department of Topographic Anatomy and Operative Surgery of the Sechenov University (Moscow/Russia) and was Visiting Professor at the Wroclaw Medical University (Wroclaw/Poland) and the Khon-Kaen University (Khon-Kaen/Thailand). He has received numerous scientific awards, including the Dr. Gerhard Mann SICCA research award from the professional organisation of ophthalmologists in Germany (Berufsverband der Augenärzte Deutschland), the Golden Lion from the German Ophthalmosurgeons, the Commemorative Medal from the Comenius University Bratislava as well as numerous awards for outstanding teaching.

His areas of focus in research concerns the surface of the eye, the protein and peptides in tears and the lacrimal system, as well as the causes of dry eyes.

Prof. Dr. med. Friedrich Paulsen

Prof. Dr. Jens Waschke
More clinical relevance in teaching

For Jens Waschke, one of the most important challenges of modern anatomy is to target the actual demands of clinical training and practice. *'The clinical aspects in the atlas direct the students within the first semester towards anatomy and show them how important the subject is for clinical practice in the future. The biggest challenge for modern anatomy is to focus on the relevant educational objectives. In our books we want to consolidate the important anatomical details, leaving out the unnecessary clinical knowledge aimed at specialists. At the start of their training, students are unable to differentiate between basic and specialist knowledge, and we need to avoid our young colleagues being overloaded instead of concentrating on the basics.'*

Jens Waschke (born 1974 in Bayreuth) studied medicine at the University of Würzburg and graduated in 2000 in Anatomy. After his AiP in Anatomy and Internal Medicine, he became qualified in 2007 in Anatomy and Cell Biology. Between 2003 and 2004 he completed a nine-month research placement in Physiology at the University of California in Davis, USA. From 2008 he held the newly founded Chair III at the University of Würzburg, before being appointed to the Ludwig-Maximilians-University in Munich, where he has been the head of Chair I at the Institute of Anatomy. He has turned down further appointments to Vienna (MUW) and Hanover (MHH).

Since 2012 he has been the head of the software company quo WADIS-Anatomie with Dr. Andreas Dietz. In 2018, Jens Waschke was chosen to be the president of the Anatomical Society and is a member of its board until 2022. In addition, he is a honorary founding member of the Anatomical Society of Ethiopia and member of the Commission of Experts of the IMPP.

In 2019, Jens Waschke published the book *Humans – Simply Genius!*, to make anatomy more easily understandable to the wider public. In 2021 he published his first anatomical crime novel *One Leg*. In his research as a cell biologist, Jens Waschke examines the mechanisms controlling the adherence between cells and the binding function of the outer and inner barriers of the human body. His main focus of interest is the mechanisms leading to the malfunctioning of cell adherence which variously cause the blister-forming skin disease pemphigus, arrhythmogenic cardiomyopathy or CROHN's disease. His goal is to understand cell adherence better and to discover new forms of treatment.

Prof. Dr. med. Jens Waschke

Prof. Dr. Thomas Klonisch

Professor Thomas Klonisch studied human medicine at the Ruhr-University Bochum and the Justus-Liebig-University (JLU) Giessen. He completed his doctoral thesis at the Institute of Biochemistry at the Faculty of Medicine of the JLU Giessen before joining the Institute of Medical Microbiology, University of Mainz (1989–1991). As an Alexander von Humboldt Fellow he joined the University of Guelph, Ontario, Canada, from 1991–1992 and, in 1993–1994, continued his research at the Ontario Veterinary College, Guelph, Ontario. From 1994–1996, he joined the immunoprotein engineering group at the Department of Immunology, University College London, UK, as a senior research fellow. From 1996–2004 he was a scientific associate at the Department of Anatomy and Cell Biology, Martin Luther University of Halle-Wittenberg, where he received his accreditation as anatomist (1999), completed his habilitation (2000), and held continuous national research funding. In 2004, he was appointed Full Professor and Head at the Department of Human Anatomy and Cell Science (HACS) at the College of Medicine, Faculty of Health Science, University of Manitoba, Winnipeg, Canada, where he was the Department Head until 2019. He remains a Professor at HACS and is currently the director of the Histology Services and Ultrastructural Imaging Platform.

His research areas include mechanisms employed by cancer stem/progenitor cells to enhance tissue invasiveness and survival strategies in response to anticancer treatments. A particular focus is the role of endocrine factors, such as the relaxin-like ligand-receptor system, in promoting carcinogenesis.

Prof. Dr. Sabine Hombach-Klonisch

Teaching clinically relevant anatomy and clinical case-based anatomy learning are the main teaching focuses of Sabine Hombach-Klonisch at the Rady Faculty of Health Sciences of the University of Manitoba. Since her appointment in 2004, Professor Hombach has been nominated annually for teaching awards by the Manitoba Medical Student Association (MMSA) and received the MMSA award for teaching in the small group setting in 2020 and 2021.

Sabine Hombach graduated from Medical School at the Justus-Liebig-University Giessen in 1991 and successfully completed her doctoral thesis in 1994. Following a career break to attend to her two children she re-engaged as a sessional lecturer at the Department of Anatomy and Cell Biology of the Martin-Luther-University Halle-Wittenberg in 1997 and received a post-doctoral fellowship from the province of Saxony-Anhalt 1998–2000. Thereafter, she joined the Department of Anatomy and Cell Biology as a scientific associate. Professor Hombach received her accreditation as anatomist in 2003 from the German Society of Anatomists and from the Medical Association of Saxony-Anhalt, and completed her habilitation at the Medical Faculty of the Martin-Luther-University Halle-Wittenberg in 2004. In 2004, Professor Hombach was appointed to the Department of Human Anatomy and Cell Science, Faculty of Medicine of the University of Manitoba. Appointed as department head in January 2020, she strongly promotes postgraduate clinical anatomy training for residents.

Her main research interests are in the field of breast and brain cancer. Her focus is to identify the molecular mechanisms that regulate metastasis and cell survival under treatment stress. She employs unique cell and animal models and human primary cells to study the influence of the tumour microenvironment on brain metastatic growth.

Preface of the 25th German edition

In the foreword to the first edition of his atlas, Johannes Sobotta wrote in May 1904: 'Many years of experience in anatomical dissection prompted the author to create a pictorial representation of the peripheral nervous system and blood vessels in the way that the student has got used to seeing the relevant parts on a dissection, i.e. showing vessels and nerves in the same area in conjunction to each other. In addition, the atlas alternately contains text and tables. The images form the core of the atlas, with additional ancillary and schematic illustrations, and the figure legends give a short and succinct clarification for quick orientation when using the book in the dissection lab.'

As with fashion, students' reading and study habits change regularly. The multimedia presence and availability of information as well as stimuli are surely the main reasons for these habits to be changing more quickly than ever before. These developments and thereby also the changing requirements students demand from the atlases and textbooks they wish to use, as well as the digital availability of the contents, need to be taken into consideration by the authors, editors and publishers. Interviews and systematic surveys with students are useful in guaging their expectations. Until now, the textbook market has also been an indicator for change: detailed textbooks claiming complete integrity are brushed aside for textbooks and lecture notes targeted at the didactic needs of the students at particular universities as well as the study content of human medicine, dentistry and biomedical sciences and the corresponding examinations involved. Equally, the illustrations in atlases such as the Sobotta, which have fascinated many generations of doctors and health professionals from all over the world with their exact and naturalistic depictions of real anatomical specimens, are sometimes regarded by students as too complicated and detailed. This realisation requires some consideration as to how to adapt the strengths of the atlas – which has developed over 25 editions into a reference work of accuracy and quality – to modern didactic concepts without comprimising its unique characteristics and originality.

Looking at it didactically, we have retained the concept of the three volumes, as used by Sobotta in his first edition: General Anatomy and Musculoskeletal System (1), Internal Organs (2) and Head, Neck and Neuroanatomy (3). We have also adopted although slightly modified the approach mentioned in the preface of the first edition of combining the figures in the atlas with explanatory text, a trend which has regained popularity. Hereby each image is accompanied by a short explanation which gives an introduction to the image and explains why the particular dissection and area were chosen. The individual chapters were systematically divided according to current study habits and various images were supplemented or replaced. Most of these new images are conceptualised in such a way that the studying of the relevant pathways supplying blood and innervation is made easier pedagogically. In addition, we have reviewed many existing figures, shortened the descriptions and have highlighted the important terms, to make the anatomical content more accessible. Numerous clinical cases are referred to, most now including illustrations, and turn the sometimes lifeless subject of anatomy into a clinical and lively one. This helps the beginner to visualize a possible future career and gives them a taste of what's to come. Introductions to the individual chapters gives a succinct overview of the contents and the most important themes, as well as presenting a relevant case in everyday clinical practice. Each chapter ends with a number of typical questions as they may be given in an oral or written anatomy exam. As with the 24th edition, every chapter contains a short introduction to the embryology of the relevant theme. Included for the first time are the lifesize poster of the skeleton and musculature of a woman and a man, as well as the instructional poster.

Two points should be taken into account:
1. The atlas in the 25th edition does not replace any accompanying textbook.
2. No matter how good the didactical concept, it cannot replace the study process, but it can at least try to make it more vivid. To study anatomy is not difficult but it is very time-consuming. Time well worth spending, as both the doctor and the patient will eventually benefit. The goal of the 25th edition of the Sobotta Atlas is not only to ease the study process but also to make it an exciting and interesting time, so that one turns to it eagerly when studying, as well as in the course of one's professional career.

Erlangen and Munich in the summer of 2022,
exactly 118 years after publication of the first German edition.

Friedrich Paulsen and Jens Waschke

Any errors?

https://else4.de/978-0-7020-6767-9

We demand a lot from our contents. Despite every precaution it is still possible that an error can slip through or that the factual contents needs updating. For all relevant errors, a correction will be provided. With this QR code, quick access is possible.

We are grateful for each and every suggestion which could help us to improve this publication. Please send your proposals, praise and criticism to the following email address: kundendienst@elsevier.com

Acknowledgements of the 25th German edition

It has again been very exciting to work on the 25th edition of the Sobotta Atlas, with which we feel increasingly closely connected.

Now more than ever, a comprehensive atlas such as the Sobotta demands a dedicated team run by a well-organised publishing company. The entire process for this 25th edition has been coordinated by the content strategist Sonja Frankl, to whom we are very grateful. Additionally, not much would have been possible without the longstanding and all-encompassing experience of Dr Andrea Beilmann, who was entrusted with many of the previous editions and who forms the foundation of the Sobotta team. We thank her warmly for all her help and support. We fondly remember the monthly telephone conferences in which Dr Beilman and Sonja Frankl were on hand to lend support with the design, bringing together their distinct and diverse working styles in a quite remarkable fashion. Along with Dr Beilmann, Sibylle Hartl coordinated the project and was responsible for the production as a whole. We thank her wholeheartedly. Without the determination and vigilance of Kathrin Nühse, this edition would not have been possible in its present form. We are further enormously grateful to Martin Kortenhaus (editing), the team at the abavo GmbH (formal image processing and setting), and Nicola Kerber (layout development), who were involved with the editorial side and in making the outcome a success.

In particular, we are grateful to our illustrators, Dr Katja Dalkowski, Anne-Kathrin Hermanns, Martin Hoffmann, Sonja Klebe and Jörg Mair, who helped us to revise many existing images as well as creating numerous new ones.

For their help in creating the clinical images, we sincerely thank: PD Dr Frank Berger, MD, Institute for Clinical Radiology at the Ludwig-Maximilians-University, Munich; Prof Dr Christopher Bohr, MD, Clinic and Polyclinic for Ear, Nose and Throat, University Hospital, Regensburg – previously UK-Erlangen/FAU; Dr Eva Louise Brahmann, MD, Clinic for Ophthalmology at the Heinrich Heine University, Düsseldorf; Prof Dr Andreas Dietz, MD, Director of the Clinic and Polyclinic for Ear, Nose and Throat, University of Leipzig; Prof Dr Arndt Dörfler, MD, Institute for Radiology, Neuroradiology, Friedrich Alexander University, Erlangen-Nuremberg; Prof Dr Gerd Geerling, MD, Clinic for Ophthalmology at the Heinrich-Heine University of Düsseldorf; Dr Berit Jordan, MD, University Clinic and Polyclinic for Neurology, Martin Luther University of Halle-Wittenberg; Prof Dr Marco Kesting, MD, Dentistry, Oral Maxillofacial Clinic, Friedrich Alexander University, Erlangen-Nuremberg; PD Dr Axel Kleespies, MD; Surgical Clinic, Ludwig-Maximilians-University, Munich; Prof Dr Norbert Kleinsasser, MD, University Clinic for Ear, Nose and Throat, Julius Maximilian University, Würzburg; PD Dr Hannes Kutta, MD, ENT Practice, Hamburg-Altona/Ottensen; Dr Christian Markus, MD, Clinic for Anaesthesiology, Julius Maximilian University, Würzburg; MTA Hong Nguyen and PD Doctor of Science Martin Schicht, Institute for Functional and Clinical Anatomy, Friedrich Alexander University at Erlangen-Nuremberg; Jörg Pekarsky, Institute for Anatomy, Functional and Clinical Anatomy, Friedrich Alexander University, Erlangen-Nuremberg; Dr Dietrich Stövesand, MD, Clinic for Diagnostic Radiology, Martin Luther University of Halle-Wittenberg; Prof Dr Jens Werner, MD, Surgical Clinic, Ludwig-Maximilians-University, Munich; Dr Tobias Wicklein, MD Dentristry, Erlangen, and Prof Dr Stephan Zierz, MD, Director of University Clinic and Polyclinic for Neurology, Martin Luther University of Halle-Wittenberg.

Finally we thank our families, who have had to share us with the Sobotta Atlas in the context of the 25th edition, as well as being on hand with advice when needed and strong support.

Erlangen and Munich, summer of 2022

Friedrich Paulsen and Jens Waschke

Adresses of the editors in chief

Prof. Dr. Friedrich Paulsen
Institute of Anatomy, Department of Functional and Clinical Anatomy
Friedrich Alexander University Erlangen-Nuremberg
Universitätsstraße 19
91054 Erlangen
Germany

Prof. Dr. Jens Waschke
Institute of Anatomy and Cell Biology, Department I
Ludwig-Maximilians-University (LMU) Munich
Pettenkoferstraße 11
80336 Munich
Germany

Adresses of the translators

Prof. Dr. Thomas Klonisch
Dept. of Human Anatomy and Cell Science
Max Rady College of Medicine, Rady Faculty of Health Sciences
University of Manitoba
130–745 Bannatyne Avenue
Winnipeg, Manitoba, R3E 0J9, Canada

Prof. Dr. Sabine Hombach-Klonisch
Dept. of Human Anatomy and Cell Science
Max Rady College of Medicine, Rady Faculty of Health Sciences
University of Manitoba
130–745 Bannatyne Avenue
Winnipeg, Manitoba, R3E 0J9, Canada

True-to-life representation is the top priority

Sabine Hildebrandt*, Friedrich Paulsen, Jens Waschke

'To practise as a doctor without profound anatomical knowledge is unthinkable. For the diagnosing, treatment and prognosis of illnesses, a detailed knowledge of the structure, positional relationships and the neurovascular pathways which supply the regions and organs of the body is central.'

Anatomical knowledge is gained through cognitive, tactile and especially visual learning processes, and can only be fully acquired when working with the human body itself. Images, graphics and three-dimensional programmes depicting the essential elements help to develop a three-dimensional perception of the relationships in the human body, and help the student to memorise and name structures.

The visual principle of learning did not always apply in anatomical teaching. The writings of the great anatomists of antiquity, such as the school of **Hippocrates of Kos** (460–370 BC) and **Galen of Pergamon** (131–200), did not include any illustrations of human anatomy, because a life-like representation of the human form in books was technically impossible; nor did these authors perform dissections on humans.[1,2,3,4] Even the reformer of anatomy, **Mondino di Luzzi** (1270–1326), had to do without illustrations. He introduced the dissection of human bodies for anatomical education in Bologna and wrote the first modern anatomy 'book' in 1316. This 77-page collection of folios became the standard reference for medical training for the next few centuries.[1,4] Images from another contemporary medical compendium were included for visual instruction; however, their lack of detail and overt inaccuracies did not add much of practical value to the volume.

The Renaissance brought an increased awareness of nature and the relevance of trueness to life in art, and in this it was **Leonardo da Vinci** (1452–1519) who emphasised the visual representation of anatomy. His depictions of human anatomy were based on his own dissections.[5] Unfortunately, he never completed his planned anatomical volume, but did leave behind his anatomical sketches. It was thus in 1543 that **Andreas Vesalius'** (1514–1564) '*De humani corporis fabrica libri septem*' became the first book to depict human anatomy entirely based on the dissection of bodies. The numerous illustrations were high-quality woodcut prints but were not coloured.[6,7] Image quality evolved over the next few centuries and reached another peak with the work of anatomist **Jean Marc Bourgery** (1797–1849) and his draftsman **Nicolas Henri Jakob** (1782–1871). Bougery and Jakob jointly created an eight-volume anatomy atlas over a period of more than 20 years. However, this work as well as the one created by Vesalius, were published in folio format and thus so expensive and unwieldy that they were – and still are – highly valued by wealthy doctors and art connoisseurs, but unsuitable for students and their foundational anatomy education. In the English-speaking world this changed in 1858, when **Henry Gray** (1827–1861) published the textbook 'Anatomy, Descriptive and Surgical'. It contained non-coloured illustrations based on dissections of the human body, and was quickly established as an affordable and popular alternative for students.[8]

Around 1900, **August Rauber** (1841–1917), along with **Friedrich Wilhelm Kopsch** (1868–1955), **Carl Heitzmann** (1836–1896), as well as **Carl Toldt** (1840–1920), **Werner Spalteholz** (1861–1940) and several other authors, created volumes on anatomy for various publishers. These atlases, sometimes in combination with a textbook, claimed to present human anatomy in full. The anatomist **Johannes Sobotta** (1869–1945), who worked in Würzburg, complained that the books were too detailed and therefore unsuitable for foundational medical education. In addition, he believed the prices for these volumes were unjustifiably high for the quality of the images. Sobotta therefore endeavored to *'produce an atlas with lifelike images and suitable for use by medical students in the dissecting room'.*[9] The publishers and editors of the Sobotta Atlas have followed this basic principle ever since.

The first edition of the Sobotta Atlas was published in 1904 by J.F. Lehmanns under the title 'Atlas of the descriptive anatomy of humans in 3 volumes' and contained 904 mostly coloured illustrations. The majority of these were created by the illustrator **Karl Hajek** (1878–1935), who thus had a large share in the quality and success of the Sobotta Atlas. The atlas seems to have had a ground-breaking effect after its publication in that it brought the further development of anatomical textbooks a big step forward.

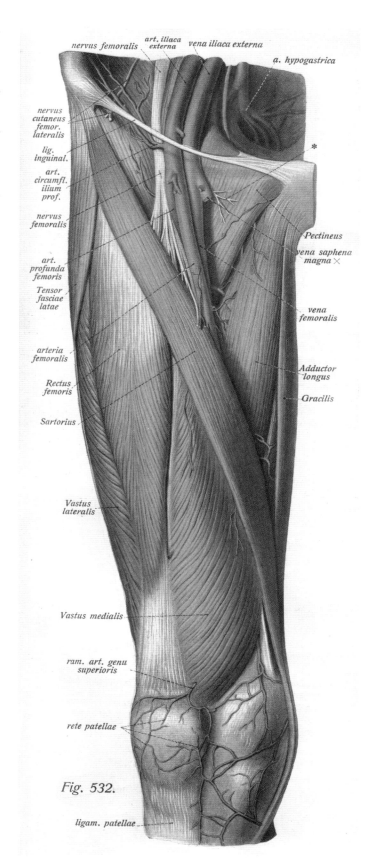

Fig. 1 Illustration of the ventral femoral musculature based on a dissection (1st edition of the Sobotta Atlas). [S700]

At the time of the first edition of the Sobotta Atlas, there were other atlases featuring muscles that were coloured, and neurovascular bundles highlighted in colour. However, it was only the Sobotta atlas which gave a complete and true-to-life colouring of the images of a situs or extremity, and this was only possible through a high-quality printing technique. This is illustrated by → Fig. 1 from the first edition with the example of the dissection of an anterior thigh. Even more than 100 years later, these images still look fresh and life-like and are therefore timeless. Many illustrations were added over the following editions, and the existing illustrations were continuously revised and adapted to match contemporary learning habits and aesthetic perceptions.

Unfortunately, we cannot mention all the illustrators over the course of 25 editions who have made the Sobotta Atlas what it is today; there are simply too many. Individual artists will therefore be singled out as being representative for all. From 1925, **Erich Lepier** (1898–1974) worked as illustrator for Urban & Schwarzenberg; first for various clinicians and then for the anatomist Eduard Pernkopf. After the Second World War, when Urban & Schwarzenberg had taken over publication of the Sobotta Atlas from J.F. Lehmanns, Lepier produced numerous illustrations for this atlas. Late in life he was awarded the title of professor because of his outstanding work.

From the 20th edition in 1993, **Sonja Klebe** contributed to the atlas and her outstanding creations need to be highlighted. The editors still work with her in a productive collaborative team, as can be seen in → Fig. 2, with an image of the topography of the head.

For later editions, images from other works by the Elsevier publishing company have also been included in the Sobotta Atlas. Since the turn of the millennium, most anatomical images from many of the publishing houses have been created digitally. Technical advances make it possible to create anatomical images in an inverse way to before. Previously, as in the Sobotta Atlas, new images were drawn exclusively using real human specimens. Schematic representations for simplification were derived by deduction.

Today, simple line drawings and schematics are first drawn up by computer programmes, to then incorporate the textures of various tissues by induction. Ultimately this produces the impression of a real representation of an anatomical specimen. The results are remarkably vivid despite being artificial. It is an attractive option for organisational as well as economic reasons. Today – in contrast to the times leading up to the postwar period – hardly any anatomical institute still employs its own illustrators, who, along with the anatomists and the dissected specimen, would create images of the quality required for the Sobotta Atlas. In addition, there are hardly any anatomists whose work time can be dedicated to producing anatomical specimens of the highest quality. Anatomists today are not only university professors and textbook

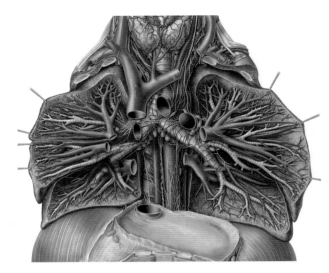

Fig. 3 Illustration of a dissection of the lungs from the Pernkopf Atlas (25th edition of the Sobotta Atlas, → Fig. 5.113). [S700-L238]/ [Q300]

authors, but scientists who conduct research and depend on performance-oriented financial resources. Due to these developments, it is next to impossible for today's anatomists to collaborate with illustrators over several months in the creation of a single optimal illustration. As a result, this manner of image creation has been almost entirely abandoned, and there are practically no representations that exceed or even compete with the images in older atlases. This is also the reason for the Sobotta Atlas to continue including images from atlases such as the Pernkopf Atlas as a model for new editions. The quality of some of the Pernkopf images is still unsurpassed, as → Fig. 3 shows, with a dissection of the lungs as an example – the editors know of no other comparable illustration of the lung structure and its associated neurovasculature that represents all vascular details, including the lymphatics, correctly.

This decision to reproduce an illustration from the Pernkopf Atlas can only be justified on the basis of a conscious examination[10] of the egregious ethical transgressions of anatomy during National Socialism (Nazi Germany), in memory of the victims of the Nazi regime whose bodies are depicted here. Since this applies to all anatomical representations in atlases that already existed and were further developed during this period, we discuss this historical background in more detail here.[11]

Anatomical work in teaching and research, as well as in the production of new teaching materials, including atlases, was and is dependent on an adequate supply of dead human bodies. Traditional legal anatomical body procurement in Germany and worldwide was based on the bodies of so-called 'unclaimed' people, i.e. those who died in public institutions and whose relatives did not claim them for a burial. It was only in the second half of the 20th century that this changed fundamentally – in Germany as in other countries – with the advent of effective body donation programmes.[12,13] Before that, the sources of anatomical body procurement primarily included psychiatric institutions, prisons, people who committed suicide and – historically the first legally regulated source – bodies of the executed. Anatomy laws were repeatedly adapted by the respective governments, including Nazi Germany.[14,15] With rare exceptions, a constant theme in the history of anatomy has been the lack of bodies for teaching and research. This changed significantly under National Socialism. In the first years after 1933 there were still the usual missives by anatomists to the authorities, complaining about the scant body supply. Very soon, however, their inquiries became specific, and they asked for access to execution sites and the bodies of the executed, or asked for the bodies of prisoners of war to be delivered to their institutes. Thus, anatomists were not only passive recipients of the bodies of Nazi victims, but actively requested them for teaching, and above all for research.[16]

In the 'Third Reich', the bodies from psychiatric hospitals included those of people murdered as part of the 'euthanasia' killing programme, as documented for various anatomical institutes.[17,18] From 1933 on there

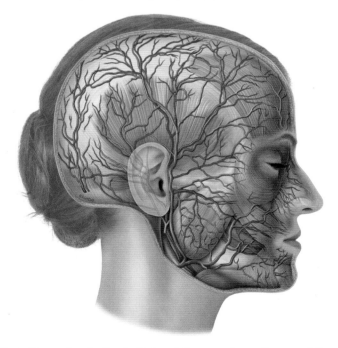

Fig. 2 Illustration by Sonja Klebe of the vascular pathways of the head (25th edition of the Sobotta Atlas, → Fig. 8.83). [S700-L238]

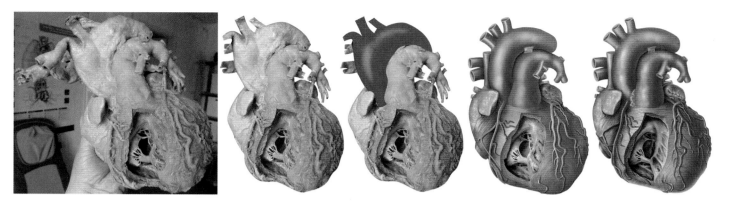

Fig. 4 Step-by-step development of one of Sonja Klebe's drawings of the topography of the heart, based on a plastinate and photos. [L238]

was also an increase in persecuted Jewish citizens among the suicides.[19] Due to the changes in Nazi legislation and the persecution of the so-called 'enemies of the German people', the number of political prisoners increased, not only in the normal penal system and in the Gestapo prisons, but above all in the constantly expanding network of concentration camps and decentralised camps for prisoners of war and forced labourers. The escalating violence and inhumane living conditions in these facilities resulted in high death rates, and the dead were delivered to many of the anatomical institutes. The number of executions after civilian and military trials also rose exponentially under the National Socialists, especially during the war years.[20] All anatomical institutes received the bodies of the executed, without exception, and regardless of the political convictions of the individual anatomists who worked with these bodies.

More than 80% of the anatomists who remained in Nazi Germany had joined the NSDAP, the Nazi party, but not all of them were such avid National Socialist ideologues as **Eduard Pernkopf** (1888–1955), the Viennese Dean of the Medical Faculty and Director of the Institute of Anatomy. He used the unrestricted access to the bodies of executed Nazi victims not primarily for scientific studies, as many of his colleagues did, but instead created the subsequent volumes of his 'Topographical Anatomy of Humans'. Together with his assistants and a group of medical illustrators, he had begun this work in the early 1930s. It is highly likely that the majority of the pictures in the atlas created during the war years show victims of the Nazi regime, because Pernkopf's institute received the bodies of more than 1,377 executed people from the Vienna prison system between 1938 and 1945, more than half of them convicted of treason.[21] Erich Lepier and his illustrator colleagues Karl Endtresser (1903–1978) and Franz Batke (1903–1983) left clear signs of their political sympathies with the Nazi regime in their signatures on images that were created during the war. Lepier often integrated a swastika in his signature, and Endtresser and Batke SS runes. These peculiarities of the atlas initially remained without comment, and the work enjoyed great popularity with anatomists, surgeons and medical illustrators alike, due to the true-to-nature details, a colour palette intensified by a new printing process, and Pernkopf's so-called 'stratigraphic' method of representation, in which a body region is presented in dissection steps from the surface to the deep layers in a sequence of dissections. After the war, Lepier copied a number of Pernkopf originals for the Sobotta Atlas to replace illustrations by Karl Hajek. Interestingly, very detailed illustrations of the body cavities and their organs which also depicted the neurovascular system were not copied. Leaving out these drawings across many editions of the Sobotta Atlas can be explained by the fact that, for many years, the relevance of neurovascular structures to the diagnostics and treatment of malignant tumours were not fully explored. As this very important function of the lymph vessels is now well-known, the current publishers

regard further appropriation of the high-quality Pernkopf images as well-justified.

Soon after the publication of the first American edition of the Pernkopf Atlas in 1963/64, questions arose about the political background of the work. The rumours were only followed up on in the 1980s with investigations by American authors, before a public debate on the ethics of the use of the Pernkopf Atlas ensued in the mid-1990s.[22] Recommendations ranged from complete removal of the atlas from libraries to its historically informed use.[23] Urban and Schwarzenberg ended the publication of the work, but this did not stop its use, especially by surgeons.[24,25] When results of the systematic study of anatomy in Nazi Germany became known to a wider audience, a new inquiry emerged about the ethical use of the Pernkopf images in special surgical situations in 2016.[26] This question found an answer, based on Jewish medical ethics, in the *Responsum Vienna Protocol* by Rabbi Joseph Polak.[27,28,29] A responsum is a traditional scholarly and legal answer to a question put to a rabbi. Rabbi Polak concludes that most authorities would certainly allow the use of the Pernkopf images if they help save human life (according to the principle of *piku'ach nefesh*). However, this use is tied to the absolute condition that it is made known to one and all what these images are. Only in this way will the dead be granted at least some of the dignity to which they are entitled.

Following the argument of the *Vienna Protocol* and the condition that the victims of National Socialism whose bodies are shown in the images of the Pernkopf Atlas are remembered explicitly, the editors see it as justifiable to include new re-drawn copies of Pernkopf images in this new edition of the Sobotta Atlas: **to save future patients through the best possible anatomical visual instruction, in memory of the victims.**

In the 25th edition, the number of images has now grown to 2,500. It remains the highest priority to continue creating images with the various illustrators and graphic artists that are in no aspect inferior to dissected specimens. → Fig. 4 shows the example of a plastinated heart from a body donor, which the illustrator Sonja Klebe used, together with photographs from different perspectives, to create a new image. The spatial depth allows for three-dimensional understanding of the anatomy. It is the result of the artist's exploration process, in which she was able to observe, 'grasp' and understand the specimen.

The editors would like to thank all the illustrators and artists involved, as well as the Elsevier publishing team, without whom the atlas would not have been possible in this form.

Boston, Erlangen and Munich, 2022

Sabine Hildebrandt*, Friedrich Paulsen and Jens Waschke

Literature

1   Persaud TVN. Early history of human anatomy. Springfield: Charles C Thomas, 1984.

2   Persaud TVN. A history of human anatomy: the post-Vesalian era. Springfield: Charles C Thomas, 1997: 298, 309.

3   Rauber A, Kopsch F. Anatomie des Menschen. 7. Aufl. Leipzig: Thieme, 1906.

4   Roberts KB, Tomlinson JDW. The fabric of the body. Oxford: OxfordUniversity Press, 1992.

5   Clayton M, Philo R. Leonardo da Vinci Anatomist. London: Royal Collection Trust, 2017.

6   Garrison DH, Hast MH. The fabric of the human body (kommentierte Übersetzung des Werks von Andreas Vesalius). Basel: Karger, 2014.

7   Vollmuth R. Das anatomische Zeitalter. München: Verlag Neuer Merkur, 2004.

8   Hayes B. The Anatomist: A True story of Gray's Anatomy. Ballantine, 2007. ISBN 978-0-345-45689-2

9   Sobotta, J. Atlas der Anatomie des Menschen. 1. Aufl. München: J. F. Lehmanns-Verlag, 1904–1907.

10 Arbeitskreis »Menschliche Präparate in Sammlungen« (2003): Empfehlungen zum Umgang mit Präparaten aus menschlichem Gewebe in Sammlungen, Museen und öffentlichen Räumen, in: Deutsches Ärzteblatt 2003; 100: A1960–A1965. As well as other points, it explains: 'If it is shown that the deceased has died because of their genealogy, ideology or political persuasion due to state-controlled and-managed acts of violence or due to the well-founded probability of this having been the case, this is seen as a grave injury to their personal dignity. If such a context of wrongdoing is established, the specimens from the collections in question will be removed and interred in a dignified manner or will cease to be used, in a comparably dignified manner.' Distinct priority is especially given to specimens from the Nazi era, 'dealing with these specimens in a specialised way – after extensive research of the source – indiscriminately removing all dissections from collections between 1933 and 1945.' For specimens with an uncertain source and date of origin, the following is recommended: 'If after a first assessment, the specimen is of unknown origin and appears to be from the 20th century, it should then be separated and be subjected to a thorough examination. If no unambiguous allocation can be made, these specimens need to be categorically interred, unless there are certain cases in which contradictory overall aspects can be presented, documented and established.'

11 A full presentation of the history of anatomy in Nazi Germany is here: Hildebrandt S. The Anatomy of Murder: Ethical Transgressions and Anatomical Science in the Third Reich. New York: Berghahn Books, 2016.

12 Garment A, Lederer S, Rogers N, et al. Let the Dead Teach the Living: The Rise of Body Bequeathal in 20th-century America. Academic Medicine 2007; 82, 1000–1005.

13 Habicht JL, Kiessling C, Winkelmann A. Bodies for anatomy education in medical schools: An overview of the sources of cadavers worldwide. Acad Med 2018; 93: 1293–1300.

14 Stukenbrock K. Der zerstückte Coerper: Zur Sozialgeschichte der anatomischen Sektionen in der frühen Neuzeit (1650–1800). Stuttgart: Franz Steiner Verlag, 2001.

15 Hildebrandt S. Capital Punishment and Anatomy: History and Ethics of an Ongoing Association. Clinical Anatomy 2008; 21: 5–14.

16 Noack T, Heyll U. Der Streit der Fakultäten. Die medizinische Verwertung der Leichen Hingerichteter im Nationalsozialismus. In: Vögele J, Fangerau H, Noack T (Hrsg.). Geschichte der Medizin – Geschichte in der Medizin. Hamburg: Literatur Verlag, 2006: 133–142.

17 Overview in: Hildebrandt S. The Anatomy of Murder: Ethical Transgressions and Anatomical Science in the Third Reich. New York: Berghahn Books, 2016.

18 Czech H, Brenner E. Nazi victims on the dissection table – the anatomical institute in Innsbruck. Ann Anat 2019; 226: 84–95.

19 Goeschel C. Suicide in Nazi Germany. Oxford: Oxford University Press, 2009.

20 Numbers in Hildebrandt 2016 , see footnote 17.

21 Angetter DC. Anatomical Science at University of Vienna 1938–45. The Lancet 2000; 355: 1445–57.

22 Weissmann G. Springtime for Pernkopf. Reprinted 1987. In: Weissmann G (ed.). They All Laughed at Christopher Columbus. New York: Times Books; Williams, 1988: 48–69.

23 Hildebrandt S. How the Pernkopf Controversy Facilitated a Historical and Ethical Analysis of the Anatomical Sciences in Austria and Germany: A Recommendation for the Continued Use of the Pernkopf Atlas. Clinical Anatomy 2006; 19: 91–100.

24 Yee A, Coombs DM, Hildebrandt S, et al. Nerve surgeons' assessment of the role of Eduard Pernkopf 's Atlas of Topographic and Applied Human Anatomy in surgical practice. Neurosurgery 2019; 84: 491–498.

25 Yee A, Li J, Lilly J, et al. Oral and maxillofacial surgeons' assessment of the role of Pernkopf's atlas in surgical practice. Ann Anat 2021; 234: 1–10.

26 Complete documentation pertaining to this enquiry and the history of the perception of the Pernkopf Atlas, as well as the 'Vienna Protocol' in: Vol. 45 No. 1 (2021): Journal of Biocommunication Special Issue on Legacies of Medicine in the Holocaust and the Pernkopf Atlas, https://journals.uic.edu/ojs/index.php/jbc/article/view/10829 (last assessed: 27. November 2021).

27 Polak J. A. Vienna Protocol for when Jewish or possibly-Jewish human remains were discovered. Wiener Klinische Wochenschrift 2018; 130: S239–S243.

28 Vienna Protocol 2017. How to deal with Holocaust era human remains: recommendations arising from a special symposium. 'Vienna Protocol' for when Jewish or Possibly-Jewish Human Remains are Discovered. Im Internet: https://journals.uic.edu/ojs/index.php/jbc/article/view/10829/9795 (last assessed: 21. October 2021).

29 Hildebrandt S, Polak J, Grodin MA, et al. The history of the Vienna Protocol. In: Hildebrandt S, Offer M, Grodin MA (eds.). Recognizing the past in the present: medicine before, during and after the Holocaust. New York: Berghahn Books, 2021: 354–372.

*   Sabine Hildebrandt, MD;
    Associate Scientific Researcher, Assistant Professor of Pediatrics, Harvard Medical School; Boston, U.S.A.

1. List of abbreviations

Singular:

			Plural:					
A.	=	Arteria	Aa.	=	Arteriae	♀	=	female
Lig.	=	Ligamentum	Ligg.	=	Ligamenta	♂	=	male
M.	=	Musculus	Mm.	=	Musculi			
N.	=	Nervus	Nn.	=	Nervi			
Proc.	=	Processus	Procc.	=	Processus			
R.	=	Ramus	Rr.	=	Rami			
V.	=	Vena	Vv.	=	Venae			
Var.	=	Variation						

Percentages:

In the light of the large variation in individual body measurements, the percentages indicating size should only be taken as approximate values.

2. General terms of direction and position

The following terms indicate the position of organs and parts of the body in relation to each other, irrespective of the position of the body (e.g. supine or upright) or direction and position of the limbs. These terms are relevant not only for human anatomy but also for clinical medicine and comparative anatomy.

General terms

anterior – posterior = in front – behind (e.g. Arteriae tibiales anterior et posterior)
ventralis – dorsalis = towards the belly – towards the back
superior – inferior = above – below (e.g. Conchae nasales superior et inferior)
cranialis – caudalis = towards the head – towards the tail
dexter – sinister = right – left (e.g. Arteriae iliacae communes dextra et sinistra)
internus – externus = internal – external
superficialis – profundus = superficial – deep (e.g. Musculi flexores digitorum superficialis et profundus)
medius, intermedius = located between two other structures (e.g. the Concha nasalis media is located between the Conchae nasales superior and inferior)
medianus = located in the midline (Fissura mediana anterior of the spinal cord). The median plane is a sagittal plane which divides the body into right and left halves.
medialis – lateralis = located near to the midline – located away from the midline of the body (e.g. Fossae inguinales medialis et lateralis)
frontalis = located in a frontal plane, but also towards the front (e.g. Processus frontalis of the maxilla)

longitudinalis = parallel to the longitudinal axis (e.g. Musculus longitudinalis superior of the tongue)
sagittalis = located in a sagittal plane
transversalis = located in a transverse plane
transversus = transverse direction (e.g. Processus transversus of a thoracic vertebra)

Terms of direction and position for the limbs

proximalis – distalis = located towards or away from the attached end of a limb or the origin of a structure (e.g. Articulationes radioulnares proximalis et distalis)

for the upper limb:
radialis – ulnaris = on the radial side – on the ulnar side (e.g. Arteriae radialis et ulnaris)

for the hand:
palmaris – dorsalis = towards the palm of the hand – towards the back of the hand (e.g. Aponeurosis palmaris, Musculus interosseus dorsalis)

for the lower limb:
tibialis – fibularis = on the tibial side – on the fibular side (e.g. Arteria tibialis anterior)

for the foot:
plantaris – dorsalis = towards the sole of the foot – towards the back of the foot (e.g. Arteriae plantares lateralis et medialis, Arteria dorsalis pedis)

3. Use of brackets

[ ]: Latin terms in square brackets refer to alternative terms as given in the Terminologia Anatomica (1998), e.g. Ren [Nephros]. To keep the legends short, only those alternative terms have been added that differ in the root of the word and are necessary to understand clinical terms, e.g. nephrology. They are primarily used in figures in which the particular organ or structure plays a central role.

( ): Round brackets are used in different ways:
– for terms also listed in round brackets in the Terminologia Anatomica, e.g. (M. psoas minor)
– for terms not included in the official nomenclature but which the editors consider important and clinically relevant, e.g. (Crista zygomaticoalveolaris)
– to indicate the origin of a given structure, e.g. R. spinalis (A. vertebralis).

4. Colour chart

Concha nasalis inferior		Os occipitale		
Mandibula		Os palatinum		
Maxilla		Os parietale		
Os ethmoidale		Os sphenoidale		
Os frontale		Os temporale		
Os lacrimale		Os zygomaticum		
Os nasale		Vomer		

In the newborn the following cranial bones are indicated by only one colour:

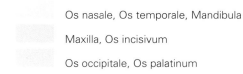

Os nasale, Os temporale, Mandibula

Maxilla, Os incisivum

Os occipitale, Os palatinum

Picture credits

The reference for all image sources in this work appears at the end of each figure legend in square brackets.
Explanation of the special characters:

[...]/[...] = after submission of
[.../...] = collaboration between author and illustrator
[...~...] = modified by author and/or illustrator
[...-...] = work combined with illustrator

All unlabelled graphics and illustrations © Elsevier GmbH, Munich. We are very grateful to all clinical colleagues named below who have made available ultrasound, computed tomographic and magnetic resonance images as well as endoscopic images and colour photos of operation sites and patients.

B500	Benninghoff-Archiv: Benninghoff A, Drenckhahn D. Anatomie, div. Bd. und Aufl. Elsevier/Urban & Fischer
B501	Benninghoff. Drenckhahn D, Waschke J. Taschenbuch Anatomie, div. Aufl. Elsevier/Urban & Fischer
C155	Földi M, Kubik S. Lehrbuch der Lymphologie. 3. A. Gustav Fischer, 1993
C185	Voss H, Herrlinger R. Taschenbuch der Anatomie. Gustav Fischer, 1963
E102-005	Silbernagl S. Taschenatlas der Physiologie. 3. A. Thieme, 2009
E107	Blechschmidt E. Die vorgeburtlichen Entwicklungsstadien des Menschen. S. Karger AG, 1961
E262-1	Rauber A, Kopsch F. Anatomie des Menschen. Band I. Thieme, 1987
E282	Kanski, J. Clinical Ophthalmology: A Systematic Approach. 5th ed. Butterworth-Heinemann, 2003
E288	Forbes C, Jackson W. Color Atlas and Text of Clinical Medicine. 3rd A. Elsevier/Mosby, 2003
E329	Pretorius ES, Solomon JA. Radiology Secrets Plus. 3rd ed. Elsevier/Mosby, 2011
E336	LaFleur Brooks, M.: Exploring Medical Language. 7th ed. Elsevier/Mosby, 2008
E339-001	Asensio JA, Trunkey DD. Current Therapy of Trauma and Surgical Critical Care. 1st ed. Elsevier/Mosby, 2008
E347-09	Moore KL, Persaud TVN, Torchia MG. The Developing Human. 9th ed. Elsevier/Saunders, 2013
E347-11	Moore KL, Persaud TVN, Torchia MG. The Developing Human. 11th ed. Elsevier/Saunders, 2020
E377	Eisenberg RL, Johnson N. Comprehensive Radiographic Pathology, Skeletal System. Elsevier/Mosby, 2012
E380	Eiff MP, Hatch RL. Fracture Management for Primary Care. 3rd ed. Elsevier/Saunders, 2012
E393	Adam A, Dixon AK. Grainger & Allison's Diagnostic Radiology. 5th ed. Elsevier/Churchill Livingstone, 2008
E402	Drake R, Vogl AW, Mitchell A. Gray's Anatomy for Students. 1st ed. Elsevier, 2005
E402-004	Drake R, Vogl AW, Mitchell A. Gray's Anatomy for Students. 4th ed. Elsevier, 2020
E404	Herring JA. Tachdjian's Pediatric Orthopaedics. 4th ed. Elsevier/Saunders, 2008.
E458	Kelley LL, Petersen C. Sectional Anatomy for Imaging Professionals. 2nd ed. Elsevier, 2007
E460	Drake R, et al. Gray's_Atlas of Anatomy. 1st ed. Elsevier, 2008
E475	Baren JM, et al. Pediatric Emergency Medicine. 1st ed. Elsevier/Saunders, 2008
E513-002	Herring W. Learning Radiology- Recognizing the Basics. 2nd ed. Elsevier/Saunders, 2012
E530	Long B, Rollins J, Smith B. Merrill's Atlas of Radiographic Positioning and Procedures. 11th ed. Elsevier/Mosby, 2007
E563	Evans R. Illustrated Orthopedic Physical Assessment. 3rd ed. Elsevier/Mosby, 2008
E602	Adams JG, et al. Emergency Medicine. Expert Consult. Elsevier/Saunders, 2008
E625	Myers E, Snyderman C. Operative Otolaryngology: Head and Neck Surgery. 3rd ed. Elsevier/Saunders, 2008
E633-002	Tillmann BN. Atlas der Anatomie. 2. A. Springer, 2010
E633-003	Tillmann BN. Atlas der Anatomie. 3. A. Springer, 2017
E684	Herrick AL, et al. Orthopaedics and Rheumatology in Focus. 1st ed. Elsevier/Churchill Livingstone, 2006
E708	Marx J, Hockberger RS, Walls RM. Rosen's Emergency Medicine 7th revised ed. Elsevier/Mosby, 2009
E748	Seidel H, et al. Mosby's Guide to Physical Examination. 7th ed. Elsevier/Mosby, 2011
E761	Fuller G, Manford MR. Neurology. An Illustrated Colour Text. 3rd ed. Elsevier/Churchill Livingstone, 2010
E813	Green M, Swiontkowski M. Skeletal Trauma in Children. 4th ed. Elsevier/Saunders, 2009
E821	Pauwels F. Gesammelte Abhandlungen zur funktionellen Anatomie des Bewegungsapparates. Springer, 1965
E838	Mitchell B, Sharma R. Embryology. An Illustrated Colour Text. 1st ed. Elsevier/Churchill Livingstone, 2005
E867	Winn HR. Youmans Neurological Surgery. 6th ed. Elsevier/Saunders, 2011
E908-003	Corne J, Pointon K. Chest X-ray Made Easy. 3rd ed. Elsevier/Churchill Livingstone, 2010
E943	Kanski J. Clinical Ophthalmology. A Systemic Approach. 6th ed. Butterworth-Heinemann, 2007
E984	Klinke R, Silbernagl S. Lehrbuch Physiologie. 5. A. Thieme; 2005
E993	Auerbach P, Cushing T, Harris NS. Auerbach's Wilderness Medicine. 7th ed. Elsevier, 2016
E1043	Radlanski RJ, Wesker KH. Das Gesicht. Bildatlas klinische Anatomie. 2. A. KVM, 2012
F201-035	Abdul-Khaliq H, Berger F. Angeborene Herzfehler: Die Diagnose wird häufig zu spät gestellt. Dtsch Arztebl 2011;108:31-2
F264-004	Hwang S. Imaging of Lymphoma of the Musculoskeletal System. Radiologic Clinics of North America 2008;46/2:75-93
F276-005	Frost A, Robinson C. The painful shoulder. Surgery 2006;24/11:363-7
F276-006	Marsh H. Brain tumors. Surgery. 2007; 25/12:526-9
F276-007	Hobbs C, Watkinson J. Thyroidectomy. Surgery 2007;25/11:474-8
F698-002	Meltzer CC, et al. Serotonin in Aging, Late-Life Depression, and Alzheimer's Disease: The Emerging Role of Functional Imaging. Neuropsychopharmacology 1998;18:407-30
F702-006	Stelzner F, Lierse W. Der angiomuskuläre Dehnverschluss der terminalen Speiseröhre. Langenbecks Arch. klin. Chir. 1968;321:35–64
F885	Senger M, Stoffels HJ, Angelov DN. Topography, syntopy and morphology of the human otic ganglion: A cadaver study. Ann Anat 2014;196: 327-35
F1062-001	Bajada S, Mofidi A, Holt M, Davies AP. Functional relevance of patellofemoral thickness before and after unicompartmental patellofemoral replacement. The Knee. 2012;19/3:155-228
F1067-001	Lee MW, McPhee RW, Stringer MD. An evidence-based approach to human dermatomes. Clin Anat 2008;21(5):363-73
F1082-001	Weed LH. Forces concerned in the absorption of cerebrospinal fluid. Am J Physiol1935;114/1:40-5
G056	Hochberg MC, et al. Rheumatology. 5th ed. Elsevier/Mosby, 2011
G123	DeLee JC, Drez D, Miller MD. DeLee & Drez's Orthopaedic Sports Medicine. 2nd ed. Elsevier/Saunders, 2003
G159	Forbes A. et al. Atlas of Clinical Gastroenterology. 3rd ed. Elsevier/Mosby, 2004
G198	Mettler F. Essentials of Radiology. 2nd ed. Elsevier/Saunders, 2005
G210	Standring S. Gray's Anatomy. 42nd ed. Elsevier, 2020

G211   Ellenbogen R, Abdulrauf S, Sekhar L. Principles of Neurological Surgery. 3rd ed. Elsevier/Saunders, 2012

G217   Waldman S. Physical Diagnosis of Pain. 2nd ed. Elsevier/Saunders, 2009

G305   Hardy M, et al.: Musculoskeletal Trauma. A guide to assessment and diagnosis. 1st ed. Elsevier/Churchill Livingstone, 2011

G322   Larsen WJ. Human embryology. 1st ed. Elsevier/Churchill Livingstone, 1993

G343   Netter FH. Atlas of Human Anatomy. 5th ed. Elsevier/Saunders, 2010

G435   Perkin GD, et al. Atlas of Clinical Neurology. 3rd ed. Elsevier/Saunders, 2011

G463   DeLee JC, Drez D, Miller MD. DeLee & Drez's Orthopaedic Sports Medicine. Principles and Practices. 3rd ed. Elsevier/Saunders, 2010

G465   Tang JB, et al. Tendon Surgery of the Hand. 1st ed. Elsevier/Saunders, 2012

G548   Swartz MH. Textbook of Physical Diagnosis. 7th ed. Elsevier, 2014

G568   Applegate E. J. The Sectional Anatomy Learning System- Concepts. 3rd ed. Elsevier/Saunders, 2009

G570   Wein AJ, et al. Campbell-Walsh Urology. 10th ed. Elsevier/Saunders, 2012

G617   Folkerth RD, Lidov H. Neuropathology. Elsevier, 2012

G645   Douglas G, Nicol F, Robertson C. Macleod's Clinical Examination. 13th ed. Elsevier/Churchill Livingstone, 2013

G704   Hagen-Ansert SL. Textbook of Diagnostic Sonography. 7th ed. Elsevier/Mosby, 2012

G716   Pagorek S, et al. Physical Rehabilitation of the Injured Athlete. 4th ed. Elsevier/Saunders, 2011

G717   Milla S, Bixby S. The Teaching Files- Pediatrics. 1st ed. Elsevier/Saunders, 2010

G718   Soto J, Lucey B. Emergency Radiology- The Requisites. 1st ed. Elsevier/Mosby, 2009

G719   Thompson SR, Zlotolow A.: Handbook of Splinting and Casting (Mobile Medicine). 1st ed. Elsevier/Mosby, 2012

G720   Slutsky DJ. Principles and Practice of Wrist Surgery. 1st ed. Elsevier/Saunders, 2010

G721   Canale ST, Beaty J. Campbell's Operative Orthopaedics (Vol.1). 11th ed. Elsevier/Mosby, 2008

G723   Rosenfeld JV. Practical Management of Head and Neck Injury. 1st ed. Elsevier/Churchill Livingstone, 2012

G724   Broder J. Diagnostic Imaging for the Emergency Physician. 1st ed. Elsevier/Saunders, 2011

G725   Waldmann S, Campbell R. Imaging of Pain. 1st ed. Elsevier/Saunders, 2011

G728   Sahrmann S. Movement System Impairment Syndromes of the Extremities, Cervical and Thoracic Spines. 1st ed. Elsevier/Mosby, 2010

G729   Browner BD, Fuller RP. Musculoskeletal Emergencies. 1st ed. Elsevier/Saunders, 2013

G744   Weir J, et al. Imaging Atlas of Human Anatomy. 4th ed. Elsevier/Mosby, 2011

G749   Le Roux P, Winn H, Newell D. Management of cerebral aneurysms. Elsevier/Saunders, 2004

G1060-001   Schünke M, Schulte E, Schumacher U. Prometheus. Allgemeine Anatomie und Bewegungsapparat. Band 1. 5. A. Thieme, 2018

G1060-002   Schünke M, Schulte E, Schumacher U. Prometheus. Innere Organe. Band 2. 5. A. Thieme, 2018

G1060-003   Schünke M, Schulte E, Schumacher U. Prometheus. Kopf, Hals, Neuroanatomie. Band 3. 5. A. Thieme, 2018

G1061   Debrunner HU. Orthopädisches Diagnostikum. 4. A. Thieme, 1982

G1062   Liniger H, Molineus G. Der Unfallmann. J.A. Barth, 1974

G1063   Vossschulte KF, et al. Lehrbuch der Chirurgie. Thieme, 1982

G1064   Schmidt H-M, Lanz U. Chirurgische Anatomie der Hand. Hippokrates, 1992

G1065   Tubiana R. The Hand, Vol. 1. Saunders, 1981

G1066   Gegenbaur C, Göpfert E. Lehrbuch der Anatomie des Menschen, Band III/1: Das Blutgefäßsystem. W. Engelmann, 1913

G1067   Baumgartl E. Das Kniegelenk. Springer, 1964

G1068   Tandler J. Lehrbuch der systematischen Anatomie, 3. Band. Das Gefäßsystem. F.C.W. Vogel, 1926

G1069   Loeweneck H, Feifel G. Bauch. In: Praktische Anatomie (begründet von von Lanz T, Wachsmuth W). Springer, 2004

G1070   Debrunner HU, Jacob AC. Biomechanik des Fußes. 2. A. Ferdinand Enke, 1998

G1071   Carpenter MB. Core Text of Neuroanatomy. 2nd ed. Williams & Wilkins, 1978

G1072   Schultze O, Lubosch W. Atlas und kurzgefasstes Lehrbuch der topographischen und angewandten Anatomie. 4. A. Lehmanns, 1935

G1073   Kubik S. Visceral lymphatic system. In: Viamonte Jr M, Rüttmann A (eds.). Atlas of Lymphography. Thieme, 1980

G1076   Schiebler TH, Korf H-W. Anatomie. 10. A. Steinkopff bei Springer, 2007

G1077   Zilles K, Rehkämper G. Funktionelle Neuroanatomie. 3. A. Springer, 1998

G1078   Stelzner F. Die anorectalen Fisteln. 3. A. Springer, 1981

G1079   Bourgery JM, Jacob NH. Atlas of Human Anatomy and Surgery. TASCHEN, 2007

G1080   Tillmann B. Farbatlas der Anatomie: Zahnmedizin – Humanmedizin. Thieme, 1997

G1081   Purves D, et al. NeuroScience. 3rd ed. Sinauer Associates Inc, 2004

G1082   von Hagens G, Whalley A, Maschke R, Kriz W. Schnittanatomie des menschlichen Gehirns. Steinkopff, 1990

G1083   Braus H, Elze C. Anatomie des Menschen, Band 3. Periphere Leitungsbahnen II, Centrales Nervensystem, Sinnesorgane. Springer, 1960

G1084   Martini FH, Timmons MJ, Tallitsch RB. Anatomie. 1. A. Pearson, 2017

G1085   Brodmann K. Vergleichende Lokalisationslehre der Großhirnrinde in ihren Prinzipien, dargestellt aufgrund des Zellenbaues. J.A. Barth, 1909

G1086   Rohen JW. Anatomie für Zahnmediziner. Schattauer, 1994

G1087   Spoendlin H. Strukturelle Organisation des Innenohres. In: Oto-Rhino-Laryngologie in Klinik und Praxis. Band 1. (Hrsg. Helms J, Herberhold C, Kastenbauer E). Thieme, 1994: 32-74

G1088   Nieuwenhuys R, Voogd J, van Huijzen C. Das Zentralnervensystem des Menschen. Ein Atlas mit Begleittext. 2. A. Springer, 1991

G1089   Berkovitz KB, et al. Oral Anatomy, Histology and Embryology. 5th ed. Elsevier/Mosby, 2017

G1091   Kandel ER, Koester JD, Mack SH, Siegelbaum SA. Principles of Neuroscience. 6th ed. McGraw Hill, 2021

G1192   O'Dowd G, Bell S, Wright S. Wheater's Pathology: A Text, Atlas and Review of Histopathology. 6th ed. Elsevier, 2019

H043-001   Mutoh K, Hidaka Y, Hirose Y, Kimura M. Possible induction of systemic lupus erythematosus by zonisamide. Pediatr Neurol 2001; 25(4):340-3

H061-001   Dodds SD, et al. Radiofrequency probe treatment for subfailure ligament injury: a biomechanical study of rabbit ACL. Clin Biomech 2004; 19(2):175-83

H062-001   Sener RN. Diffusion MRI: apparent diffusion coefficient (ADC) values in the normal brain and a classification of brain disorders based on ADC values. Comput Med Imaging Graph 2001; 25(4):299-326

H063-001   Heller AC, Kuether T, Barnwell SL, Nesbit G, Wayson KA. Spontaneous brachial plexus hemorrhage-case report. Surg Neurol 2000; 53(4):356-9

H064-001   Philipson M, Wallwork N. Traumatic dislocation of the sternoclavicular joint. Orthopaedics and Trauma 2012; 26(6):380-4

H081   Yang B, et al. A Case of Recurrent In-Stent Restenosis with Abundant Proteoglycan Component. Korean Circulation 2003; 33(9):827-31

H084-001   Custodio C, et al. Neuromuscular Complications of Cancer and Cancer Treatments. Physical Med Rehabilitation Clin North America 2008; 19(1):27-45

H102-002   Armour JA, et al. Gross and microscopic anatomy of the human intrinsic cardiac nervous system. Anat Rec 1997; 247:289–98

H230-001	Boyden EA. The anatomy of the choledochoduodenal junction in man. Surg Gynec Obstet 1957; 104:641–52
H233-001	Perfetti R, Merkel P. Glucagon-like peptide-1: a major regulator of pancreatic b-cell function. Eur J Endocrinol 2000; 143:717–25.
H234-001	Braak H. Architectonics as seen by lipofuscin stains. In: Peters A, Jones EG (eds.): Cerebral Cortex. Cellular Components of the Cerebral Cortex. Cellular Components of the Cerebral Cortex, Vol I. Plenum Press, 1984:59–104
J787	Colourbox.com
J803	Biederbick & Rumpf, Adelsdorf, Germany
K383	Cornelia Krieger, Hamburg, Germany
L106	Henriette Rintelen, Velbert, Germany
L126	Dr. med. Katja Dalkowski, Buckenhof, Germany
L127	Jörg Mair, München, Germany
L131	Stefan Dangl, München, Germany
L132	Michael Christof, Würzburg, Germany
L141	Stefan Elsberger, Planegg, Germany
L157	Susanne Adler, Lübeck, Germany
L190	Gerda Raichle, Ulm, Germany
L231	Stefan Dangl, München, Germany
L238	Sonja Klebe, Löhne, Germany
L240	Horst Ruß, München, Germany
L266	Stephan Winkler, München, Germany
L271	Matthias Korff, München, Germany
L275	Martin Hoffmann, Neu-Ulm, Germany
L280	Johannes Habla, München, Germany
L281	Luitgard Kellner, München, Germany
L284	Marie Davidis, München, Germany
L285	Anne-Katrin Hermanns, „Ankats Art", Maastricht, Netherlands
L303	Dr. med. Andreas Dietz, Konstanz, Germany
L316	Roswitha Vogtmann, Würzburg, Germany
L317	H.-C. Thiele, Gießen, Germany
L318	Tamas Sebesteny, Bern, Suisse
L319	Marita Peter, Hannover, Germany
M282	Prof. Dr.med. Detlev Drenckhahn, Würzburg, Germany
M492	Prof. Dr. med. Peter Kugler, Würzburg, Germany
M580	Prof. Dr. med. W. Kriz, Heidelberg, Germany
M1091	Prof. Dr. Reinhard Pabst, Hannover, Germany
O534	Prof. Dr. Arnd Dörfler, Erlangen, Germany
O548	Prof. Dr. med Andreas Franke, Kardiologie, Klinikum Region Hannover, Germany
O1107	Dr. Helmuth Ferner- Privatklinik Döbling, Wien, Austria
O1108	Prof. Hans-Rainer Duncker, Gießen, Germany
O1109	August Vierling (1872–1938), Heidelberg, Germany
P310	Prof. Dr. med. Friedrich Paulsen, Erlangen, Germany
P498	Prof. Dr. med. Philippe Pereira, SLK-Kliniken, Klinik für Radiologie, Heilbronn, Germany
Q300	Pernkopf-Archiv: Pernkopf E. Atlas der topgraphischen und angewandten Anatomie des Menschen, div. Bd. und Aufl. Elsevier/Urban & Fischer
R110-20	Rüther W, Lohmann C. Orthopädie und Unfallchirurgie. 20. A. Elsevier, 2014
R170-5	Welsch U, Kummer W, Deller T. Histologie – Das Lehrbuch: Zytologie, Histologie und mikroskopische Anatomie. 5. A. Elsevier/Urban & Fischer, 2018
R234	Bruch H-P, Trentz O. Berchtold Chirurgie. 6. A. Elsevier/Urban & Fischer, 2008
R235	Böcker W, Denk H, Heitz P, Moch H. Pathologie. 4. A. Elsevier/Urban & Fischer, 2008
R236	Classen M, Diehl V, Kochsiek K. Innere Medizin. 6. A. Elsevier/Urban & Fischer, 2009
R242	Franzen A. Kurzlehrbuch Hals-Nasen-Ohren-Heilkunde 3. A. Elsevier/Urban & Fischer, 2007
R247	Deller T, Sebesteny T. Fotoatlas Neuroanatomie. 1. A. Elsevier/Urban & Fischer, 2007
R252	Welsch U. Atlas Histologie. 7. A. Elsevier/Urban & Fischer, 2005
R254	Garzorz N. Basics Neuroanatomie. 1. A. Elsevier/Urban & Fischer, 2009
R261	Sitzer M, Steinmetz H. Neurologie. 1. A. Elsevier/Urban & Fischer, 2011
R306	Illing St, Classen M. Klinikleitfaden Pädiatrie.8. A. Elsevier/Urban & Fischer, 2009
R314	Böckers T, Paulsen F, Waschke J. Sobotta Lehrbuch Anatomie. 2. A. Elsevier/Urban & Fischer, 2019
R316-007	Wicke L. Atlas der Röntgenanatomie. 7. A. Elsevier/Urban & Fischer, 2005
R317	Trepel M. Neuroanatomie. 5. A. Elsevier/Urban& Fischer, 2011
R331	Fleckenstein P, Tranum-Jensen J. Röntgenanatomie. 1. A. Elsevier/Urban & Fischer, 2004
R333	Scharf H-P, Rüter A. Orthopädie und Unfallchirurgie. 2. A. Elsevier/Urban & Fischer, 2018
R349	Raschke MJ, Stange R. Alterstraumatologie – Prophylaxe, Therapie und Rehabilitation 1. A. Elsevier/Urban & Fischer, 2009,
R388	Weinschenk S. Handbuch Neuraltherapie. Diagnostik und Therapie mit Lokalanästhetika. 1. A. Elsevier/Urban & Fischer, 2010
R389	Gröne B. Schlucken und Schluckstörungen: Eine Einführung. 1. A. Elsevier/Urban & Fischer, 2009
R419	Menche N. Biologie- Anatomie- Physiologie. 9. A. Elsevier/Urban & Fischer, 2020
R449	Hansen JT. Netter's Clinical Anatomy. 4th ed. Elsevier/Urban & Fischer, 2018
R476	Kienzle-Müller B, Wilke-Kaltenbach G. Babies in Bewegung. 4. A. Elsevier, 2020
S002-5	Lippert H. Lehrbuch Anatomie. 5. A. Elsevier/Urban & Fischer, 2000
S002-7	Lippert H. Lehrbuch Anatomie. 7. A. Elsevier/Urban & Fischer, 2006
S008-4	Kauffmann GW, Sauer R, Weber WA. Radiologie. 4. A. Elsevier/Urban & Fischer, 2008
S100	Classen M, et al. Differentialdiagnose Innere Medizin 1. A. Urban & Schwarzenberg, 1998
S124	Breitner B. Chirurgische Operationslehre, Band III, Chirurgie des Abdomens. 2. A. Urban & Schwarzenberg, 1996
S130-6	Speckmann E-J, Hescheler J, Köhling R. Physiologie. 6. A. Elsevier/Urban & Fischer, 2013
S133	Wheater PR, Burkitt HG, Daniels VG. Funktionelle Histologie. 2. A. Urban & Schwarzenberg, 1987.
S700	Sobotta-Archiv: Sobotta. Atlas der Anatomie des Menschen, div. Aufl. Elsevier/Urban & Fischer
S701	Sobotta-Archiv: Hombach-Klonisch S, Klonisch T, Peeler J. Sobotta. Clinical Atlas of Human Anatomy. 1st ed. Elsevier/Urban & Fischer, 2019
S702	Sobotta-Archiv: Böckers T, Paulsen F, Waschke J. Sobotta. Lehrbuch Anatomie, div. Aufl. Elsevier/Urban & Fischer
T127	Prof. Dr. Dr. Peter Scriba, München, Germany
T419	Jörg Pekarsky, Institut für Anatomie LST II, Universität Erlangen-Nürnberg, Germany
T534	Prof. Dr. med. Matthias Sitzer, Klinik für Neurologie, Klinikum Herford, Germany
T663	Prof. Dr. Kurt Fleischhauer, Hamburg, Germany
T719	Prof. Dr. Norbert Kleinsasser, HNO-Klinik, Universitätsklinikum Würzburg, Germany
T720	PD Dr. med. Hannes Kutta, Universitätsklinikum Hamburg-Eppendorf, Germany
T786	Dr. Stephanie Lescher, Institut für Neuroradiologie, Klinikum der Goethe-Universität, Frankfurt, Prof. Joachim Berkefeld, Institut für Neuroradiologie, Klinikum der Goethe-Universität, Frankfurt, Germany
T832	PD Dr. Frank Berger, Institut für Klinische Radiologie der LMU, München, Germany
T863	C. Markus, Uniklinik Würzburg, Germany
T867	Prof. Dr. Gerd Geerling, Universitätsklinikum Düsseldorf, Germany
T872	Prof. Dr. med. Micheal Uder, Universitätsklinikum Erlangen, Germany
T882	Prof. Dr. med Christopher Bohr, Universitätsklinikum Regensburg, Germany
T884	Tobias Wicklein, Erlangen, Germany
T887	Prof. Dr. med Stephan Zierz, Dr. Jordan, Uniklinik Halle, Germany

T893   Prof. Galanski, Dr. Schäfer, Abteilung Diagnostische Radiologie, Med. Hochschule Hannover, Germany

T894   Prof. Gebel, Abteilung Gastroenterologie und Hepatologie, Med. Hochschule Hannover, Germany

T895   Dr. Greeven, St.-Elisabeth-Krankenhaus, Neuwied, Germany

T898   Prof. Jonas, Urologie, Med. Hochschule Hannover, Germany

T899   Prof. Kampik, Prof. Müller, Augenklinik, Universität München, Germany

T900   Dr. Kirchhoff, Dr. Weidemann, Abteilung Diagnostische Radiologie, Med. Hochschule Hannover, Germany

T901   Dr. Meyer, Abteilung Gastroenterologie und Hepatologie, Med. Hochschule Hannover, Germany

T902   Prof. Pfeifer, Radiologie Innenstadt, Institut für radiologische Diagnostik, Universität München, Germany

T903   Prof. Possinger, Prof. Bick, Medizinische Klinik und Poliklinik II mit Schwerpunkt Onkologie und Hämatologie, Charité Campus Mitte, Berlin, Germany

T904   Prof. Ravelli (verstorben), ehem. Institut für Anatomie, Universität Innsbruck, Austria

T905   Prof. Reich, Klinik für Mund-Kiefer-Gesichtschirurgie, Universität Bonn, Germany

T906   Prof. Reiser, Dr. Wagner, Institut für radiologische Diagnostik, LMU, München, Germany

T907   Dr. Scheibe, Chirurgische Abteilung, Rosman-Krankenhaus Breisach, Germany

T908   Prof. Scheumann, Klinik für Viszeral- und Transplantationschirurgie, Hannover, Germany

T909   Prof. Schillinger, Frauenklinik, Universität Freiburg, Germany

T910   Prof. Schliephake, Mund-Kiefer-Gesichtschirurgie, Universität Göttingen, Germany

T911   Prof. Schlösser, Zentrum Frauenheilkunde, Med. Hochschule Hannover, Germany

T912   cand. med. Carsten Schröder, Kronshagen, Germany

T916   PD Dr. Vogl, Radiologische Poliklinik, Universität München, Germany

T917   Prof. Witt, Klinik für Neurochirurgie, Universität München, Germany

T975   Dr. Noam Millo, Department of Radiology, Health Sciences Centre, University of Manitoba, Canada

T1129   Prof. Dr. med. Dr. med. dent. Marco Kesting, Erlangen, Germany

T1157   Priv. Doz. Dr. R. Fuhrmann, Bad Neustadt a. d. Saale, Germany

T1188   Prof. Dr. med. Horst-Werner Korf, Frankfurt, Germany

T1189   Prof. Dr. med. Esther Asan, Julius-Maximilians-Universität Würzburg, Germany

T1190   Prof. Dr. Dr. Robert Nitsch, WWU, Münster, Germany

T1191   Prof. Dr. Dr. Dr. Günter Rager, Fribourg, Suisse

X338   Visible Human Data® Project, US National Library of Medicine

X389   Kummer B. Funktionelle Anatomie des Vorfußes. Verhandl Deutsch Orthop Ges. 53. Kongr. Hamburg 1966, Enke, 1987:482–93

Table of content

Head

Eye

Ear

Neck

Brain and spinal cord

Head

8

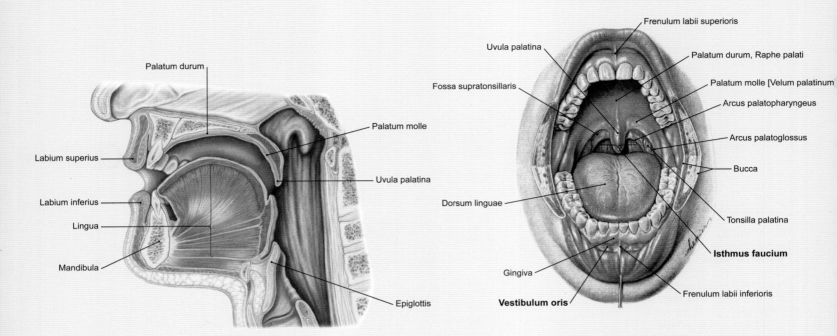

Overview

The **head (caput)** is flexibly connected to the torso (trunk, Truncus) via the neck area. This allows one to direct the sensory organs of the head towards environmental stimuli without having to move the whole body. The bony skeleton of the head is the **skull (cranium).** Its posterior section, called the neurocranium, encloses essential parts of the central nervous system (brain), while its front section, the viscerocranium, encloses the highly specialised organs of sensory perception with their greatly varying functions: the **eye** (organ of sight), the **ear** (organ of hearing and balance), the **nose** (organ of smell) and the **oral cavity** and **pharynx** (organs of taste). The respiratory tract starts in the nasal cavity and upper part of the pharynx, while the oral cavity and middle section of the pharynx mark the beginning of the digestive tract. We therefore use our heads both for **food intake and spatial orientation.** Our mouth, pharynx and masticatory apparatus along with our nose and sinuses – significantly contribute to the shape of our face. We humans additionally use the oral cavity and its organs for **articulation – enabling speech and singing.** The **mimetic muscles,** which do not have their own fascia, insert directly into the skin of the head, thus enabling unique facial expressions to aid our communication with the rest of the world. The boundary between the head and neck area are marked from the back to the front by the Protuberantia occipitalis externa at the back of the skull, the base of the ears and the Mandibula.

Main topics

After working through this chapter, you should be able to:

- describe the cranial bones and cranial development;
- name sutures and fontanelles, including closure;
- describe the basic structure of the skull, its bones and their positional relationship to each other;
- identify the neurocranium, viscerocranium, internal surface of the cranial base and cranial fossae, and explain their structure;
- name the main passageways and structures, foramina, fissures and fossae on the inner and outer surfaces of the cranial base;
- describe the insertion, origin, function and innervation of the muscles of facial expression;
- describe the structure, blood supply, lymphatic drainage and innervation of the scalp;
- name and locate key landmarks in the different areas (face, lateral facial region), systematically identify them and be able to describe the topographical route of neurovascular pathways in the areas, as well as name and visualise in three dimensions the anatomical structures deep within the lateral facial region that are not visible from the outside;
- name the main topographical features and explain their clinical relevance;
- outline the origin, route and fibre quality, and the innervation areas of the twelve cranial nerves (→ Chapter 12);
- describe the general embryological development of the nose and sinuses;
- describe the external structure of the nose, the bony and cartilaginous structure of the nasal skeleton, and the boundaries of the nasal cavities and their dimension;

- describe the blood supply and innervation of the entire nose with respect to its clinical relevance;
- demonstrate the olfactory epithelium and how it is connected to the anterior cranial fossa;
- describe the position, bony structures and openings of the sinuses, and their topographical relationship to other structures;
- explain the embryological development of the oral cavity, masticatory apparatus, tongue, palate and salivary glands;
- describe all structures of the oral cavity, their neurovascular supply, and the routes of nerves and vessels;
- describe the topography and the interrelationship of the structures and organs to each other and to the neighbouring regions, and their functions;
- explain the dental development and the detailed structure of the different teeth, including the different stages of dentition;
- describe the structure and function of the Articulatio temporomandibularis, and the position, function, blood supply and innervation of the masticatory muscles;
- outline the structure, position, function, innervation, vascular supply and lymphatic drainage of the tongue, palate and salivary glands;
- provide an exact explanation of the blood supply to the Tonsilla palatina;
- outline the topography of the floor of the mouth including its compartments, the muscles involved, and the blood supply, innervation and lymphatic drainage.

Clinical relevance

In order not to lose touch with prospective everyday clinical life with so many anatomical details, the following describes a typical case that shows why the content of this chapter is so important.

Facial paralysis

Case study
In the summer, a 22-year-old trainee visits his GP stating that for several days now he has had increasing problems moving the right side of his face and has had problems when trying to drink. In addition, saliva has been drooling constantly from the corner of his mouth. Sounds also seem louder on the right side. Otherwise, the patient appears to be healthy. He has not had any recent fever, headaches, painful limbs, any flu bouts or a tick bite. His medical history is normal. The young man is not on any medication and does not take drugs. He only drinks alcohol occasionally and in moderate amounts; he does not smoke. His family medical history is also normal.

Result of examination
The first impression and diagnosis of the patient's face as he comes into the examination room is that of facial paralysis. The right side of his face is visibly 'drooping' (→ Fig. a). The nasolabial fold on the right side has disappeared. When requested, the patient cannot frown, smile, whistle a tune or puff out his cheek on the right side. His attempt to close his eyes results in lagophthalmos (his right eye remains open) and in BELL's phenomenon.

 BELL's phenomenon: the eyeball automatically turns upwards when closing the eyelid. As the lid cannot be closed, only the white sclera of the eye remains visible.

The doctor tests the facial nerve sensitivity by brushing the patient's cheek, and finds it to be intact. Because the patient cannot frown on the affected side, the doctor comes to a preliminary diagnosis: idiopathic (no identified cause) peripheral (infranuclear) facial paralysis.

 People with central facial paralysis can still wrinkle their foreheads.

The GP refers the patient to an ENT specialist.

The ENT specialist also notes a complete right-sided peripheral facial paralysis. The patient's outer ear and facial soft tissue are normal, and his ear canal and eardrum show no signs of irritation on either side. His parotid saliva shows no signs of irritation. The palpation of his neck and face gives no indication of any tumour or infection.

Diagnostic procedure
The ENT specialist conducts an audiometry, which shows no evidence of hearing loss. To exclude other more serious causes (e.g. a tumour), he orders an MRI of the head, blood tests, an electroneurography (ENoG) and an electromyography (EMG). The blood test results are all normal, which therefore rules out zoster oticus, a herpes simplex infection and borreliosis. The ENoG and EMG reveal no signs of major nerve damage. After examination by a neurologist, neurological symptoms can also be ruled out. The MRI image shows a slight swelling of the N. facialis [VII] inside the bony canal.

Diagnosis
Idiopathic, right-sided peripheral facial paralysis.

 In up to 70 % of all cases a peripheral facial paralysis is idiopathic.

Treatment
An outpatient treatment with cortisone infusion quickly shows results; the facial movements have already begun to return to normal by the third day. The part of the nerve innervating the forehead is the only part of the nerve still not working at this stage.

Further development
An outpatient follow-up examination four weeks later confirms that his facial movements are perfectly symmetrical again.

Dissection lab
Look out for the following branches of the N. facialis: N. petrosus major, Chorda tympani and N. stapedius.

Back in the clinic
Although the patient's facial (mimetic) muscles become increasingly mobile during his cortisone treatment, he has noticed that his right eye always waters when he is eating, so he goes to visit his GP again. The doctor tells him that this so-called 'crocodile tears syndrome' is also referred to as gustatory hyperlacrimation. This harmless syndrome occasionally occurs in the regenerative processes after a facial paralysis. Affected patients experience increased lacrimation (shedding of tears) on one side when eating. Because the regenerating parasympathetic gustatory nerve fibres are growing into the lacrimal gland (Glandula lacrimalis), this results in faulty misconnection and misrouting of the nerve fibres. If the patient suffers greatly with strong subjective symptoms, Botulinum injections can be attempted as a treatment option.

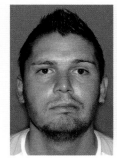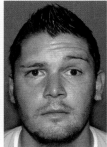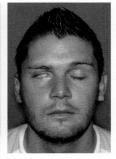

Fig. a Left: patient during examination; Centre: patient when asked to wrinkle his forehead; Right: patient when asked to close his eyes. [S700-T887]

Regions of the head and neck

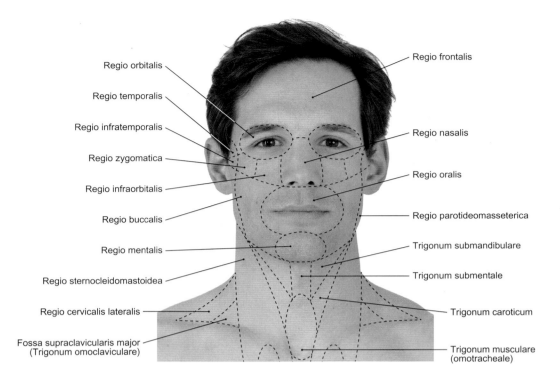

Regio orbitalis

Regio temporalis

Regio infratemporalis

Regio zygomatica

Regio infraorbitalis

Regio buccalis

Regio mentalis

Regio sternocleidomastoidea

Regio cervicalis lateralis

Fossa supraclavicularis major
(Trigonum omoclaviculare)

Regio frontalis

Regio nasalis

Regio oralis

Regio parotideomasseterica

Trigonum submandibulare

Trigonum submentale

Trigonum caroticum

Trigonum musculare
(omotracheale)

Fig. 8.1 Regions of the head and neck, Regiones capitis et colli;
frontal view. [S700-J803]
The **head** is conventionally subdivided into the following topographical
regions:
* Regio frontalis
* Regio temporalis
* Regio orbitalis
* Regio nasalis

* Regio infraorbitalis
* Regio zygomatica
* Regio oralis
* Regio buccalis
* Regio mentalis
* Regio parietalis
* Regio occipitalis
* Regio parotideomasseterica.

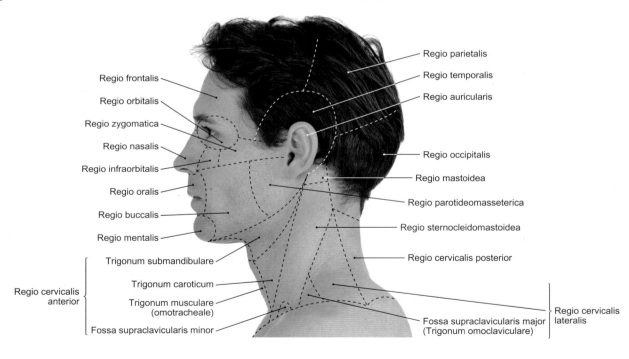

Regio frontalis

Regio orbitalis

Regio zygomatica

Regio nasalis

Regio infraorbitalis

Regio oralis

Regio buccalis

Regio mentalis

Trigonum submandibulare

Regio cervicalis
anterior

Trigonum caroticum

Trigonum musculare
(omotracheale)

Fossa supraclavicularis minor

Regio parietalis

Regio temporalis

Regio auricularis

Regio occipitalis

Regio mastoidea

Regio parotideomasseterica

Regio sternocleidomastoidea

Regio cervicalis posterior

Regio cervicalis
lateralis

Fossa supraclavicularis major
(Trigonum omoclaviculare)

Fig. 8.2 Regions of the head and neck, Regiones capitis et colli;
lateral view. [S700-J803]
The **neck** is conventionally subdivided into the following topographical
regions:
* Regio cervicalis anterior, consisting of the Trigonum submandibulare,
Trigonum caroticum and Trigonum musculare (omotracheal)

* Regio sternocleidomastoidea with Fossa supraclavicularis minor
* Regio cervicalis lateralis with Trigonum omoclaviculare
* Regio cervicalis posterior.

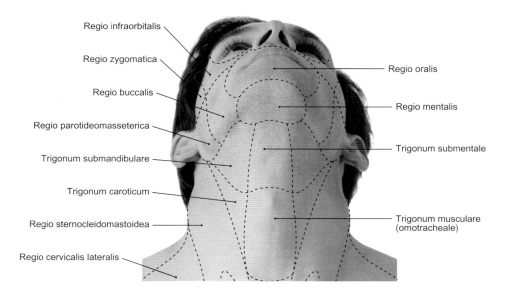

Regio infraorbitalis

Regio zygomatica

Regio buccalis

Regio parotideomasseterica

Trigonum submandibulare

Trigonum caroticum

Regio sternocleidomastoidea

Regio cervicalis lateralis

Regio oralis

Regio mentalis

Trigonum submentale

Trigonum musculare (omotracheale)

Fig. 8.3   Regions of the head and neck, Regiones capitis et colli; anterolateral view. [S700-J803]

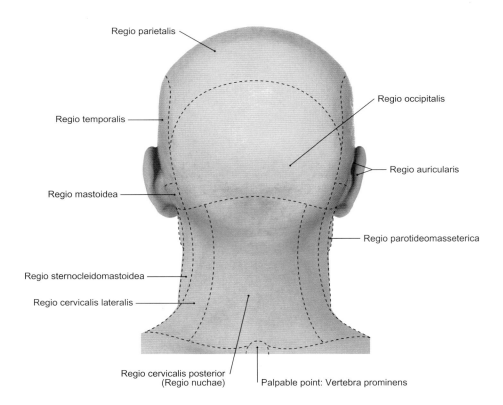

Regio parietalis

Regio temporalis

Regio mastoidea

Regio sternocleidomastoidea

Regio cervicalis lateralis

Regio occipitalis

Regio auricularis

Regio parotideomasseterica

Regio cervicalis posterior (Regio nuchae)

Palpable point: Vertebra prominens

Fig. 8.4   Regions of the head and neck, Regiones capitis et colli; posterior view. [S700-J803/L271]
The posterior region of the neck is often also referred to as the nuchal region.

Facial morphometry and proportions

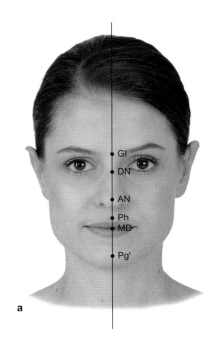

a

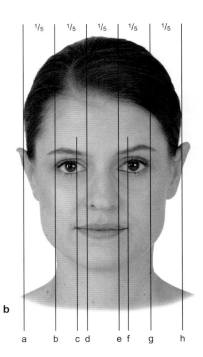

b

a   b   c d   e f   g   h

Fig. 8.5a and b   Facial morphometry and proportions; frontal view; vertical proportions. [S700-J803]/[E1043]

a In ideally proportioned faces, the midline of the face runs directly through the glabella (Gl), the bridge of the nose (Dorsum nasi, DN), the tip of the nose (Apex nasi, AN), the philtrum (Ph) and the soft tissue of the pogonion (Pg'). The centre of the dental arch (Medietas dentium, MD) also aligns with this midline.

b If perfectly symmetrical, the face can be divided by vertical lines into five equal parts. These lines run along the outer edge of the auricles (a, h), and pass through the lateral (b, g) and medial (d, e) corners of the eyes. The corners of the mouth (c, f) generally align vertically with the medial rim of the iris.

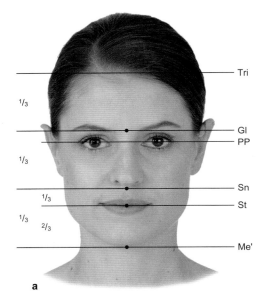

a

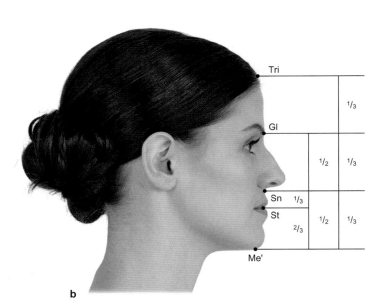

b

Fig. 8.6a and b   Facial morphometry and proportions; transverse proportions. [S700-J803]/[E1043]

a Frontal view.

b Lateral view.

If perfectly symmetrical, the face can be divided by horizontal lines into three equal parts. Equal distances between the hairline (trichion, Tri) and the glabella (Gl), between the glabella and the subnasion (Sn), and be-

tween the subnasion and the chin (Menton, Me') allow the division into the upper face, midface and lower face. The lower face is further divided into thirds by the line where the upper lip and lower lip meet (St). One third is located above the line between the two lips, while the chin region takes up the lower two-thirds. The transverse mid-pupillary line (PP) can also be used for orientation if both eyes are exactly at the same height.

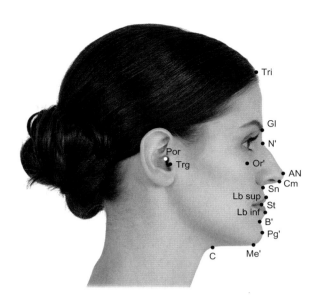

Fig. 8.7 Most common measuring points of the face; lateral view.
[S700-J803]/[E1043]

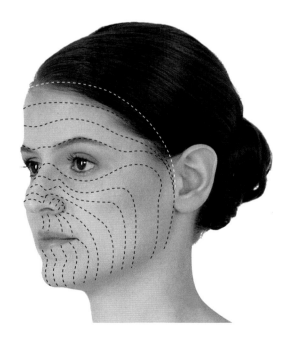

Fig. 8.8 Tension lines of the skin of the face; frontal view from the right side. [S700-J803]/[E1043]

With any facial surgical operations involving incisions in the skin, attention must be paid to the tension lines, which are created by the direction of the collagen fibrils and the position of the mimetic muscles. Incisions along these lines and wrinkles are the best option as they reduce the tension in the skin to a minimum, and thus minimise the scar formation.

Abbreviation	Measuring point	Explanation
Tri	Trichion	Hairline
Gl	Glabella	Raised area of the Os frontale between the eyebrows
N'	Soft tissue nasion	Lowest point between the nose and forehead
Or'	Soft tissue orbital point	Lowest point of the curved edge of the orbit
AN	Apex nasi	Tip of nose
Cm	Columella	Bridge of tissue that separates the nostrils
Sn	Subnasion	
Lb sup	Labrale superius	Foremost point of the upper lip
St	Stomium	Contact area between the two lips
Lb Inf	Labrale inferius	Foremost point of the lower lip
B'	Soft tissue labio-mental point	Lowest point of the labiomental fold
Pg'	Soft tissue pogo-nion	
Me'	Soft tissue chin	Furthest caudal point of the soft tissue of the chin contour
C	Cervical point	Transition point where the submental contour meets the contour of the neck
Por	Porion	Opening of the ear canal
Trg	Tragion	Protruding edge of the tragus

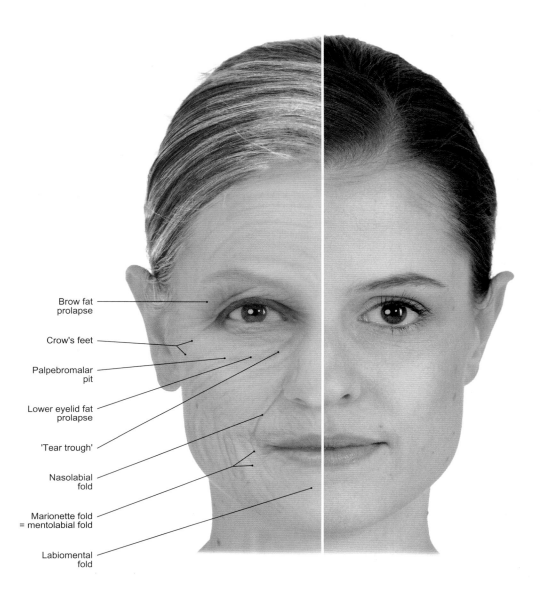

Brow fat
prolapse

Crow's feet

Palpebromalar
pit

Lower eyelid fat
prolapse

'Tear trough'

Nasolabial
fold

Marionette fold
= mentolabial fold

Labiomental
fold

Fig. 8.9 Ageing of the face; frontal view. [S700-J803/L271]/[E1043]
Increasing age brings complex changes not only to the skin of the face, but to all other tissues such as bone, muscle or subcutaneous fat deposits (subcutaneous fat compartments) as well. This is due to ageing processes that are specific to each region of the face, and progress at very different rates depending on the individual. They can be influenced by many environmental factors (e. g. UV radiation, smoking). The ageing process, which is slow but inexorable, has a visible effect on the skin: more and more wrinkles are formed, and gravity forces make the skin and the subcutaneous connective tissue sag. This is particularly evident on the eyelids and at the corners of the mouth.

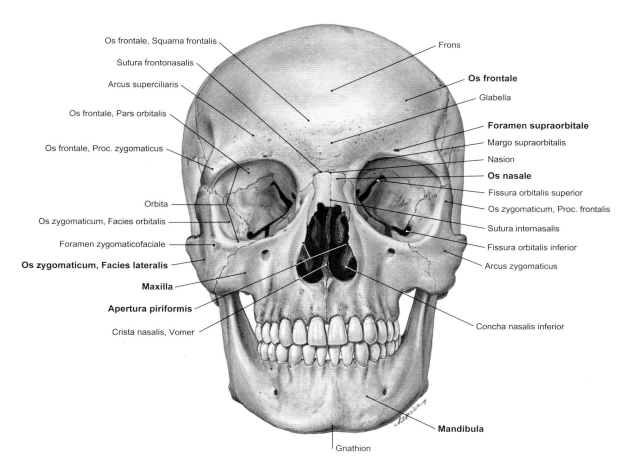

Os frontale, Squama frontalis

Sutura frontonasalis

Arcus superciliaris

Os frontale, Pars orbitalis

Os frontale, Proc. zygomaticus

Orbita

Os zygomaticum, Facies orbitalis

Foramen zygomaticofaciale

Os zygomaticum, Facies lateralis

Maxilla

Apertura piriformis

Crista nasalis, Vomer

Frons

Os frontale

Glabella

Foramen supraorbitale

Margo supraorbitalis

Nasion

Os nasale

Fissura orbitalis superior

Os zygomaticum, Proc. frontalis

Sutura internasalis

Fissura orbitalis inferior

Arcus zygomaticus

Concha nasalis inferior

Mandibula

Gnathion

Fig. 8.10 Skull, cranium; frontal view. [S700]
From bottom to top: the lower jaw (Mandibula), the two halves of the upper jaw (Maxillae), the nasal bones (Ossa nasalia) between the upper jaw and orbit (Orbita) and, above the Orbita, the Os frontale.
The **Os frontale** consists of four parts (→ Fig. 8.28). Above the upper margin of each orbit (Margo supraorbitalis), the protruding Arcus superciliaris (superciliary arch) can be felt. A continuation of the Os frontale extends medially downwards to form in part the medial margin of the

orbit. Laterally, the Proc. zygomaticus meets the Proc. frontalis of the Os zygomaticum. Both form the lateral margin of the orbit.
The **Os zygomaticum** constitutes the major part of the lateral and lower margins of the orbit.
The nasal bone **(Os nasale)** connects with the Os frontale at the frontonasal suture on both sides, while the internasal suture connects the two nose bones themselves.

Structure and function

The skull bones cover the brain (neurocranium, blue) and forms the bony foundation of the face (viscerocranium or splanchnocranium, orange)(→ figure). Based on morphological criteria, the skull is divided into the calvaria (top part of the skull) and the skull base. The bones of the **neurocranium** are: 1. Os ethmoidale (ethmoid bone), 2. upper part of the Os frontale (frontal bone), 3. Os sphenoidale (sphenoidal bone), 4. Os temporale (paired temporal bone), 5. Os parietale (paired parietal bone), 6. Os occipitale (occipital bone).
The **viscerocranium** is composed of: 1. the lower part of the Os frontale (frontal bone), 2. maxilla (paired, includes the Os incisivum which is fused with the maxilla bones prenatally), 3. Os zygomaticum (paired zygomatic bone), 4. Mandibula (mandible), 5. Os nasale (paired nasal bone), 6. Os concha inferius (paired inferior concha),

7. Os lacrimale (paired lacrimal bone), 8. Os palatinum (paired palatine bone), 9. Vomer.

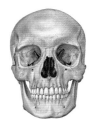

[S700-L127]

Clinical remarks

Central midface fractures occur most frequently as a result of traffic accidents. They are categorised according to LE FORT (→ figure) as:
• **LE FORT I:** isolated disjunction fracture of the Proc. alveolaris
• **LE FORT II:** disjunction fracture of the maxilla in the area of the mid-orbital floor, possibly involving the Os ethmoidale, the anterior cranial base and/or the Os nasale
• **LE FORT III:** complete disjunction fracture of the facial skeleton from the neurocranium

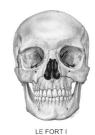

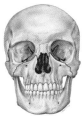

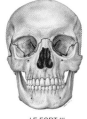

LE FORT I

LE FORT II

LE FORT III

[S700]

Skeleton and joints

Cranial bones

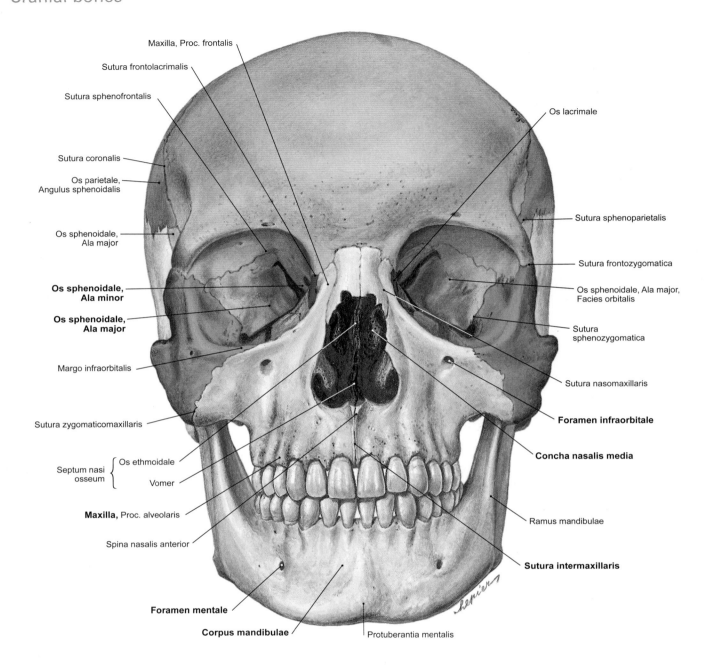

Maxilla, Proc. frontalis

Sutura frontolacrimalis

Sutura sphenofrontalis

Os lacrimale

Sutura coronalis

Os parietale,
Angulus sphenoidalis

Sutura sphenoparietalis

Os sphenoidale,
Ala major

Sutura frontozygomatica

**Os sphenoidale,
Ala minor**

Os sphenoidale, Ala major,
Facies orbitalis

**Os sphenoidale,
Ala major**

Sutura
sphenozygomatica

Margo infraorbitalis

Sutura nasomaxillaris

Sutura zygomaticomaxillaris

Foramen infraorbitale

Septum nasi osseum { Os ethmoidale

Concha nasalis media

Vomer

Maxilla, Proc. alveolaris

Spina nasalis anterior

Ramus mandibulae

Sutura intermaxillaris

Foramen mentale

Corpus mandibulae

Protuberantia mentalis

Fig. 8.11 Cranial bones, Ossa cranii; frontal view; for colour chart, see p. XIII. [S700]

The upper jaw or maxillary bone **(Maxilla)** is located between the orbit and the oral cavity. The maxilla forms part of the lower and the medial margins of the orbit and borders laterally on the Os zygomaticum. The Proc. frontalis of the maxilla connects with the Os frontale. In the body of the maxilla, below the lower orbital margin, is the Foramen infraorbitale. There is a bony projection in the midline, the Spina nasalis anterior.

Below this is the Proc. alveolaris, which forms the lower edge of the upper jaw and holds the teeth.

The lower jaw or mandible **(Mandibula)** consists of the Corpus and Rami mandibulae, both of which converge at the Angulus mandibulae. The Corpus mandibulae holds the teeth. Underneath that is the Basis mandibulae, the protrusion at the midline of the Protuberantia mentalis. The Foramen mentale is also visible.

Clinical remarks

Fractures of the nasal bone or other bone/cartilage of the nose are among the most common fractures in the facial area. We distinguish between closed and open nasal fractures; in the latter, the bone is exposed as a result of injury to the skin and soft tissue. The

nasal septum and Conchae nasales can also be fractured as a result. Fractures of the bone/cartilage of the nose are typical injuries resulting from violent physical disputes, car accidents, martial arts such as karate and boxing, and a variety of team sports.

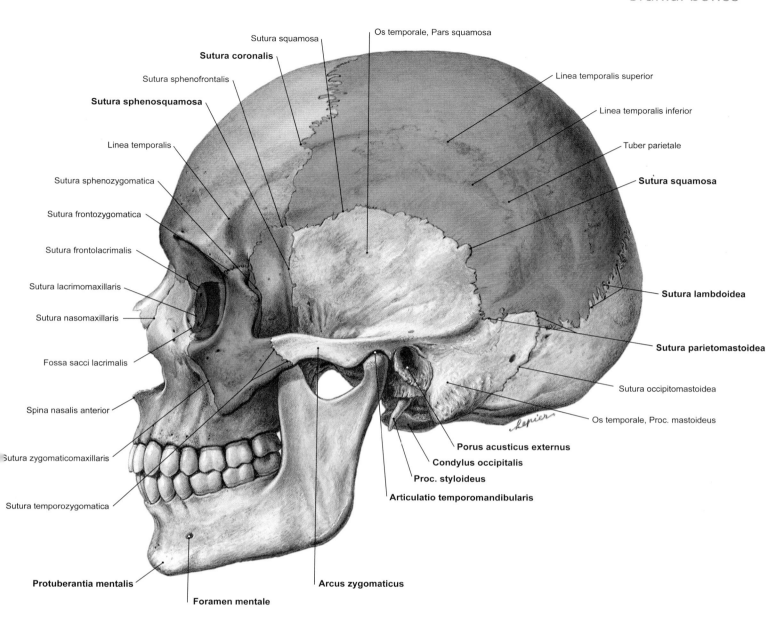

Sutura squamosa
Sutura coronalis
Sutura sphenofrontalis
Sutura sphenosquamosa
Linea temporalis
Sutura sphenozygomatica
Sutura frontozygomatica
Sutura frontolacrimalis
Sutura lacrimomaxillaris
Sutura nasomaxillaris
Fossa sacci lacrimalis
Spina nasalis anterior
Sutura zygomaticomaxillaris
Sutura temporozygomatica
Protuberantia mentalis
Foramen mentale
Arcus zygomaticus
Os temporale, Pars squamosa
Linea temporalis superior
Linea temporalis inferior
Tuber parietale
Sutura squamosa
Sutura lambdoidea
Sutura parietomastoidea
Sutura occipitomastoidea
Os temporale, Proc. mastoideus
Porus acusticus externus
Condylus occipitalis
Proc. styloideus
Articulatio temporomandibularis

Fig. 8.12 Cranial bones, Ossa cranii; lateral view; for colour chart, see p. XIII. [S700]

The lateral view displays parts of the Ossa frontale, parietale, occipitale, sphenoidale and temporale, parts of the viscerocranium (Os nasale, Os lacrimale, maxilla and Os zygomaticum) and the lateral aspect of the lower jaw (Mandibula).

Within the viscerocranium, the **Os nasale** borders the Os frontale cranially and the maxilla posteriorly. The upper part of the Os lacrimale forms the Fossa sacci lacrimalis between the maxilla and the Os ethmoidale. The Proc. alveolaris of the maxilla contains the upper teeth. Medially, the **maxilla** connects with the Os frontale and laterally with the Os zygomaticum. At the front there is a bony projection, the Spina nasalis anterior. The **Os zygomaticum** gives the cheek area its contour. The head of the Mandibula (Caput mandibulae) articulates with the temporal bone in the Articulatio temporomandibularis.

The upper frontal aspect of the **Os frontale** connects with the parietal bone (Os parietale) and the sphenoidal bone (Os sphenoidale) along the Sutura coronalis. The Os parietale borders the occipital bone (Os occipitale) along the Sutura lambdoidea. The Pars squamosa of the Os temporale forms the major part of the lateral wall of the skull.

The Os temporale and Os zygomaticum form the Arcus zygomaticus, which bridges the Fossa temporalis.

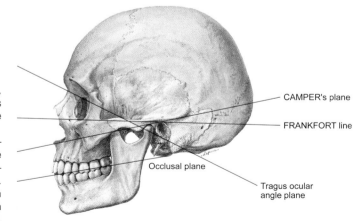

CAMPER's plane
FRANKFORT line
Occlusal plane
Tragus ocular angle plane

Fig. 8.13 Planes of reference for the jaw. [S700]
FRANKFORT horizontalline: plane between the lower edge of the orbit and the upper edge of the Meatus acusticus externus
CAMPER's plane: between the lowest point of the Spina nasalis anterior and the highest point of the Meatus acusticus externus
Occlusal plane: runs parallel to the CAMPER's plane
Basion-nasion plane: between the medial angle of the eye and the tragus

Skeleton and joints

Cranial bones

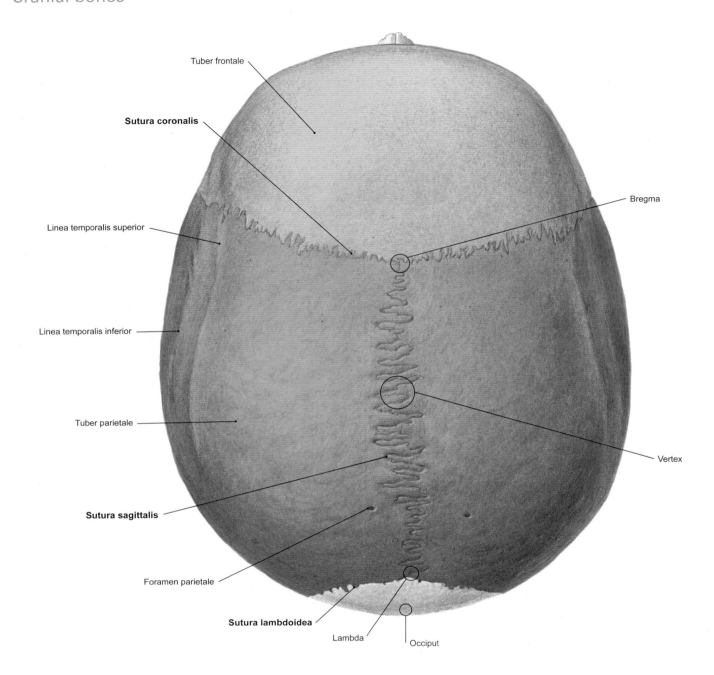

Tuber frontale

Sutura coronalis

Bregma

Linea temporalis superior

Linea temporalis inferior

Tuber parietale

Vertex

Sutura sagittalis

Foramen parietale

Sutura lambdoidea

Lambda

Occiput

Fig. 8.14 Cranial bones, Ossa cranii; view from above; for colour chart, see p. XIII. [S700]
A view of the upper part of the skull (skull cap, calvaria) reveals the Os frontale, the Ossa parietalia, and the Os occipitale. The Os frontale and Ossa parietalia are bordered by the **Sutura coronalis.** The two Ossa parietalia are bordered by the **Sutura sagittalis.** The Os occipitale is connected, along with the two Ossa parietalia, to the **Sutura lambdoidea.** The point of contact of the Sutura coronalis and the Sutura sagittalis is called the **Bregma,** and the point at which the Suturae sagittalis and lambdoidea meet, is called the **Lambda.** In the dorsal part of the Ossa parietalia, directly adjacent to the Sutura sagittalis, are pairs of Foramina parietalia for the passage of the Vv. emissariae.

Clinical remarks

A violent impact with a great external force can often cause **skull fractures.** It is possible to differentiate between the following: **linear fractures** with a clear fracture line, **split skull fractures** with multiple bony fragments (impression fractures in which bony parts point inwards which can cause a compression or tear of the dura mater as well as an injury to brain tissue), sutural **diastases** (widening of sutures) and **fractures of the base of the skull.** Any fracture associated with a rupture/laceration of the scalp or linked to the sinuses or the middle ear is regarded as an open fracture requiring surgical treatment due to the potential risk of infection.

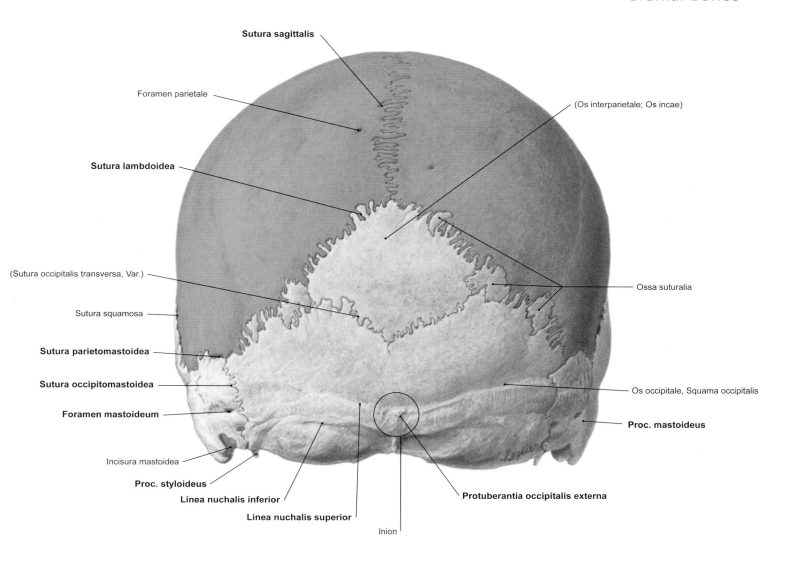

Sutura sagittalis

Foramen parietale

(Os interparietale; Os incae)

Sutura lambdoidea

(Sutura occipitalis transversa, Var.)

Ossa suturalia

Sutura squamosa

Sutura parietomastoidea

Sutura occipitomastoidea

Os occipitale, Squama occipitalis

Foramen mastoideum

Proc. mastoideus

Incisura mastoidea

Proc. styloideus

Linea nuchalis inferior

Protuberantia occipitalis externa

Linea nuchalis superior

Inion

Fig. 8.15   Cranial bones, Ossa cranii; posterior view; for colour chart, see p. XIII. [S700]
This view from the posterior aspect shows the Os temporale, Os parietale and Os occipitale. Laterally, the **Os temporale** can be seen with the Proc. mastoideus on both sides. At the lower medial edge of the Proc. mastoideus is the Incisura mastoidea, a notch where the Venter posterior of the M. digastricus inserts.
In this posterior view, both of the **Ossa parietalia** can be seen, which meet in the midline via the Sutura sagittalis, and posteriorly border the Os occipitale via the Sutura lambdoidea, and laterally and externally border the temporal bones via the Suturae parietomastoideae.

A large portion of the posterior skull is formed by the **Os occipitale.** Its central structure is the Squama occipitalis. Frequently, structural variants called sutural bones (Ossa suturalia) can be found in the area of the Sutura lambdoidea. The Os occipitale has a bony landmark, the Protuberantia occipitalis externa, which is usually easily palpable. Its furthest protruding point is called the inion. Laterally, the protuberance continues on both sides in the arch-shaped Linea nuchalis superior, a bony ridge for the attachment of the autochthonous back muscles. Approximately 2–2.5 cm below the Protuberantia occipitalis externa are the arch-shaped ridges of the Linea nuchalis inferior, serving as attachment sites for further muscles.

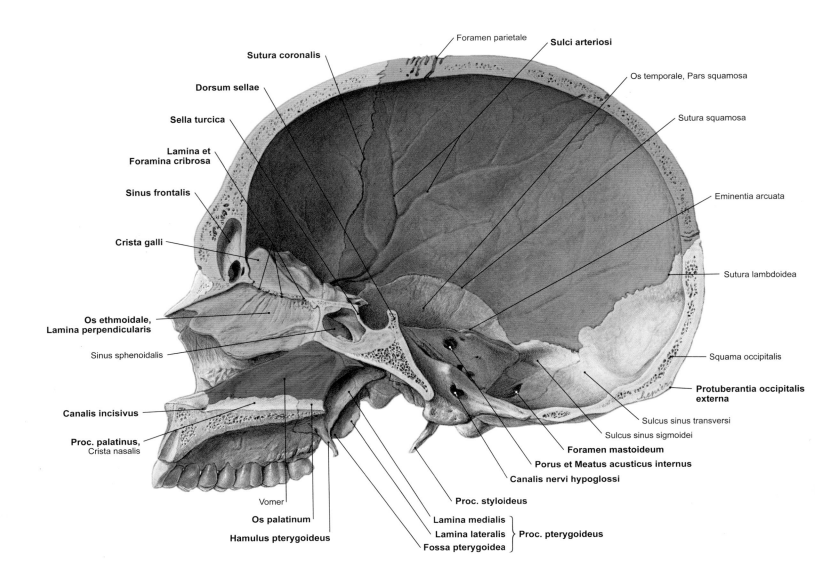

Foramen parietale
Sulci arteriosi
Sutura coronalis
Os temporale, Pars squamosa
Dorsum sellae
Sutura squamosa
Sella turcica
Lamina et Foramina cribrosa
Sinus frontalis
Eminentia arcuata
Crista galli
Sutura lambdoidea
Os ethmoidale, Lamina perpendicularis
Sinus sphenoidalis
Squama occipitalis
Canalis incisivus
Protuberantia occipitalis externa
Proc. palatinus, Crista nasalis
Sulcus sinus transversi
Sulcus sinus sigmoidei
Foramen mastoideum
Porus et Meatus acusticus internus
Canalis nervi hypoglossi
Vomer
Proc. styloideus
Os palatinum
Lamina medialis
Hamulus pterygoideus
Lamina lateralis ⎫ Proc. pterygoideus
Fossa pterygoidea ⎭

Fig. 8.16 Cranial bones, Ossa cranii, right side; medial view; for co-lour chart, see p. XIII. [S700]

The cranial cavity comprises the calvaria, as well as the base of the skull formed by the anterior, middle and posterior cranial fossae. The cranial cavity surrounds the brain with its meninges and encloses the proximal portion of the cranial nerves, including the blood vessels and the ve-nous sinuses. On the internal surface of the cranium, the arterial grooves (Sulci arteriosi) can be seen, made visible by the pulsing of the A. meningea media. At the transition to the viscerocranium, the Lamina perpendicularis of the Os ethmoidale and the vomer connect to the bony nasal septum. The hard palate is formed by the Proc. palatinus of the maxilla and by the Os palatinum.

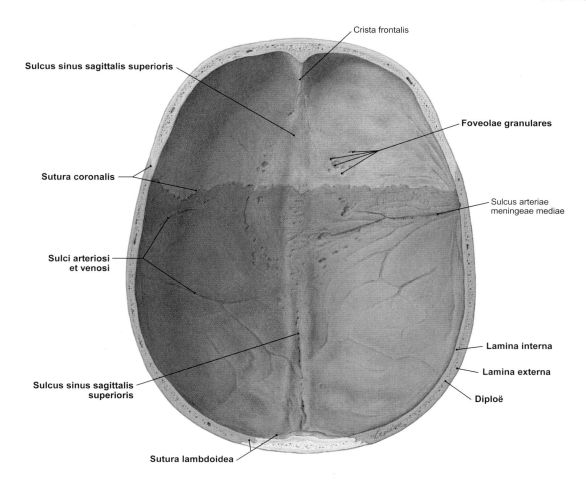

Crista frontalis

Sulcus sinus sagittalis superioris

Foveolae granulares

Sutura coronalis

Sulcus arteriae meningeae mediae

Sulci arteriosi et venosi

Lamina interna

Lamina externa

Sulcus sinus sagittalis superioris

Diploë

Sutura lambdoidea

Fig. 8.17   Calvaria; view from the inside; for colour chart, see p. XIII. [S700]
On the inside of the calvaria, the Suturae coronalis between the Os frontale and Ossa parietalia can be seen, and the Sutura lambdoidea between the Ossa parietalia and the Os occipitale. Further along, the Crista frontalis is visible on the inside of the Os frontale, which serves to connect the Falx cerebri (duplication of tight connective tissue; separates the two cerebral hemispheres). The Crista frontalis transitions into the Sulcus sinus sagittalis superioris (groove of the Sinus sagittalis superior) which becomes wider and deeper towards the posterior part. It extends across the Sutura lambdoidea to the Os occipitale.

Bilaterally and along the entire length of the Sulcus sinus sagittalis superioris, there are irregularly grouped small depressions (Foveolae granulares), in which the cauliflower-like Granulationes arachnoideae (PACCHIONIAN granulations) are found. In the lateral parts of the cranial bones, numerous grooves can be seen (Sulci arteriosi et venosi).
The **bones** of the **calvaria** possess a special **structure.** They consist of a thick outer and a thin inner compact layer, the Lamina externa and Lamina interna (Lamina vitrea), and a thin layer of spongiosa, known as diploë.

Clinical remarks

An external impact to the head can cause **skull fractures** (→ figures).

1. **Linear fractures** show clear fracture lines (1) extending through the entire thickness of the skull and mostly do not include a shift in bones.
2. Closed **depressed fractures** (2) include several bone fragments pointing inwards. Frequently, the dura mater is injured which is an indication for surgical intervention. Otherwise, these fractures heal very well on their own without special treatment.
3. Open depressed fractures are another type and include a simultaneous injury to the scalp (3). If the underlying dura mater ruptured as well, this qualifies as an open brain trauma. In both cases, intervention by a neurosurgeon or ENT physician is necessary, depending on a possible involvement of the sinuses and/or ear which increases the risk of infection.
4. **Diastatic fractures,** also named 'growing fractures', (4) occur in babies and toddlers, aligning with or perpendicular to sutures, and can cause widening of the sutures.
5. **Skull base fractures** (not shown). The very fine Lamina interna of the skull cap is frequently traumatised during **bending fractures of the skull.** When branches of the A. meningea media are injured along their pathway in the Sulcus arteriae meningeae mediae of

the Lamina interna, an epidural haematoma can develop (see Clinical remarks → Fig. 12.74).

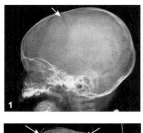
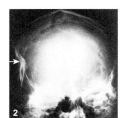
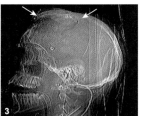
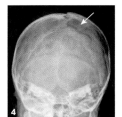

1 [G305], 2 [G198], 3 [G211], 4 [G305]

Internal surface of the cranial base

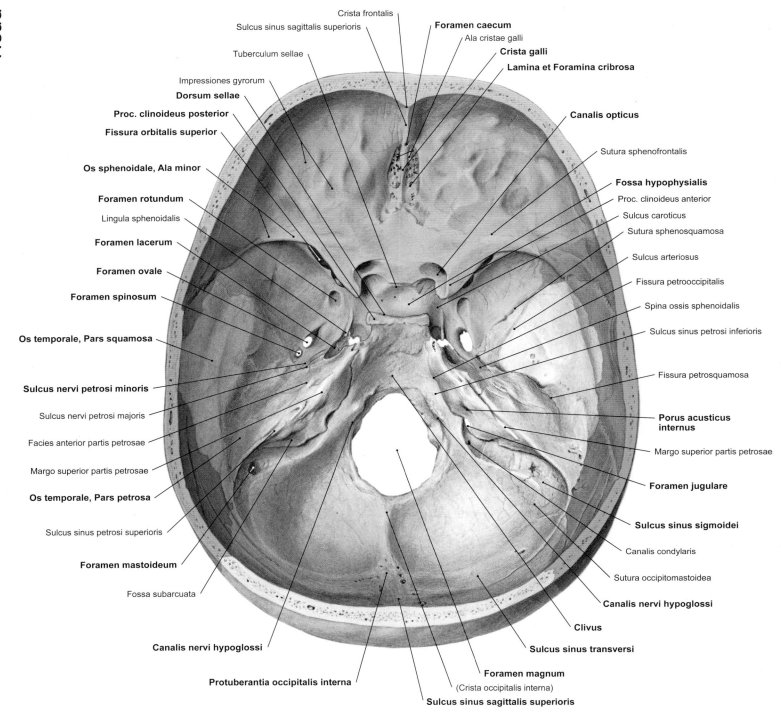

Crista frontalis
Sulcus sinus sagittalis superioris
Tuberculum sellae
Impressiones gyrorum
Dorsum sellae
Proc. clinoideus posterior
Fissura orbitalis superior
Os sphenoidale, Ala minor
Foramen rotundum
Lingula sphenoidalis
Foramen lacerum
Foramen ovale
Foramen spinosum
Os temporale, Pars squamosa
Sulcus nervi petrosi minoris
Sulcus nervi petrosi majoris
Facies anterior partis petrosae
Margo superior partis petrosae
Os temporale, Pars petrosa
Sulcus sinus petrosi superioris
Foramen mastoideum
Fossa subarcuata
Canalis nervi hypoglossi
Protuberantia occipitalis interna

Foramen caecum
Ala cristae galli
Crista galli
Lamina et Foramina cribrosa
Canalis opticus
Sutura sphenofrontalis
Fossa hypophysialis
Proc. clinoideus anterior
Sulcus caroticus
Sutura sphenosquamosa
Sulcus arteriosus
Fissura petrooccipitalis
Spina ossis sphenoidalis
Sulcus sinus petrosi inferioris
Fissura petrosquamosa
Porus acusticus internus
Margo superior partis petrosae
Foramen jugulare
Sulcus sinus sigmoidei
Canalis condylaris
Sutura occipitomastoidea
Canalis nervi hypoglossi
Clivus
Sulcus sinus transversi
Foramen magnum
(Crista occipitalis interna)
Sulcus sinus sagittalis superioris

Fig. 8.18 Internal surface of the cranial base, Basis cranii interna; view from above; for colour chart, see p. XIII. [S700]

The anterior (Fossa cranii anterior), middle (Fossa cranii media) and posterior cranial fossae (Fossa cranii posterior) form the internal surface of the cranial base.

The Ossa frontale, ethmoidalia and sphenoidale make up the floor of the **anterior cranial fossa,** which lies above the nasal cavity and the eye sockets. In the anterior cranial fossa are the Foramen caecum, the Crista galli (attachment point of the Falx cerebri) and on both sides the Lamina cribrosa. Posterior to the Ossa frontale and ethmoidalia, the Corpus and the Alae minores of the Os sphenoidale form the base of

the anterior cranial fossa. The Corpus also forms the border to the middle cranial fossa.

The **middle cranial fossa** is formed by the Ossa sphenoidale and temporalia. Its floor is elevated in the midline, where it continues into the Corpus of the Os sphenoidale. The lateral portion forms fossae and are all part of the Ala major of the Os sphenoidale and the Pars squamosa of the Os temporale. Located in the middle cranial fossa are, on both sides of the saddle-shaped Sella turcica with the Fossa hypophysialis, the Canalis opticus, the Fissura orbitalis superior, and the Foramina rotundum, ovale, spinosum and lacerum. The posterior aspect of the middle cranial fossa is formed by the Facies anterior partis petrosae.

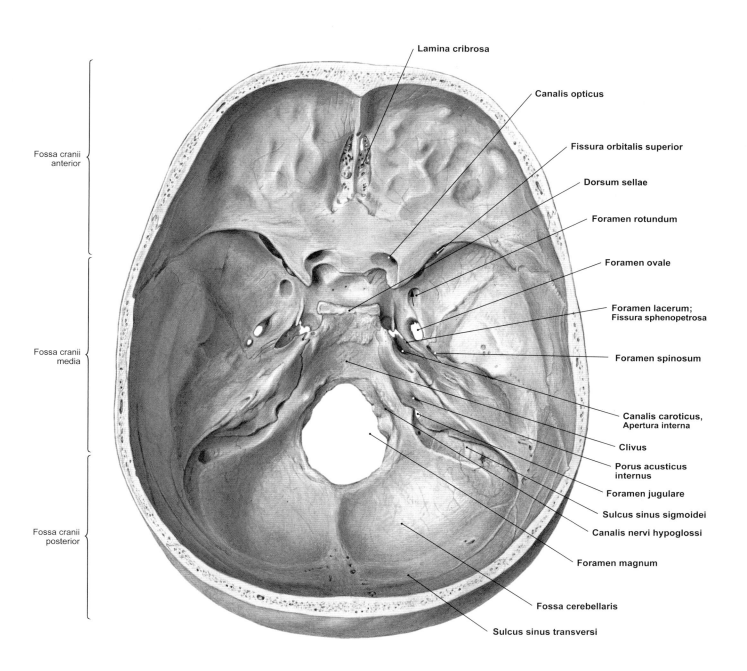

Fossa cranii anterior

Fossa cranii media

Fossa cranii posterior

Lamina cribrosa

Canalis opticus

Fissura orbitalis superior

Dorsum sellae

Foramen rotundum

Foramen ovale

Foramen lacerum; Fissura sphenopetrosa

Foramen spinosum

Canalis caroticus, Apertura interna

Clivus

Porus acusticus internus

Foramen jugulare

Sulcus sinus sigmoidei

Canalis nervi hypoglossi

Foramen magnum

Fossa cerebellaris

Sulcus sinus transversi

Fig. 8.19 Internal surface of the cranial base, Basis cranii interna; view from above. [S700]

Of the three cranial fossae, the **posterior cranial fossa** is the biggest. It is mainly formed by the Ossa temporalia and the Os occipitale and to a lesser extent by the Os sphenoidale and the Ossa parietalia.

In the midline, its anterior margin is formed by the Dorsum sellae and the Clivus. The Clivus is a bony surface sloping from the Dorsum sellae to the Foramen magnum. It consists of parts of the Corpus of the Os sphenoidale and the Pars basilaris of the Os occipitale. Dorsally, the

posterior cranial fossa is mainly confined by the Sulcus sinus transversi. The Foramen magnum is the largest opening of the posterior cranial fossa.

Additional structures of the posterior cranial fossa include the Canalis nervi hypoglossi, the Porus acusticus internus and the Foramen jugulare. The Sulcus sinus sigmoidei leads laterally to the Foramen jugulare. The central depression of the posterior cranial fossa is the Fossa cerebellaris.

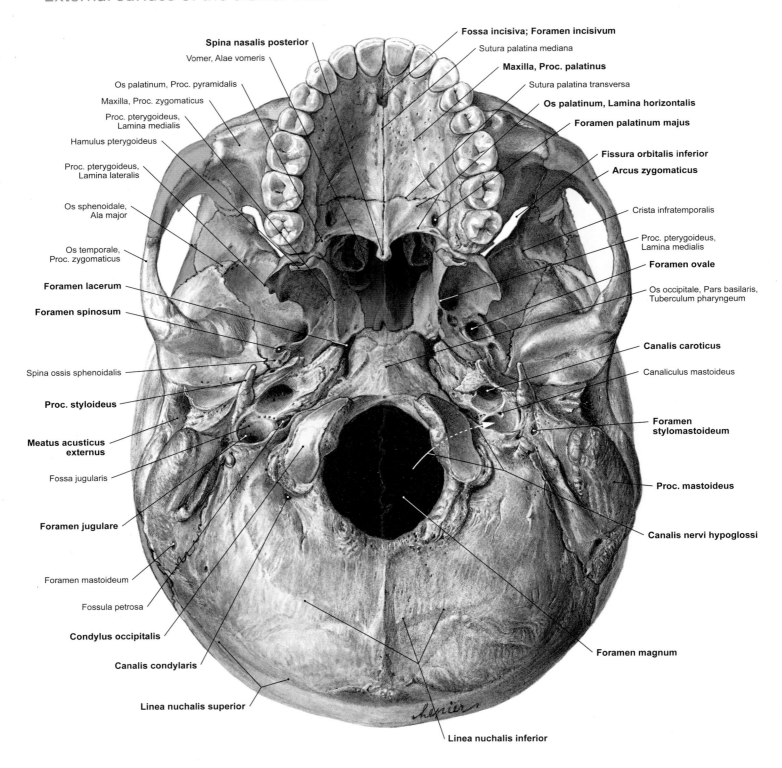

Spina nasalis posterior
Vomer, Alae vomeris
Os palatinum, Proc. pyramidalis
Maxilla, Proc. zygomaticus
Proc. pterygoideus, Lamina medialis
Hamulus pterygoideus
Proc. pterygoideus, Lamina lateralis
Os sphenoidale, Ala major
Os temporale, Proc. zygomaticus
Foramen lacerum
Foramen spinosum
Spina ossis sphenoidalis
Proc. styloideus
Meatus acusticus externus
Fossa jugularis
Foramen jugulare
Foramen mastoideum
Fossula petrosa
Condylus occipitalis
Canalis condylaris
Linea nuchalis superior

Fossa incisiva; Foramen incisivum
Sutura palatina mediana
Maxilla, Proc. palatinus
Sutura palatina transversa
Os palatinum, Lamina horizontalis
Foramen palatinum majus
Fissura orbitalis inferior
Arcus zygomaticus
Crista infratemporalis
Proc. pterygoideus, Lamina medialis
Foramen ovale
Os occipitale, Pars basilaris, Tuberculum pharyngeum
Canalis caroticus
Canaliculus mastoideus
Foramen stylomastoideum
Proc. mastoideus
Canalis nervi hypoglossi
Foramen magnum
Linea nuchalis inferior

Fig. 8.20 External surface of the cranial base, Basis cranii externa; view from below; for colour chart, see p. XIII. [S700]

At the front, the cranial base extends up to the middle incisors, laterally to the Proc. mastoideus and Arcus zygomaticus, respectively, and at the back to the Lineae nuchales superiores. The cranial base is divided into three compartments:

- anterior compartment, with maxillary teeth and palate
- middle compartment, posterior to the palate up to the anterior margin of the Foramen magnum
- posterior compartment from the anterior margin of the Foramen magnum to the Lineae nuchales superiores.

Anterior cranial base: encompasses the hard palate (→ Fig. 8.31).

Middle cranial base: the anterior part of the middle compartment consists of the vomer and Os sphenoidale; the posterior part is formed by the Ossa temporalia and Os occipitale. The Os sphenoidale, which is above the vomer and in the midline at the front, contributes to the Pars posterior of the bony nasal septum.

The Os sphenoidale is composed of a central Corpus and the paired Alae majores and Alae minores (not visible from below).

Immediately behind the Corpus of the Os sphenoidale, the Pars basilaris of the Os occipitale represents the beginning of the posterior part of the middle cranial base. The Pars basilaris extends up to the Foramen magnum. At this point, the Tuberculum pharyngeum protrudes as a projection, to which parts of the pharynx are attached at the base of the skull (continuation → Fig. 8.21).

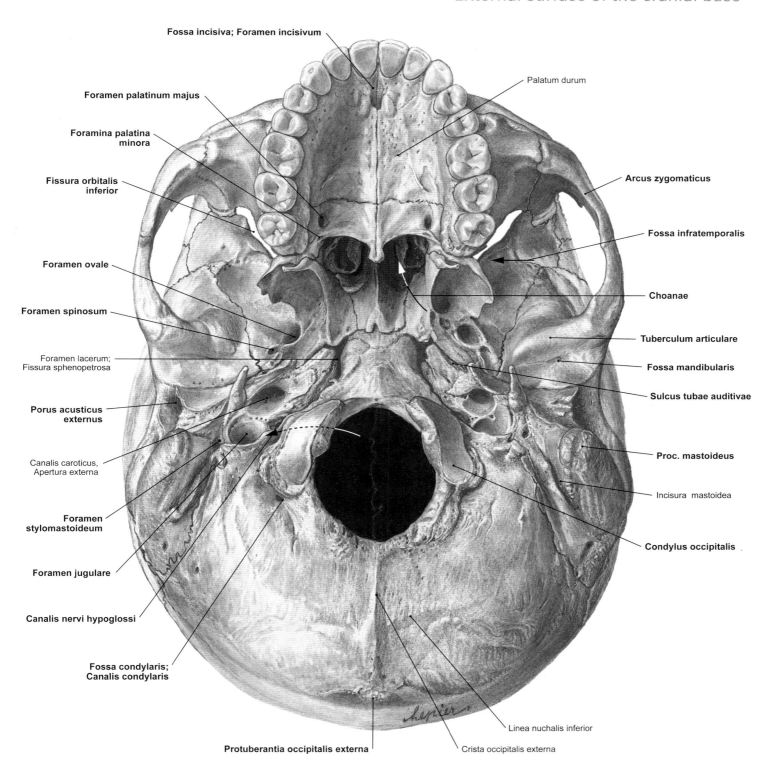

Fossa incisiva; Foramen incisivum

Foramen palatinum majus

Foramina palatina minora

Fissura orbitalis inferior

Foramen ovale

Foramen spinosum

Foramen lacerum; Fissura sphenopetrosa

Porus acusticus externus

Canalis caroticus, Apertura externa

Foramen stylomastoideum

Foramen jugulare

Canalis nervi hypoglossi

Fossa condylaris; Canalis condylaris

Protuberantia occipitalis externa

Palatum durum

Arcus zygomaticus

Fossa infratemporalis

Choanae

Tuberculum articulare

Fossa mandibularis

Sulcus tubae auditivae

Proc. mastoideus

Incisura mastoidea

Condylus occipitalis

Linea nuchalis inferior

Crista occipitalis externa

Fig. 8.21 External surface of the cranial base, Basis cranii externa; view from below. [S700]

Middle cranial base (continuation of → Fig. 8.20): the Sulcus tubae auditivae is positioned at the border between the Ala major of the Os sphenoidale and the Pars petrosa of the Os temporale and forms the entrance into the bony part of the Tuba auditiva (→ Fig. 10.20, → Fig. 10.21). The bony canal continues through the Pars petrosa of the Os temporale to the tympanic cavity. Located laterally is the Pars squamosa of the Os temporale which is involved in the formation of the Articulatio temporomandibularis. The Fossa mandibularis is part of the Facies articularis of the Articulatio temporomandibularis. The Tuberc-

ulum articulare is located at the anterior margin of the Fossa mandibularis (→ Fig. 8.58, → Fig. 8.66).

Posterior cranial base: the posterior compartment extends from the anterior margin of the Foramen magnum to the Lineae nuchales superiores and consists of parts of the Os occipitale and the Ossa temporalia. The paired Pars lateralis has a Condylus occipitalis on either side to articulate with the atlas. Located behind each condyle is the Fossa condylaris, which contains the Canalis condylaris; the Canalis nervi hypoglossi runs above the condyle. Immediately lateral thereof is the Foramen jugulare.

Skeleton and joints

Passageways of the external surface of the cranial base

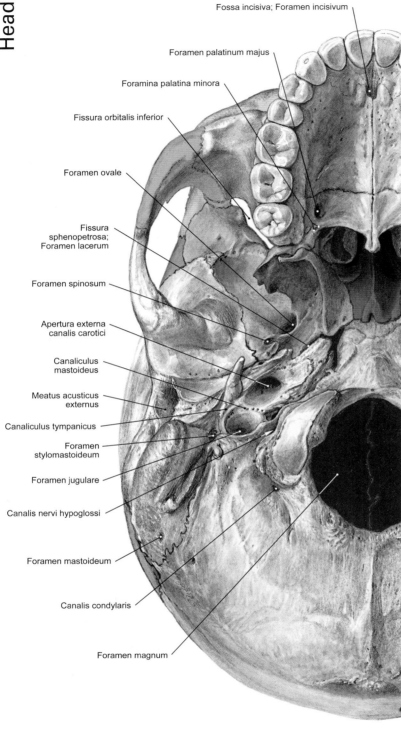

Fossa incisiva; Foramen incisivum

Foramen palatinum majus

Foramina palatina minora

Fissura orbitalis inferior

Foramen ovale

Fissura sphenopetrosa; Foramen lacerum

Foramen spinosum

Apertura externa canalis carotici

Canaliculus mastoideus

Meatus acusticus externus

Canaliculus tympanicus

Foramen stylomastoideum

Foramen jugulare

Canalis nervi hypoglossi

Foramen mastoideum

Canalis condylaris

Foramen magnum

Fig. 8.22 External surface of the cranial base, Basis cranii externa; with foramina; view from below; for colour chart, see p. XIII. [S700]

Foramina of the external surface of the cranial base and their content	
Foramen	**Content**
Foramen incisivum	N. nasopalatinus (N. maxillaris [V/2])
Foramen palatinum majus	• N. palatinus major (N. maxillaris [V/2]) • A. palatina major (A. palatina descendens)
Foramina palatina minora	• Nn. palatini minores (N. maxillaris [V/2]) • Aa. palatinae minores (A. palatina descendens)
Fissura orbitalis inferior	• A. infraorbitalis (A. maxillaris) • V. ophthalmica inferior • N. infraorbitalis (N. maxillaris [V/2]) • N. zygomaticus (N. maxillaris [V/2])
Foramen rotundum (→ Fig. 8.18)	N. maxillaris [V/2]
Foramen ovale	• N. mandibularis [V/3] • Plexus venosus foraminis ovalis
Foramen spinosum	• R. meningeus (N. mandibularis [V/3]) • A. meningea media (A. maxillaris)
Fissura sphenopetrosa, Foramen lacerum	• N. petrosus minor (N. glossopharyngeus [IX]) • N. petrosus major (N. facialis [VII]) • N. petrosus profundus (Plexus caroticus internus)
Apertura externa canalis carotici and Canalis caroticus	• A. carotis interna, Pars petrosa • Plexus venosus caroticus internus • Plexus caroticus internus (Truncus sympathicus, Ganglion cervicale superius)
Foramen stylomastoideum	N. facialis [VII]
Foramen jugulare	Anterior area: • Sinus petrosus inferior • N. glossopharyngeus [IX] Posterior area: • A. meningea posterior (A. pharyngea ascendens) • Sinus sigmoideus (Bulbus superior venae jugularis) • N. vagus [X] • R. meningeus (N. vagus [X]) • N. accessorius [XI]
Canaliculus mastoideus	R. auricularis nervi vagi (N. vagus [X])
Canaliculus tympanicus	• N. tympanicus • A. tympanica inferior
Canalis nervi hypoglossi	• N. hypoglossus [XII] • Plexus venosus canalis nervi hypoglossi
Canalis condylaris	V. emissaria condylaris
Foramen magnum	• Meninges • Plexus venosus vertebralis internus (Sinus marginalis) • Aa. vertebrales (Aa. subclaviae) • A. spinalis anterior (Aa. vertebrales) • Medulla oblongata/Medulla spinalis • Radices spinales (N. accessorius [XI])

Clinical remarks

In the case of **fractures of the cranial base,** the fracture lines often run through the openings of the cranial base. The penetrating nerves and blood vessels can thereby be injured. Nerve lesions and bleeding therefore frequently occur. Similarly, fractures of the frontal and sphenoidal sinuses, as well as of the ethmoidal cells, are possible (leakage of cerebrospinal fluid from the nose). With lateral fractures, the Os temporale is often affected (leakage of cerebrospinal fluid from the ear).

Foramina of the internal surface of the cranial base and their content

Foramen	Content
Lamina cribrosa	• Nn. olfactorii [I] • A. ethmoidalis anterior (A. ophthalmica)
Canalis opticus	• N. opticus [II] • A. ophthalmica (A. carotis interna) • Meninges; Vaginae nervi optici
Fissura orbitalis superior	Medial area: • N. nasociliaris (N. ophthalmicus [V/1]) • N. oculomotorius [III] • N. abducens [VI] Lateral area: • N. trochlearis [IV] common trunk of: – N. frontalis (N. ophthalmicus [V/1]) – N. lacrimalis (N. ophthalmicus [V/1]) • R. orbitalis (A. meningea media) • V. ophthalmica superior
Foramen rotundum	N. maxillaris [V/2]
Foramen ovale	• N. mandibularis [V/3] • Plexus venosus foraminis ovalis
Foramen spinosum	• R. meningeus (N. mandibularis [V/3]) • A. meningea media (A. maxillaris)
Fissura sphenopetrosa, Foramen lacerum	• N. petrosus minor (N. glossopharyngeus [IX]) • N. petrosus major (N. facialis [VII]) • N. petrosus profundus (Plexus caroticus internus)
Apertura interna canalis carotici and Canalis caroticus	• A. carotis interna, Pars petrosa • Plexus venosus caroticus internus • Plexus caroticus internus (Truncus sympathicus, Ganglion cervicale superius)
Porus and Meatus acusticus internus	• N. facialis [VII] • N. vestibulocochlearis [VIII] • A. labyrinthi (A. basilaris) • Vv. labyrinthi
Foramen jugulare	Anterior area: • Sinus petrosus inferior • N. glossopharyngeus [IX] Posterior area: • A. meningea posterior (A. pharyngea ascendens) • Sinus sigmoideus (Bulbus superior venae jugularis) • N. vagus [X] • N. accessorius [XI] • R. meningeus (N. vagus [X])
Canalis nervi hypoglossi	• N. hypoglossus [XII] • Plexus venosus canalis nervi hypoglossi
Canalis condylaris	V. emissaria condylaris
Foramen magnum	• Meninges • Plexus venosus vertebralis internus (Sinus marginalis) • Aa. vertebrales (Aa. subclaviae) • A. spinalis anterior (Aa. vertebrales) • Medulla oblongata/Medulla spinalis • Radices spinales (N. accessorius [XI])

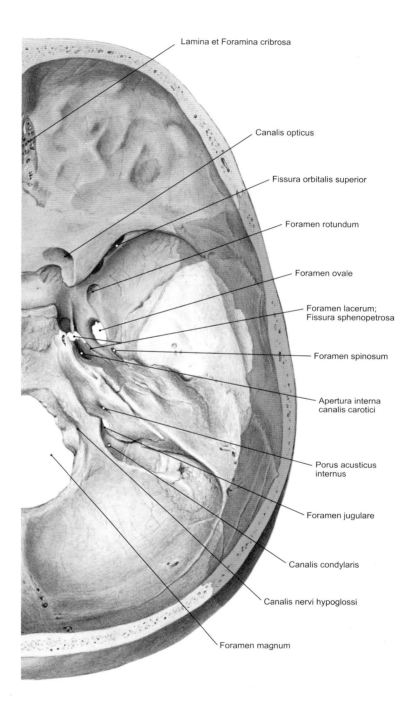

Lamina et Foramina cribrosa

Canalis opticus

Fissura orbitalis superior

Foramen rotundum

Foramen ovale

Foramen lacerum; Fissura sphenopetrosa

Foramen spinosum

Apertura interna canalis carotici

Porus acusticus internus

Foramen jugulare

Canalis condylaris

Canalis nervi hypoglossi

Foramen magnum

Fig. 8.23   Internal surface of the cranial base, Basis cranii interna; with foramina; view from above; for colour chart, see p. XIII. [S700]

Development of the skull

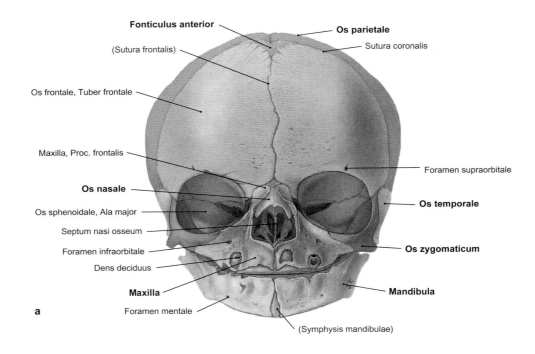

Fonticulus anterior

(Sutura frontalis)

Os frontale, Tuber frontale

Maxilla, Proc. frontalis

Os nasale

Os sphenoidale, Ala major

Septum nasi osseum

Foramen infraorbitale

Dens deciduus

Maxilla

Foramen mentale

Os parietale

Sutura coronalis

Foramen supraorbitale

Os temporale

Os zygomaticum

Mandibula

(Symphysis mandibulae)

a

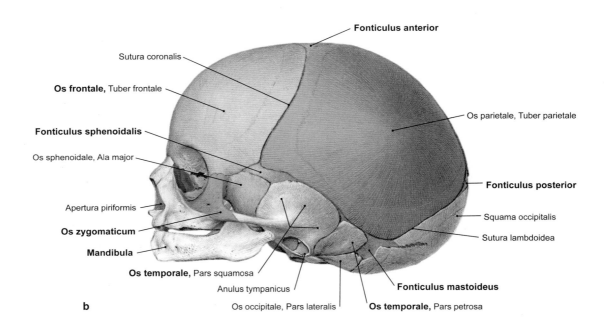

Fonticulus anterior

Sutura coronalis

Os frontale, Tuber frontale

Fonticulus sphenoidalis

Os sphenoidale, Ala major

Apertura piriformis

Os zygomaticum

Mandibula

Os temporale, Pars squamosa

Anulus tympanicus

Os occipitale, Pars lateralis

Os temporale, Pars petrosa

Fonticulus mastoideus

Sutura lambdoidea

Squama occipitalis

Fonticulus posterior

Os parietale, Tuber parietale

b

Fig. 8.24a and b   Cranium of a newborn; for colour chart, see p. XIII. [S700-L238]
a Frontal view.
b Lateral view.
At birth, a newborn has six fontanelles, two unpaired (Fonticuli anterior and posterior) and two paired (Fonticuli sphenoidales and mastoidei). During the **birth process,** the cranial sutures and fontanelles serve as

reference structures for assessing the position and presentation of the child's head. The posterior fontanelle is the leading part of the head in a normal presentation of the fetus.
Together with the cranial sutures, the fontanelles ensure limited skull deformation during the birth process. The acceleration of growth after birth results in a rapid reduction of the fontanelles, which will be closed by the third year of life.

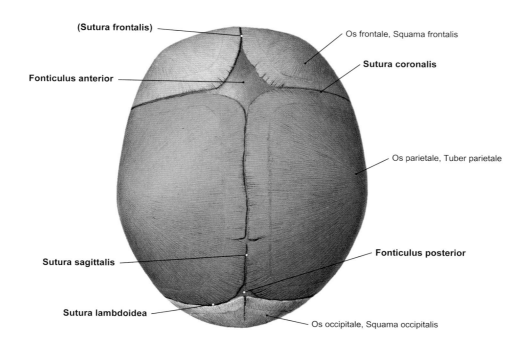

(Sutura frontalis)

Os frontale, Squama frontalis

Fonticulus anterior

Sutura coronalis

Os parietale, Tuber parietale

Sutura sagittalis

Fonticulus posterior

Sutura lambdoidea

Os occipitale, Squama occipitalis

Fig. 8.25 Cranium of a newborn; view from above; for colour chart, see p. XIII. [S700]
At birth, the bony plates of the skull cap (calvaria) are still separated by the interstitial tissue located in the cranial sutures (Suturae). The sutures are widened to fontanelles (Fonticuli) in regions where more than two bones meet. Over the course of life, most sutures, fonticuli and synchondroses ossify. Important sutures are the Suturae lambdoidea **(lambdoid suture)**, frontalis **(frontal suture)**, sagittalis **(sagittal suture)** and coronalis **(coronal suture)**, which continue closing, up to the age of 50 (the frontal suture closes between the first and second years of life).

Fontanelles		
Fontanelle	**Number**	**Closure [LM = month of life]**
Fonticulus anterior (large fontanelle)	1	approx. 36th LM
Fonticulus posterior (small fontanelle)	1	approx. third LM
Fonticulus sphenoidalis (anterior lateral fontanelle)	paired	approx. sixth LM
Fonticulus mastoideus (posterior lateral fontanelle)	paired	approx. 18th LM

Head

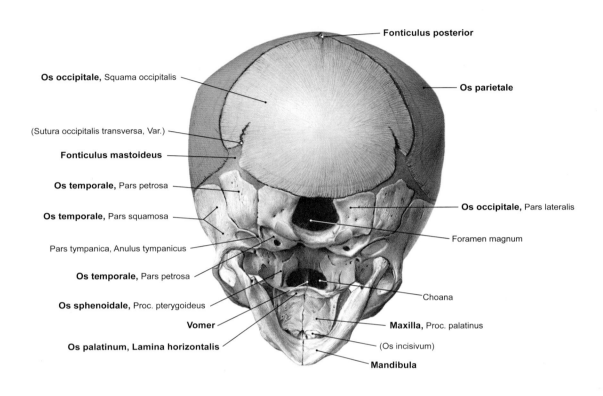

Fonticulus posterior

Os occipitale, Squama occipitalis

Os parietale

(Sutura occipitalis transversa, Var.)

Fonticulus mastoideus

Os temporale, Pars petrosa

Os temporale, Pars squamosa

Os occipitale, Pars lateralis

Pars tympanica, Anulus tympanicus

Foramen magnum

Os temporale, Pars petrosa

Os sphenoidale, Proc. pterygoideus

Choana

Vomer

Maxilla, Proc. palatinus

Os palatinum, Lamina horizontalis

(Os incisivum)

Mandibula

Fig. 8.26 Cranium of a newborn; anterior view from below; for colour chart, see p. XIII. [S700]
The development of the skull partially follows an intramembranous (desmal) mode, and partially an endochondral mode of osteogenesis (→ table). The primordial substance collectively consists of the mesenchyme derived from the paraxial cranial mesenchyme, the prechordal mesoderm, the occipital somites and the neural crest. At the time of birth, some cranial bones are linked by cartilaginous joints (Articulationes cartilagineae; Synchondroses cranii).

Ossification mode of the cranial bones			
	Viscerocranium	**Neurocranium**	**Auditory ossicles**
Desmal	Mandibula up to the Proc. condylaris, Maxilla, Os zygomaticum, Os palatinum, Os nasale, vomer, Os lacrimale	Lamina medialis of the Proc. pterygoideus of the Os sphenoidale, Pars squamosa of the Os temporale, Squama occipitalis, Os frontale, Os parietale	
Endochondral	Proc. condylaris of the Mandibula, Os ethmoidale, Concha nasalis inferior	Os sphenoidale up to the Lamina medialis of the Proc. pterygoideus, Pars petrosa and Pars tympanica of the Os temporale, Pars lateralis and Pars basilaris of the Os occipitale	
MECKEL's cartilage			Malleus, incus
REICHERT's cartilage		Proc. styloideus of the Os temporale	Stapes

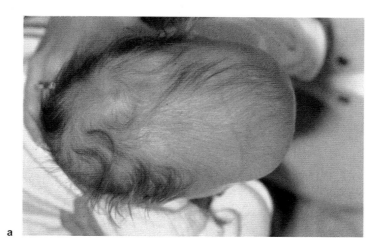

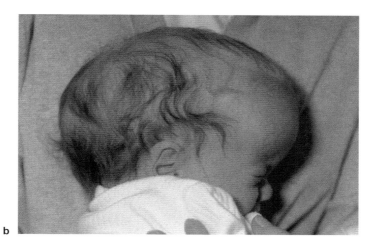

Fig. 8.27a and b   Craniostenoses; child with scaphocephaly.
[E347-09]
a View from above.

b View from the right.
This malformation results in the premature closure of the Sutura sagittalis. The cranial calotte is overly extended.

Clinical remarks

Disturbances in bone growth are referred to as dysostoses. **Craniosynostoses** are malformations resulting from the premature closure of one or more sutures. The premature closure of the Sutura sagittalis results in the extension of the skull in the frontal and occipital regions. The skull becomes longer and narrower **(scaphocephaly)**. The premature closure of the Sutura coronalis leads to the formation of a pointed skull **(oxycephaly** or **turricephaly)**. If the premature closure of the Suturae coronalis and lambdoidea occurs on one side only, this results in an asymmetrical craniosynostosis **(plagiocephaly)**. A failure in brain growth results in a **microcephaly.** Because the skull growth adapts to the brain growth, the entire neurocranium remains small. Children with microcephaly are intellectually disabled.

Head

Frontal bone and ethmoidal bone

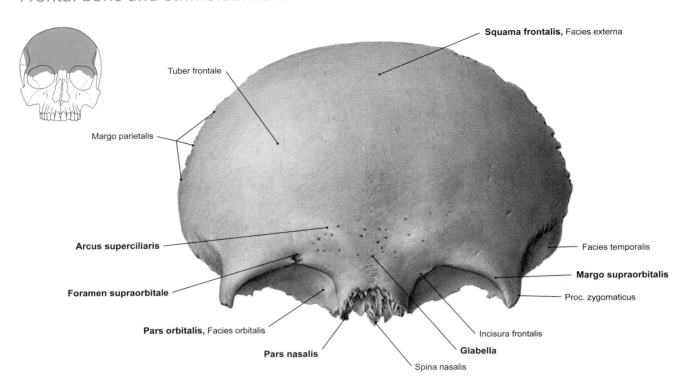

Squama frontalis, Facies externa

Tuber frontale

Margo parietalis

Arcus superciliaris

Foramen supraorbitale

Pars orbitalis, Facies orbitalis

Pars nasalis

Spina nasalis

Glabella

Incisura frontalis

Proc. zygomaticus

Margo supraorbitalis

Facies temporalis

Fig. 8.28 Frontal bone, Os frontale; frontal view; for colour chart, see p. XIII. [S700]
The Os frontale is the bone of the calvaria which is furthest to the front. It forms part of the walls of the orbital and nasal cavities. The unpaired Os frontale is divided into **four parts:**
* the unpaired Pars squamosa (Squama frontalis)
* the paired Pars orbitalis and
* the unpaired Pars nasalis.

Above the upper margin of the orbit (Margo supraorbitalis), a prominent Arcus superciliaris protrudes on both sides, usually more prominent in men than in women. In the midline between the two arches, the bone is flat and creates the glabella (area between the eyebrows). A Foramen supraorbitale is usually formed at the medial upper margin of the orbit; very occasionally it is an Incisura frontalis.

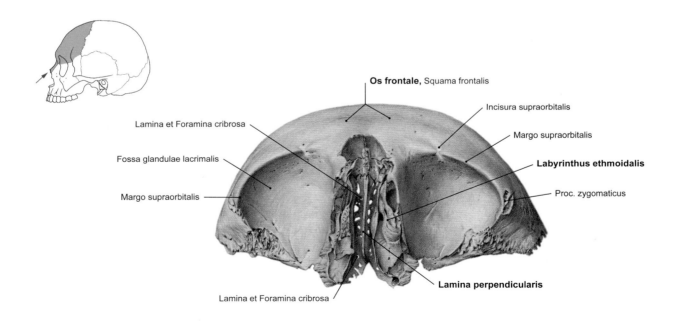

Os frontale, Squama frontalis

Incisura supraorbitalis

Margo supraorbitalis

Labyrinthus ethmoidalis

Proc. zygomaticus

Lamina perpendicularis

Lamina et Foramina cribrosa

Fossa glandulae lacrimalis

Margo supraorbitalis

Lamina et Foramina cribrosa

Fig. 8.29 Frontal bone, Os frontale, ethmoidal bone, Os ethmoidale, and nasal bones, Ossa nasalia; view from below; for colour chart, see p. XIII. [S700]

Medially in front and below, the Os ethmoidale and Ossa nasalia, which are connected to the Os frontale, form parts of the nasal skeleton. The Sinus frontalis is located in the Os frontale.

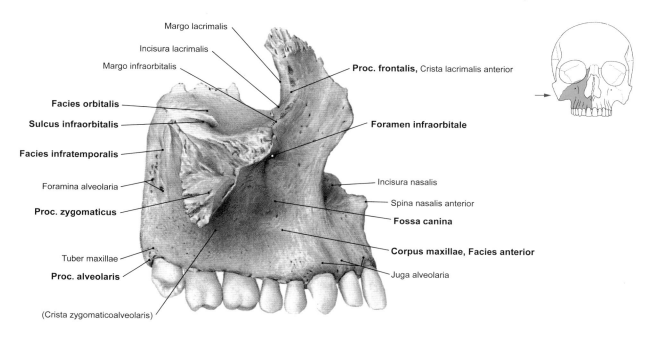

Margo lacrimalis
Incisura lacrimalis
Margo infraorbitalis
Facies orbitalis
Sulcus infraorbitalis
Facies infratemporalis
Foramina alveolaria
Proc. zygomaticus
Tuber maxillae
Proc. alveolaris
(Crista zygomaticoalveolaris)
Proc. frontalis, Crista lacrimalis anterior
Foramen infraorbitale
Incisura nasalis
Spina nasalis anterior
Fossa canina
Corpus maxillae, Facies anterior
Juga alveolaria

Fig. 8.30 Maxilla, right side; lateral view. [S700]
The upper jaw can be divided into the body of the maxilla (Corpus maxillae), the frontal process (Proc. frontalis, which is connected to the Os frontale), the zygomatic process (Proc. zygomaticus, which forms the Arcus zygomaticus with the Os zygomaticum), the palate process (Proc. palatinus, anterior portion of the bony palate, → Fig. 8.31) and the

Proc. alveolaris. The latter forms the lower margin of the maxilla and contains tooth sockets (Alveoli dentales) for the roots of the teeth. The prominent anterior rims of the dental alveoli are known as Juga alveolaria. In the Corpus maxillae, just below the lower orbital margin, is the Foramen infraorbitale.

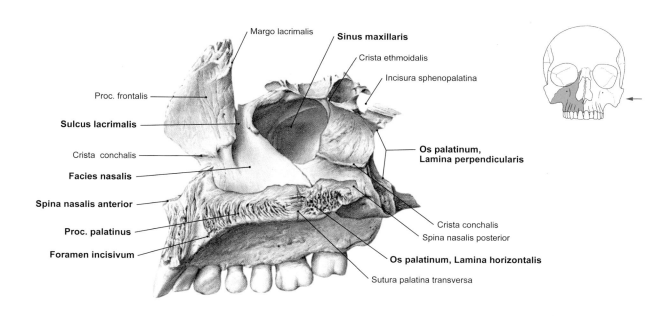

Margo lacrimalis
Sinus maxillaris
Crista ethmoidalis
Incisura sphenopalatina
Proc. frontalis
Sulcus lacrimalis
Crista conchalis
Facies nasalis
Spina nasalis anterior
Proc. palatinus
Foramen incisivum
Os palatinum, Lamina perpendicularis
Crista conchalis
Spina nasalis posterior
Os palatinum, Lamina horizontalis
Sutura palatina transversa

Fig. 8.31 Maxilla and palatine bone, Os palatinum, right side; medial view when looking at the Sinus maxillaris; for colour chart, see p. XIII. [S700]
Posterior to the maxilla lies the Os palatinum which is composed of two plates: the **Lamina horizontalis** creates the Pars posterior of the palate

(Palatum osseum), and the **Lamina perpendicularis** extends vertically upwards (perpendicular to the Lamina horizontalis) and is the posterior medial margin of the Sinus maxillaris.

Nasal cavity

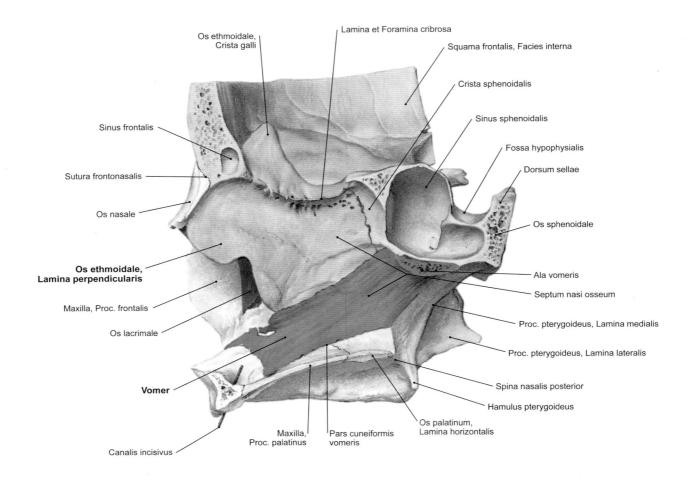

Os ethmoidale, Crista galli
Lamina et Foramina cribrosa
Squama frontalis, Facies interna
Crista sphenoidalis
Sinus frontalis
Sinus sphenoidalis
Fossa hypophysialis
Sutura frontonasalis
Dorsum sellae
Os nasale
Os sphenoidale
Os ethmoidale, Lamina perpendicularis
Ala vomeris
Septum nasi osseum
Maxilla, Proc. frontalis
Proc. pterygoideus, Lamina medialis
Os lacrimale
Proc. pterygoideus, Lamina lateralis
Spina nasalis posterior
Vomer
Hamulus pterygoideus
Os palatinum, Lamina horizontalis
Maxilla, Proc. palatinus
Pars cuneiformis vomeris
Canalis incisivus

Fig. 8.32 Bony nasal septum, Septum nasi osseum; lateral view; for colour chart, see p. XIII. [S700]
The bony nasal septum is formed by the Lamina perpendicularis of the Os ethmoidale and by the vomer.
The **Os ethmoidale** is situated between the Os frontale and the maxilla and is also connected to the Ossa nasalia, lacrimalia, sphenoidale and palatina. It forms the Crista galli above. Perforated with multiple holes, the Lamina cribrosa forms the roof of the nasal cavity and forms part of the floor of the anterior cranial fossa. The Lamina perpendicularis of the

Os ethmoidale is located below the Crista galli, dividing the bony labyrinth of the Os ethmoidale into a right and left part, and constitutes the upper part of the bony nasal septum.
The **vomer** forms the largest part of the bony nasal septum. The flat trapezoid bone is connected above to the Lamina perpendicularis of the Os ethmoidale and via the Ala vomeris at the back to the Os sphenoidale. Below, the Pars cuneiformis vomeris borders the Proc. palatinus of the maxilla, and the Lamina horizontalis of the Os palatinum.

Clinical remarks

A **nasal septum deviation** can be the result of a blow to the nose or by falling onto the nose, or is otherwise caused by a developmental deformity of the facial bones. More than 60 % of the population has at least a mild septum deviation. Nasal septum deviations primarily hinder nasal breathing. If this is the case, the inhaled air cannot be warmed up, cleaned and moistened. The obstruction to nasal breath-

ing leads to increased mouth breathing with snoring and/or increased risk of inflammation. Since the paranasal sinuses are no longer sufficiently ventilated, this can lead to sinusitis with a postnasal drip and inflammations of the larynx and bronchi. Later in life, cardiovascular diseases can result from the lack of oxygen.

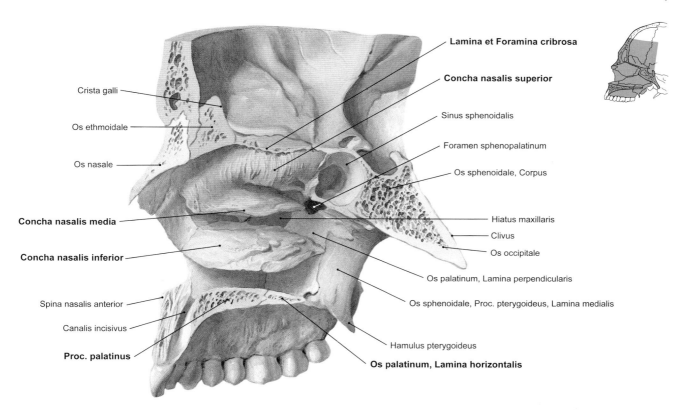

Fig. 8.33 Lateral wall of the nasal cavity, Cavitas nasi, right side; view from the left; for colour chart, see p. XIII. [S700]
The view of the lateral nasal wall shows that the Lamina cribrosa of the Os ethmoidale forms the roof, and also forms the upper nasal concha (Concha nasalis superior) and the middle nasal concha (Concha nasalis media). The upper nasal passage (Meatus nasi superior) is located between the two nasal conchae. Below them, the Concha nasalis inferior is an independent bone.

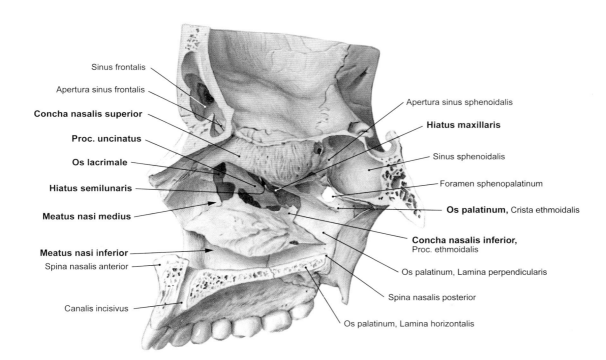

Fig. 8.34 Lateral wall of the nasal cavity, Cavitas nasi, right side; medial view after removal of the middle nasal concha; for colour chart, see p. XIII. [S700]
Below the middle nasal concha is a thin lamellar bone, the **Proc. uncinatus,** which forms part of the Os ethmoidale, but does not completely close the medial wall of the Sinus maxillaris. There are numerous openings above and below the Proc. uncinatus. One of these is the Hiatus maxillaris.

The **maxilla** and the **Os palatinum** create the floor and parts of the lateral wall (floor: Lamina horizontalis; lateral wall: Lamina perpendicularis). The **Os lacrimale** is also part of the lateral wall and forms part of the anterior margin of the Sinus maxillaris. The Concha nasalis inferior is attached to the maxilla, palatine and lacrimal bone. It divides the lateral nasal wall into an overlying middle nasal passage (Meatus nasi medius) and an underlying lower nasal passage (Meatus nasi inferior).

Hard palate

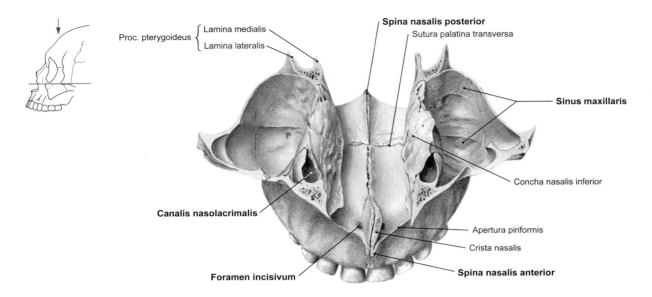

Proc. pterygoideus { Lamina medialis / Lamina lateralis

Spina nasalis posterior

Sutura palatina transversa

Sinus maxillaris

Concha nasalis inferior

Canalis nasolacrimalis

Apertura piriformis

Crista nasalis

Foramen incisivum

Spina nasalis anterior

Fig. 8.35 Hard palate, Palatum durum; maxillary sinus, Sinus maxillaris, and inferior nasal concha, Concha nasalis inferior; view from above; for colour chart, see p. XIII. [S700]
The hard palate represents a horizontal bony plate created by the maxilla and the Os palatinum. It separates the oral and nasal cavities from

each other. A connection exists via the Foramina incisiva. This illustration shows the floor of the nasal cavity. The Sinus maxillares can be found laterally.

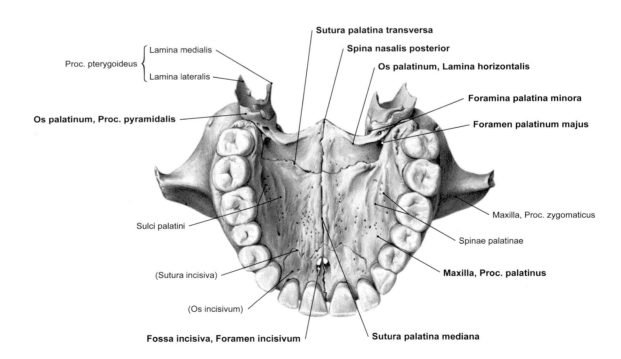

Proc. pterygoideus { Lamina medialis / Lamina lateralis

Sutura palatina transversa

Spina nasalis posterior

Os palatinum, Lamina horizontalis

Foramina palatina minora

Foramen palatinum majus

Os palatinum, Proc. pyramidalis

Sulci palatini

Maxilla, Proc. zygomaticus

Spinae palatinae

Maxilla, Proc. palatinus

(Sutura incisiva)

(Os incisivum)

Fossa incisiva, Foramen incisivum

Sutura palatina mediana

Fig. 8.36 Hard palate, Palatum durum; view from below; for colour chart, see p. XIII. [S700]
The hard palate is part of the **anterior cranial base.** The teeth are attached to the two maxillary alveolar arches, which enclose the hard palate at the front and laterally. It consists rostrally of the Procc. palatini of the maxillae and posteriorly of the Laminae horizontales of the Ossa palatina. The **Procc. palatini** are connected in the midline via the Sutura palatina mediana, and posteriorly they border the two Ossa palatina via the Sutura palatina transversa. The **Laminae horizontales** of the Ossa

palatina make contact with each other in the midline via the Sutura interpalatina (continuation of the Sutura palatina mediana).
Behind the incisors, in the frontal part of the midline, is the **Fossa incisiva,** which transitions into the Foramen incisivum and the Canales incisivi. Close to the lateral posterior margin of the hard palate, on both sides, is a **Foramen palatinum majus,** which transitions into the Canalis palatinus majus, as well as the **Foramina palatina minora.** They are located in the Proc. pyramidalis of the Os palatinum and transition into the Canales palatini minores. In the midline, the **Spina nasalis posterior** protrudes backwards as a pointed process of the hard palate.

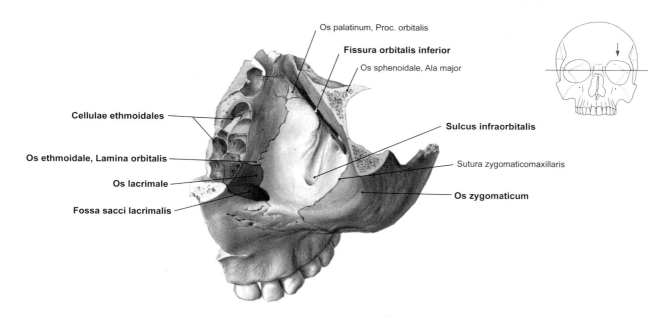

Os palatinum, Proc. orbitalis

Fissura orbitalis inferior

Os sphenoidale, Ala major

Cellulae ethmoidales

Os ethmoidale, Lamina orbitalis

Os lacrimale

Fossa sacci lacrimalis

Sulcus infraorbitalis

Sutura zygomaticomaxillaris

Os zygomaticum

Fig. 8.37 Floor of the orbit, Paries inferior orbitae, left side; view from above; for colour chart, see p. XIII. [S700]
The floor of the orbit forms the roof of the Sinus maxillaris. Inside it is the Sulcus infraorbitalis, which becomes a bony canal passing anteriorly below the floor of the orbit and opens into the Foramen infraorbitale. It contains the N. infraorbitalis and the infraorbital vessels. Laterally, the floor of the orbit is formed by the Os zygomaticum, with medial participation of the Proc. orbitalis of the Os palatinum, the Lamina orbitalis of the Os ethmoidale and the Os lacrimale. The latter, along with the maxilla, forms the Fossa sacci lacrimalis in which the lacrimal sac can be found. For the orbital cavity → Fig. 9.7 to → Fig. 9.11.

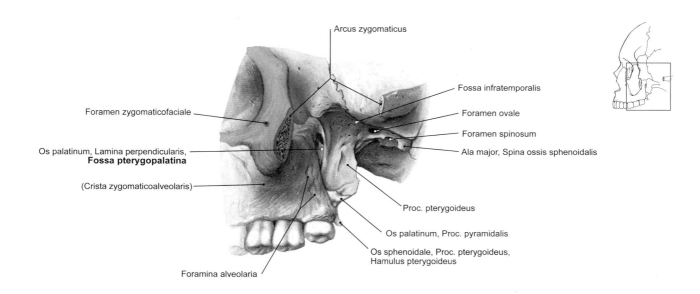

Arcus zygomaticus

Fossa infratemporalis

Foramen ovale

Foramen spinosum

Ala major, Spina ossis sphenoidalis

Foramen zygomaticofaciale

Os palatinum, Lamina perpendicularis,
Fossa pterygopalatina

(Crista zygomaticoalveolaris)

Proc. pterygoideus

Os palatinum, Proc. pyramidalis

Os sphenoidale, Proc. pterygoideus,
Hamulus pterygoideus

Foramina alveolaria

Fig. 8.38 Pterygopalatine fossa, Fossa pterygopalatina, left side; lateral view; for colour chart, see p. XIII. [S700]
The Fossa pterygopalatina is the medial continuation of the Fossa infratemporalis and is bordered by the maxilla, Os palatinum and Os sphenoidale. It forms a **switching point** between the middle cranial fossa and the orbit and nose. It serves as a conduit for many nerves and blood vessels which supply the structures in these cavities (→ Fig. 8.156 to → Fig. 8.160).
Access to the pterygopalatine fossa within the context of tumour surgery in this region is generally achieved laterally, e.g. in the case of a nasopharyngeal fibroma.

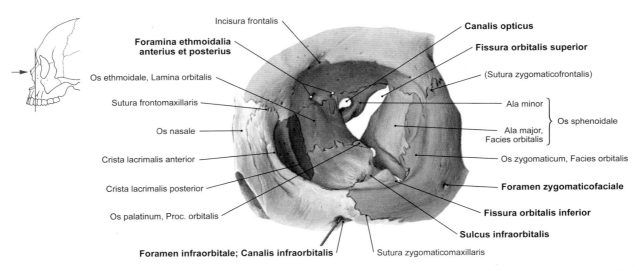

Fig. 8.39 Orbit, Orbita, left side; frontal view; probe in the Canalis infraorbitalis; for colour chart, see p. XIII. [S700]
The Orbita is bordered by the Ossa frontale, ethmoidale, lacrimale, palatinum, sphenoidale, zygomaticum and the maxilla. The Fissurae orbitales superior and inferior, the Canalis opticus and the Foramina ethmoidalia anterius and posterius serve as openings into the Orbita. The Sulcus infraorbitalis is located in the posterior part of the floor of the Orbita, which continues anteriorly as Canalis infraorbitalis and opens into the Foramen infraorbitale below the inferior orbital margin. Laterally, the Foramen zygomaticofaciale is usually found in the Os zygomaticum. For the orbital cavity, → Fig. 9.7 to → Fig. 9.11.

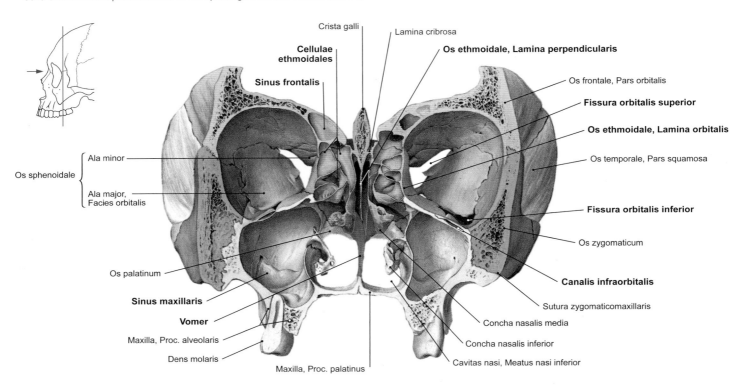

Fig. 8.40 Viscerocranium; frontal section at the level of the orbits; frontal view; for colour chart, see p. XIII. [S700]
The unpaired Os ethmoidale contains the anterior and posterior ethmoidal cells **(Cellulae ethmoidales).** The Lamina perpendicularis of the Os ethmoidale lies immediately beneath the Crista galli, separates the bony labyrinth of the Os ethmoidale into a right and a left half, and forms the upper part of the bony nasal septum. The vomer joins its posterior aspect. The thin **Lamina orbitalis** forms the lateral walls of the Cellulae ethmoidales as well as the major part of the medial wall of the orbit, which is known as the **Lamina papyracea.** Directly below the Orbita is the Sinus maxillaris. The Canalis infraorbitalis can be found in its roof, which is also the floor of the Orbita. The level of the Lamina cribrosa is significantly lower than the roof of the Orbita. For the orbital cavity, → Fig. 9.7 to → Fig. 9.11.

Clinical remarks

Due to the paper-thin Lamina orbitalis (Lamina papyracea) of the Os ethmoidale between the orbit and the **ethmoidal cells, inflammations** of the latter can easily spread to the orbit and cause an orbital phlegmon. In → Fig. 8.40, the close proximity of the root of a molar tooth to the Sinus maxillaris can be seen. Inflammations of the second premolars and/or the first molars can lead to an odontogenic inflammation of the Sinus maxillaris (Sinusitis maxillaris).

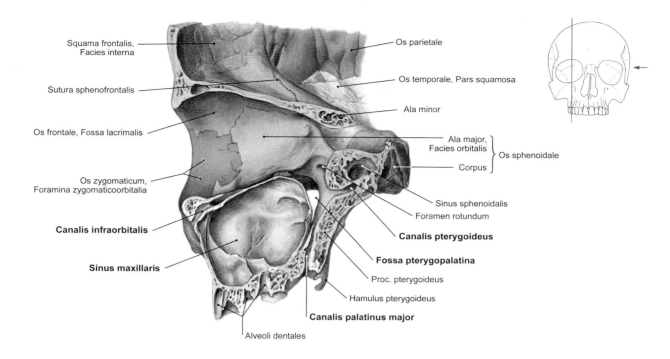

Squama frontalis, Facies interna

Sutura sphenofrontalis

Os frontale, Fossa lacrimalis

Os zygomaticum, Foramina zygomaticoorbitalia

Canalis infraorbitalis

Sinus maxillaris

Os parietale

Os temporale, Pars squamosa

Ala minor

Ala major, Facies orbitalis } Os sphenoidale

Corpus

Sinus sphenoidalis

Foramen rotundum

Canalis pterygoideus

Fossa pterygopalatina

Proc. pterygoideus

Hamulus pterygoideus

Canalis palatinus major

Alveoli dentales

Fig. 8.41 Lateral wall of the orbit, Paries lateralis orbitae, right side; medial view; for colour chart, see p. XIII. [S700]
The lateral wall of the orbit is formed by the Ossa zygomaticum, frontale, sphenoidale and the maxilla. The Canalis infraorbitalis is depicted clearly in the anterior third of the orbital floor, as well as the very thin bony layer separating the orbit from the Sinus maxillaris. Posteriorly, the

Fossa pterygopalatina closes the Sinus maxillaris, which has a lateral connection to the Fossa infratemporalis, a superior connection to the Orbita, and an inferior connection via the Canalis palatinus majus to the oral cavity. From a posterior cranial position, the Canalis pterygoideus exits into the Fossa pterygopalatina.

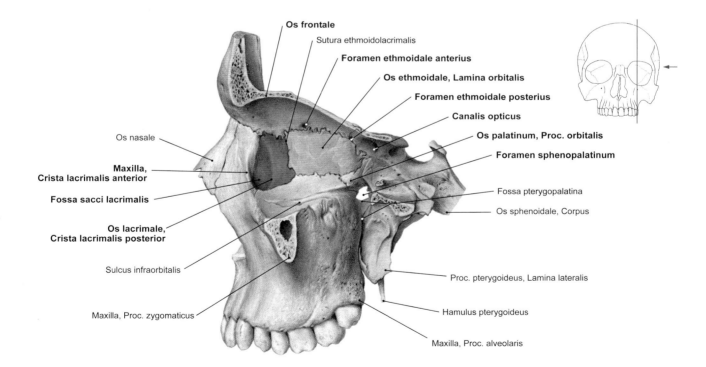

Os frontale

Sutura ethmoidolacrimalis

Foramen ethmoidale anterius

Os ethmoidale, Lamina orbitalis

Foramen ethmoidale posterius

Canalis opticus

Os palatinum, Proc. orbitalis

Foramen sphenopalatinum

Os nasale

Maxilla, Crista lacrimalis anterior

Fossa sacci lacrimalis

Os lacrimale, Crista lacrimalis posterior

Sulcus infraorbitalis

Maxilla, Proc. zygomaticus

Fossa pterygopalatina

Os sphenoidale, Corpus

Proc. pterygoideus, Lamina lateralis

Hamulus pterygoideus

Maxilla, Proc. alveolaris

Fig. 8.42 Medial wall of the orbit, Paries medialis orbitae, left side; lateral view; for colour chart, see p. XIII. [S700]
The Os lacrimale, the maxilla, and the Os frontale form the anterior part of the medial wall of the orbit, whereas the Lamina orbitalis of the Os ethmoidale (Lamina papyracea), the Proc. orbitalis of the Os palatinum, and the Os sphenoidale are placed between the Os frontale and the

maxilla in the posterior part. Both the anterior Crista lacrimalis of the maxilla and the posterior Crista lacrimalis of the Os lacrimale confine a depression (Fossa sacci lacrimalis) for the lacrimal sac. Located in the medial wall of the orbit are the Foramina ethmoidalia anterius and posterius and the Canalis opticus. Just above the Fossa pterygopalatina is the Foramen sphenopalatinum.

Head

Sphenoidal bone

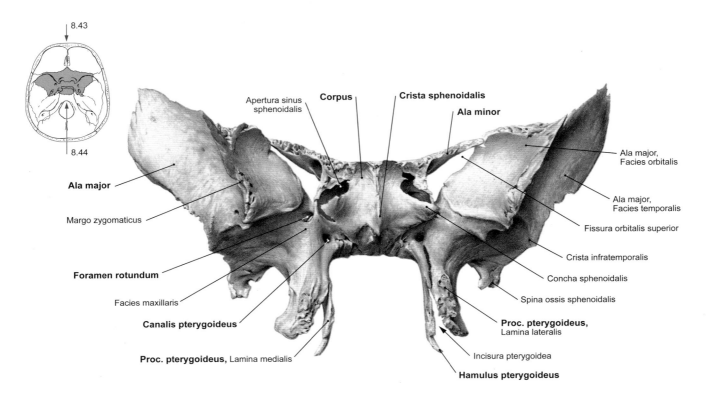

Fig. 8.43   Sphenoidal bone, Os sphenoidale; frontal view. [S700]
The unpaired Os sphenoidale is a bone connecting the viscerocranium and the neurocranium. From the Corpus of the Os sphenoidale, two pairs of wings (Alae) extend outwards laterally. At the top are the **Alae minores,** and below are the **Alae majores.** Extending downwards are the **pterygoid processes (Procc. pterygoidei).** In the centre of the Os sphenoidale are the sphenoidal sinuses **(Sinus sphenoidales).** The Crista sphenoidalis subdivides the anterior part of the Corpus into two halves.

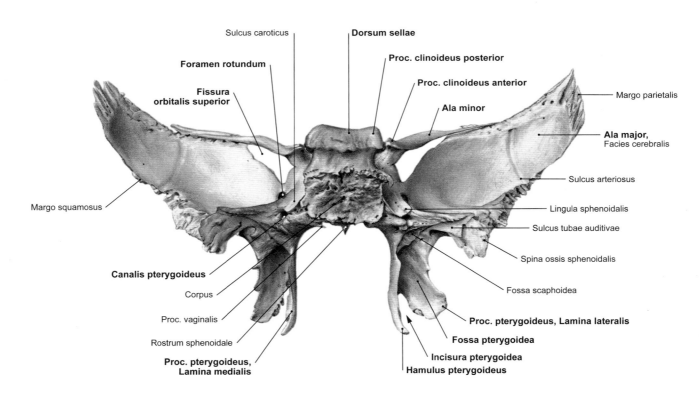

Fig. 8.44   Sphenoidal bone, Os sphenoidale; posterior view. [S700]
The Ala minor and Ala major of the Os sphenoidale confine the **Fissura orbitalis superior.** The Proc. pterygoideus is divided on each side into a smaller Lamina medialis and a larger Lamina lateralis, which between them enclose the Fossa pterygoidea and are separated by the **Incisura (Fissura) pterygoidea.** The Lamina medialis continues caudally into the **Hamulus pterygoideus.** At its base, the Canalis pterygoideus pierces the Os sphenoidale and opens into the Fossa pterygopalatina.

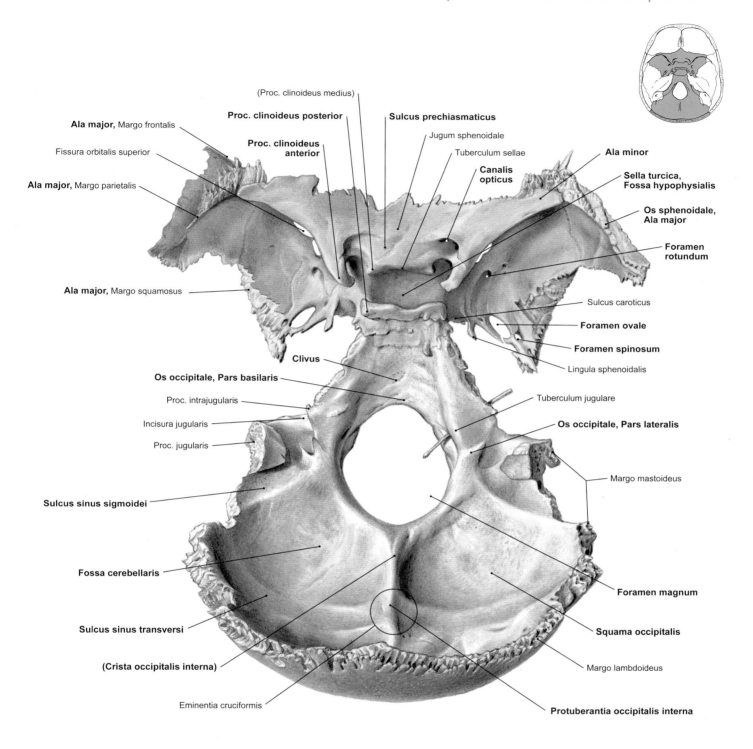

(Proc. clinoideus medius)

Proc. clinoideus posterior

Sulcus prechiasmaticus

Ala major, Margo frontalis

Jugum sphenoidale

Proc. clinoideus anterior

Tuberculum sellae

Fissura orbitalis superior

Ala minor

Canalis opticus

Ala major, Margo parietalis

Sella turcica, Fossa hypophysialis

Os sphenoidale, Ala major

Foramen rotundum

Ala major, Margo squamosus

Sulcus caroticus

Foramen ovale

Foramen spinosum

Clivus

Lingula sphenoidalis

Os occipitale, Pars basilaris

Tuberculum jugulare

Proc. intrajugularis

Os occipitale, Pars lateralis

Incisura jugularis

Proc. jugularis

Margo mastoideus

Sulcus sinus sigmoidei

Fossa cerebellaris

Foramen magnum

Sulcus sinus transversi

Squama occipitalis

(Crista occipitalis interna)

Margo lambdoideus

Eminentia cruciformis

Protuberantia occipitalis interna

Fig. 8.45 Sphenoidal bone, Os sphenoidale, and occipital bone, Os occipitale; view from above; for colour chart, see p. XIII. [S700]
The centre of the **Os sphenoidale** is composed of the **Sella turcica** and the Fossa hypophysialis. The Tuberculum sellae, which laterally continues the middle clinoid process on each side, forms the anterior margin of the Fossa hypophysialis. The Sulcus prechiasmaticus and the Jugum sphenoidale are located in front of the Tuberculum sellae. The clivus forms the posterior portion of the Sella turcica, of which the upper edge is laterally raised to the Proc. clinoideus posterior. The Ala minor is pierced at its anterior margin by the Canalis opticus in the area of the Sella turcica. The Foramina rotundum, ovale and spinosum pierce the Ala major bilaterally in an anterior cranial to posterior caudal direction.

The unpaired **Os occipitale** consists of the Squama occipitalis with two Partes laterales and a Pars basilaris. These four parts confine the **Foramen magnum.** On the inner surface of the Squama occipitalis, the Sulcus sinus sagittalis superioris and the grooves of the Sinus transversi meet at the Protuberantia occipitalis interna. In addition, the Sulcus sinus sigmoidei and the Sulcus sinus occipitalis can also be seen on the inner surface on the right and left. Above and below the Protuberantia occipitalis, the inner surface of the Squama occipitalis forms the Fossa cerebralis and the Fossa cerebellaris, respectively. Together with the Corpus of the Os sphenoidale, the Pars basilaris of the Os occipitale generates the Clivus.

Head

Temporal bone

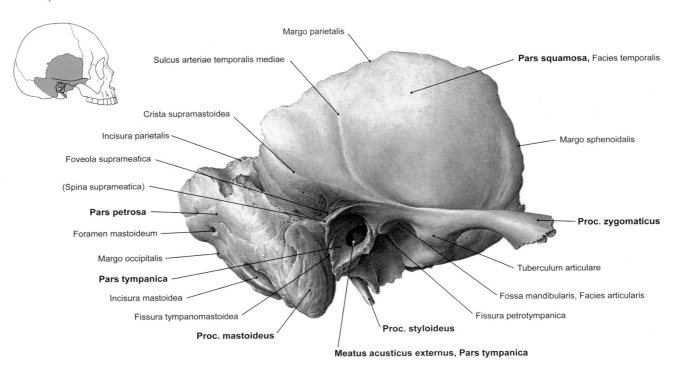

Margo parietalis

Sulcus arteriae temporalis mediae

Pars squamosa, Facies temporalis

Crista supramastoidea

Margo sphenoidalis

Incisura parietalis

Foveola suprameatica

(Spina suprameatica)

Pars petrosa

Proc. zygomaticus

Foramen mastoideum

Margo occipitalis

Tuberculum articulare

Pars tympanica

Fossa mandibularis, Facies articularis

Incisura mastoidea

Fissura petrotympanica

Fissura tympanomastoidea

Proc. styloideus

Proc. mastoideus

Meatus acusticus externus, Pars tympanica

Fig. 8.46 Temporal bone, Os temporale, right side; lateral view. [S700]

The paired Os temporale belongs to both the neurocranium and the viscerocranium. It is part of the lateral wall and the base of the cranium. A distinction is made between the Pars squamosa, the Pars tympanica and the Pars petrosa.

The **Pars squamosa,** which is scale-like, borders the Os parietale on the Margo parietalis. In front and above the meatus, the Proc. zygomaticus protrudes and is directed forward.

The **Pars petrosa** borders the Ossa parietale and occipitale. Its central outer opening is the Meatus acusticus externus. Located at its poste-

rior caudal aspect is the Proc. mastoideus. The middle and inner ear are located within the Pars petrosa (not visible). Access routes are the internal acoustic meatus (Meatus acusticus internus, → Fig. 8.23), the Foramen stylomastoideum (→ Fig. 8.22) and the Canalis musculotubarius (→ Fig. 10.28 and → Fig. 10.40).

The **Pars tympanica** forms the bony wall of the external acoustic meatus. It is a ring-shaped structure lying on the Partes squamosa and petrosa. The Pars tympanica borders the Meatus acusticus externus at its frontal, caudal, and posterior sides and extends to the tympanic membrane (→ Fig. 10.14 and → Fig. 10.22).

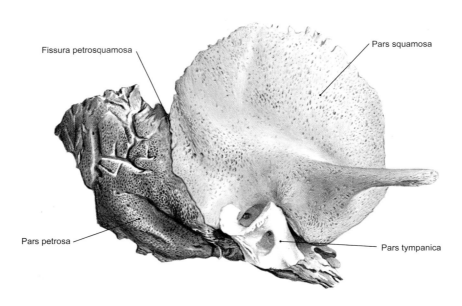

Fissura petrosquamosa

Pars squamosa

Pars petrosa

Pars tympanica

Fig. 8.47 Temporal bone, Os temporale, of a newborn, right side; lateral view; schematic representation; for colour chart, see p. XIII. [S700]

The illustration shows the different parts of the Os temporale: Pars squamosa, Pars petrosa and Pars tympanica.

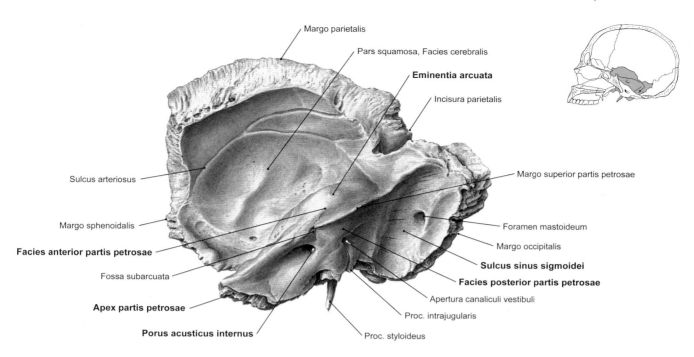

Margo parietalis
Pars squamosa, Facies cerebralis
Eminentia arcuata
Incisura parietalis
Margo superior partis petrosae
Sulcus arteriosus
Foramen mastoideum
Margo occipitalis
Margo sphenoidalis
Sulcus sinus sigmoidei
Facies anterior partis petrosae
Facies posterior partis petrosae
Fossa subarcuata
Apertura canaliculi vestibuli
Apex partis petrosae
Proc. intrajugularis
Porus acusticus internus
Proc. styloideus

Fig. 8.48 Temporal bone, Os temporale, right side; inner aspect. [S700]
The Pars petrosa is shaped like a pyramid, the tip of which (Apex partis petrosae) is aligned medially forwards and the base of which is facing the Proc. mastoideus. The Facies anterior is directed towards the middle cranial fossa, and protrudes as Eminentia arcuata; in the Facies pos-

terior, the **Porus acusticus internus** is the entrance to the Meatus acusticus internus. The Facies posterior of the Pars petrosa is deepened by the Sulcus sinus sigmoidei. This is also where the **Foramen mastoideum** is found. On the inside (Facies cerebralis) of the Pars squamosa, the Sulci arteriosi of the A. meningea media can be seen.

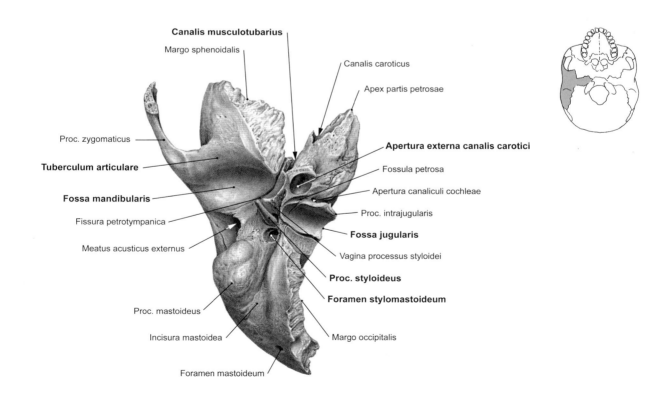

Canalis musculotubarius
Margo sphenoidalis
Canalis caroticus
Apex partis petrosae
Proc. zygomaticus
Apertura externa canalis carotici
Tuberculum articulare
Fossula petrosa
Fossa mandibularis
Apertura canaliculi cochleae
Fissura petrotympanica
Proc. intrajugularis
Meatus acusticus externus
Fossa jugularis
Vagina processus styloidei
Proc. styloideus
Foramen stylomastoideum
Proc. mastoideus
Incisura mastoidea
Margo occipitalis
Foramen mastoideum

Fig. 8.49 Temporal bone, Os temporale, right side; inferior view. [S700]
The Facies inferior of the Os temporale deepens towards the **Fossa jugularis,** which borders the Foramen jugulare together with the Os occipitale. At the notch (Incisura) between the Pars squamosa and the Pars

petrosa, the Canalis musculotubarius begins. In addition, the Apertura externa canalis carotici and the Proc. styloideus can be seen. The **Foramen stylomastoideum** opens to the lateral posterior side. Just before the external ear canal, the Pars squamosa forms the **Fossa mandibularis,** which is rostrally surrounded by the Tuberculum articulare.

Skeleton and joints

Head

Mandible

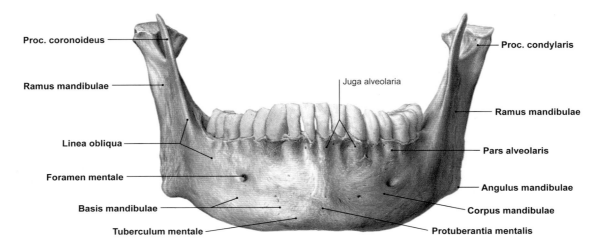

- Proc. coronoideus
- Ramus mandibulae
- Linea obliqua
- Foramen mentale
- Basis mandibulae
- Tuberculum mentale
- Juga alveolaria
- **Proc. condylaris**
- **Ramus mandibulae**
- **Pars alveolaris**
- **Angulus mandibulae**
- **Corpus mandibulae**
- **Protuberantia mentalis**

Fig. 8.50 Mandible, Mandibula; frontal view. [S700]
The unpaired Mandibula consists of a body (Corpus mandibulae) and two rami (Rami mandibulae). Each ramus divides into a **Proc. coronoideus** and a **Proc. condylaris**. The Corpus mandibulae consists of the Basis and the Pars alveolaris, which are separated from the Proc. coro-

noideus by the Linea obliqua descending obliquely towards the front. At the front of the Pars alveolaris is the chin (Menta) with the Protuberantia mentalis, the bilateral tubercles of the chin (Tubercula mentalia) and the Foramina mentalia.

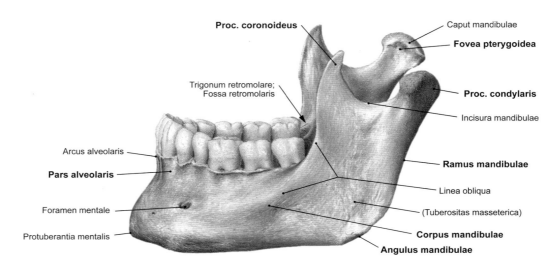

- **Proc. coronoideus**
- Trigonum retromolare; Fossa retromolaris
- Arcus alveolaris
- **Pars alveolaris**
- Foramen mentale
- Protuberantia mentalis
- Caput mandibulae
- **Fovea pterygoidea**
- **Proc. condylaris**
- Incisura mandibulae
- **Ramus mandibulae**
- Linea obliqua
- (Tuberositas masseterica)
- **Corpus mandibulae**
- **Angulus mandibulae**

Fig. 8.51 Mandible, Mandibula; lateral view. Corpus mandibulae and Ramus mandibulae merge at the **Angulus mandibulae.** [S700]

The Proc. condylaris carries the **Caput mandibulae.**

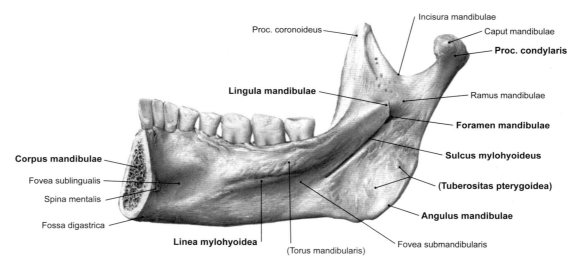

- Proc. coronoideus
- **Lingula mandibulae**
- **Corpus mandibulae**
- Fovea sublingualis
- Spina mentalis
- Fossa digastrica
- **Linea mylohyoidea**
- Incisura mandibulae
- Caput mandibulae
- **Proc. condylaris**
- Ramus mandibulae
- **Foramen mandibulae**
- **Sulcus mylohyoideus**
- **(Tuberositas pterygoidea)**
- **Angulus mandibulae**
- Fovea submandibularis
- (Torus mandibularis)

Fig. 8.52 Mandible, Mandibula; inner aspect of the mandibular arch. [S700]
The **Foramen mandibulae** is located on the inner surface of the Ramus mandibulae. In front of the foramen, the **Linea mylohyoidea** forms a

'terraced' ledge, which serves as the point of attachment for the M. mylohyoideus and which marks the level of the floor of the mouth.

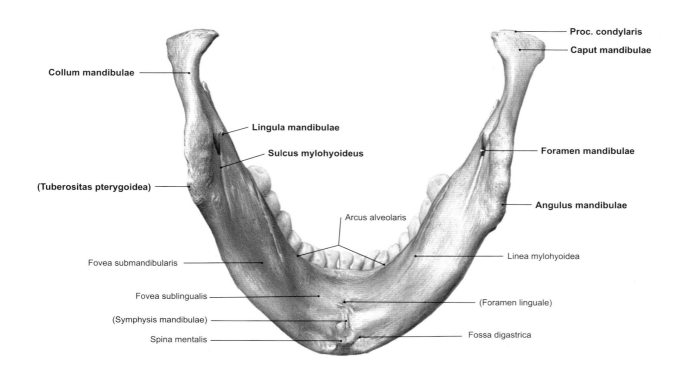

Fig. 8.53 Mandible, Mandibula; inferior view. [S700]
The Spina mentalis is located on the inside of the Mandibula close to the midline. Laterally and below this, the bone deepens into the Fossa

digastrica, and above the Spina mentalis, into the Fovea sublingualis and the Fovea submandibularis on each side. The **Tuberositas ptery-goidea** is found on the inside of the Angulus mandibulae.

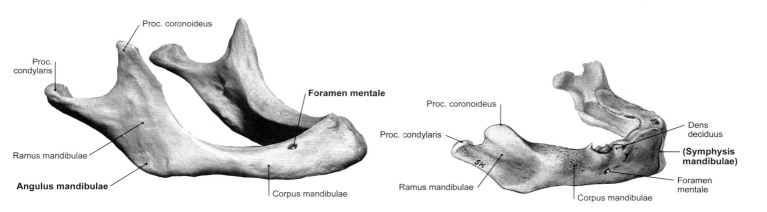

Fig. 8.54 Mandible, Mandibula, of an old man. [S700]
Loss of teeth – particularly at an advanced age – results in a **regression of the Pars alveolaris** of the Mandibula. This can progress until the Foramen mentale becomes located at the upper edge of the toothless Mandibula. The **Angulus mandibulae** of a toothless jaw is much wider than one with dentition.

Fig. 8.55 Mandible, Mandibula, of a newborn. [S700-L238]
In newborns, the two mandibular segments are still connected via the **Symphysis mandibulae.** The angle between the Corpus and Ramus mandibulae is still very large.

Clinical remarks

After fractures of the nose, fractures of the mandible also occur frequently due to its exposed position. Due to the U-shaped form, various types of mandibular fractures can occur, in particular at the level of the canines and the third molar teeth. Extravasated blood from the Mandibula collects in the loose tissue of the floor of the mouth, resulting in tiny spotty patches of bleeding under the skin (ecchymosis), which is a typical sign of a mandibular fracture.

When lost teeth are not replaced, **tooth loss** will lead to degeneration of the Pars alveolaris mandibulae in the affected area. Adapting a dental prosthesis is very challenging in the case of a largely regressed Pars alveolaris and often only successful after reconstructing the bone structure.

Temporomandibular joint

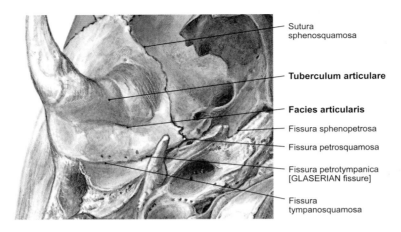

Sutura sphenosquamosa

Tuberculum articulare

Facies articularis

Fissura sphenopetrosa

Fissura petrosquamosa

Fissura petrotympanica [GLASERIAN fissure]

Fissura tympanosquamosa

Fig. 8.56 Glenoid fossa and articular protrusion of the temporo-mandibular joint, Articulatio temporomandibularis, right side; inferior view. For colour chart, see p. XIII. [S700]
The illustration shows the Facies articularis of the Fossa mandibularis, which is normally coated with hyaline articular cartilage. At the front is the Tuberculum articulare, which is likewise coated with hyaline cartilage. In the posterior third of the Fossa mandibularis, the Pars squamo-sa is connected to the Pars petrosa of the Os temporale, and the Os temporale is medially adjacent to the Os sphenoidale. **Three fissures** exist in this area:
- laterally and externally, the Fissura tympanosquamosa can be seen
- in the middle lies the Fissura petrotympanica
- medially runs the Fissura sphenopetrosa, from which the Chorda tympani leaves the cranial base.

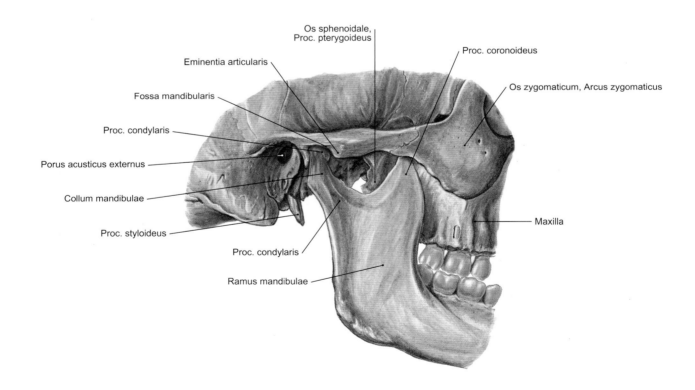

Os sphenoidale, Proc. pterygoideus

Proc. coronoideus

Eminentia articularis

Os zygomaticum, Arcus zygomaticus

Fossa mandibularis

Proc. condylaris

Porus acusticus externus

Collum mandibulae

Maxilla

Proc. styloideus

Proc. condylaris

Ramus mandibulae

Fig. 8.57 Temporomandibular joint, Articulatio temporomandibularis, right side; lateral view. [S700-L285]
The Proc. condylaris of the Mandibula is located in the Fossa mandibularis of the Os temporale. In front of the condyle is the Eminentia articularis, and behind it, the bony part of the Meatus acusticus externus. Above the Fossa mandibularis is the middle cranial fossa.

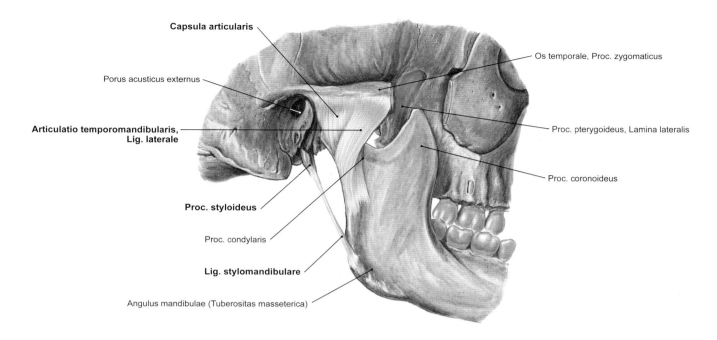

Capsula articularis

Porus acusticus externus

Articulatio temporomandibularis,
Lig. laterale

Proc. styloideus

Proc. condylaris

Lig. stylomandibulare

Angulus mandibulae (Tuberositas masseterica)

Os temporale, Proc. zygomaticus

Proc. pterygoideus, Lamina lateralis

Proc. coronoideus

Fig. 8.58 Temporomandibular joint, Articulatio temporomandibularis, right side; lateral view. [S700-L285]
The temporomandibular joint is enclosed by a wide joint capsule (Capsula articularis) that extends in a funnel-shaped manner from the Os temporale to the Proc. condylaris. The joint capsule is reinforced laterally and anteriorly by the Lig. laterale, which runs obliquely downwards from the Arcus zygomaticus to the Collum mandibulae. At the inside of the joint (not shown), connective tissue generates the variable Lig. me-

diale. The Lig. laterale and Lig. mediale (insofar as they are formed) are involved in the articulation and inhibit marginal movements, particularly backwards. The Lig. laterale also stabilises the condyle on the working side. From the Proc. styloideus, the **Lig. stylomandibulare** runs to the posterior rim of the Ramus mandibulae. It is usually weak and, together with the **Lig. sphenomandibulare,** resists further movements of the lower jaw at a position close to the maximal opening of the mouth (→ Fig. 8.60).

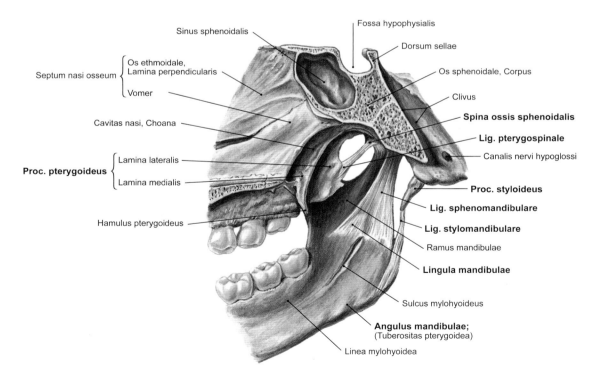

Sinus sphenoidalis

Septum nasi osseum { Os ethmoidale, Lamina perpendicularis / Vomer

Cavitas nasi, Choana

Proc. pterygoideus { Lamina lateralis / Lamina medialis

Hamulus pterygoideus

Fossa hypophysialis

Dorsum sellae

Os sphenoidale, Corpus

Clivus

Spina ossis sphenoidalis

Lig. pterygospinale

Canalis nervi hypoglossi

Proc. styloideus

Lig. sphenomandibulare

Lig. stylomandibulare

Ramus mandibulae

Lingula mandibulae

Sulcus mylohyoideus

Angulus mandibulae;
(Tuberositas pterygoidea)

Linea mylohyoidea

Fig. 8.59 Lig. stylomandibulare and Lig. sphenomandibulare, right side; medial view. [S700]
Both ligaments affect the **kinematics** of the Articulatio temporomandibularis but are not associated with the joint capsule.
The powerful **Lig. sphenomandibulare** originates at the Spina ossis sphenoidalis and runs between the Mm. pterygoidei lateralis and medialis to the Lingula mandibulae. Here it inserts in a fan-shaped manner above the Foramen mandibulae. The **Lig. stylomandibulare** which

comes from the Proc. styloideus inserts at the Angulus mandibulae. Together, both ligaments inhibit the **opening movements** of the lower jaw at the maximal opening position of the mouth.
Without a connection to the temporomandibular joint and without any impact on its kinematics, the **Lig. pterygospinale** runs from the Spina ossis sphenoidalis to the Lamina lateralis of the Proc. pterygoideus. This ligament has a **stabilising** function.

Skeleton and joints

Temporomandibular joint

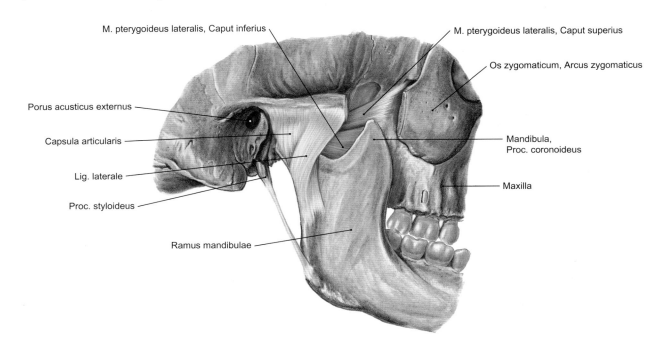

M. pterygoideus lateralis, Caput inferius

M. pterygoideus lateralis, Caput superius

Porus acusticus externus

Os zygomaticum, Arcus zygomaticus

Capsula articularis

Mandibula,
Proc. coronoideus

Lig. laterale

Maxilla

Proc. styloideus

Ramus mandibulae

Fig. 8.60   Temporomandibular joint, Articulatio temporomandibularis, right side; lateral view. [S700-L285]

The M. pterygoideus lateralis is connected directly to the temporomandibular joint. Its two muscular parts run towards the anterior portion of the joint capsule. They are located medially behind the Lig. laterale.

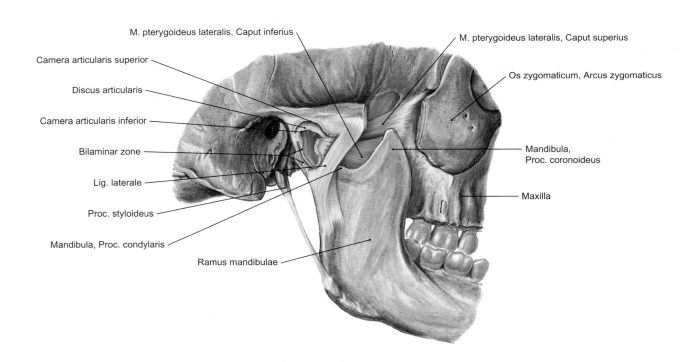

M. pterygoideus lateralis, Caput inferius

M. pterygoideus lateralis, Caput superius

Camera articularis superior

Discus articularis

Os zygomaticum, Arcus zygomaticus

Camera articularis inferior

Bilaminar zone

Mandibula,
Proc. coronoideus

Lig. laterale

Maxilla

Proc. styloideus

Mandibula, Proc. condylaris

Ramus mandibulae

Fig. 8.61   Temporomandibular joint, Articulatio temporomandibularis, right side; lateral view. [S700-L285]
Upon partial removal of the lateral part of the capsule and parts of the Lig. laterale, it becomes apparent that the Caput superius of the M. pterygoideus lateralis, which originates from the Ala major of the Os sphenoidale, penetrates the anterior part of the joint capsule above the Pars inferior. It inserts into the Discus articularis of the Articulatio tem-

poromandibularis, as well as into the Proc. condylaris. The Caput inferius of the M. pterygoideus lateralis originates at the outer surface of the Lamina lateralis of the Proc. pterygoideus of the Os sphenoidale, and penetrates the joint capsule from the front beneath the tendon of the Caput superius of the M. pterygoideus lateralis, and inserts completely into the Proc. condylaris.

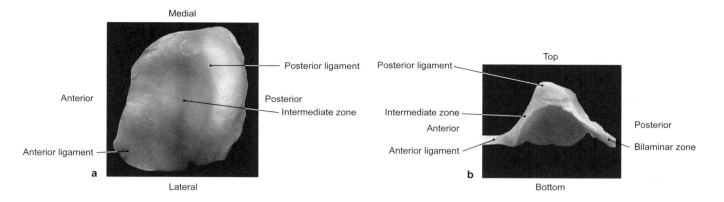

Medial
Anterior
Posterior ligament
Posterior
Intermediate zone
Anterior ligament
a
Lateral

Top
Posterior ligament
Intermediate zone
Anterior
Anterior ligament
Posterior
Bilaminar zone
b
Bottom

Fig. 8.62a and b   Articular disc, Discus articularis, of the Articulatio temporomandibularis. [S700]
a View from above.
b Lateral view.

From the front to the back, the Discus articularis consists of an anterior ligament (connective tissue), an intermediate zone (fibrous cartilage), a posterior ligament (connective tissue), and a bilaminar zone (connective tissue). The intermediate zone is particularly thin in the lateral portion. The Discus articularis is fused on all sides to the joint capsule.

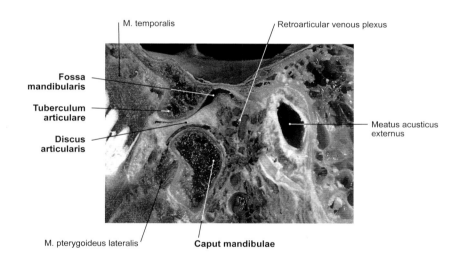

M. temporalis
Retroarticular venous plexus
Fossa mandibularis
Tuberculum articulare
Discus articularis
Meatus acusticus externus
M. pterygoideus lateralis
Caput mandibulae

Fig. 8.63   Temporomandibular joint, Articulatio temporomandibularis; sagittal section through the joint area with injected veins; lateral view. [S700]
The bilaminar zone between the Tuberculum articulare and Caput mandibulae is visible. The bone between the middle cranial fossa and the

Fossa mandibularis is thin. Between the tracts of connective tissue in the bilaminar zone lies a distinct **retroarticular venous plexus.** There is a close relationship to the external auditory canal (Meatus acusticus externus).

Clinical remarks

If the Mandibula suffers a violent impact, this often leads to a fracture of the Collum mandibulae **(Collum fracture)**. These intra- or extracapsular fractures can occur with or without dislocation. In addition, bleeding from the retroarticular venous plexus (→ Fig. 8.63) can contribute to the pain sensations in the Meatus acusticus externus. Anterior dislocation of the mandibular condyles are most frequent (→ figure). However, uni- and bilaterally posterior, lateral or superior dislocations can occur as well.
The Articulatio temporomandibularis is a diarthrosis and is similar to large joints of the limbs, and can be afflicted by the same pathology, e.g. osteoarthritis or rheumatoid arthritis. An **osteoarthritis of the temporomandibular joint** tends to cause defects in the lateral part of the Discus articularis.

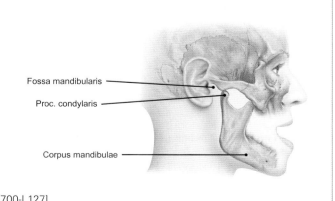

Fossa mandibularis
Proc. condylaris
Corpus mandibulae

[S700-L127]

Skeleton and joints

Temporomandibular joint

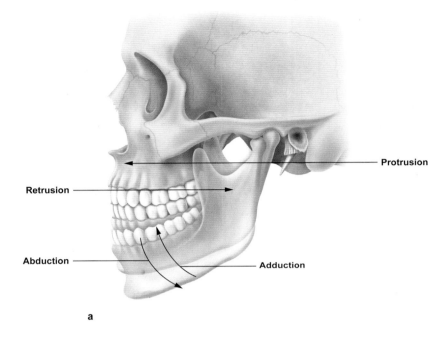

Protrusion

Retrusion

Abduction

Adduction

a

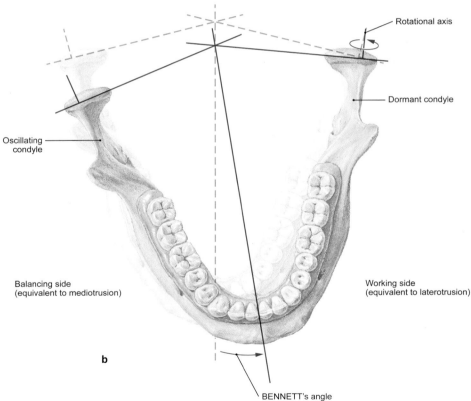

Rotational axis

Dormant condyle

Oscillating
condyle

Balancing side
(equivalent to mediotrusion)

Working side
(equivalent to laterotrusion)

b

BENNETT's angle

Fig. 8.64a and b Movements of the temporomandibular joint, Articulatio temporomandibularis; left side.
a Lateral view. Independent movements in one of the joints are not possible because both temporomandibular joints are linked via the Mandibula. The temporomandibular joints permit two main functions during chewing: elevation **(adduction)** and lowering **(abduction)** of the lower jaw as well as grinding movements. In addition to abduction and adduction, the forward movement **(protrusion)** and backward movement **(retrusion),** as well as grinding movements (moving sideways – **laterotrusion and mediotrusion)** constitute the movement patterns of the Articulatio temporomandibularis. The masticatory muscles are variously involved in the movements. [S700-L275]

b Grinding movements of the mandible, Mandibula, in the left temporomandibular joint; view from above. The Articulatio temporomandibularis is a bicondylar joint; movements on one side always affect the other side. In the case of grinding movements, the **dormant condyle** (shown here on the left on the **working side**) rotates around an almost vertical axis via the Caput mandibulae, while the **oscillating condyle** (shown here on the right on the **balancing side**) oscillates forwards and medially at the same time (translation movement). The **BENNETT's angle** describes the extent (amplitude) of the mandibular oscillation. On the working side, the Mandibula performs a laterotrusion, and on the balancing side, a mediotrusion. [S700-L127]

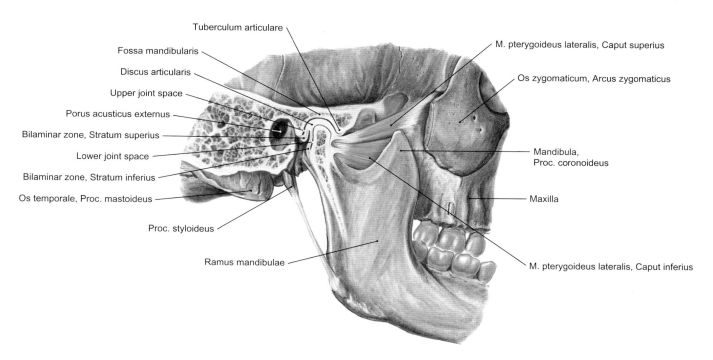

Fig. 8.65 Temporomandibular joint, Articulatio temporomandibularis, right side; sagittal section, lateral view. [S700-L285]
When the mouth is closed with intercuspidating rows of teeth (resting position), the Proc. condylaris with the Discus articularis is located in the Fossa mandibularis. As the Discus articularis is fused on all sides to the joint capsule, a larger superior joint chamber (between the Fossa mandibularis and the Discus) and a smaller inferior joint chamber (between the Discus and Proc. condylaris) are formed. Therefore, it is called

a bithalamic joint (consisting of two chambers). At the posterior aspect, the superior ligament (Stratum superius) and the inferior ligament (Stratum inferius) of the bilaminar zone of the Discus articularis can be recognised. The Stratum superius is short and stretchy. It runs to the Fissurae petrotympanica and tympanosquamosa and is closely positioned to the Chorda tympani of the N. facialis [VII] (→ Fig. 8.95). The tighter Stratum inferius inserts much further below and behind between the Caput and Collum mandibulae.

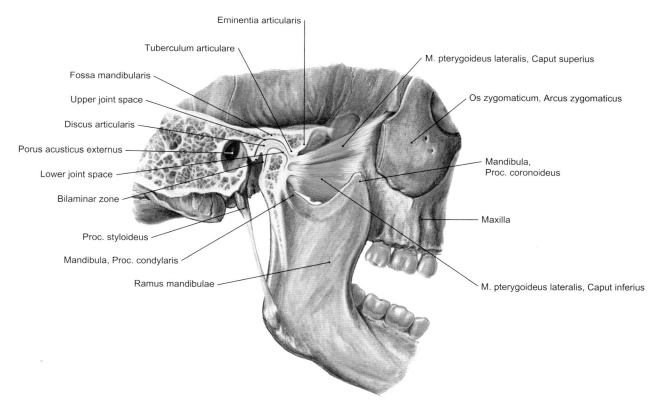

Fig. 8.66 Temporomandibular joint, Articulatio temporomandibularis, right side; sagittal section, lateral view. [S700-L285]
When the mouth opens up to 15°, rotation of the condyle occurs around its transverse axis. Through the tension of the Lig. laterale, and the

traction of the Caput superius of the M. pterygoideus lateralis, the condyle is also drawn forwards onto the Tuberculum articulare when the mouth is opened more than 15°.

Temporomandibular joint, X-ray imaging

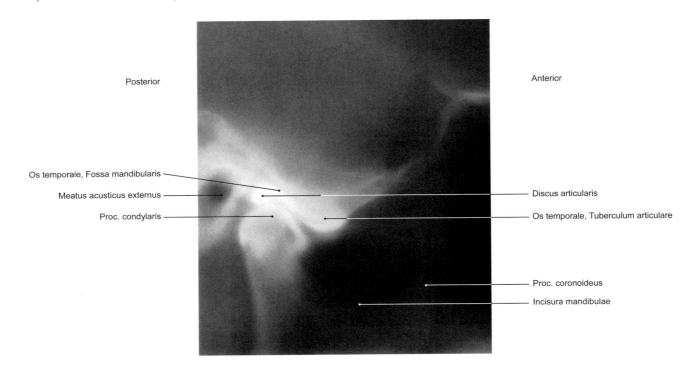

Posterior   Anterior

Os temporale, Fossa mandibularis ⎯

Meatus acusticus externus ⎯⎯⎯⎯⎯   ⎯ Discus articularis

Proc. condylaris ⎯⎯⎯⎯⎯⎯   ⎯ Os temporale, Tuberculum articulare

                                                                        ⎯ Proc. coronoideus
                                                                        ⎯ Incisura mandibulae

Fig. 8.67   Temporomandibular joint, Articulatio temporomandibularis; X-ray image in lateral projection; mouth closed. [S700-T905]

With a closed mouth and relaxed masticatory muscles, the Proc. condylaris lies in the Fossa mandibularis.

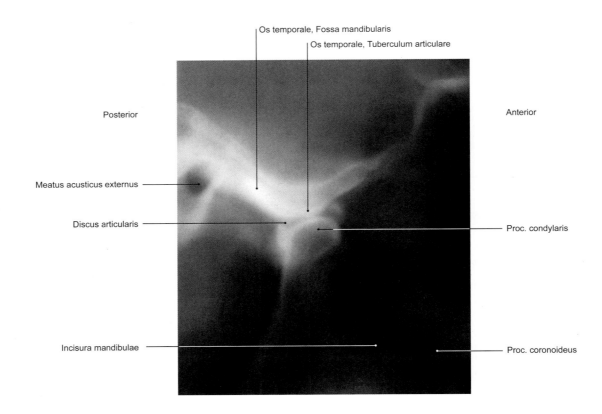

Os temporale, Fossa mandibularis

Os temporale, Tuberculum articulare

Posterior   Anterior

Meatus acusticus externus ⎯⎯⎯⎯

Discus articularis ⎯⎯⎯⎯⎯   ⎯ Proc. condylaris

Incisura mandibulae ⎯⎯⎯⎯⎯   ⎯ Proc. coronoideus

Fig. 8.68   Temporomandibular joint, Articulatio temporomandibularis; X-ray image in lateral projection; mouth open. [S700-T905]

With an open mouth, the Discus articularis and the Proc. condylaris will slide forward onto the Tuberculum articulare.

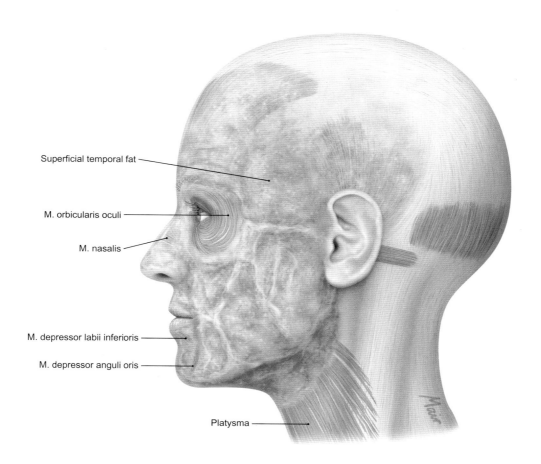

Superficial temporal fat

M. orbicularis oculi

M. nasalis

M. depressor labii inferioris

M. depressor anguli oris

Platysma

Fig. 8.69 Subcutaneous fat layer of the face; lateral view.
[S700- J803/L127]/[E1043]
After removal of the facial skin, the distribution of the superficial subcutaneous fat layer can be seen. The shaping of the adipose tissue varies greatly in each individual and depends highly on the nutritional status; it adds to the individuality of the face. Only on the M. orbicularis oculi and in the region of the nose is there very little subcutaneous fat. The adipose tissue is divided by connective tissue septa into compart-

ments (→ Fig. 8.70). The connective tissue septa are stretched out between the skin, the loose connective tissue, the mimetic muscles and the 'superficial muscular aponeurotic system' (SMAS), which consists of the fasciae of the Glandula parotidea (Fascia parotidea), of the M. masseter (Fascia masseterica), of the M. buccinator (Fascia buccopharyngea) and of the M. temporalis (Fascia temporalis), forming a layer of remarkable tensile strength. The SMAS extends up to the scalp.

Subcutaneous adipose tissue

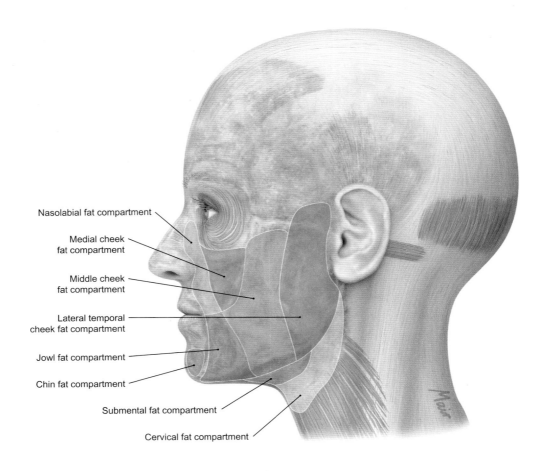

Nasolabial fat compartment

Medial cheek
fat compartment

Middle cheek
fat compartment

Lateral temporal
cheek fat compartment

Jowl fat compartment

Chin fat compartment

Submental fat compartment

Cervical fat compartment

Fig. 8.70 Subcutaneous fat compartments; lateral view. [S700-L127]/[E1043]
Presentation of the topography of the connective tissue septa of the 'superficial muscular aponeurotic system' (SMAS) as well as coloured representation of the various subcutaneous fat compartments underneath the Arcus zygomaticus.

Clinical remarks

The **SMAS (superficial muscular aponeurotic system)** is crucial in plastic surgery for **face lifts** (rhytidectomy). Via an arc-shaped incision in front of the auricle, the SMAS can be dissected and detached from the surrounding structures. A customised cut of the part close to the ear can be made to reduce it, and the edge of the cut can be sewn up again by pulling it towards the auricle. In this way the facial skin is tightened (→ figure).

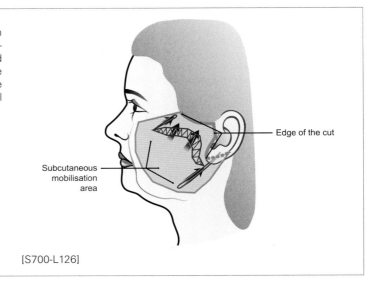

Edge of the cut

Subcutaneous
mobilisation
area

[S700-L126]

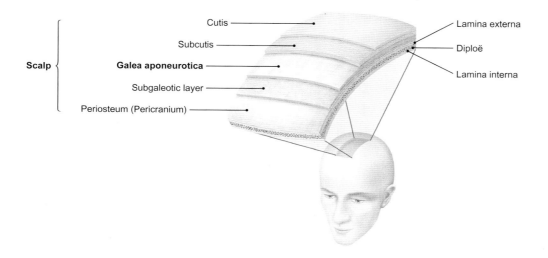

Fig. 8.71 Structure of the scalp; frontal and cranial oblique view. [S700-L127]
The functional unit of skin, subcutis and tendinous epicranial aponeurosis (Galea aponeurotica) overlying the calvaria is referred to as the scalp. It consists of **five layers** which can be remembered by using the mnemonic **SCALP.**

- S = skin (cutis)
- C = connective tissue (subcutis)
- A = aponeurosis (Aponeurosis epicranialis, Galea aponeurotica with M. epicranius)
- L = loose connective tissue (subgaleotic layer)
- P = pericranium (periosteum of the cranium).

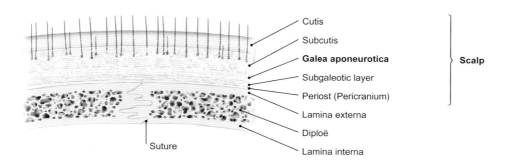

Fig. 8.72 Structure of the scalp; sagittal section. [S700-L127]
The total thickness of the scalp is approx. 5 mm. The cutis is rough in the area covered with hair and contains many hair shafts, sebaceous glands and sweat glands. In the subcutis are the corresponding papillae, hair follicles and hair roots. It consists for the most part of dense connective tissue, which anchors the skin in the Galea aponeurotica. In addition, blood vessels and nerves run here. In bald areas, the cutis and subcutis are thinner. The Galea aponeurotica is an expansive tendon to which the paired Venter frontalis and Venter occipitalis of the M. epicranius (M. occipitofrontalis) are attached, as well as the variably occurring M. temporoparietalis on each side. The Galea aponeurotica and subcutis are firmly connected by retinacula. The loose connective tissue (subgaleotic layer) connects the Galea aponeurotica with the pericranium. The pericranium of the calvaria is firmly fused to the external lamina of the facial bones and the connective tissue of the cranial sutures.

Clinical remarks

During the birth process, the stress on the child's skull when passing through the birth canal is high. Especially in the occipital and parietal areas, it can lead to serous and sometimes blood-tinged oedema which is known as **scalp swelling (Caput succedaneum).** Bleeding under the periosteum (subperiostal bleeding) remains limited to individual bones of the calvaria **(cephalic haematoma),** since the periosteum is very strongly adherent in the area of the cranial sutures. If long hair is caught in a rotating machine, it could be torn off together with the scalp **(scalping injury).** Health and safety therefore prescribes the use of headgear in the proximity of such machines. The easily detachable nature of the scalp is useful in surgical procedures carried out on the brain where the scalp, by means of a 'temple cut' (from one auricle to the other) can be removed towards the front and towards the back from the periosteum. After the surgery, the scalp is moved back into place and sewn on. Due to the strong connective tissue, injured blood vessels in the subcutis remain open with only poor retraction. **Bleeding** after injury is therefore often extensive.

Head

Facial muscles

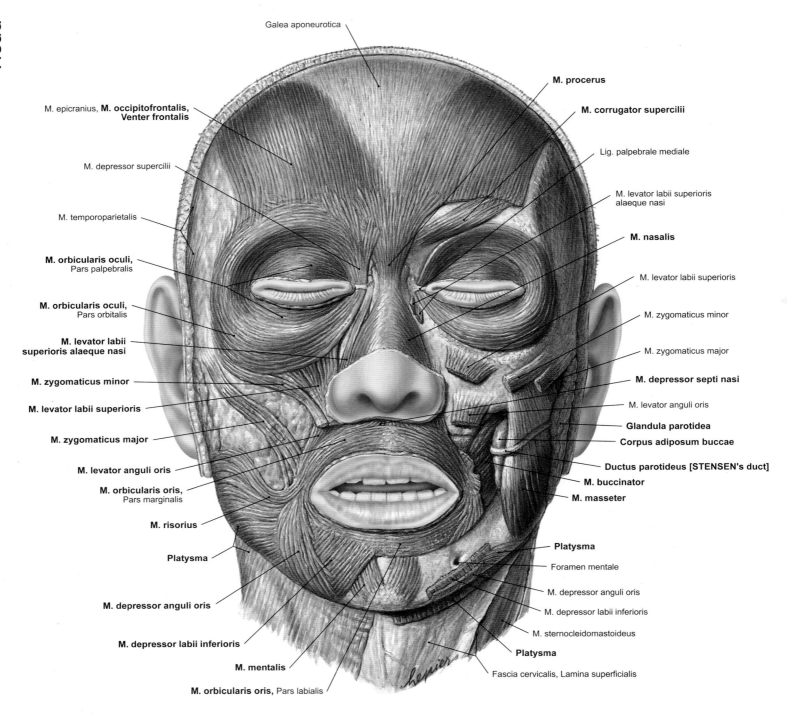

Galea aponeurotica

M. procerus

M. corrugator supercilii

M. epicranius, **M. occipitofrontalis,**
Venter frontalis

Lig. palpebrale mediale

M. depressor supercilii

M. levator labii superioris
alaeque nasi

M. temporoparietalis

M. nasalis

M. orbicularis oculi,
Pars palpebralis

M. levator labii superioris

M. orbicularis oculi,
Pars orbitalis

M. zygomaticus minor

M. levator labii
superioris alaeque nasi

M. zygomaticus major

M. depressor septi nasi

M. zygomaticus minor

M. levator anguli oris

M. levator labii superioris

Glandula parotidea

M. zygomaticus major

Corpus adiposum buccae

M. levator anguli oris

Ductus parotideus [STENSEN's duct]

M. orbicularis oris,
Pars marginalis

M. buccinator

M. masseter

M. risorius

Platysma

Foramen mentale

Platysma

M. depressor anguli oris

M. depressor anguli oris

M. depressor labii inferioris

M. sternocleidomastoideus

M. depressor labii inferioris

Platysma

M. mentalis

Fascia cervicalis, Lamina superficialis

M. orbicularis oris, Pars labialis

Fig. 8.73   Facial muscles, Mm. faciei, and masticatory muscles,
Mm. masticatorii; frontal view. [S700]
The mimetic muscles are, as the name indicates, responsible for facial
expressions, as well as creating the individual facial physiognomy of a
person. The muscles in the region of the eyes have important protective
functions, while the muscles in the region of the mouth serve the food
uptake and articulation.
Visible on both sides of the face are the Venter frontalis of the M. occipitofrontalis (M. epicranius), the Partes orbitalis and palpebralis of the
M. orbicularis oculi (Pars lacrimalis, → Fig. 9.26), the M. corrugator supercilii, M. procerus, Mm. nasalis, depressor septi nasi, levator labii
superioris alaeque nasi, the M. orbicularis oris with the Pars labialis and
Pars marginalis, the M. buccinator, the Mm. zygomatici major and minor, the Mm. risorius, levator labii superioris, levator anguli oris, depres-

sor anguli oris, depressor labii inferioris and mentalis, as well as the
platysma projecting into the neck area.
Of the masticatory muscles, the only one to be seen in the left half of
the face is the M. masseter, across which the Ductus parotideus (STE-
NON duct, STENSEN's duct) runs. The duct runs from the Glandula parotidea anteriorly and bends around the frontal edge of the M. masseter, almost at a right angle, in order to enter into the M. buccinator.
A buccal fat pad (Corpus adiposum buccae, BICHAT's fat pad) is located
between the M. masseter and M. buccinator and contributes to the
contour of the cheek area. With the exception of the M. buccinator, the
facial muscles do not possess a fascia. The fascia of the M. buccinator,
the M. masseter and the Glandula parotidea have been removed.

→ T 1.1, T 1.3–T 1.6, T 6

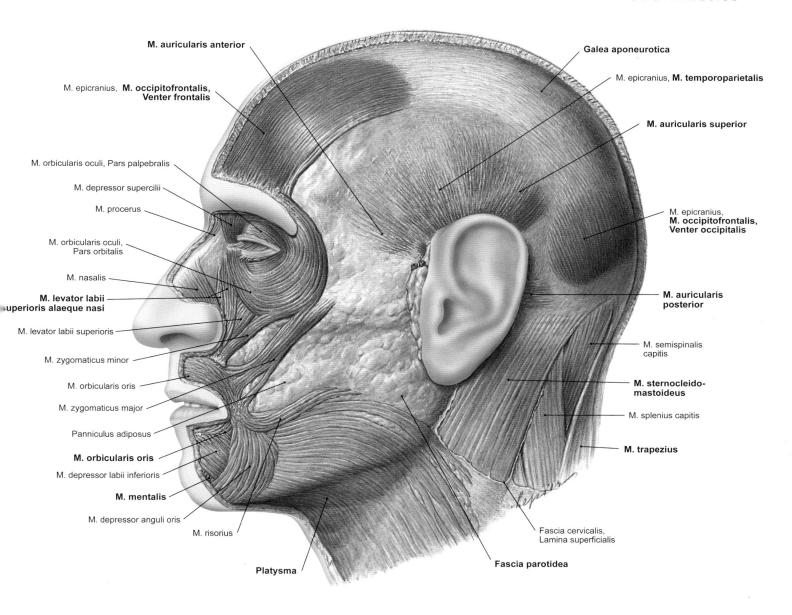

M. auricularis anterior

M. epicranius, **M. occipitofrontalis, Venter frontalis**

M. orbicularis oculi, Pars palpebralis

M. depressor supercilii

M. procerus

M. orbicularis oculi, Pars orbitalis

M. nasalis

M. levator labii superioris alaeque nasi

M. levator labii superioris

M. zygomaticus minor

M. orbicularis oris

M. zygomaticus major

Panniculus adiposus

M. orbicularis oris

M. depressor labii inferioris

M. mentalis

M. depressor anguli oris

M. risorius

Platysma

Galea aponeurotica

M. epicranius, **M. temporoparietalis**

M. auricularis superior

M. epicranius, **M. occipitofrontalis, Venter occipitalis**

M. auricularis posterior

M. semispinalis capitis

M. sternocleido-mastoideus

M. splenius capitis

M. trapezius

Fascia cervicalis, Lamina superficialis

Fascia parotidea

Fig. 8.74 Facial muscles, Mm. faciei, left side; lateral view. [S700]
In addition to the muscles labelled in → Fig. 8.73, the view from the side shows the Venter occipitalis of the M. occipitofrontalis (M. epicranius) and the **Galea aponeurotica** extending between the Venter frontalis and Venter occipitalis. Located above the ear and also projecting into the Galea aponeurotica is the M. temporoparietalis (also a part of the

M. epicranius) which originates from the Fascia temporalis. In addition, further mimetic muscles such as the Mm. auriculares anterior, superior and posterior can be seen. In the neck area, parts of the M. sternocleidomastoideus, the M. trapezius and some intrinsic muscles are visible.

→ T 1

Clinical remarks

Paralysis of the M. orbicularis oculi, associated with a paresis of the N. facialis [VII] (facial paralysis), results in an inability to actively close the eyelid, causing it to stay open during sleep (paralytic **lagophthalmos,** → Fig. 12.152). The lower eyelid has no tension and hangs down limply **(paralytic ectropion).** The lacrimal fluid can no longer be discharged via the Canaliculus inferior and flows over the everted lower eyelid (excessive watering of the eye, **epiphora**). The

inability to blink leads to the drying out of the cornea with inflammation **(keratitis)** and opacity of the cornea.
The age-related flaccid weakness of the lower eyelid is described as a **senile ectropion.**
Paralysis of the M. orbicularis oris (also in the context of facial paralysis) results in speech disabilities. The corner of the mouth hangs down so that saliva involuntarily flows from the mouth.

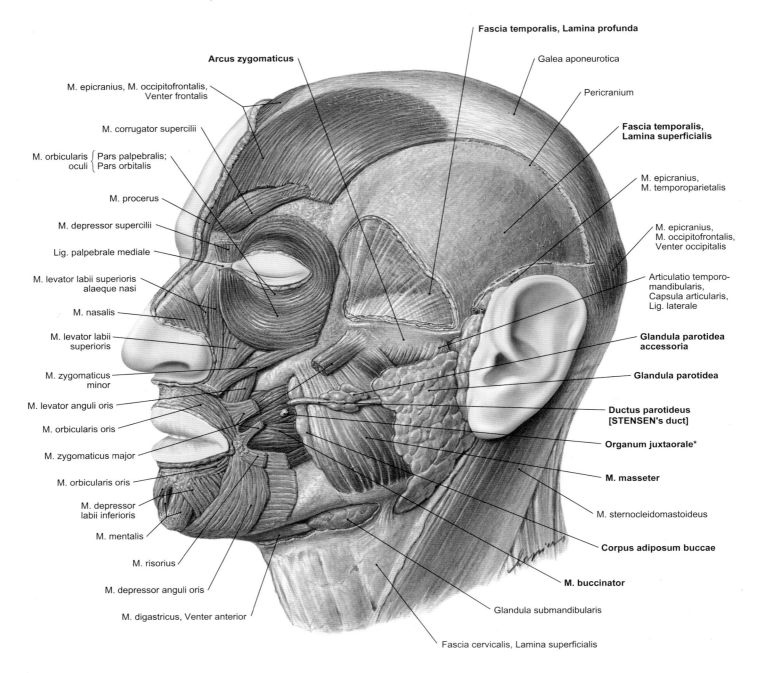

Fascia temporalis, Lamina profunda

Galea aponeurotica

Pericranium

Arcus zygomaticus

Fascia temporalis, Lamina superficialis

M. epicranius, M. occipitofrontalis, Venter frontalis

M. epicranius, M. temporoparietalis

M. corrugator supercilii

M. epicranius, M. occipitofrontalis, Venter occipitalis

M. orbicularis { Pars palpebralis;
oculi { Pars orbitalis

Articulatio temporo-mandibularis, Capsula articularis, Lig. laterale

M. procerus

M. depressor supercilii

Lig. palpebrale mediale

Glandula parotidea accessoria

M. levator labii superioris alaeque nasi

Glandula parotidea

M. nasalis

M. levator labii superioris

Ductus parotideus [STENSEN's duct]

M. zygomaticus minor

Organum juxtaorale*

M. levator anguli oris

M. orbicularis oris

M. masseter

M. zygomaticus major

M. orbicularis oris

M. sternocleidomastoideus

M. depressor labii inferioris

M. mentalis

Corpus adiposum buccae

M. risorius

M. depressor anguli oris

M. buccinator

M. digastricus, Venter anterior

Glandula submandibularis

Fascia cervicalis, Lamina superficialis

Fig. 8.75 Facial muscles, Mm. faciei, and masticatory muscles, Mm. masticatorii; oblique lateral view. [S700]

The fascia of the M. buccinator and the M. masseter, as well as the Fascia parotidea and, in some cases, the Lamina superficialis of the Fascia cervicalis, are removed. As a result, the corresponding muscles, the Glandula parotidea extending to the neck area, and the Glandula submandibularis become visible.

The main excretory duct of the Glandula parotidea, the Ductus parotideus (STENON duct, STENSEN's duct), emerges from the gland at the anterior pole and runs horizontally from the posterior side of the **M. masseter** forwards and then bends inwards, almost at a right angle, to the anterior margin of the M. masseter in order to penetrate the **M. buccinator.** Between the M. buccinator and M. masseter lies the Corpus adiposum buccae (BICHAT's fat pad). Next to the Ductus parotideus is accessory glandular tissue (Glandula parotidea accessoria). On the M. buccinator, the juxtaoral organ (* organ of CHIEVITZ) lies close to the

site where the Ductus parotideus penetrates the M. buccinator. It is approx. 5×3 mm and is an epithelial organ in the cheek, embedded in connective tissue rich in nerves and cells, and surrounded by a perineural sheath. Its function is not conclusively established; it is assumed, however, that it effects dynamic changes when chewing, swallowing, sucking and speaking, and among other things, helps prevent one from biting one's cheek when chewing.

In the temporal region, the M. parietoparietalis of the M. epicranius has been removed. This reveals the Lamina superficialis of the Fascia temporalis.

Above the Arcus zygomaticus, a part of the Lamina superficialis along with the underlying temporal fat pad (Corpus adiposum temporale) is removed so that the deep layer (Lamina profunda) of the Fascia temporalis can be seen, as well as the M. temporalis gleaming through it.

→ T 1, T 6

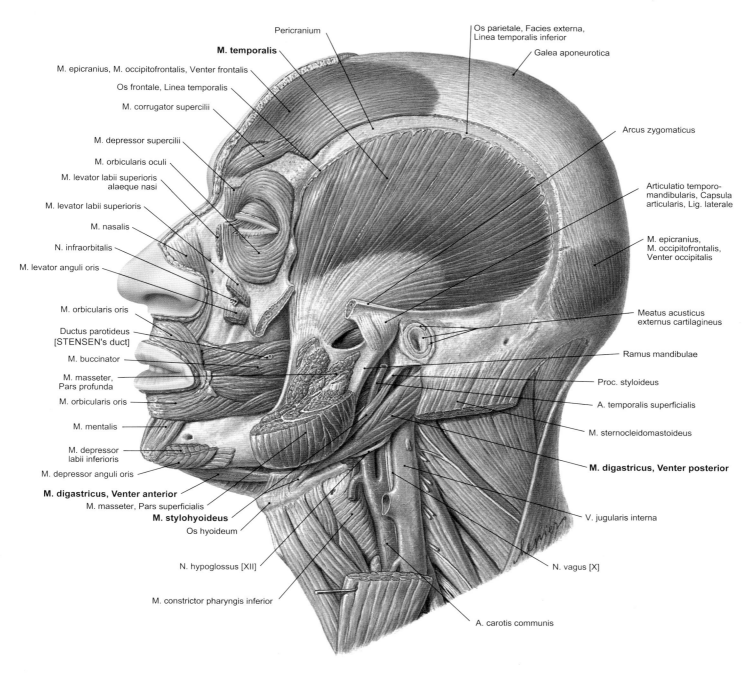

Pericranium

M. temporalis

M. epicranius, M. occipitofrontalis, Venter frontalis

Os frontale, Linea temporalis

M. corrugator supercilii

M. depressor supercilii

M. orbicularis oculi

M. levator labii superioris alaeque nasi

M. levator labii superioris

M. nasalis

N. infraorbitalis

M. levator anguli oris

M. orbicularis oris

Ductus parotideus [STENSEN's duct]

M. buccinator

M. masseter, Pars profunda

M. orbicularis oris

M. mentalis

M. depressor labii inferioris

M. depressor anguli oris

M. digastricus, Venter anterior

M. masseter, Pars superficialis

M. stylohyoideus

Os hyoideum

N. hypoglossus [XII]

M. constrictor pharyngis inferior

Os parietale, Facies externa, Linea temporalis inferior

Galea aponeurotica

Arcus zygomaticus

Articulatio temporo-mandibularis, Capsula articularis, Lig. laterale

M. epicranius, M. occipitofrontalis, Venter occipitalis

Meatus acusticus externus cartilagineus

Ramus mandibulae

Proc. styloideus

A. temporalis superficialis

M. sternocleidomastoideus

M. digastricus, Venter posterior

V. jugularis interna

N. vagus [X]

A. carotis communis

Fig. 8.76 Facial muscles, Mm. faciei, and masticatory muscles, Mm. masticatorii, left side; oblique lateral view. [S700]
Upon removal of the superficial and deep laminae of the Fascia temporalis and the partial removal of the Arcus zygomaticus and parts of the M. masseter, the **M. temporalis** becomes visible.
The origin of the M. temporalis is shown along the Linea temporalis inferior of the Facies externa of the Os parietale, and the Facies temporalis of the Os frontale. The muscle fibres converge into a flat tendon, which disappears behind the Arcus zygomaticus into the Fossa infratemporalis and extends to the Proc. coronoideus.

Origins of the M. temporalis:
* Linea temporalis inferior of the Facies externa of the Os parietale
* Facies temporalis of the Os frontale
* Facies temporalis, Pars squamosa of the Os temporale
* Facies temporalis of the Os zygomaticum
* Facies temporalis of the Os sphenoidale to the Crista infratemporalis.
The illustration also shows some of the Mm. suprahyoidei (M. digastricus with Venter anterior and Venter posterior, M. stylohyoideus).

→ T 1, T 6

Clinical remarks

Swelling of the Glandula parotidea (e.g. in the case of a parotitis epidemic [mumps], Clinical remarks for → Fig. 8.190) is often very painful when chewing due to the close proximity to the masticatory muscles and because it shares a common fascia (Fascia parotideomasseterica) with the M. masseter. The pain is often referred/conducted into the external acoustic meatus (pain from pressure on the tragus).
In the case of severe emaciation, e.g. in the final stages of malignant tumour diseases **(cancer cachexia)** or in an advanced stage of HIV, the BICHAT's fat pad of the cheek wastes away, leaving the patient with sunken cheeks.

Masticatory muscles

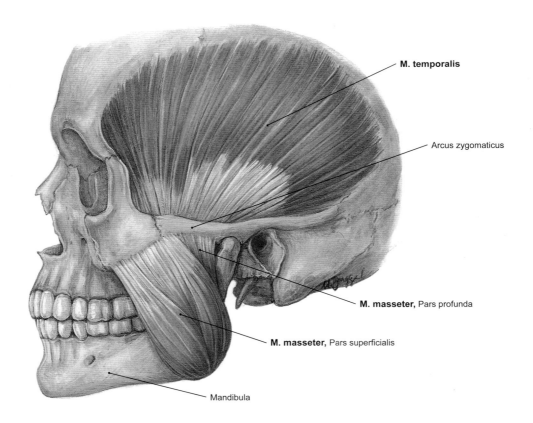

M. temporalis

Arcus zygomaticus

M. masseter, Pars profunda

M. masseter, Pars superficialis

Mandibula

Fig. 8.77 M. masseter and M. temporalis, left side; lateral view. [S700]

The **M. masseter** consists of a Pars superficialis and a Pars profunda.

→ T 6

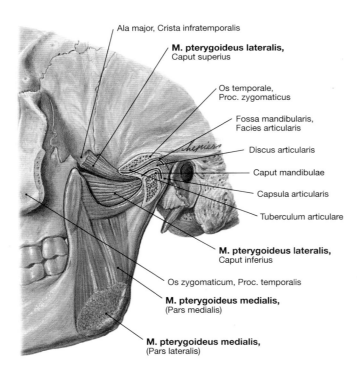

Ala major, Crista infratemporalis

M. pterygoideus lateralis, Caput superius

Os temporale, Proc. zygomaticus

Fossa mandibularis, Facies articularis

Discus articularis

Caput mandibulae

Capsula articularis

Tuberculum articulare

M. pterygoideus lateralis, Caput inferius

Os zygomaticum, Proc. temporalis

M. pterygoideus medialis, (Pars medialis)

M. pterygoideus medialis, (Pars lateralis)

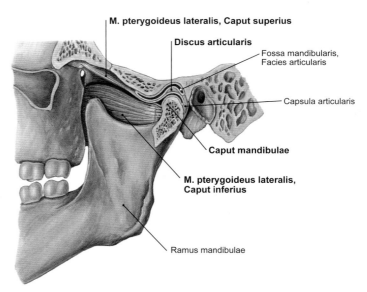

M. pterygoideus lateralis, Caput superius

Discus articularis

Fossa mandibularis, Facies articularis

Capsula articularis

Caput mandibulae

M. pterygoideus lateralis, Caput inferius

Ramus mandibulae

Fig. 8.78 Temporomandibular joint, Articulatio temporomandibularis, M. pterygoideus medialis and M. pterygoideus lateralis, left side; lateral view. [S700]
The M. pterygoideus medialis consists of a Pars medialis and a Pars lateralis.

→ T 6

Fig. 8.79 Temporomandibular joint, Articulatio temporomandibularis, and relationship with the M. pterygoideus lateralis, left side; lateral view. [S700]
The M. pterygoideus lateralis consists of a Caput superius and a Caput inferius (→ Fig. 8.78).

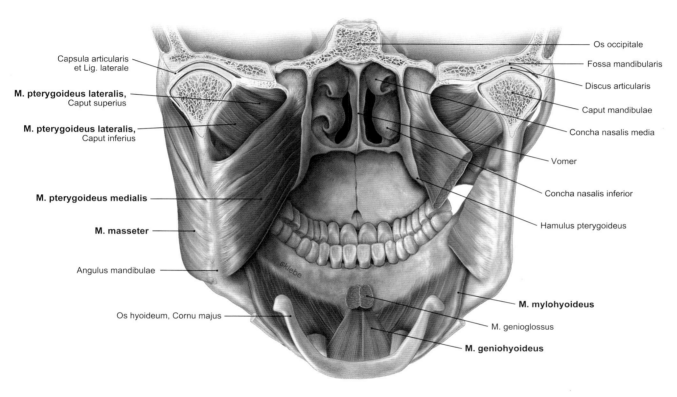

Capsula articularis et Lig. laterale

M. pterygoideus lateralis, Caput superius

M. pterygoideus lateralis, Caput inferius

M. pterygoideus medialis

M. masseter

Angulus mandibulae

Os hyoideum, Cornu majus

Os occipitale

Fossa mandibularis

Discus articularis

Caput mandibulae

Concha nasalis media

Vomer

Concha nasalis inferior

Hamulus pterygoideus

M. mylohyoideus

M. genioglossus

M. geniohyoideus

Fig. 8.80 Masticatory muscles, Mm. masticatorii; frontal section at the level of the Articulatio temporomandibularis; posterior view. [S700-L238]
The insertion sites of the M. masseter and M. pterygoideus medialis to both sides of the Angulus mandibulae are shown. The Mandibula is suspended by these muscles similar to a swing (shown on the left side).

→ T 6

Clinical remarks

Trismus manifests itself as an inability to open the mouth. It is caused by abscesses in the fascial compartments of the masticatory muscles. **Lockjaw,** the inability to close the mouth, is differentiated from trismus and is usually triggered by a very strong yawn or extreme opening of the mouth, although it can also be the result of an accident.

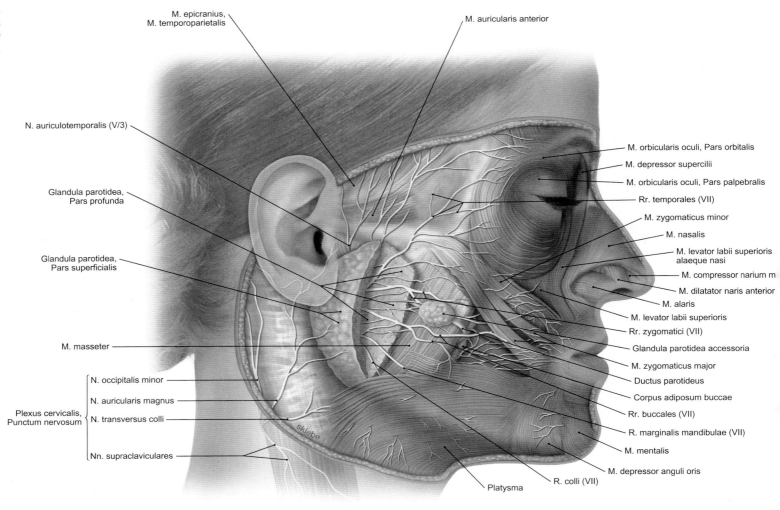

M. epicranius,
M. temporoparietalis

M. auricularis anterior

N. auriculotemporalis (V/3)

Glandula parotidea,
Pars profunda

Glandula parotidea,
Pars superficialis

M. masseter

Plexus cervicalis,
Punctum nervosum

N. occipitalis minor

N. auricularis magnus

N. transversus colli

Nn. supraclaviculares

M. orbicularis oculi, Pars orbitalis

M. depressor supercilii

M. orbicularis oculi, Pars palpebralis

Rr. temporales (VII)

M. zygomaticus minor

M. nasalis

M. levator labii superioris
alaeque nasi

M. compressor narium m

M. dilatator naris anterior

M. alaris

M. levator labii superioris

Rr. zygomatici (VII)

Glandula parotidea accessoria

M. zygomaticus major

Ductus parotideus

Corpus adiposum buccae

Rr. buccales (VII)

R. marginalis mandibulae (VII)

M. mentalis

M. depressor anguli oris

R. colli (VII)

Platysma

Fig. 8.81   Vessels and nerves of the head and neck, lateral super-ficial regions, right side; lateral view. [S700-L238]
The terminal branches of the **N. facialis [VII]** are superficial nerves which arise from the Plexus intraparotideus (Rr. temporales, Rr. zygomatici, Rr. buccales, Rr. marginales mandibulares and R. colli n. facialis) located within the parotid gland (anterior section of the superficial part removed).

The **N. auriculotemporalis,** which originates from the N. trigeminus [V], ascends in front of the outer ear. The neck and occipital region receive branches from the **Plexus cervicalis** for sensory innervation, most of which originate from the Punctum nervosum (ERB's point) on the back of the M. sternocleidomastoideus: N. transversus colli, N. auricularis magnus, N. occipitalis minor and Nn. supraclaviculares.

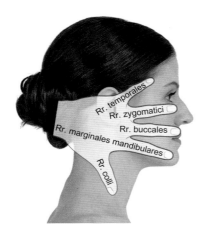

Rr. temporales

Rr. zygomatici

Rr. buccales

Rr. marginales mandibulares

Rr. colli

Fig. 8.82   Terminal branches of the N. facialis [VII], lateral superficial regions, right side; lateral view. [S700-J803/L126]
Spreading the fingers of a hand on the side of the face simulates the pathway of the terminal branches of the N. facialis [VII] as they emerge from the Plexus intraparotideus.

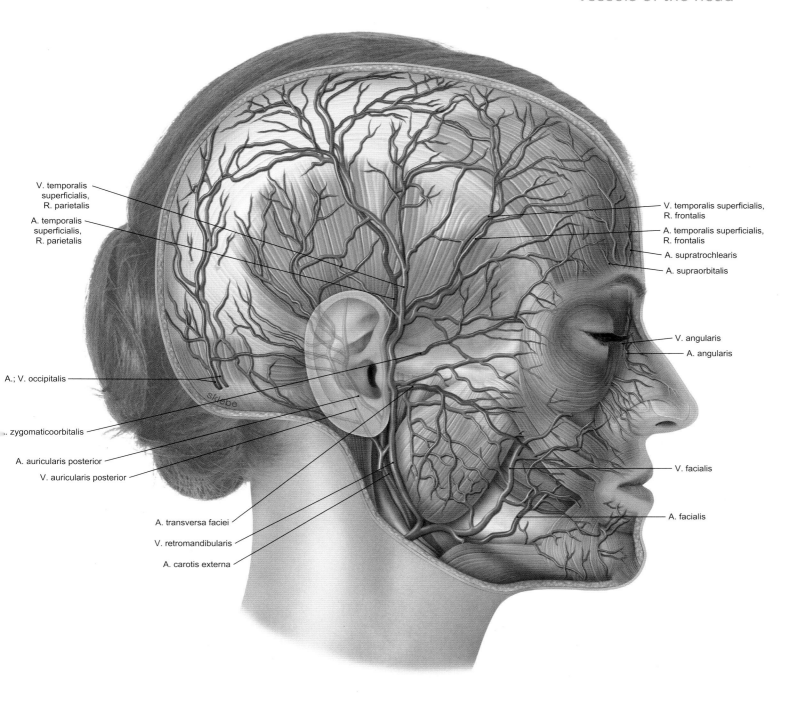

V. temporalis
superficialis,
R. parietalis

A. temporalis
superficialis,
R. parietalis

A.; V. occipitalis

.. zygomaticoorbitalis

A. auricularis posterior

V. auricularis posterior

A. transversa faciei

V. retromandibularis

A. carotis externa

V. temporalis superficialis,
R. frontalis

A. temporalis superficialis,
R. frontalis

A. supratrochlearis

A. supraorbitalis

V. angularis

A. angularis

V. facialis

A. facialis

Fig. 8.83   Vessels of the head, lateral superficial regions, right side; lateral view. [S700-L238]
Upon removal of the Glandula parotidea, the pathway of the branches originating from the **A. carotis externa** and the veins draining into the V. retromandibularis become visible. Additionally, the A. and V. facialis are visible as they pass around the mandibular. At this location, the arterial pulse can be palpated. Just below the eye, the A. and V. facialis continue as the A. and V. angularis, anastomosing with branches of the A. ophthalmica and V. ophthalmica superior in the orbital cavity.

Clinical remarks

Operations or incision injuries to the Glandula parotidea can lead to a **disruption of the intraparotid branches of the N. facialis [VII],** with partial paralysis of mimetic muscles (peripheral facial paralysis or partial paralysis).

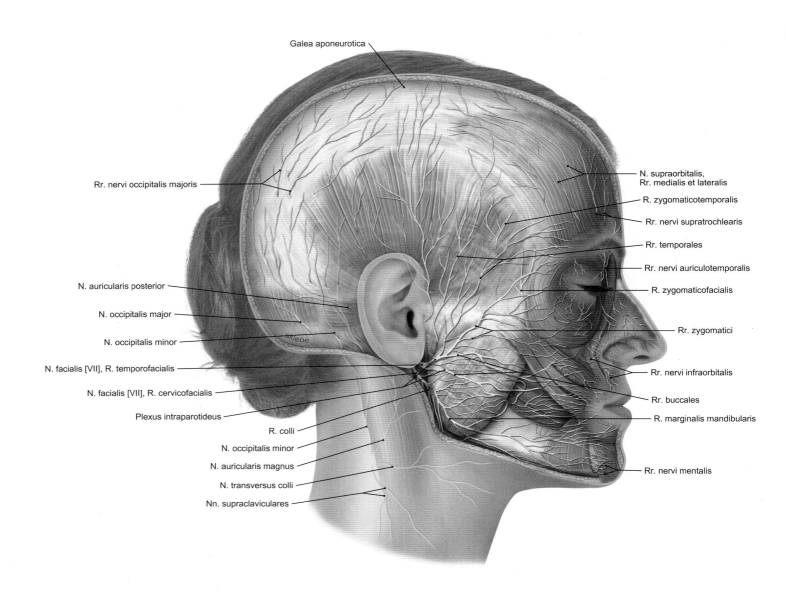

Galea aponeurotica

N. supraorbitalis,
Rr. medialis et lateralis

R. zygomaticotemporalis

Rr. nervi supratrochlearis

Rr. temporales

Rr. nervi auriculotemporalis

R. zygomaticofacialis

Rr. zygomatici

Rr. nervi infraorbitalis

Rr. buccales

R. marginalis mandibularis

Rr. nervi mentalis

Rr. nervi occipitalis majoris

N. auricularis posterior

N. occipitalis major

N. occipitalis minor

N. facialis [VII], R. temporofacialis

N. facialis [VII], R. cervicofacialis

Plexus intraparotideus

R. colli

N. occipitalis minor

N. auricularis magnus

N. transversus colli

Nn. supraclaviculares

Fig. 8.84   Nerves of the head, lateral superficial regions, right side; lateral view. [S700-L238]
Upon removal of the Glandula parotidea, the origin of the terminal branches of the N. facialis, provided by the **Plexus intraparotideus,** become clearly visible. In addition, the origin of the terminal branches of the N. facialis come into view. The **terminal sensory branches of the N. trigeminus [V]** can also be seen.

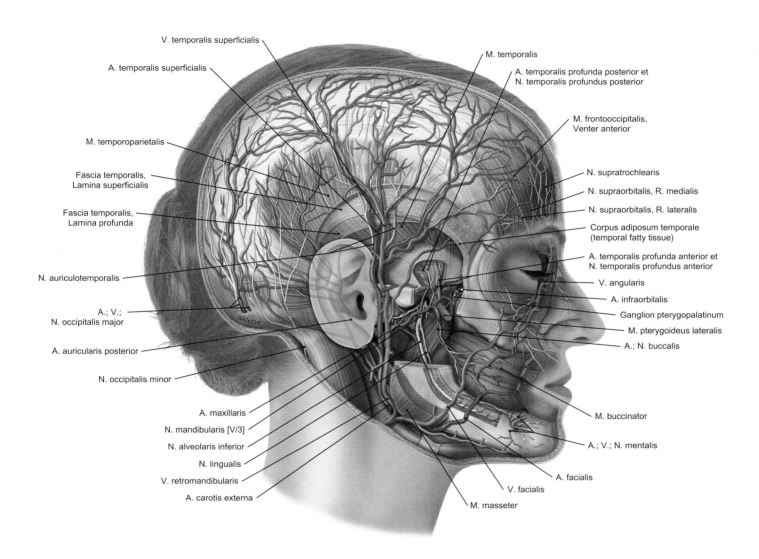

V. temporalis superficialis

A. temporalis superficialis

M. temporoparietalis

Fascia temporalis,
Lamina superficialis

Fascia temporalis,
Lamina profunda

N. auriculotemporalis

A.; V.;
N. occipitalis major

sklebe

A. auricularis posterior

N. occipitalis minor

A. maxillaris

N. mandibularis [V/3]

N. alveolaris inferior

N. lingualis

V. retromandibularis

A. carotis externa

M. masseter

V. facialis

A. facialis

M. temporalis

A. temporalis profunda posterior et
N. temporalis profundus posterior

M. frontooccipitalis,
Venter anterior

N. supratrochlearis

N. supraorbitalis, R. medialis

N. supraorbitalis, R. lateralis

Corpus adiposum temporale
(temporal fatty tissue)

A. temporalis profunda anterior et
N. temporalis profundus anterior

V. angularis

A. infraorbilalis

Ganglion pterygopalatinum

M. pterygoideus lateralis

A.; N. buccalis

M. buccinator

A.; V.; N. mentalis

**Fig. 8.85 Vessels and nerves of the head, lateral deep regions,
right side;** lateral view. [S700-L238]
Upon removal of the Glandula parotidea, the structures of the **Fossa
retromandibularis** in the deep lateral head region become visible. The
A. carotis externa, along with the V. retromandibularis and the N. auriculotemporalis, run in the Fossa retromandibularis, and branches into
the Aa. occipitalis, auricularis posterior, maxillaris, and temporalis superficialis, as well as into smaller branches. The M. temporalis has been
cut free of its fascia at the level of the upper margin of the auricle, its
insertion point at the Proc. coronoideus has been removed and the in-
serting tendon has been fenestrated to demonstrate the Nn. temporalis

profundi and Aa. temporalis profundi as they enter this muscle. In the
section of muscle above it, the M. temporalis is visibly covered by two
layers of fascia with adipose tissue in-between them (temporal fat pad).
In the lower facial region, all muscles of facial expression have been
removed, and the Canalis mandibulae in its entire intraosseous length
from the Foramen mandibulae to the Foramen mentale has been
opened up to visualise the N. and V. alveolaris inferior embedded within
this canal.
On top of the M. buccinator, the sensory N. buccalis, a branch of the
N. mandibularis [V/3], is visible.

Head

8

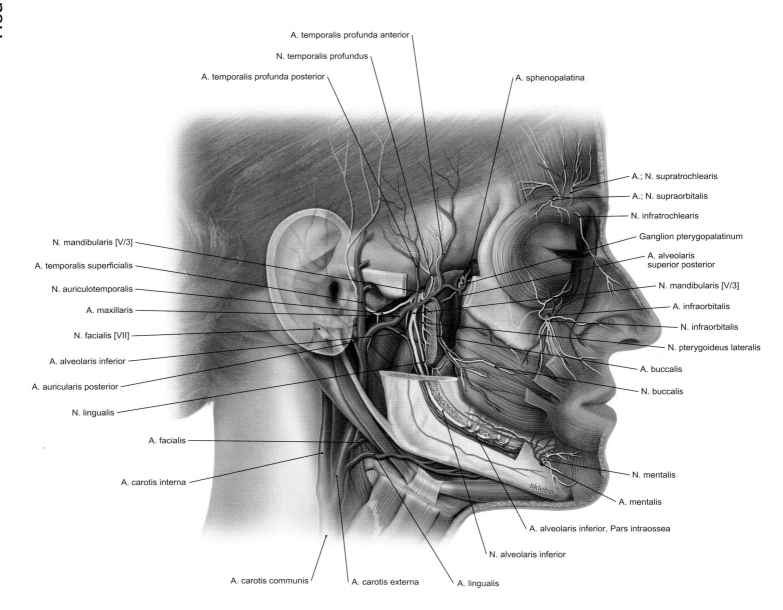

A. temporalis profunda anterior

N. temporalis profundus

A. temporalis profunda posterior

A. sphenopalatina

A.; N. supratrochlearis

A.; N. supraorbitalis

N. infratrochlearis

Ganglion pterygopalatinum

A. alveolaris superior posterior

N. mandibularis [V/3]

A. infraorbitalis

N. infraorbitalis

N. pterygoideus lateralis

A. buccalis

N. buccalis

N. mandibularis [V/3]

A. temporalis superficialis

N. auriculotemporalis

A. maxillaris

N. facialis [VII]

A. alveolaris inferior

A. auricularis posterior

N. lingualis

A. facialis

A. carotis interna

sklebe

N. mentalis

A. mentalis

A. alveolaris inferior, Pars intraossea

N. alveolaris inferior

A. carotis communis

A. carotis externa

A. lingualis

Fig. 8.86 Arteries and nerves of the head, lateral deep regions, right side; lateral view. [S700-L238]

In most cases, the **A. maxillaris** runs beneath the Ramus mandibulae and only rarely laterally thereof (→ Fig. 8.87). The artery continues between the masticatory muscles, providing them with blood, and sends branches to the M. buccinator and the Mandibula, before its terminal branches reach the orbit, nose, maxilla and palate. The **A. carotis externa** and its branches pass through the Fossa retromandibularis. The A. facialis covering the opened Corpus mandibulae has been removed.

Also visible are the **sensory terminal branches of the N. trigeminus [V]**, respectively emerging from its three parts:
• Nn. supraorbitalis and supratrochlearis (from the N. ophthalmicus [V/1])
• N. infraorbitalis (from the N. maxillaris [V/2])
• N. mentalis (from the N. mandibularis [V/3]).

In addition, several branches derived from the N. mandibularis [V/3] are shown, including the N. alveolaris inferior running within the Mandibula.

6%

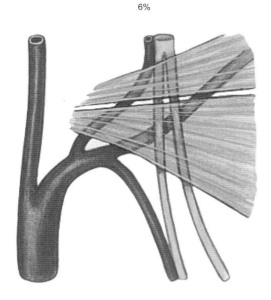

a

3%

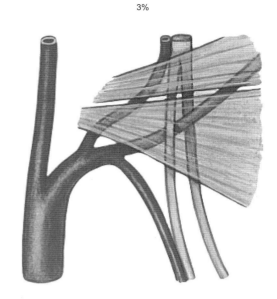

b

4%

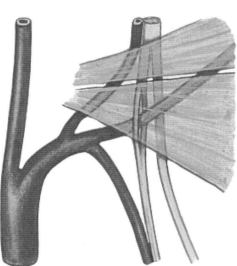

c

18%

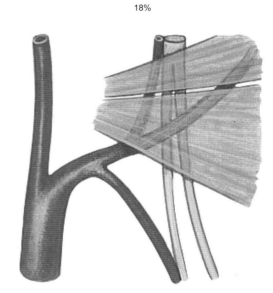

d

Branches of the A. maxillaris	
Segment	**Branches**

Pars retromandibularis	• A. auricularis profunda
	• A. tympanica anterior
	• A. alveolaris inferior
	  – Rr. dentales
	  – Rr. peridentales
	  – R. mentalis
	  – R. mylohyoideus
	• A. meningea media
	• A. pterygomeningea

Pars intermuscularis	• A. masseterica • A. temporalis profunda anterior • A. temporalis profunda posterior • Rr. pterygoidei • A. buccalis

Pars sphenopalatina	• A. alveolaris superior posterior
	  – Rr. dentales
	  – Rr. peridentales
	• A. infraorbitalis
	  – Aa. alveolares superiores anteriores
	    – Rr. dentales
	    – Rr. peridentales
	• A. canalis pterygoidei
	• A. palatina descendens
	• A. sphenopalatina

Fig. 8.87a–d   Variants of the pathways of the A. maxillaris. [S700]
a Pathway of the A. maxillaris medially of the M. pterygoideus lateralis, and medially of the N. lingualis and the N. alveolaris inferior
b Pathway of the A. maxillaris between the N. lingualis and N. alveolaris inferior
c Pathway of the A. maxillaris through a loop of the N. alveolaris inferior
d A. meningea media, branching off distally to the outlet of the A. alveolaris inferior.

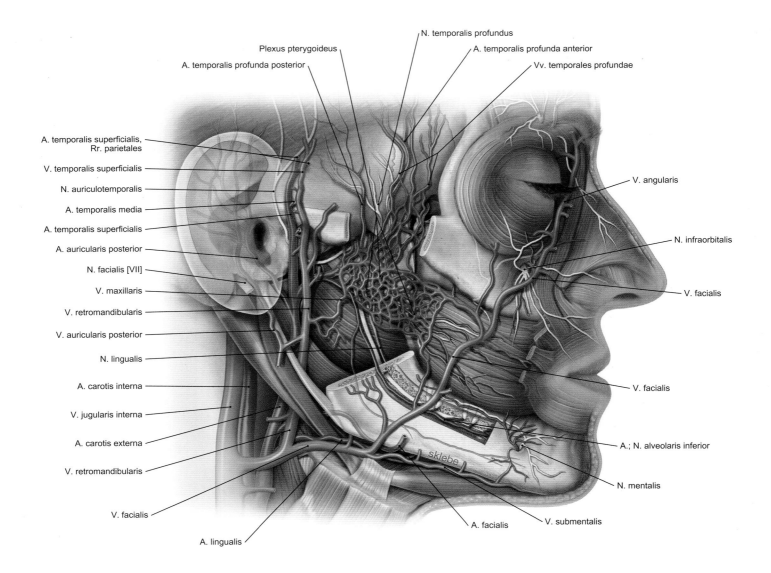

N. temporalis profundus

Plexus pterygoideus

A. temporalis profunda posterior

A. temporalis profunda anterior

Vv. temporales profundae

A. temporalis superficialis, Rr. parietales

V. temporalis superficialis

N. auriculotemporalis

A. temporalis media

A. temporalis superficialis

A. auricularis posterior

N. facialis [VII]

V. maxillaris

V. retromandibularis

V. auricularis posterior

N. lingualis

A. carotis interna

V. jugularis interna

A. carotis externa

V. retromandibularis

V. facialis

A. lingualis

V. angularis

N. infraorbitalis

V. facialis

V. facialis

A.; N. alveolaris inferior

N. mentalis

A. facialis

V. submentalis

sklebe

Fig. 8.88   Vessels and nerves of the head, lateral deeper regions, right side; lateral view. [S700-L238]
Upon removal of the greater part of the Glandula parotis, the lateral deeper head region reveals structures within the **Fossa retromandibularis.**
Beneath the Mm. digastricus and stylohyoideus, the Aa. carotides interna and externa ascend. The **A. carotis externa,** along with the V. retromandibularis and the N. auriculotemporalis, runs in the retromandibular fossa and divides into the Aa. occipitalis, auricularis posterior, maxillaris and temporalis superficialis, as well as numerous small branches. In the lower facial region, all the mimetic muscles on the Mandibula have been removed. The intraosseous Canalis mandibularis from the Foramen mandibulae to the Foramen mentale is opened up to expose the **N. alveolaris inferior** and its eponymous artery. At the Foramen mentale, the nerve becomes the **N. mentalis.**

Below the Orbita, a part of the A. facialis has been removed. The sensory **N. buccalis,** a branch of the N. mandibularis [V/3], is visible on the M. buccinator.
Below the auricle, the truncated **N. facialis [VII]** is still visible. Shortly after exiting the Foramen stylomastoideum, this cranial nerve releases branches to the M. digastricus, Venter posterior (R. digastricus) and to the M. stylohyoideus (R. stylohyoideus) as well as to the mimic muscles of the ear (N. auricularis posterior, not shown).
Venous blood in the region of the masticatory muscles is drained via the **Plexus pterygoideus** and for the most part reaches the V. mandibularis. The Plexus pterygoideus connects with the V. facialis via the V. profunda faciei and has connections to the Sinus cavernosus via the V. ophthalmica inferior.

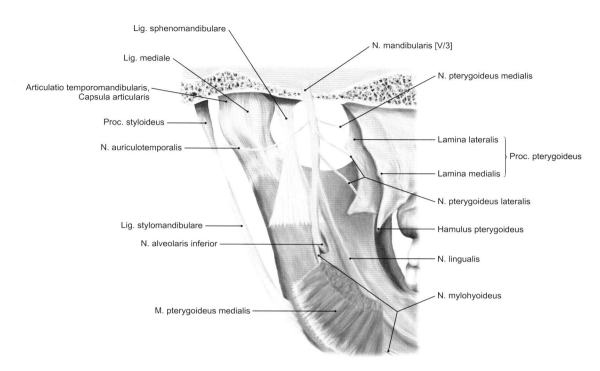

Fig. 8.89 Branches of the N. mandibularis [V/3], right side; medial view. [S700-L284]/[E1043]

The branching of the N. mandibularis [V/3] (→ Fig. 12.141) into the **N. lingualis** and **N. alveolaris inferior** normally occurs between the Lig. sphenomandibulare and the Pars medialis of the M. pterygoideus medialis. The N. alveolaris inferior then runs laterally to enter the Canalis mandibularis lateral of the Lig. sphenomandibulare.

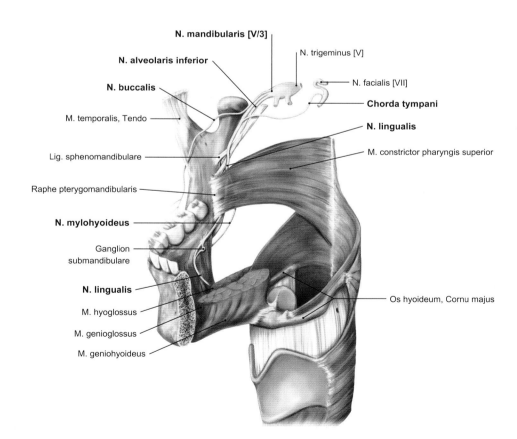

Fig. 8.90 Branches of the N. mandibularis [V/3], right side; frontal view from the left side. [S700-L266]

Branching off the N. mandibularis [V/3], the **N. lingualis** approaches the tongue from the lateral side. Shortly after branching off from the N. mandibularis [V/3], the Chorda tympani joins it, branching off the N. facialis [VII] in the Canalis facialis. The Chorda tympani guides para-sympathetic fibres to the Ganglion submandibulare, as well as the gustatory fibres for the anterior two-thirds of the tongue. The figure displays the 'high branching point' of the N. mandibularis [V/3], which divides into the N. alveolaris inferior and N. lingualis shortly after exiting from the Ganglion trigeminale.

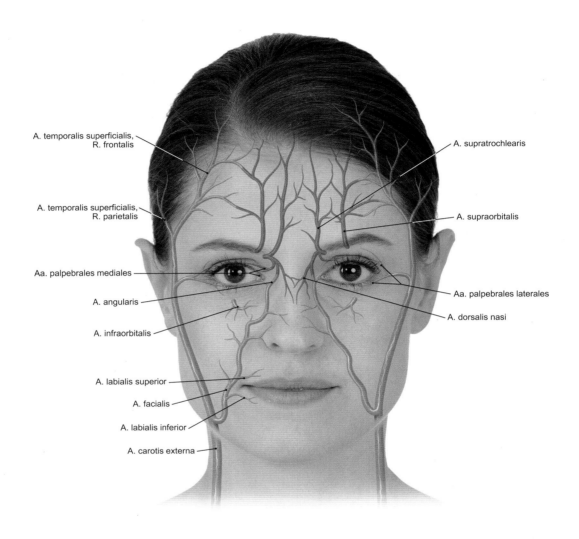

A. temporalis superficialis,
R. frontalis

A. temporalis superficialis,
R. parietalis

Aa. palpebrales mediales

A. angularis

A. infraorbitalis

A. labialis superior

A. facialis

A. labialis inferior

A. carotis externa

A. supratrochlearis

A. supraorbitalis

Aa. palpebrales laterales

A. dorsalis nasi

Fig. 8.91 Branches of the A. carotis externa (red) and the A. carotis interna (brown) in the facial region; anterior view. [S700-J803/L127]

There are several anastomoses between the A. carotis externa and the A. carotis interna.

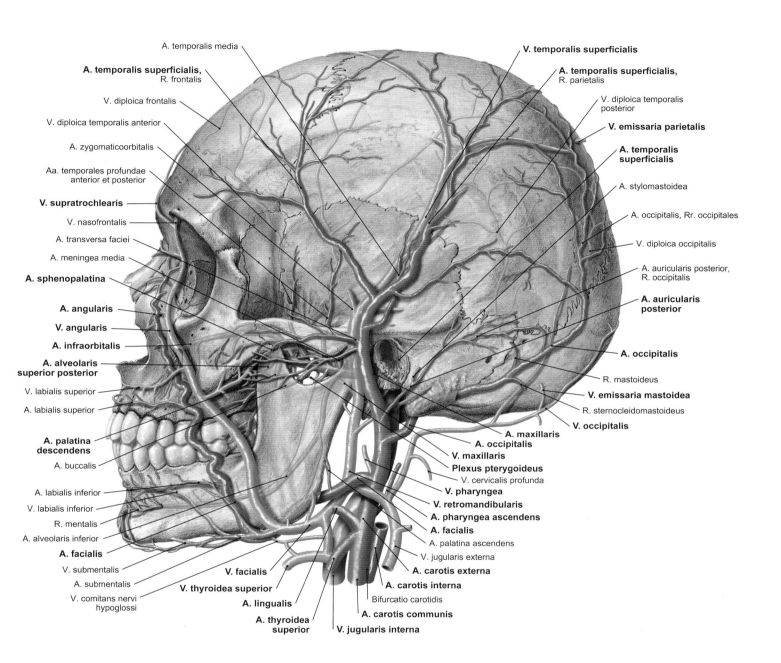

A. temporalis media

A. temporalis superficialis,
R. frontalis

V. diploica frontalis

V. diploica temporalis anterior

A. zygomaticoorbitalis

Aa. temporales profundae
anterior et posterior

V. supratrochlearis

V. nasofrontalis

A. transversa faciei

A. meningea media

A. sphenopalatina

A. angularis

V. angularis

A. infraorbitalis

**A. alveolaris
superior posterior**

V. labialis superior

A. labialis superior

**A. palatina
descendens**

A. buccalis

A. labialis inferior

V. labialis inferior

R. mentalis

A. alveolaris inferior

A. facialis

V. submentalis

A. submentalis

V. comitans nervi
hypoglossi

V. facialis

V. thyroidea superior

A. lingualis

**A. thyroidea
superior**

V. jugularis interna

V. temporalis superficialis

A. temporalis superficialis,
R. parietalis

V. diploica temporalis
posterior

V. emissaria parietalis

**A. temporalis
superficialis**

A. stylomastoidea

A. occipitalis, Rr. occipitales

V. diploica occipitalis

A. auricularis posterior,
R. occipitalis

**A. auricularis
posterior**

A. occipitalis

R. mastoideus

V. emissaria mastoidea

R. sternocleidomastoideus

V. occipitalis

A. maxillaris

A. occipitalis

V. maxillaris

Plexus pterygoideus

V. cervicalis profunda

V. pharyngea

V. retromandibularis

A. pharyngea ascendens

A. facialis

A. palatina ascendens

V. jugularis externa

A. carotis externa

A. carotis interna

Bifurcatio carotidis

A. carotis communis

Fig. 8.92 A. carotis externa, and V. jugularis interna, left side; lateral view. [S700-L127]

The main trunks of these vessels are in close proximity to each other; the pathway of the branches, particularly those of the veins, is highly variable.

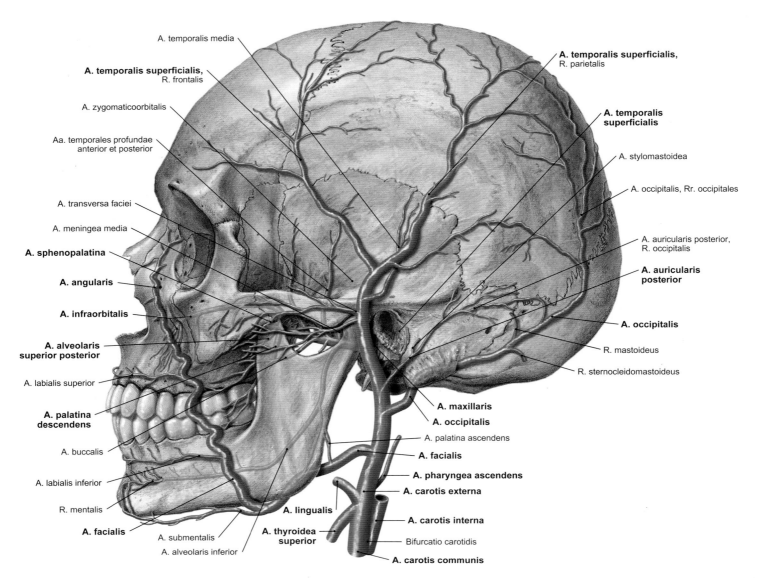

Fig. 8.93   A. carotis externa, external carotid artery, left side; lateral view. [S702]

When branching off the A. carotis communis, the A. carotis externa divides into **branches** corresponding to the order given in the → table.

Branches of the A. carotis externa			

1. A. thyroidea superior
 	
• R. infrahyoideus
• A. laryngea superior
• R. cricothyroideus
• R. sternocleido-mastoideus
• Rr. glandulares
	4. A. facialis
	
	• A. palatina ascendens
	• R. tonsillaris
	• A. submentalis
	• Rr. glandulares
	• A. labialis inferior
	• A. labialis superior
	  – R. septi nasi
	• R. lateralis nasi
	• A. angularis
		7. A. temporalis superficialis
		
		• R. parotideus
		• A. transversa faciei
		• Rr. auriculares anteriores
		• A. zygomaticoorbitalis
		• A. temporalis media
		• R. frontalis
		• R. parietalis
			8. A. maxillaris *(continuation)*
			
			• A. alveolaris superior posterior ⎫
			  – Rr. dentales
			  – Rr. peridentales
			• A. infraorbitalis
			  – Aa. alveolares superiores anteriores
			• A. palatina descendens
			  – A. palatina major
			  – Aa. palatinae minores
			    – R. pharyngeus
			• A. sphenopalatina ⎬ Pars ptery-gopalatina
			  – Aa. nasales posteriores laterales
			  – Rr. septales posteriores
			  – A. nasopalatina ⎭

2. A. pharyngea ascendens
 	
• Rr. tonsillares
• Rr. pharyngeales
• A. tympanica inferior
• A. meningea posterior
	5. A. occipitalis
	
	• R. mastoideus
	• R. auricularis
	• Rr. sternocleidomastoi-dei
	• Rr. occipitales
	• R. meningeus (Var.)
	• R. descendens
		8. A. maxillaris
		
		• A. alveolaris inferior ⎫
		  – R. mentalis ⎬ Pars mandi-bularis
		• A. meningea media ⎪
		  – A. tympanica superior
		  – A. auricularis profunda
		  A. tympanica anterior ⎭
		• A. masseterica ⎫
		• Aa. temporales profundae posterior et anterior ⎬ Pars ptery-goidea
		• Rr. pterygoidei
		  – A. buccalis ⎭
			The terminal branches of the A. maxillaris are the A. infraorbitalis, A. sphenopalatina, A. alveolaris superior posterior and the A. palatina descendens.

3. A. lingualis • Rr. dorsales linguae • A. sublingualis • A. profunda linguae	**6. A. auricularis posterior** • A. stylomastoidea – A. tympanica posterior • R. auricularis • R. occipitalis • R. parotideus		

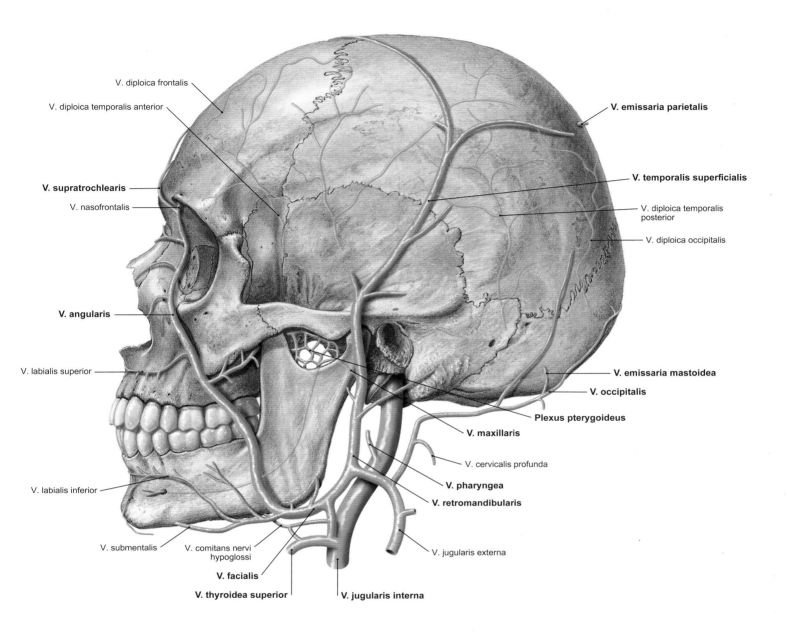

V. diploica frontalis

V. diploica temporalis anterior

V. emissaria parietalis

V. supratrochlearis

V. temporalis superficialis

V. nasofrontalis

V. diploica temporalis posterior

V. diploica occipitalis

V. angularis

V. labialis superior

V. emissaria mastoidea

V. occipitalis

Plexus pterygoideus

V. maxillaris

V. cervicalis profunda

V. pharyngea

V. retromandibularis

V. labialis inferior

V. jugularis externa

V. submentalis

V. comitans nervi hypoglossi

V. facialis

V. thyroidea superior

V. jugularis interna

Fig. 8.94 Internal jugular vein, V. jugularis interna, left side; lateral view. [S700]
The V. jugularis interna begins as an extended continuation of the Sinus sigmoideus at the base of the skull. This vein drains the blood from the skull, brain and facial regions, and areas of the neck. It receives tributaries from the superficial head region via the Vv. facialis, lingualis, pharyngea, occipitalis, thyroidea superior, thyroidea media and via the Vv. emissariae.

Clinical remarks

The pulse of the V. jugularis **(jugular pulse)** provides useful information on the venous blood pressure, and the wave-like characteristic of the jugular pulse reflects the function of the right heart.
An inflammation in the facial area can result in germs (e.g. from squeezing a pimple) reaching the intraorbital veins (V. ophthalmica superior) and the Sinus cavernosus. This is particularly the case for the 'triangle of danger' (→ figure), which extends from the corners of the mouth via the back of the nose to the area between the eyebrows. In the small veins of this facial area, especially those of the V. angularis to the intraorbital veins (V. ophthalmica superior), the direction of blood flow and lack of valves provides a connection to the venous Sinus durae matris and from here to the Sinus cavernosus. Here, the infection can cause a life-threatening thrombophlebitis and thrombosis of the Sinus cavernosus with meningitis and a possible brain abscess.

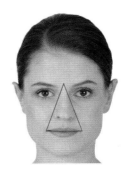

[S700-J803]

N. facialis [VII]

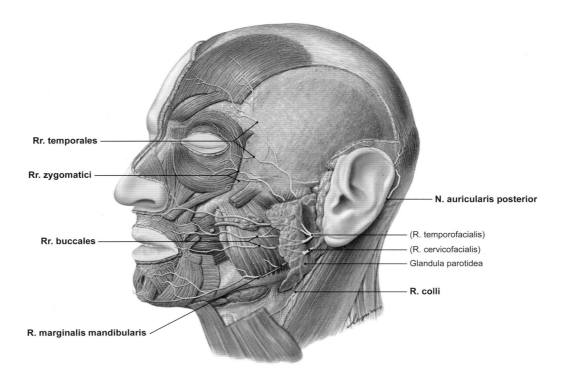

Rr. temporales

Rr. zygomatici

Rr. buccales

R. marginalis mandibularis

N. auricularis posterior

(R. temporofacialis)
(R. cervicofacialis)
Glandula parotidea

R. colli

Fig. 8.95   Terminal branches of the N. facialis [VII] in the face, left side; lateral view. [S700]
Within the Glandula parotidea, the N. facialis [VII] (→ Fig. 12.149) forms the parotid plexus, which for practical clinical reasons is divided into a R. temporofacialis (Pars temporofacialis) and a R. cervicofacialis (Pars cervicofacialis). These two parts generate the terminal branches of the N. facialis [VII]: the Rr. temporales, zygomatici, buccales, marginales mandibulares and colli. The outgoing N. auricularis posterior, also seen as a terminal branch of the N. facialis [VII], runs dorsally behind the auricle.

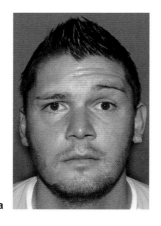

a

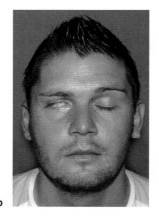

b

Fig. 8.96a and b   Peripheral paralysis of the N. facialis [VII], right side. [S700-T887]
a When the patient is asked to raise his eyebrows, only the left side of the forehead displays wrinkles (loss of function of the M. occipitofrontalis as sign of a peripheral facial paralysis).

b When the patient is asked to shut both eyes, he does not manage it on the side with the damaged N. facialis (lagophthalmos). The eyeball automatically turns upwards when closing the eyes. Because the eyelid on the affected side fails to close properly, the white sclera becomes visible (BELL's palsy).

Clinical remarks

In the case of a **peripheral facial paralysis** (→ Fig. 12.152) the second motor neuron of this nerve pathway is affected; the lesion can be located anywhere between the Nucleus nervi facialis and its peripheral branches. It can in particular be caused by viral infections or a nerve injury during surgery on the Glandula parotidea. The so-called central (supranuclear) damage of the N. facialis [VII] **(central facial paralysis)** is a result of lesions of the first motor neurons. The cause is usually bleeding or infarction in the region of the corticonuclear tract of the inner capsule of the contralateral side. Since the central area for the temporal branches of the N. facialis [VII] receives a contralateral as well as an ipsilateral influx, the muscles of the forehead and the M. orbicularis oculi can still be contracted on both sides in the upper eyelid area. However, on the contralateral side, the muscles innervated by the Rr. zygomatici, buccales, marginales mandibulares and colli are paralysed (so-called lower facial paralysis).

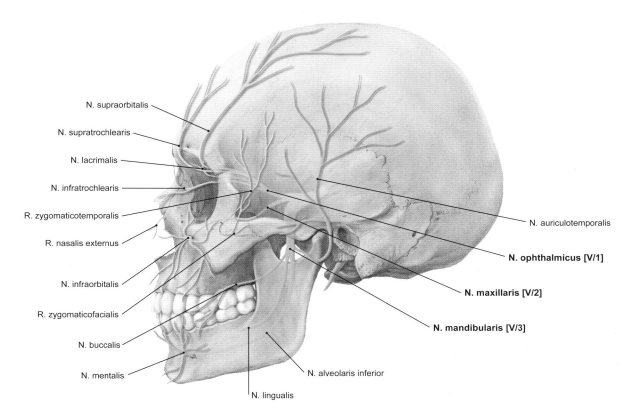

Fig. 8.97 Branches of the N. trigeminus [V], left side; lateral view. [S700-L284]

Upon exiting the cranium, the three major branches of the N. trigeminus [V] – N. ophthalmicus [V/1], N. maxillaris [V/2], and N. mandibularis [V/3] – subdivide into smaller branches in a specific topographical order. Visible branches of the **N. ophthalmicus [V/1]** are the Nn. supraorbitalis, supratrochlearis, lacrimalis, infratrochlearis and the R. nasalis exter-

nus. Branches of the N. infraorbitalis and the N. zygomaticus (with its Rr. zygomaticotemporalis and zygomaticofacialis) can here be seen emerging from the **N. maxillaris [V/2].** The Nn. buccalis, lingualis, alveolaris inferior and auriculotemporalis branch off from the **N. mandibularis [V/3].** After leaving the Canalis mandibularis, the terminal branch of the N. alveolaris inferior is the N. mentalis.

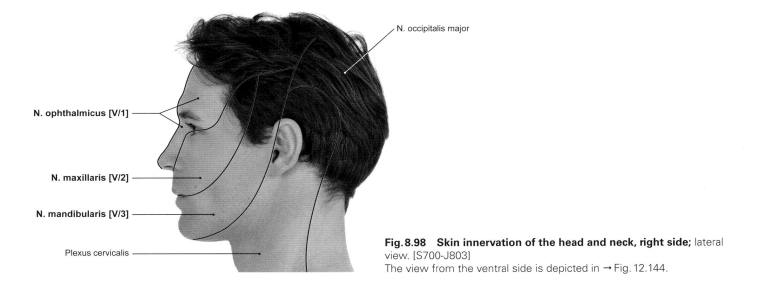

Fig. 8.98 Skin innervation of the head and neck, right side; lateral view. [S700-J803]

The view from the ventral side is depicted in → Fig. 12.144.

Clinical remarks

In the course of a clinical examination of the cranial nerves, the N. trigeminus [V] is checked by exerting manual pressure on its three exit points **(trigeminal pressure points),** which should normally not be painful: it is checked at the Foramen supraorbitale/Incisura supraorbitalis, the Foramen infraorbitale and the Foramen mentale.

Trigeminal neuralgia (tic douloureux) is a complex and particularly painful dysfunction of the sensory trigeminal root. Typically located in the innervation areas of the N. mandibularis [V/3] and the N. maxillaris [V/2], the facial pain can be intense and occur quite suddenly. It can often be triggered by touching the corresponding area of the face.

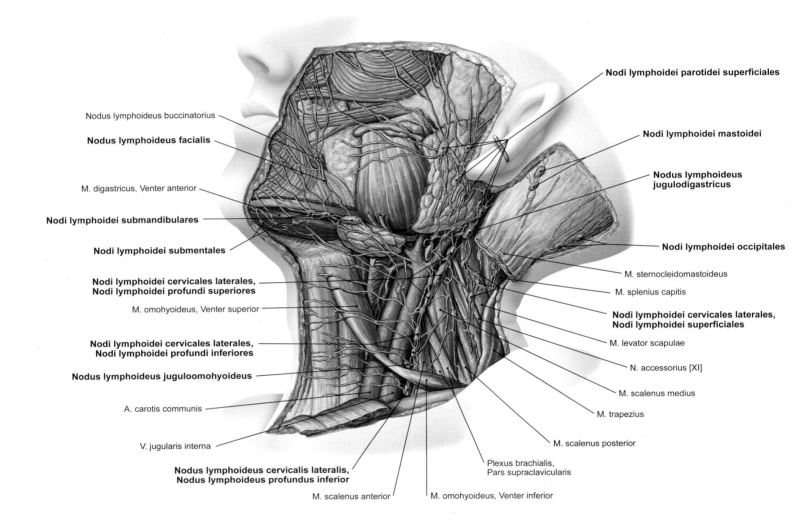

Nodi lymphoidei parotidei superficiales

Nodus lymphoideus buccinatorius

Nodus lymphoideus facialis

Nodi lymphoidei mastoidei

M. digastricus, Venter anterior

Nodus lymphoideus jugulodigastricus

Nodi lymphoidei submandibulares

Nodi lymphoidei submentales

Nodi lymphoidei occipitales

Nodi lymphoidei cervicales laterales, Nodi lymphoidei profundi superiores

M. sternocleidomastoideus

M. splenius capitis

M. omohyoideus, Venter superior

Nodi lymphoidei cervicales laterales, Nodi lymphoidei superficiales

M. levator scapulae

Nodi lymphoidei cervicales laterales, Nodi lymphoidei profundi inferiores

N. accessorius [XI]

Nodus lymphoideus juguloomohyoideus

M. scalenus medius

A. carotis communis

M. trapezius

V. jugularis interna

M. scalenus posterior

Nodus lymphoideus cervicalis lateralis, Nodus lymphoideus profundus inferior

Plexus brachialis, Pars supraclavicularis

M. scalenus anterior

M. omohyoideus, Venter inferior

Fig. 8.99 Superficial lymph vessels, Vasa lymphatica superficialia, and lymph nodes, Nodi lymphoidei, of the head and neck of a child, left side; lateral view. [S700]

The lymph of the face, scalp and occiput region is drained **regionally** to the Nodi lymphoidei submentales, submandibulares, parotidei, mastoidei and occipitales. From here, the lymphatic drainage continues into the superficial (**Nodi lymphoidei cervicales laterales superficiales**) and the deep (**Nodi lymphoidei cervicales laterales profundi superiores and inferiores,** → Fig. 11.93) lateral cervical lymph nodes.

The Nodus lymphoideus jugulodigastricus is an important deep cervical lymph node between the anterior margin of the M. sternocleidomastoideus and the mandibular angle at the lower edge of the Glandula parotidea.

The Nodi lymphoidei parotidei are divided into the superficial (**Nodi lymphoidei parotidei superficiales**) and deep lymph nodes (**Nodi lymphoidei parotidei profundi**). The latter include the Nodi lymphoidei preauriculares, infraauriculares and intraglandulares. In addition, there are single facial lymph nodes (**Nodi lymphoidei faciales**) (Nodi lymphoidei buccinatorius, nasolabialis, malaris, mandibularis) and lymph nodes of the tongue (Nodi lymphoidei linguales).

Lymph nodes of the head (Nodi lymphoidei capitis)
• Nodi lymphoidei occipitales
• Nodi lymphoidei mastoidei
• Nodi lymphoidei parotidei superficiales
• Nodi lymphoidei parotidei profundi
– Nodi lymphoidei preauriculares
– Nodi lymphoidei infraauriculares
– Nodi lymphoidei intraglandulares
• Nodi lymphoidei faciales
– Nodus lymphoideus buccinatorius
– Nodus lymphoideus nasolabialis
– Nodus lymphoideus malaris
– Nodus lymphoideus mandibularis
• Nodi lymphoidei submentales
• Nodi lymphoidei submandibulares
• Nodi lymphoidei linguales

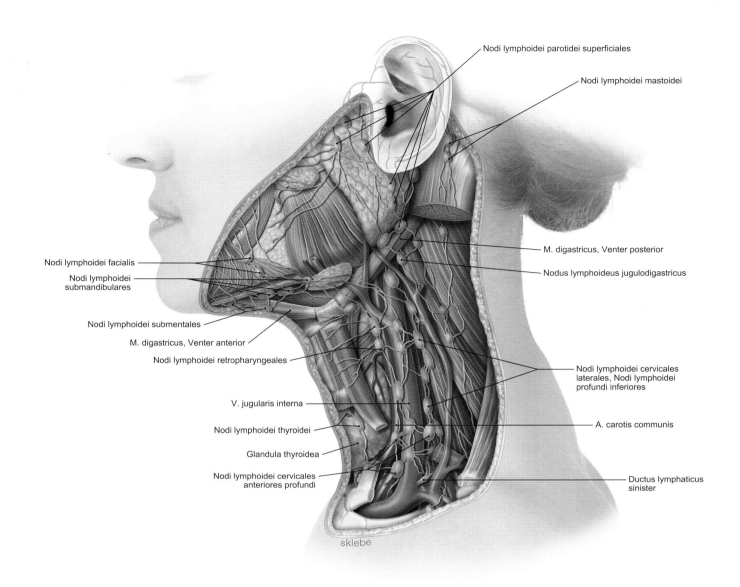

Nodi lymphoidei parotidei superficiales

Nodi lymphoidei mastoidei

M. digastricus, Venter posterior

Nodus lymphoideus jugulodigastricus

Nodi lymphoidei facialis

Nodi lymphoidei submandibulares

Nodi lymphoidei submentales

M. digastricus, Venter anterior

Nodi lymphoidei retropharyngeales

Nodi lymphoidei cervicales laterales, Nodi lymphoidei profundi inferiores

V. jugularis interna

A. carotis communis

Nodi lymphoidei thyroidei

Glandula thyroidea

Nodi lymphoidei cervicales anteriores profundi

Ductus lymphaticus sinister

sklebe

Fig. 8.100 Superficial lymph vessels, Vasa lymphatica superficialia, and lymph nodes, Nodi lymphoidei of the face, and deep cervical lymph nodes, Nodi lymphoidei cervicales profundi, right side; lateral view. [S700-L238]

As in children (→ Fig. 8.99), the lymph fluids in the adult are drained from the face, scalp and occipital region to the Nodi lymphoidei submentales, submandibulares, parotidei, mastoidei and occipitales.

The anterior cervical lymph nodes (Nodi lymphoidei cervicales anteriores) as well as the lateral cervical lymph nodes (Nodi lymphoidei cervicales laterales) are divided into superficial and deep lymph nodes.

The **anterior** deep cervical lymph nodes (Nodi lymphoidei cervicales anteriores profundi) include the Nodi lymphoidei infrahyoidei with the

Nodi lymphoidei prelaryngei, the Nodi lymphoidei thyroidei, Nodi lymphoidei pretracheales, Nodi lymphoidei paratracheales and Nodi lymphoidei retropharyngeales.

The **lateral** deep cervical lymph nodes (Nodi lymphoidei cervicales laterales profundi) include a **superior group** (Nodi lymphoidei profundi superiores) consisting of the Nodus lymphoideus jugulodigastricus, Nodus lymphoideus lateralis and Nodus lymphoideus anterior, as well as an **inferior group** consisting of the Nodus lymphoideus juguloomohyoideus, Nodus lymphoideus lateralis and Nodi lymphoidei anteriores. There are also Nodi lymphoidei supraclaviculares and Nodi lymphoidei accessorii (along the N. accessorius [XI]) with Nodi lymphoidei retropharyngeales.

Nasal skeleton

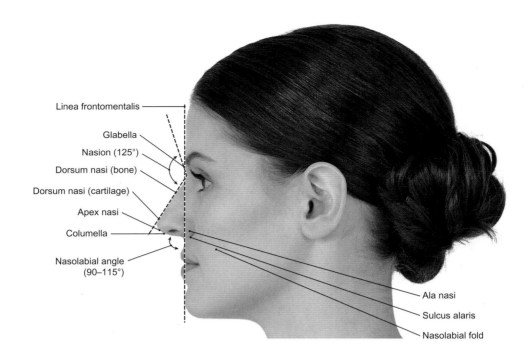

Linea frontomentalis

Glabella

Nasion (125°)

Dorsum nasi (bone)

Dorsum nasi (cartilage)

Apex nasi

Columella

Nasolabial angle
(90–115°)

Ala nasi

Sulcus alaris

Nasolabial fold

Fig. 8.101 External nose with aesthetic nasolabial angles and orientation points; view from the left side. [S700-J803]
The external nose has a great impact on the shape of the face. A distinction is made between:
- Base (or root) of nose (Radix nasi) above the philtrum (Sulcus nasolabialis)

- Dorsum of nose (Dorsum nasi)
- Left and right alae of nose (Alae nasi dextra and sinistra)
- Tip of nose (Apex nasi)
- Membranous part of the nasal septum (Pars membranacea septi nasi, Columella, Pars mobilis septi)
- Nostril (Naris, paired).

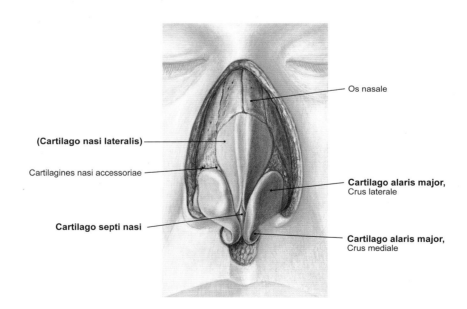

Os nasale

(Cartilago nasi lateralis)

Cartilagines nasi accessoriae

Cartilago alaris major,
Crus laterale

Cartilago septi nasi

Cartilago alaris major,
Crus mediale

Fig. 8.102 Nasal skeleton; frontal view. [S700]
The nasal skeleton consists of a bony and a cartilaginous portion. The cartilaginous portion is attached to the Apertura piriformis between the Os nasale and maxilla via the associated connective tissue. The individual elements consist of hyaline cartilage and are linked via connective tissue. The roof is formed by the **upper lateral or triangular cartilage**

(Cartilago nasi lateralis, Cartilago triangularis), and the ala is formed by **cartilage** from the **tip of the nose or major alar cartilage** (Cartilago alaris major) with a Crus laterale and a Crus mediale. On each side there are often two smaller **alar cartilages** (Cartilagines alares minores). Below and centrally, the nasal skeleton is supported by the cartilaginous portion of the nasal septum (Cartilago septi nasi).

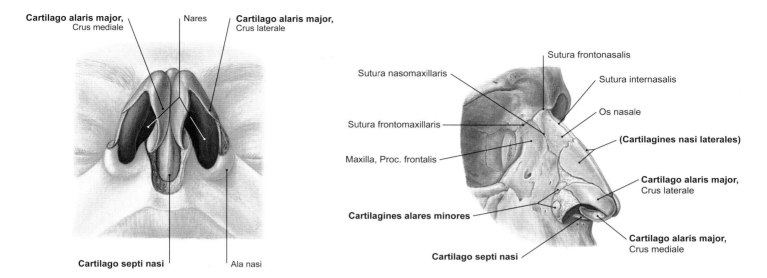

Fig. 8.103   Nasal cartilages, Cartilagines nasi; view from below. [S700]
The view from below shows the nasal orifices (Nares) which are delineated by the crura (Crus mediale and Crus laterale) of the greater alar cartilage (Cartilago alaris major). At the bottom in the centre, the bony nasal septum (Cartilago septi nasi) can be seen.

Fig. 8.104   Nasal skeleton; frontal view from the right. [S700]
The cartilaginous nasal skeleton is fixed at the Apertura piriformis with connective tissue. The Cartilagines nasi laterales, alares majores, alares minores and the Cartilago septi nasi can be seen. Connective tissue is found in cartilage-free areas.

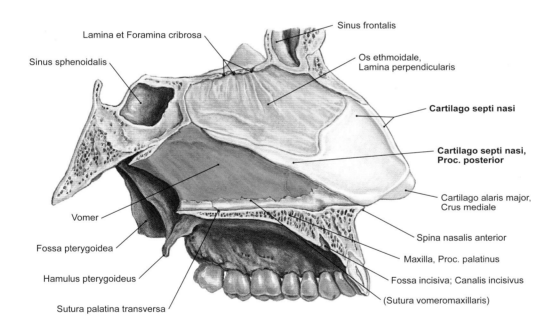

Fig. 8.105   Nasal septum, Septum nasi; view from the right side; for colour chart, see p. XIII. [S700]
The nasal septum is formed at the front by the Cartilago septi nasi which extends with a long Proc. posterior between the bony nasal septum

(above), consisting of the Lamina perpendicularis of the Os ethmoidale and the vomer (below).

Clinical remarks

Frequently used clinical terms are: **columella** (Pars anterior of the nasal septum between the tip of the nose and the philtrum), **keystone area** (where the Os nasale overlaps the lateral cartilages), **soft triangle** (skin area at the upper rim of the nostril, close to the point where the Crus mediale bends to become the Crus laterale; this **cartilage-free area** is composed exclusively of a skin duplication), **supratip area** (on the bridge of the nose just above the tip), and

weak triangle (similar to the supratip area, as the bridge of the nose is exclusively formed here by the septum). These areas are considered to be potential danger points for plastic surgery.
In the case of a **nasal septal haematoma** (e.g. with a nasal fracture), immediate relief is required in the form of a puncture and, if necessary, with an incision and nasal tamponade, otherwise the septum cartilage is at risk of being destroyed.

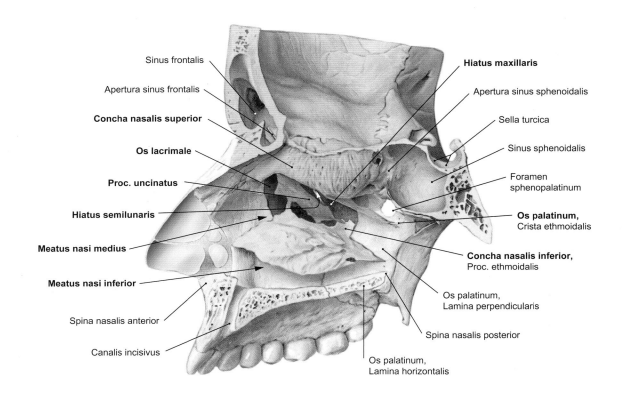

Sinus frontalis

Apertura sinus frontalis

Concha nasalis superior

Os lacrimale

Proc. uncinatus

Hiatus semilunaris

Meatus nasi medius

Meatus nasi inferior

Spina nasalis anterior

Canalis incisivus

Hiatus maxillaris

Apertura sinus sphenoidalis

Sella turcica

Sinus sphenoidalis

Foramen
sphenopalatinum

Os palatinum,
Crista ethmoidalis

Concha nasalis inferior,
Proc. ethmoidalis

Os palatinum,
Lamina perpendicularis

Spina nasalis posterior

Os palatinum,
Lamina horizontalis

Fig. 8.106 Bony structures of the lateral wall of the nose, Cavitas nasi, without middle nasal concha; view from the left side; for colour chart, see p. XIII. [S700]
The lateral wall of the nasal cavity has a complex and variable structure. The most predominant topography is shown. The bony elements are:
• Frontal:
  – Os nasale
  – Facies nasalis maxillae
  – Os lacrimale.

• In the middle:
  – Corpus maxillae with Hiatus maxillaris
  – Os ethmoidale with Proc. uncinatus (a thin lamellar bone), the bony wall to the anterior and posterior ethmoidal cells (Cellulae ethmoidales anteriores and posteriores) and the superior and middle nasal conchae (Conchae nasales superior and media). The middle nasal concha is not shown (→ Fig. 8.107).
  – Concha nasalis inferior.
• Posterior:
  – Lamina perpendicularis of the Os palatinum
  – Lamina medialis of the Proc. pterygoideus ossis sphenoidalis.

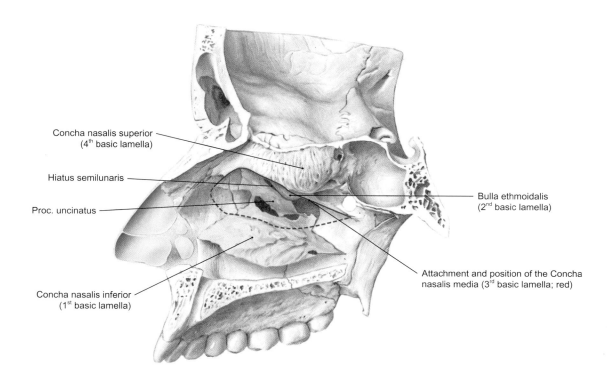

Concha nasalis superior
(4ᵗʰ basic lamella)

Hiatus semilunaris

Proc. uncinatus

Concha nasalis inferior
(1ˢᵗ basic lamella)

Bulla ethmoidalis
(2ⁿᵈ basic lamella)

Attachment and position of the Concha
nasalis media (3ʳᵈ basic lamella; red)

Fig. 8.107 Bony structures of the lateral wall of the nose, Cavitas nasi, without middle nasal concha; view from the left side. [S700]
The relatively complex anatomy of the Hiatus semilunaris and the area surrounding it below the middle nasal concha is known as the **osteomeatal complex.** Hereby, access to the Sinus maxillaris (via the Hiatus maxillaris) is usually only partially closed by three structures:

- **Proc. uncinatus** – a thin lamellar bone of the Os ethmoidale, which partially closes the Hiatus maxillaris. It forms part of the medial wall of the Sinus maxillaris. At the superior edge of the Proc. uncinatus, a crescent-shaped smooth cleft called the **Hiatus semilunaris** re-

mains. Below the Proc. uncinatus there are usually also some openings that are normally covered by the nasal mucosa, but may also remain as openings. They are referred to as the anterior and posterior fontanelles.

- In front of and below the Proc. uncinatus it is bordered by the Os lacrimale and the Concha nasalis inferior.
- From behind and above, a frequently enlarged or pronounced anterior ethmoidal cell protrudes into and in front of the Hiatus maxillaris, which is called the **Bulla ethmoidalis.** It confines the Hiatus semilunaris from behind and above.

Clinical remarks

From a surgical perspective, a distinction is made between the four **basic lamellae (BL)** of the lateral nasal wall. This relates to the bony lamellae, which are found within the Os ethmoidale as embryological residues: first BL – Proc. uncinatus; second BL – Bulla ethmoidalis; third BL – Concha nasalis media; fourth BL – Concha nasalis superior.

The structures of the **osteomeatal complex** are extraordinarily important in clinical terms, not only with regard to ventilation, but also for the drainage of the paranasal sinuses. In **endonasal sinus surgery,** this is the central surgical access route, e.g. in the treatment of chronic sinusitis or polyposis nasi.

Nasal cavity

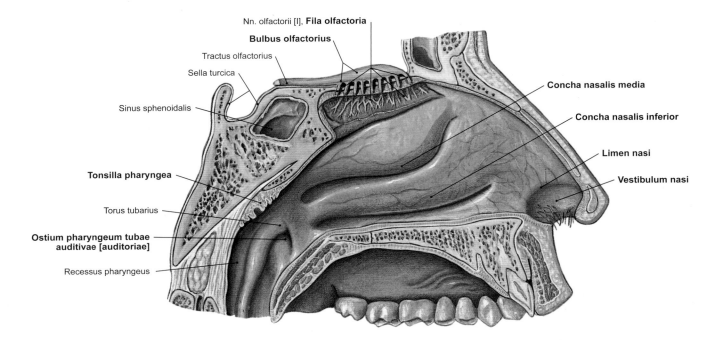

Nn. olfactorii [I], **Fila olfactoria**

Bulbus olfactorius

Tractus olfactorius

Sella turcica

Sinus sphenoidalis

Tonsilla pharyngea

Torus tubarius

Ostium pharyngeum tubae auditivae [auditoriae]

Recessus pharyngeus

Concha nasalis media

Concha nasalis inferior

Limen nasi

Vestibulum nasi

Fig. 8.108 Lateral wall of the nasal cavity, Cavitas nasi, left side; view from the right side. [S700]

The lateral nasal wall is largely occupied by the lower nasal concha (**Concha nasalis inferior**) and the middle nasal concha (**Concha nasalis media**). The upper nasal concha (Concha nasalis superior) is small. It is related to the olfactory epithelium of the roof of the nose. Here, the Fila olfactoria of the Bulbus olfactorius pass through the Lamina cribrosa and

extend into the neighbouring mucosa, including the mucosa of the upper nasal concha.

The **Vestibulum nasi** is lined by keratinising stratified squamous epithelium, which transitions at the Limen nasi via nonkeratinised stratified squamous epithelium into ciliated pseudostratified columnar epithelium. The Concha nasalis inferior projects to the Ostium pharyngeum of the Tuba auditiva. Above it, the Tonsilla pharyngea sits at the roof of the pharynx.

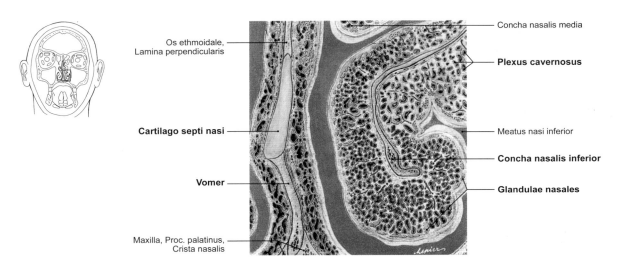

Os ethmoidale, Lamina perpendicularis

Cartilago septi nasi

Vomer

Maxilla, Proc. palatinus, Crista nasalis

Concha nasalis media

Plexus cavernosus

Meatus nasi inferior

Concha nasalis inferior

Glandulae nasales

Fig. 8.109 Inferior nasal concha, Concha nasalis inferior, left side; frontal section at the level of the initial part of the Proc. posterior of the Cartilago septi nasi; frontal view. [S700]

This section demonstrates the thin bony skeleton of the Concha nasalis inferior, which is covered by a vascular plexus (Plexus cavernosus) com-

posed of a network of specialised arteries and veins. Located on the surface of the nasal concha is the ciliated epithelium with embedded serous glands (Glandulae nasales).

Clinical remarks

A characteristic feature of the nasal mucosa is a dense subepithelial plexus of venous sinusoids. Depending on the level of swelling, approx. 35 % of the nasal mucosa is composed of vascular plexuses. The highest density of venous sinusoids is found in the lower and middle nasal conchae, as well as in the KIESSELBACH's area of the nasal septum.

In approx. 80 % of people, a so-called **nasal cycle** can be detected. The nasal mucosa of both nasal passages swells and subsides for two to seven hours with alternating airway resistance during nasal breathing in a ratio of 1:3, but without changing overall resistance.

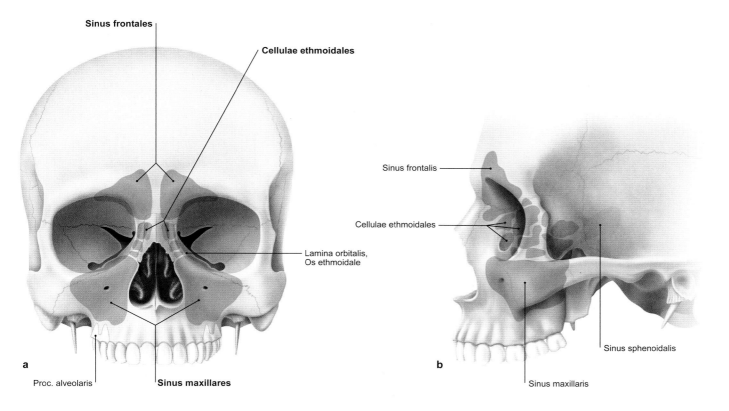

a

Sinus frontales

Cellulae ethmoidales

Lamina orbitalis,
Os ethmoidale

Proc. alveolaris

Sinus maxillares

b

Sinus frontalis

Cellulae ethmoidales

Sinus sphenoidalis

Sinus maxillaris

Fig. 8.110a and b   Projection of the sinuses onto the skull. [S700-L275]
a Frontal view.
b Lateral view.

As the formation of the sinuses is extremely variable, individual cavities can be missing.

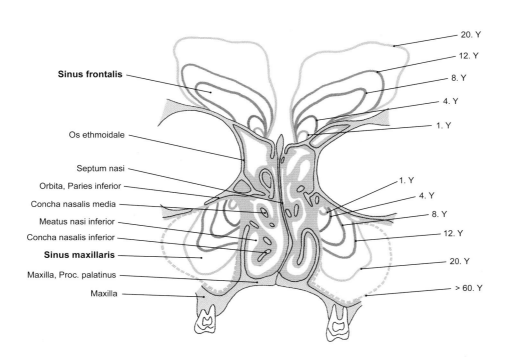

Sinus frontalis

Os ethmoidale

Septum nasi

Orbita, Paries inferior

Concha nasalis media

Meatus nasi inferior

Concha nasalis inferior

Sinus maxillaris

Maxilla, Proc. palatinus

Maxilla

20. Y

12. Y

8. Y

4. Y

1. Y

1. Y

4. Y

8. Y

12. Y

20. Y

> 60. Y

Fig. 8.111   Development of the maxillary and frontal sinuses.
[S700-L238] Y: year of life.

The Sinus frontalis forms and reaches the rim of the Orbita by approx. the age of five.

Orifices of the sinuses

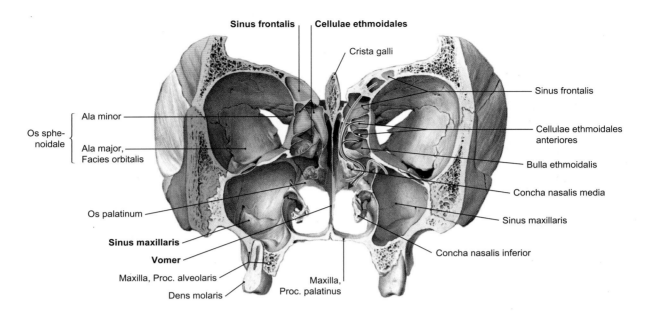

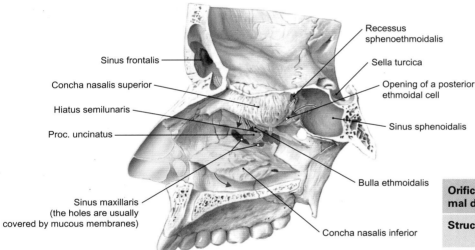

Fig. 8.112 Bony topography (right calvaria) and orifices of the paranasal sinuses (left calvaria); frontal section through the viscerocranium; for colour chart, see p. XIII. [S700]
The Sinus frontalis (green), the anterior ethmoidal cells (Cellulae ethmoidales anteriores, purple) and the Sinus maxillaris (blue) open via the

Hiatus semilunaris into the middle nasal passage. On the left side of the skull, the close relationship between the root of the tooth and the Sinus maxillaris can be seen in the section here made through the maxilla.

Fig. 8.113 Orifices of the paranasal sinuses and the Ductus nasolacrimalis in the lateral nasal wall. View from the left side. [S700]
Arrows: brown = Ductus nasolacrimalis; green = Sinus frontalis; purple = anterior ethmoidal cells; blue = Sinus maxillaris; orange = posterior ethmoidal cells; red = Sinus sphenoidalis.
The Sinus sphenoidalis has a close topographical relationship to the Sella turcica, in which the pituitary gland (Glandula pituitaria) is located. The Ductus nasolacrimalis opens into the lower nasal passage via the Plica lacrimalis (HASNER's valve). The middle nasal concha is not shown. As a result, the Hiatus semilunaris is visible. The Bulla ethmoidalis lies above it and the Proc. uncinatus lies below it. Behind the upper nasal concha, the Recessus sphenoethmoidalis is located at the orifice of the Sinus sphenoidalis (Apertura sinus sphenoidalis, red arrow).

Orifice points of the paranasal sinuses and the nasolacrimal ducts			
Structure	**Lower nasal passage**	**Middle nasal passage**	**Upper nasal passage**
Ductus nasofrontalis	x		
Sinus frontalis		x	
Cellulae ethmoidales anteriores		x	
Cellulae ethmoidales posteriores			x
Sinus maxillaris		x	
Sinus sphenoidalis			x

Clinical remarks

The **Sinus sphenoidalis** may extend into large parts of the sphenoidal bone. In the case of surgical interventions, extensive pneumatisation of the Sinus sphenoidalis can endanger the A. carotis interna

(Tuberculum arteriae carotidis internae) and the N. opticus [II] because of their close relationship to the lateral sinus wall.

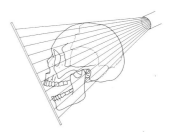

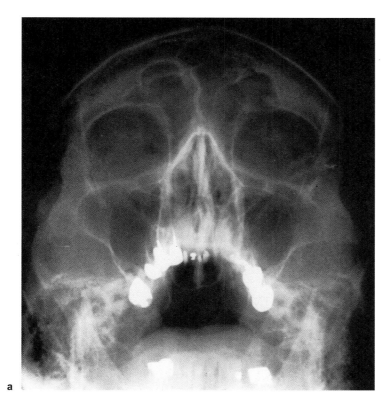

a

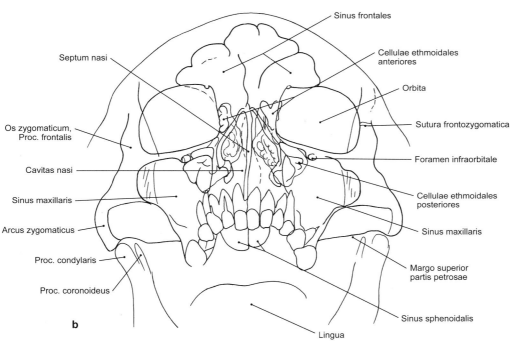

Sinus frontales

Septum nasi

Cellulae ethmoidales anteriores

Orbita

Os zygomaticum, Proc. frontalis

Sutura frontozygomatica

Cavitas nasi

Foramen infraorbitale

Sinus maxillaris

Cellulae ethmoidales posteriores

Arcus zygomaticus

Sinus maxillaris

Proc. condylaris

Margo superior partis petrosae

Proc. coronoideus

Sinus sphenoidalis

b

Lingua

Fig. 8.114a and b   Paranasal sinuses, Sinus paranasales; X-ray image of the skull with opened mouth in postero-anterior (PA) projection. [S700-T895]

Clinical remarks

Conventional X-ray images are useful for rapid orientation on the sinus system, but are increasingly rarely carried out. They have been replaced by computed tomography (CT) and magnetic resonance imaging (MRI) to assess the need for surgical intervention.
Sinusitis is a common disease. In children, it is most often due to an inflammation of the ethmoidal cells, while in adults the Sinus maxillaris is most frequently affected. Inflammation of the ethmoidal cells can penetrate the thin Lamina orbitalis (papyracea) of the Os ethmoidale into the Orbita, or can spread in the posterior region of the ethmoidal cells or the Sinus maxillaris into the Canalis opticus and damage the optic nerve.

Topography of the sinuses

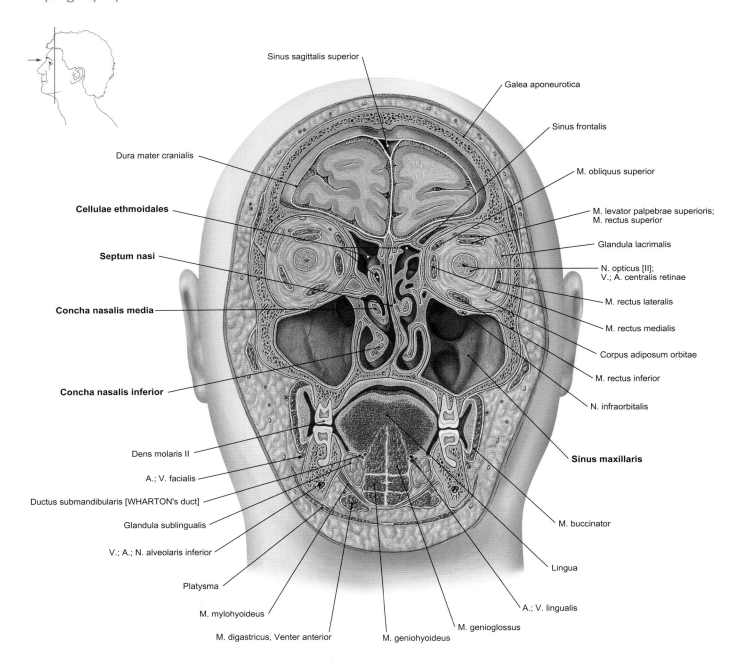

Sinus sagittalis superior

Galea aponeurotica

Sinus frontalis

Dura mater cranialis

M. obliquus superior

M. levator palpebrae superioris;
M. rectus superior

Cellulae ethmoidales

Glandula lacrimalis

Septum nasi

N. opticus [II];
V.; A. centralis retinae

Concha nasalis media

M. rectus lateralis

M. rectus medialis

Corpus adiposum orbitae

Concha nasalis inferior

M. rectus inferior

N. infraorbitalis

Dens molaris II

Sinus maxillaris

A.; V. facialis

Ductus submandibularis [WHARTON's duct]

Glandula sublingualis

M. buccinator

V.; A.; N. alveolaris inferior

Platysma

Lingua

M. mylohyoideus

A.; V. lingualis

M. digastricus, Venter anterior

M. geniohyoideus

M. genioglossus

Fig. 8.115 Frontal section through the head at the level of the second upper molar; frontal view. [S700-L238]
This section emphasises the individual bilateral differences in the formation of the paranasal sinuses. The Sinus maxillares are formed differently on both sides and have variable chambers. The nasal septum is shifted to the left (nasal septum deviation). As a result, the lower and middle nasal conchae are developed more strongly on the right than on the left. The ethmoidal cells are also formed differently on the right and left. On the left side, in the supraorbital region, parts of the Sinus frontalis are visible.

Clinical remarks

With a **nasal septum deviation,** nasal breathing may be so severely restricted that headaches, hyposmia or even anosmia may occur. Formation of the paranasal sinuses is extremely variable. There are interindividual and lateral differences, including a complete lack of individual sinuses **(aplasia).**

However, individual sinuses can reach extreme sizes. If the Sinus frontalis extends in an occipital direction well beyond the orbital roof **(Recesses supraorbitalis),** the clinician refers to it as a dangerous frontal sinus. An inflammatory process of the frontal sinus can transcend the thin bony barrier and spread into the anterior cranial fossa, leading to meningitis, epidural abscesses or even brain abscesses.

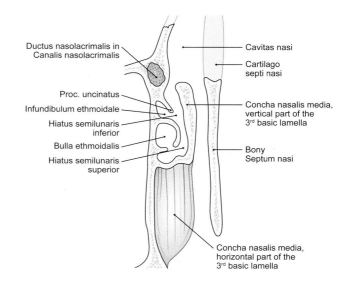

Fig. 8.116 Topography of the sinuses. Horizontal section through the nasal septum and osteomeatal complex of the left side of the nose just above the Concha nasalis inferior. [S700-L126]
The Ductus nasolacrimalis has close topographical relationships to the Sinus maxillaris laterally, and to the sinuses medially. The Proc. uncinatus, Hiatus semilunaris and Bulla ethmoidalis are located (from front to back) just behind the anterior tip of the middle turbinate.

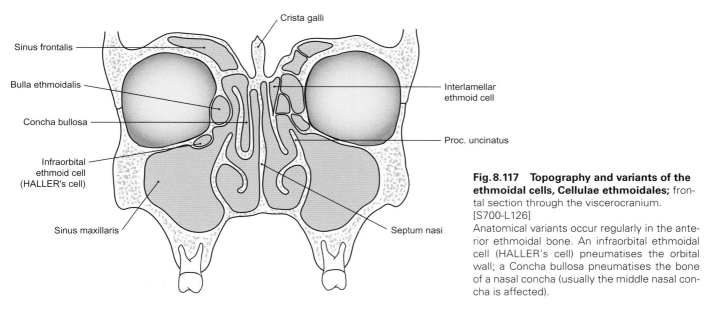

Fig. 8.117 Topography and variants of the ethmoidal cells, Cellulae ethmoidales; frontal section through the viscerocranium. [S700-L126]
Anatomical variants occur regularly in the anterior ethmoidal bone. An infraorbital ethmoidal cell (HALLER's cell) pneumatises the orbital wall; a Concha bullosa pneumatises the bone of a nasal concha (usually the middle nasal concha is affected).

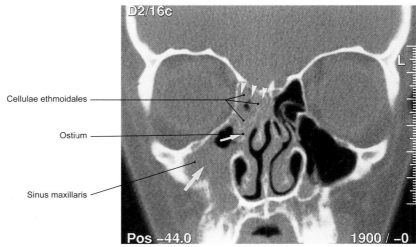

Fig. 8.118 Chronic sinusitis; coronal computed tomography (CT) scan of the paranasal sinuses. [S700-T720]
White arrows indicate a swelling of the inflamed mucosa in the right Sinus maxillaris and the ostium, while white arrowheads point to a swelling of the ethmoidal cells.

Clinical remarks

The middle nasal meatus is the endonasal access route in paranasal surgery for the treatment of a chronic inflammation of the frontal or maxillary sinus and anterior ethmoidal cells. One-sided **inflamma-** **tion of the Sinus maxillaris** is often odontogenic (maxillary odontogenic sinusitis). Commonly, the cause is an inflammation of the second premolar or the first molar (→ Fig. 8.40).

Topography of the sinuses

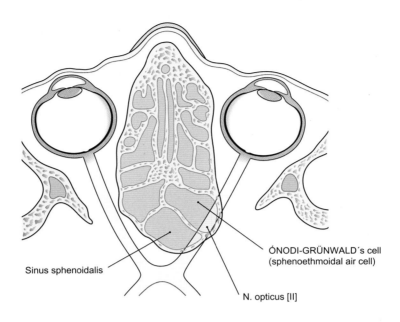

Sinus sphenoidalis

ÓNODI-GRÜNWALD´s cell
(sphenoethmoidal air cell)

N. opticus [II]

Fig. 8.119 Topography and variants of the ethmoidal cells, Cellulae ethmoidales; horizontal section through the Os ethmoidale at the level of the Canalis opticus. [S702-L126]

If an ÓNODI-GRÜNWALD´s cell develops, the Sinus sphenoidalis lies partially below this posterior sphenoidal cell. It is often closely situated to the N. opticus [II].

Sinuses – clinical terms	
Agger nasi	An anterior ethmoidal cell in front of and above the attachment of the middle nasal concha
Atrium meatus medii	Region in front of the middle nasal passage above the head of the Concha nasalis inferior
Bulla ethmoidalis	An anterior ethmoidal cell above the Hiatus semilunaris, which is usually present, but can also be missing
Fontanelle	Accessory opening in the medial wall of the Sinus maxillaris that is covered by a mucous membrane
Basic lamellae	Lamellae within the Os ethmoidale as embryological residues. **Four basic lamellae** (BL) can be distinguished: • First BL: Proc. uncinatus • Second BL: Bulla ethmoidalis • Third BL: Concha nasalis media • Fourth BL: Concha nasalis superior
HALLER's cell	An ethmoidal cell which pneumatises the lower orbital wall (infraorbital cell)
Hiatus maxillaris	A large opening of the Sinus maxillaris into the nasal cavity, which is partially closed by the Proc. uncinatus of the Os ethmoidale, as well as by the mucous membrane
Hiatus semilunaris	A crescent-shaped cleft up to 3 cm wide between the Bulla ethmoidalis and the upper free margin of the Proc. uncinatus; the Hiatus semilunaris provides access to the Infundibulum ethmoidale
Infundibulum ethmoidale	Space delineated by the Proc. uncinatus, the Lamina papyracea and the Bulla ethmoidalis
ÓNODI-GRÜNWALD's cell	A posterior ethmoidal cell which protrudes posteriorly via the Sinus sphenoidalis
Osteomeatal complex	General term for the complicated anatomy of the Hiatus semilunaris and its surroundings
Proc. uncinatus	A thin lamellar bone of the Os ethmoidale participating in the formation of the medial wall of the Sinus maxillaris and confining the Hiatus semilunaris at its anteroposterior aspect
Recessus frontalis	Cleavage space or gap connecting the frontal sinus and nasal cavity (Ductus nasofrontalis, Canalis nasofrontalis)
Sulcus olfactorius	A groove or canal between the anterior attachment of the Concha nasalis media at the cranial base and the roof of the nose

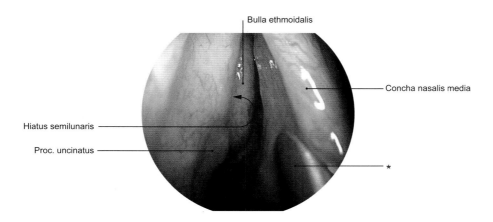

Bulla ethmoidalis

Concha nasalis media

Hiatus semilunaris

Proc. uncinatus

*

Fig. 8.120   Nasal cavity, Cavitas nasi, left side; transnasal endoscopy with a 30° endoscope. [S700-T720]

The examiner views the head of the middle nasal concha (Concha nasalis media).
* Antrum curette

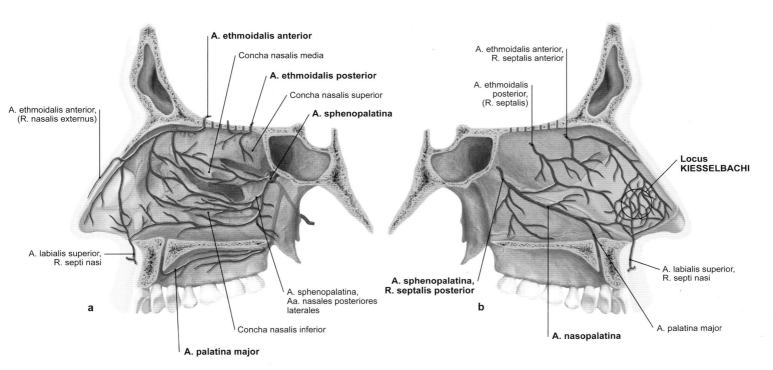

A. ethmoidalis anterior

Concha nasalis media

A. ethmoidalis posterior

Concha nasalis superior

A. sphenopalatina

A. ethmoidalis anterior,
(R. nasalis externus)

A. labialis superior,
R. septi nasi

a

A. sphenopalatina,
Aa. nasales posteriores
laterales

Concha nasalis inferior

A. palatina major

A. ethmoidalis anterior,
R. septalis anterior

A. ethmoidalis
posterior,
(R. septalis)

Locus
KIESSELBACHI

A. sphenopalatina,
R. septalis posterior

b

A. nasopalatina

A. labialis superior,
R. septi nasi

A. palatina major

Fig. 8.121a and b   Arteries of the nasal cavity. [S700-L284]
a Lateral wall of the right half of the nasal cavity.
b Nasal septum of the right half of the nasal cavity.
The nose receives its arterial blood supply from the A. carotis externa and A. carotis interna.

- A. carotis interna: the **Aa. ethmoidales anterior** and **posterior** run from the ophthalmic artery through the anterior and posterior Os ethmoidale to reach the lateral nasal wall and the nasal septum.

- A. carotis externa: as a terminal branch of the A. maxillaris, the **A. sphenopalatina** enters the nasal cavity via the Foramen sphenopalatinum. Anastomoses take place between the blood vessels of the lip and the facial artery. On the nasal septum, the **A. nasopalatina** branches off the A. sphenopalatina, which enters the oral cavity via the Canalis incisivus and anastomoses with the A. palatina major. Along with the Aa. ethmoidales anterior and posterior, the A. nasopalatina feeds the KIESSELBACH's plexus, which is an arteriovenous plexus.

Clinical remarks

The most frequent location for **nasal bleeding** (epistaxis) is the KIESSELBACH's plexus at the nasal septum.
Fractures of the base of the skull in the area of the Lamina cribrosa can cause ruptures of the Aa. ethmoidales anterior and/or posterior with consecutive nosebleeds.

If, in the event of life-threatening bleeding, a nasal tamponade is not successful, the A. sphenopalatina must be ligated.

Head

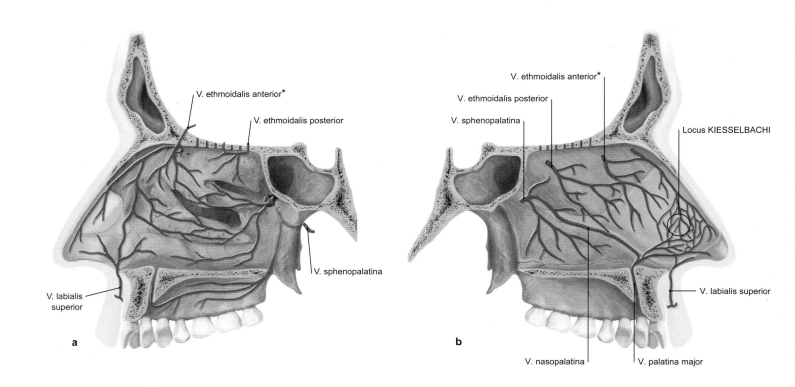

Fig. 8.122a and b Veins of the nasal cavity, Cavitas nasi. [S700-L284]
a Lateral wall of the right half of the nasal cavity.
b Nasal septum of the right half of the nasal cavity.
The blood is drained via the **Vv. ethmoidales anterior** and **posterior** to the Sinus cavernosus at the base of the skull, via the **V. sphenopalati-** na to the Plexus pterygoideus in the Fossa infratemporalis, and via the connection with the **Vv. labiales** into the V. facialis.

* connecting vein to the Sinus sagittalis superior via the Foramen cae-cum (only present during childhood)

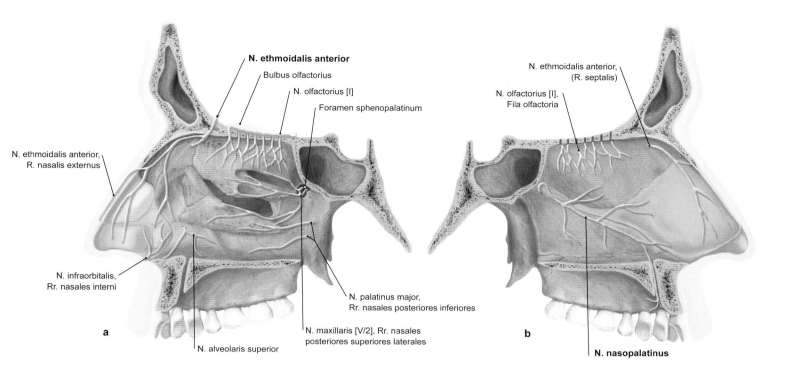

N. ethmoidalis anterior
Bulbus olfactorius
N. olfactorius [I]
Foramen sphenopalatinum

N. ethmoidalis anterior,
R. nasalis externus

N. infraorbitalis,
Rr. nasales interni

a

N. alveolaris superior

N. palatinus major,
Rr. nasales posteriores inferiores

N. maxillaris [V/2], Rr. nasales
posteriores superiores laterales

N. ethmoidalis anterior,
(R. septalis)

N. olfactorius [I],
Fila olfactoria

b

N. nasopalatinus

Fig. 8.123a and b Innervation of the nasal cavity, Cavitas nasi.
[S700-L284]
a Lateral wall of the right half of the nasal cavity.
b Nasal septum of the right half of the nasal cavity.
The sensory innervation of the nasal mucosa is provided by branches of
the N. trigeminus [V]: N. ophthalmicus [V/1] → N. ethmoidalis anterior

and N. maxillaris [V/2] → Rr. nasales, N. nasopalatinus. The olfactory epithelium is innervated by the **N. olfactorius [I]**. Along the nasal septum
runs the **N. nasopalatinus,** which passes through the Canalis incisivus
and innervates the mucosa of the hard palate in the area at the back of
the incisors up to the canine tooth.

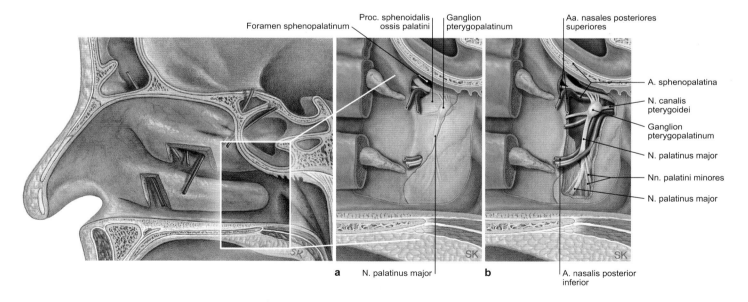

Foramen sphenopalatinum

Proc. sphenoidalis
ossis palatini

Ganglion
pterygopalatinum

Aa. nasales posteriores
superiores

A. sphenopalatina

N. canalis
pterygoidei

Ganglion
pterygopalatinum

N. palatinus major

Nn. palatini minores

N. palatinus major

a   N. palatinus major

b

A. nasalis posterior
inferior

Fig. 8.124a and b Fossa pterygopalatina; medial view, lateral wall
of the right half of the nasal cavity. [S700-L238]
a Mucous membrane severed and bent rostrally, with the Ganglion pterygopalatinum and the N. palatinus major shown transparently.

b Lateral wall of the open Fossa pterygopalatina.
Visible within the Fossa pterygopalatina are the Ganglion pterygopalatinum and those neurovascular bundles running within.

Clinical remarks

The sensory innervation of the nasal mucosa is extremely good. Any
manipulation inside the nose can therefore be extremely painful.
Damage (rupture) of the Fila olfactoria within the context of a traumatic brain injury may result in **anosmia** (the patient loses the sense of
smell).

Tearing (rupture) of the dura mater can cause a **rhinorrhoea of cerebrospinal fluid.** A clear transparent fluid (CSF, cerebrospinal fluid)
seeps out of the patient's nose. The diagnosis can be confirmed by
the detection of glucose with a glucose test strip. Due to the risk of
infection, surgical care is urgently needed.

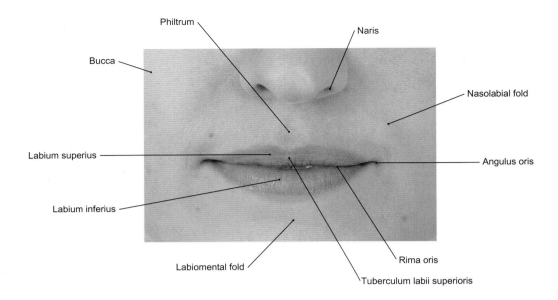

Bucca

Philtrum

Naris

Nasolabial fold

Labium superius

Angulus oris

Labium inferius

Labiomental fold

Rima oris

Tuberculum labii superioris

Fig. 8.125 Oral fissure, Rima oris; frontal view. [S700-J803]
The entrance to the mouth is closed by the lips. Since the epithelium of the lips is thin and not pigmented, and the connective tissue papillae that are richly vascularised with capillaries are located close to the free surface, the blood in the papillae shimmers through the skin and causes the red colour of the lips (vermilion). The margin of the upper lip has a depression lying below the columella of the nose, the philtrum, which ends as a lip protuberance or torus, the Tuberculum labii superioris.

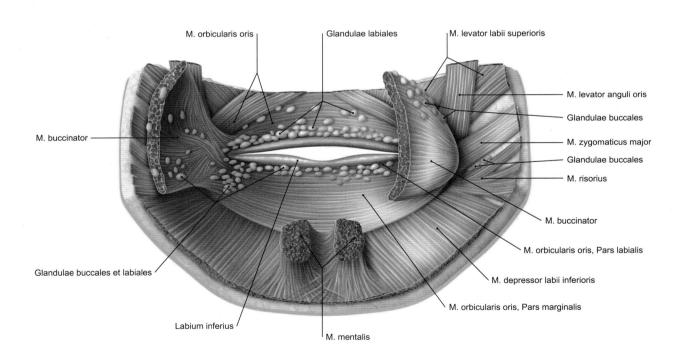

M. orbicularis oris

Glandulae labiales

M. levator labii superioris

M. levator anguli oris

Glandulae buccales

M. zygomaticus major

Glandulae buccales

M. risorius

M. buccinator

M. orbicularis oris, Pars labialis

M. depressor labii inferioris

M. orbicularis oris, Pars marginalis

M. buccinator

Glandulae buccales et labiales

Labium inferius

M. mentalis

Fig. 8.126 Muscles of the oral region, Regio oralis; intraoral view.
The mucosa is removed; small salivary glands are partially preserved. [S700-L275]
The base of the lips is the Pars labialis of the transversely striated M. orbicularis oris. Its Pars marginalis bends outwards below the prolabium and under the skin, and branches out into other mimetic muscles. In the submucosa, below the M. orbicularis oris, are lots of small, mixed seromucous salivary glands (Glandulae labiales). In contrast, the small Glandulae buccales around the M. buccinator produce a mucoserous secretion.

→ T 1.5

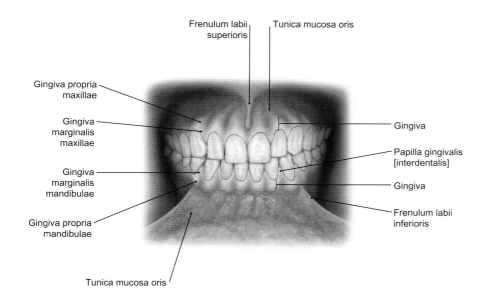

Frenulum labii superioris

Tunica mucosa oris

Gingiva propria maxillae

Gingiva marginalis maxillae

Gingiva marginalis mandibulae

Gingiva propria mandibulae

Tunica mucosa oris

Gingiva

Papilla gingivalis [interdentalis]

Gingiva

Frenulum labii inferioris

Fig. 8.127 Oral vestibule, Vestibulum oris, with gums, Gingiva, and oral mucosa, Mucosa oralis; frontal view. [S702-L266]/[G1089]
The lips are stabilised with connective tissue. The upper lip is fixed via the Frenulum labii superioris, which runs in the midline. The lower lip is fixed via the paired Frenulum labii inferioris, which passes on both sides to the oral mucosa, usually between the canines and first premolars.

The gums extend up to the cervix of the teeth as the Gingiva marginalis, which is movable and forms the Sulcus gingivalis between the teeth. The non-movable Gingiva propria connects to the Gingiva marginalis and covers the Proc. alveolaris of the maxilla and Mandibula, respectively. It continues into the oral mucosa.

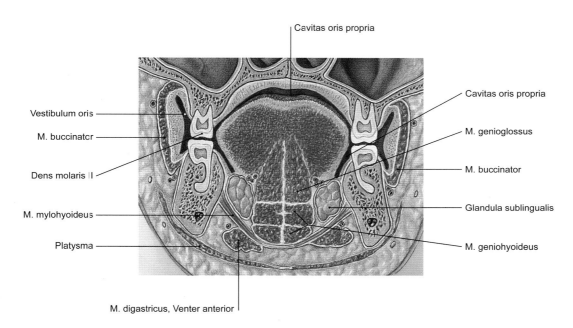

Cavitas oris propria

Vestibulum oris

M. buccinator

Dens molaris II

M. mylohyoideus

Platysma

M. digastricus, Venter anterior

Cavitas oris propria

M. genioglossus

M. buccinator

Glandula sublingualis

M. geniohyoideus

Fig. 8.128 Frontal section through the oral cavity, Cavitas oris, at the level of the second molars; frontal view. [S700-L238]
The oral vestibule (Vestibulum oris) is confined at the front by the lips, on both sides by the cheeks, as well as inside and outside by the Procc.

alveolares and the teeth. The mouth cavity is the Cavitas oris propria. With a closed mouth, it is almost completely filled by the tongue. Its roof is formed by the palate, and its floor is the floor of the mouth.

Clinical remarks

To create a genetic fingerprint, e.g. in the context of testing a biological relationship (paternity test) or to detect criminal offences, a **mouth swab** is taken. For this purpose, a sterile buccal swab is used to obtain mucosal cells from the inside of the cheek, from which DNA is then extracted and analysed.
Keratinisation disorders with cellular and epithelial atypia of the usually pink oral mucosa lead to white mucosal changes **(leukoplakia).**

If they cannot be wiped off, they are referred to as **precarcinoma,** which are classified as premalignant diseases of the oral mucosa and require immediate histopathological evaluation and, if necessary, surgical removal. If, on the other hand, the white plaques can be wiped away, they are usually due to **fungal infections** (most commonly *Candida albicans*), which can be treated with medication.

Mouth and oral cavity

Oral cavity

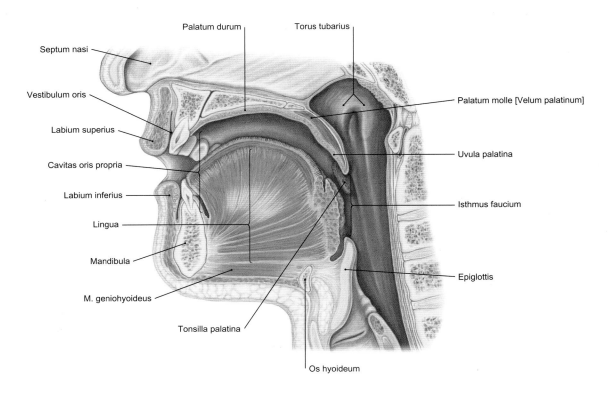

Fig. 8.129 Oral cavity, Cavitas oris, right side; view from the left. Median sagittal section. [S700-L285]
The Cavitas oris propria is filled by the body of the tongue. It is confined by the teeth at the front and on both sides, and above by the hard and soft palate. Below, the tongue lies on the floor of the mouth. Anterior parts of the tongue muscles are fixed at the Mandibula.

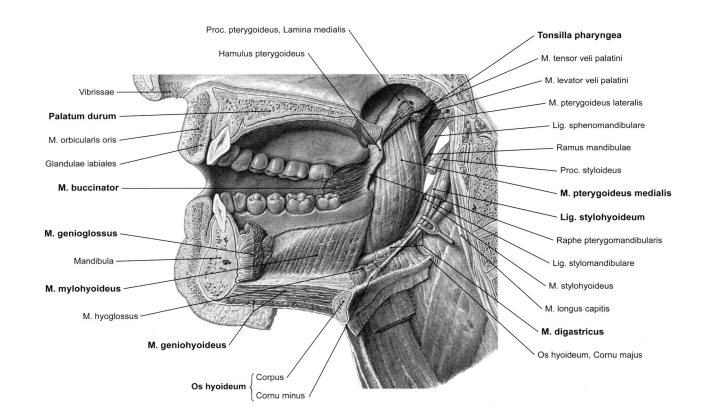

Fig. 8.130 Oral cavity, Cavitas oris, right side; view from the left. The sagittal section is at the level of the first incisors. [S700]
The oral cavity is confined on its sides by the cheeks, at the top by the palate, and at the bottom by the muscles of the floor of the mouth.

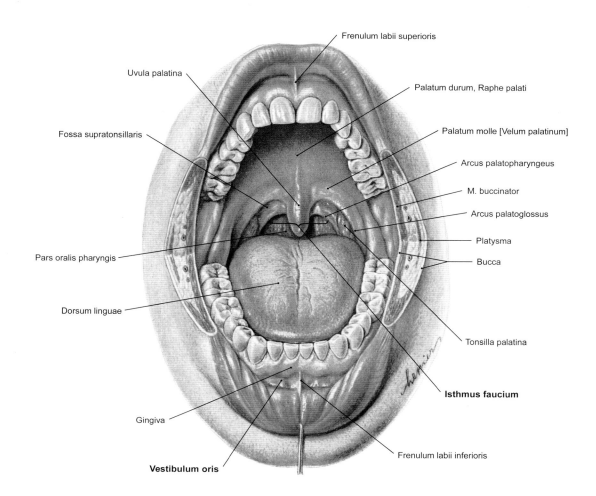

Frenulum labii superioris

Uvula palatina

Palatum durum, Raphe palati

Palatum molle [Velum palatinum]

Fossa supratonsillaris

Arcus palatopharyngeus

M. buccinator

Arcus palatoglossus

Platysma

Pars oralis pharyngis

Bucca

Dorsum linguae

Tonsilla palatina

Isthmus faucium

Gingiva

Frenulum labii inferioris

Vestibulum oris

Fig. 8.131 Oral cavity, Cavitas oris; frontal view. The mouth is open. [S700]

The oral opening (Rima oris) represents the entrance to the digestive tract and the oral cavity. This is divided into the oral vestibule (Vestibulum oris) and the actual mouth, called the Cavitas oris propria. The **Vestibulum oris** is bordered externally by the lips and cheeks and internally by the Procc. alveolares and the teeth. When the teeth are occluded, there is a connection to the oral cavity behind the last tooth (Spatium retromolare). In the region of the oropharyngeal isthmus **(Isthmus faucium),** the oral cavity becomes the Pars oralis of the pharynx (oropharynx). Opening into the Vestibulum oris and the Cavitas oris propria are numerous (500–1,000) small excretory ducts and three paired large salivary glands. The inside of the oral cavity is filled for the most part by the tongue (Corpus linguae).

Dental arches

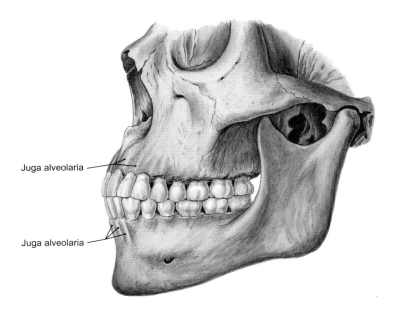

Juga alveolaria

Juga alveolaria

Fig. 8.132 Superior and inferior dental arches, Arcus dentales maxillaris [superior] and mandibularis [inferior]; in the viscerocranium of a 28-year-old; teeth in occlusion position; lateral view. [S700]
In the Proc. alveolaris, the roots of the teeth produce ridge-shaped, vertically extending protrusions (Juga alveolaria). The teeth of the upper jaw are in the **occlusion position** above those of the lower jaw. They are arranged and fit together in such a way that the cusp of a tooth comes to rest in the fissure of the two opposite teeth (interlocking cusp-fissures). In the **upper jaw,** each quadrant consists of a central incisor and a smaller lateral incisor, which often have pronounced marginal edges. The canine has the longest root and only one cusp. The two premolars have two cusps; the (distal) second premolar is usually a little bit smaller. The largest tooth is the first molar. It is marked by a mesiopalatinal cusp. The second molar is similar to the first, but is smaller. The third molar (wisdom tooth, Dens serotinus) is designed very differently and can also be missing (either not developed or not erupted). In the **lower jaw,** incisors and canine teeth are smaller. There are also two premolars. The first molar usually has five cusps, the second molar has four, and the third molar (wisdom tooth, Dens serotinus), as in the upper jaw, is very variable in terms of formation and can also be missing.

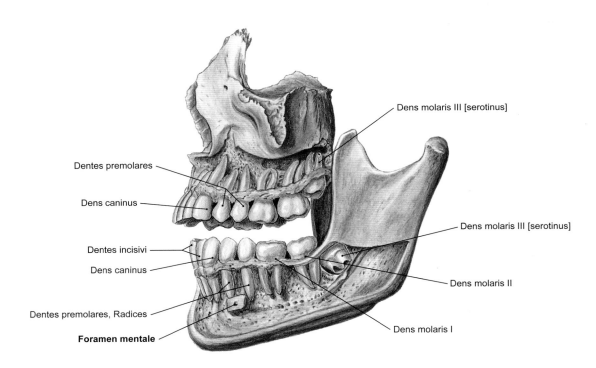

Dens molaris III [serotinus]

Dentes premolares

Dens caninus

Dens molaris III [serotinus]

Dentes incisivi

Dens caninus

Dens molaris II

Dentes premolares, Radices

Foramen mentale

Dens molaris I

Fig. 8.133 Maxilla, and mandible, Mandibula, of a 20-year-old person. [S700]
Completion of the permanent dentition results in up to 32 permanent teeth (Dentes permanentes). The third molar (Dens molaris tertius, wisdom tooth, Dens serotinus) has not yet erupted in the Mandibula. It can be regressed or has not been developed at all (aplasia). Usually, the molar teeth erupt approx. seven months earlier in girls than in boys. In both sexes, the molar teeth in the lower jaw erupt earlier than molar teeth in the maxilla. The roots of the deciduous teeth require another 16 to 26 months to develop; the roots of the permanent teeth are fully developed only after another 1.7 to 3.5 years.

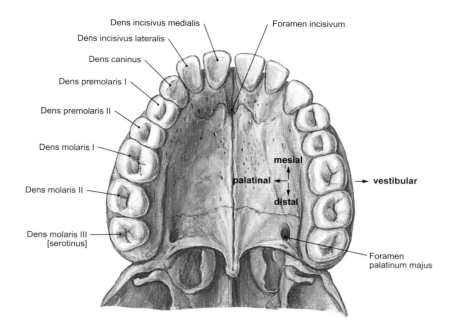

Fig. 8.134 Maxillary dental arch, Arcus dentalis maxillaris [superior]. [S700]

The teeth (Dentes) are arranged in two dental arches, the upper (Arcus dentalis maxillaris or superior) and the lower dental arch (Arcus dentalis mandibularis or inferior), and are anchored in the upper and lower jaw.

The dentition is **heterodontic** in humans; the teeth are shaped differently with distinct features, and thereby are categorised as incisors (Incisivi), canines (Canini), premolars (Premolares) and molars (Molares). Incisors and canine teeth are also called front teeth, whereas premolars and molars are lateral teeth.

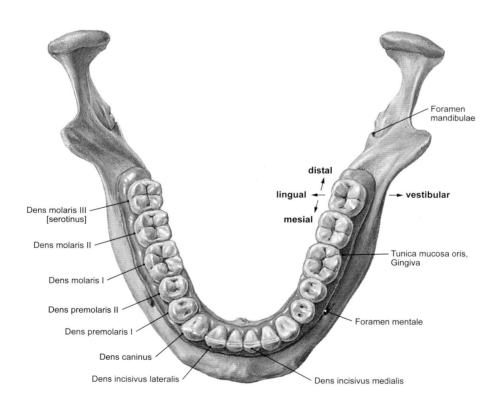

Fig. 8.135 Mandibular dental arch, Arcus dentalis mandibularis [inferior]. [S700]

With one exception, the arrangement of teeth in the lower dental arch is similar to that in the upper dental arch. For a precise indication of the 'oral' topographical relationships, 'palatinal' is the term used in the upper jaw and 'lingual' in the lower jaw. The **gingiva** is part of the oral mucosa, covers the Proc. alveolaris and also covers the alveolar bone as

well as the interdental bony septa. Furthermore, it wraps around the cervix of the tooth and continues at the Margo gingivalis into the oral mucosa. The gingiva supports the anchorage of the teeth and stabilises their position in the alveolar bone (Pars fixa gingivae); as part of the oral mucosa, the gingiva marginalis forms the junctional epithelium attached to the dental surfaces.

Mouth and oral cavity

Structure of the teeth

Fig. 8.136 Incisor tooth, Dens incisivus.
[S700-L126]
On each tooth, a distinction is made between the crown (Corona dentis), the neck or cervix (Cervix dentis) and the root (Radix dentis). The **dental crown** is the visible part of the tooth. It sticks out above the gums (Gingiva) and is covered by enamel (Enamelum). The **root of the tooth** is placed in the tooth socket (Alveolus dentalis), which is the root compartment, a depression in the Proc. alveolaris of the maxilla or mandible; the root is covered by cement (Cementum). Periodontal fibres (periodontium, desmodontium) anchor the root of the tooth in the alveolar bone. The **dental cervix** is the area where the enamel and cement are adjacent to each other. This is where the gingiva is attached to the tooth.

The lowest point of the root is the **root apex** (Apex radicis dentis). The dental papilla (Papilla dentis) is perforated in the Foramen apicis by the root canal (Canalis radicis dentis), through which vessels and nerves enter the Cavitas dentis, consisting of the Cavitas pulparis and the Cavitas coronae.

The **dental pulp** (Pulpa dentis) consists of connective tissue, containing blood vessels, lymph vessels and nerves, and thus nourishes the tooth. Here, too, a distinction is made between the root pulp (Pulpa radicularis) and the crown pulp (Pulpa coronalis). Collectively, the cement, desmodontium, alveolar bone, and parts of the gingiva are referred to as the parodontium.

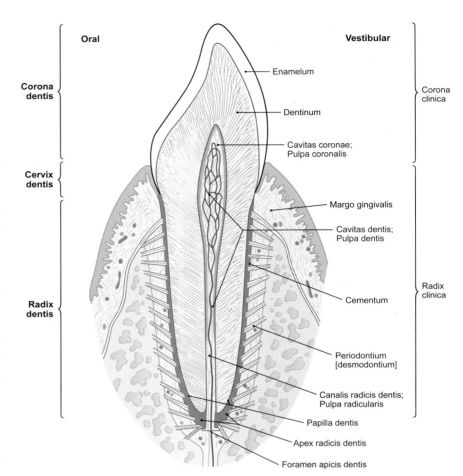

Fig. 8.137 Permanent canine tooth, Dens caninus permanens. [S700]
Example of a tooth with one root.

Fig. 8.138 Second deciduous molar tooth, Dens molaris deciduus. [S700]
Example of a tooth with two roots.

Fig. 8.139 First molar tooth, Dens molaris primus. [S700]
Occlusal surface of a molar tooth with the individual parts labelled.

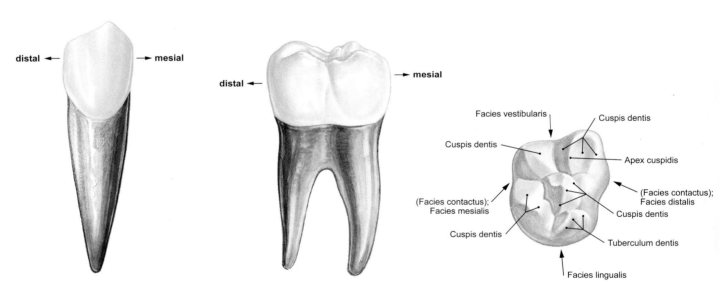

Structure and function

Form, arrangement and orientation rules
The **labelling of the surfaces** of the teeth is from the midline outwards. The part closest to the midline is referred to as mesial, and the part furthest away as distal. Neighbouring structures to the teeth are defined as **surfaces** (Facies). The number, dimension, and form of the roots (Radices) are functionally adapted to the dental crown.

The morphology of the roots of individual teeth in deciduous dentition is different and variable to those in permanent dentition. Teeth with a single root are the incisors, canines and premolars. Teeth with two roots are the first upper premolars and the lower molars. Teeth with three roots are the upper molars.

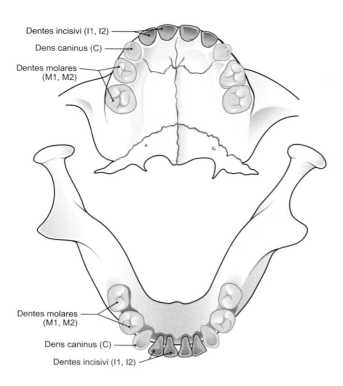

Dentes incisivi (I1, I2)
Dens caninus (C)
Dentes molares (M1, M2)

Dentes molares (M1, M2)
Dens caninus (C)
Dentes incisivi (I1, I2)

Fig. 8.140 Teeth, first dentition, deciduous teeth, Dentes decidui; view from below onto the maxilla and from above onto the Mandibula. [S700-L126]

The deciduous teeth consist of 4 x 5 = 20 teeth, Dentes: 4 x 2 incisors, Dentes incisivi (purple); 4 x 1 canines, Dens caninus (blue); 4 x 2 molars, Dentes molares (green).

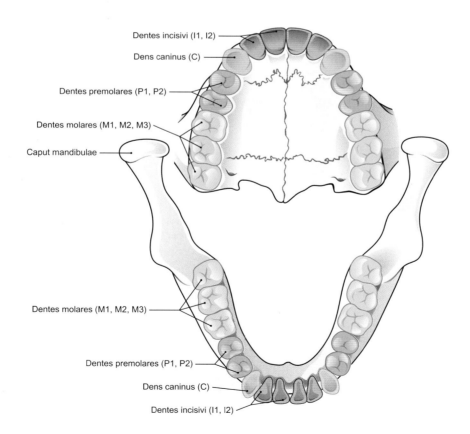

Dentes incisivi (I1, I2)
Dens caninus (C)
Dentes premolares (P1, P2)
Dentes molares (M1, M2, M3)
Caput mandibulae

Dentes molares (M1, M2, M3)
Dentes premolares (P1, P2)
Dens caninus (C)
Dentes incisivi (I1, I2)

Fig. 8.141 Teeth, second dentition, permanent teeth, Dentes permanentes; view from below onto the maxilla and from above onto the Mandibula. [S700-L126]

The permanent teeth consist of 4 x 8 = 32 teeth, Dentes: 4 x 2 incisors, Dentes incisivi (purple); 4 x 1 canines, Dens caninus (blue); 4 x 2 premolars, Dentes premolares (red); 4 x 3 molars, Dentes molares (green).

Milk teeth

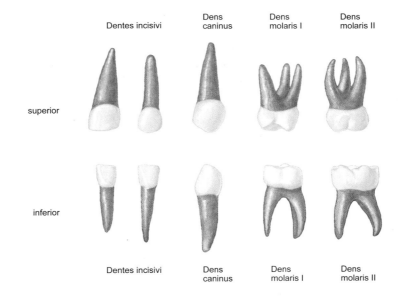

Fig. 8.142   Milk or deciduous teeth, Dentes decidui, of a three-year-old child; vestibular view. [S700]
Tooth development begins prior to birth. Teething starts about six months after birth with the first deciduous (milk) teeth, Dentes decidui, breaking through in the oral cavity. A complete set of 20 deciduous teeth is usually present by the age of 30 months. These teeth remain until about the age of six years when they are gradually replaced by permanent teeth, Dentes permanentes.
Although the deciduous teeth are temporary, they should be well taken care of because these teeth only have a thin enamel layer and are therefore vulnerable to tooth decay (caries). Because their pulpa cavities are larger, they are more sensitive than permanent teeth.

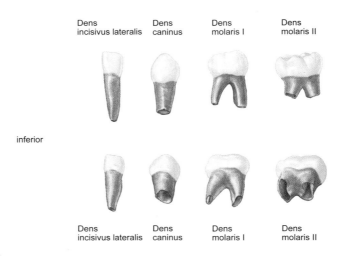

Fig. 8.143   Deciduous teeth, Dentes decidui, of a two-year-old child; upper row, vestibular view; lower row, view from below at an oblique angle. [S700]

The medial incisors are not presented here. One can see that in a two-year-old child the root formation has not yet been completed in many teeth. This process is only complete after dental eruption.

Clinical remarks

Dental formula
There is an internationally accepted dental formula which is applied by all disciplines of dental medicine (→ formula). In doing so, each half of a jaw **(quadrant)** is given a number. Starting from the midline, **teeth** of the permanent and deciduous dentition are numbered consecutively from one to eight (permanent dentition) and from one to five (deciduous dentition), respectively. The number of the quadrant is followed by the number of the tooth. For example, the digits 11 (called 'one-one') describe the first incisor in the right upper jaw of the permanent dentition; the digits 52 (called 'five-two') describe the second incisor in the right upper jaw of the deciduous dentition.

Teeth numbering chart for adult teeth

Maxilla

right	18 17 16 15 14 13 12 11	21 22 23 24 25 26 27 28	left
	48 47 46 45 44 43 42 41	31 32 33 34 35 36 37 38	

Mandibula

Teeth numbering chart for deciduous (primary) teeth

Maxilla

right	55 54 53 52 51	61 62 63 64 65	left
	85 84 83 82 81	71 72 73 74 75	

Mandibula

[S700]

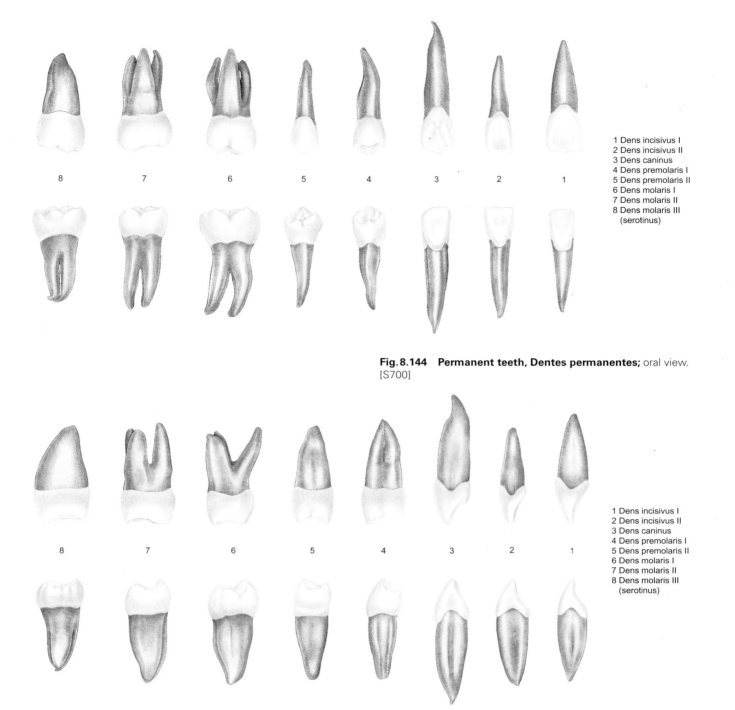

1 Dens incisivus I
2 Dens incisivus II
3 Dens caninus
4 Dens premolaris I
5 Dens premolaris II
6 Dens molaris I
7 Dens molaris II
8 Dens molaris III
  (serotinus)

Fig. 8.144 Permanent teeth, Dentes permanentes; oral view. [S700]

1 Dens incisivus I
2 Dens incisivus II
3 Dens caninus
4 Dens premolaris I
5 Dens premolaris II
6 Dens molaris I
7 Dens molaris II
8 Dens molaris III
  (serotinus)

Fig. 8.145 Permanent teeth, Dentes permanentes; distal view. [S700]
Starting at the age of six years, dentition results in the loss of the first deciduous teeth, Dentes decidui. This creates space for the permanent teeth, Dentes permanentes. Like the deciduous teeth, the permanent teeth are formed prenatally and have developed into mature teeth inside the jaw. They now start breaking through one by one into the oral cavity. The new teeth facilitate this dentition process by secreting substances that slowly dissolve the roots of the milk teeth. Over time, the deciduous teeth become loose and eventually fall out. Their place is then occupied by the permanent teeth.

Normally, the lower incisors and the so-called **six-year-molars** erupt first; the latter are the first permanent molars (Dens molaris I, number 6 in the adult tooth chart). These molars stabilise the upper and lower jaw to ensure a good bite position. Next, the lateral incisors and premolars erupt. At 11–13 years of age, the canines and a second set of molars, the **12-year-molars** (Dens molaris II, number 7 in the adult tooth chart), erupt. The last set of permanent teeth are the wisdom teeth (Dens molaris III [serotinus], number 8 in the adult tooth chart) which may or may not erupt at approx. 17 years of age.

Clinical remarks

In clinical terms, the back teeth are referred to as molars and those in front of them as premolars. Since the teeth are the most imperishable parts of the human body and therefore particularly durable, they play an important role in **forensic medicine** for the identification of victims.

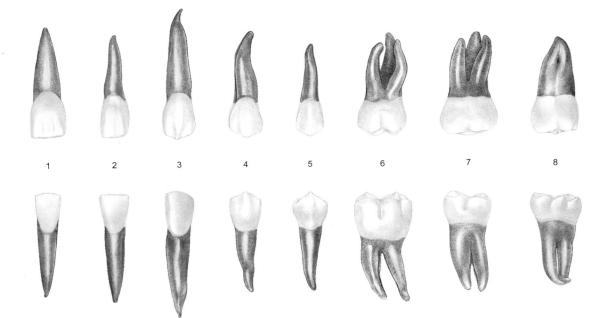

Fig. 8.146 Permanent teeth, Dentes permanentes; vestibular view.
[S700]

1 Dens incisivus I
2 Dens incisivus II
3 Dens caninus
4 Dens premolaris I
5 Dens premolaris II
6 Dens molaris I
7 Dens molaris II
8 Dens molaris III
   (serotinus)

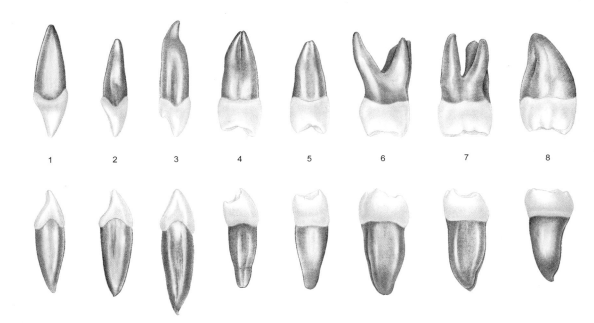

Fig. 8.147 Permanent teeth, Dentes permanentes; mesial view.
[S700]

1 Dens incisivus I
2 Dens incisivus II
3 Dens caninus
4 Dens premolaris I
5 Dens premolaris II
6 Dens molaris I
7 Dens molaris II
8 Dens molaris III
   (serotinus)

Clinical remarks

- Environmental and genetic factors can influence the **development of the teeth.** Resulting dental anomalies can affect the size, shape and number of teeth.
- The administration of **tetracyclines** (an antibiotic) during dental development can result in discolouration of the teeth and enamel defects.

- Also significant is discolouration of the teeth and enamel defects caused by high doses of fluorides in the form of tablets **(dental fluorosis).**
- Enamel defects can also be caused by a vitamin D deficiency **(rickets).**
- Remnants of the dental lamina can remain as SERRE's bodies, as can remnants of the epithelial root sheath as so-called epithelial cell rests of MALASSEZ, and both can generate cysts.

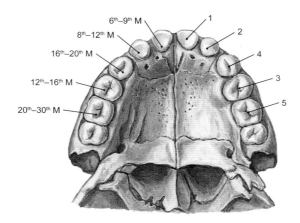

6th–9th M
8th–12th M
16th–20th M
12th–16th M
20th–30th M
1
2
4
3
5

Fig. 8.148 Upper jaw, Maxilla, with deciduous teeth, Dentes decidui, and first permanent teeth; left: average time of eruption in months (M); right: sequence of tooth eruption. [S700]
The development of permanent teeth (replacement teeth) and deciduous (milk) teeth is similar but happens at different times. The time of eruption and the sequence at which milk teeth appear in the oral cavity is subject to significant interindividual differences. By 30 months, the milk teeth have usually all appeared.

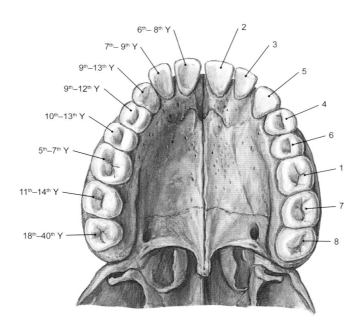

6th–8th Y
7th–9th Y
9th–13th Y
9th–12th Y
10th–13th Y
5th–7th Y
11th–14th Y
18th–40th Y
2
3
5
4
6
1
7
8

Fig. 8.149 Upper jaw, Maxilla, with permanent teeth, Dentes permanentes; left: average time of eruption in years (Y); right: sequence of tooth eruption. [S700]
With the exception of the molar teeth, the deciduous dentition (first dentition with 20 teeth) is similar to the permanent dentition (second dentition with 32 teeth). The sequence of eruption of the permanent molars is always the same: first molars at the age of six years **(six-year molars)**, second molars at 12 years, and third molars at approx. 17 years or later.

Clinical remarks

The term **parodontopathies** refers to diseases of the periodontium. Parodontosis is a chronic degenerative form of periodontal disease and results in an increased tooth mobility and tooth loss with subsequent atrophy of the Proc. alveolaris caused by the decline of the **periodontal support system.** The systemic administration of fluoride ions during the formation of the hard substance in permanent teeth sometimes leads to the formation of **fluorapatite** instead of hydroxyapatite. Fluorapatite is less soluble in acid and thus increases resistance to caries.

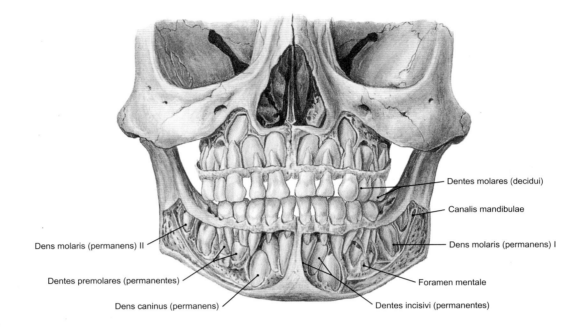

Fig. 8.150   **Upper jaw, Maxilla, and lower jaw, Mandibula, of a five-year-old child,** with milk teeth and primordium of permanent teeth, frontal view. [S700]
Human dentition is diphyodont; there are two successive sets of teeth, known as the deciduous and permanent dentitions. First, the 20 milk teeth (Dentes decidui) develop in children. Development and eruption of the first and second dentitions and the body growth are synchronised in a chronological manner. Resorption of the roots of the milk teeth occurs at different points in time.

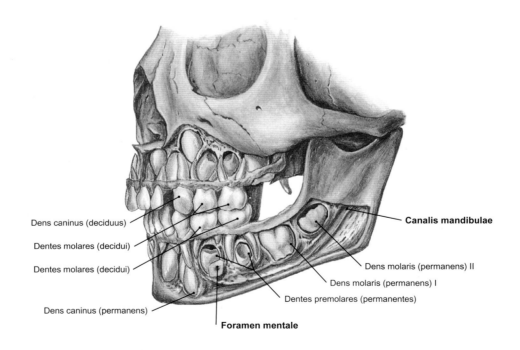

Fig. 8.151   **Upper jaw, Maxilla, and lower jaw, Mandibula, of a five-year-old child,** with milk teeth and primordium of permanent teeth, lateral view. [S700]

The primordium of the third molar (Dens molaris permanens III) is not visible.

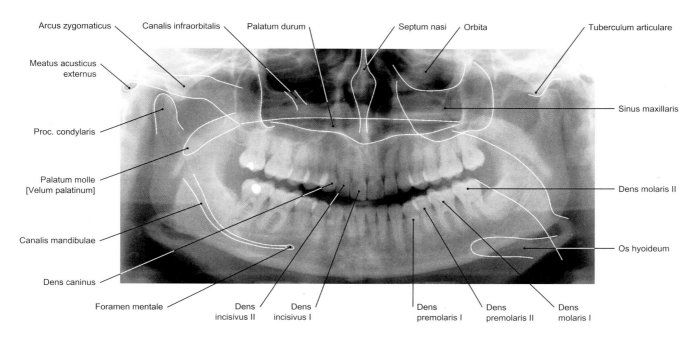

Arcus zygomaticus
Canalis infraorbitalis
Palatum durum
Septum nasi
Orbita
Tuberculum articulare

Meatus acusticus externus

Sinus maxillaris

Proc. condylaris

Dens molaris II

Palatum molle [Velum palatinum]

Canalis mandibulae

Os hyoideum

Dens caninus

Foramen mentale
Dens incisivus II
Dens incisivus I
Dens premolaris I
Dens premolaris II
Dens molaris I

Fig. 8.152 Upper jaw, Maxilla, and lower jaw, Mandibula, without wisdom teeth; panoramic X-ray image. [S700]

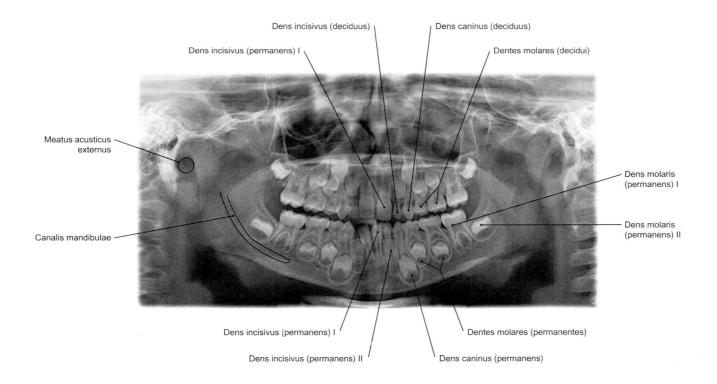

Dens incisivus (deciduus)
Dens caninus (deciduus)

Dens incisivus (permanens) I
Dentes molares (decidui)

Meatus acusticus externus

Dens molaris (permanens) I

Canalis mandibulae

Dens molaris (permanens) II

Dens incisivus (permanens) I
Dentes molares (permanentes)

Dens incisivus (permanens) II
Dens caninus (permanens)

Fig. 8.153 Upper jaw, Maxilla, and lower jaw, Mandibula, of a five-year-old child; panoramic X-ray image. [S700-T884]

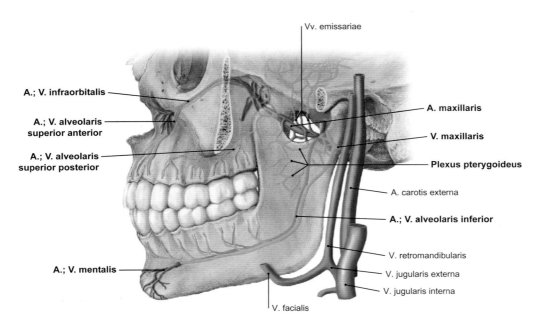

Vv. emissariae

A.; V. infraorbitalis

A.; V. alveolaris superior anterior

A.; V. alveolaris superior posterior

A. maxillaris

V. maxillaris

Plexus pterygoideus

A. carotis externa

A.; V. alveolaris inferior

V. retromandibularis

A.; V. mentalis

V. jugularis externa

V. jugularis interna

V. facialis

Fig. 8.154 Blood supply to the teeth. [S700-L284]
The upper lateral teeth are supplied by the A. maxillaris via the **A. alveolaris superior posterior,** and the upper front teeth by the **A. infraorbitalis.** Teeth and gingiva of the lower jaw are supplied by the **A. alveolaris inferior,** which runs in the Canalis mandibularis. The veins accompanying the arteries drain the blood into the **Plexus pterygoideus.**

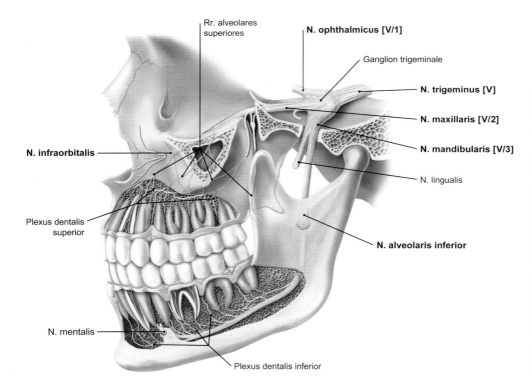

Rr. alveolares superiores

N. ophthalmicus [V/1]

Ganglion trigeminale

N. trigeminus [V]

N. maxillaris [V/2]

N. infraorbitalis

N. mandibularis [V/3]

N. lingualis

Plexus dentalis superior

N. alveolaris inferior

N. mentalis

Plexus dentalis inferior

Fig. 8.155 Innervation of the teeth, left side; lateral view. [S700-L275]
The N. maxillaris [V/2] and N. mandibularis [V/3] of the N. trigeminus [V] provide the sensory innervation for the teeth. The **maxillary teeth** are innervated by the Plexus dentalis superior, which is composed of the Rr. alveolares superiores posteriores, medii and anteriores of the Nn. alveolares superiores of the N. infraorbitalis. The **teeth of the mandible** are innervated by the Plexus dentalis inferior, which is formed from the N. alveolaris inferior and divides into Rr. dentales inferiores. In addition, the anterior teeth of the Mandibula are reached by the N. mentalis. The innervation of the gingiva is even more complex than the sensory innervation of the teeth (→ Fig. 8.165).

Clinical remarks

Because of the individual differences in the shape of the third molar (**wisdom tooth,** Dens serotinus, Dens molaris permanens III) and the Mandibula, the decision to leave in place or remove the wisdom teeth is dependent on the specific conditions with each patient (→ Fig. a). Orthodontists use **braces** as a temporary measure to adjust and correct the position of the teeth to ensure correct bite symmetry and improved dental health (→ Fig. b).

a Panoramic X-ray image of the upper and lower jaw of an adult; 1. incisor I; 2: incisor II; 3: canine; 4: premolar I; 5: premolar II; 6: molar I; 7. molar II; 8: molar III (wisdom tooth)
b Braces on the upper and lower teeth of an adult.
[S700-T1129]

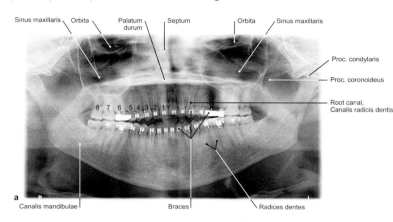

Sinus maxillaris | Orbita | Palatum durum | Septum | Orbita | Sinus maxillaris
Proc. condylaris
Proc. coronoideus
Root canal, Canalis radicis dentis
8 7 6 5 4 3 2 1
a
Canalis mandibulae | Braces | Radices dentes

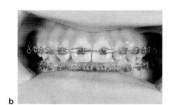

b

Clinical remarks

Fractures of the Mandibula are frequent. Due to the U-shaped structure of the Mandibula, various types of fractures can occur, in particular at the level of the canines and the third molars (arrows in → figure). At the site of the fracture, extravasated blood from ruptured blood vessels collects in the loose connective tissue on the floor of the mouth and causes small spots of bleeding under the skin **(ecchymoses),** which is a typical sign of a mandibular fracture.

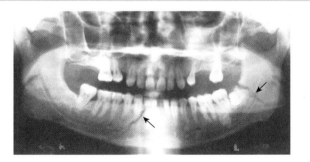

[E393]

Clinical remarks

Because the **teeth and gingiva of the maxilla** are innervated by different nerve branches, a local infiltration anaesthesia has to be applied tooth by tooth. For the **teeth of the Mandibula,** a nerve block is used. The N. alveolaris inferior is hereby anaesthetised shortly before it enters the Canalis mandibularis. Because the N. lingualis is also anaesthetised, this leads to a sensory block in the ipsilateral half of the tongue with the exception of the tip of the tongue. The chin and parts of the lower lip are also numb since the terminal branch of the N. alveolaris inferior is also anaesthetised.

The local infiltration anaesthesia targets the branches of the N. infraorbitalis [V/2] and the N. alveolaris inferior [V/3]. The goal is to anaesthetise defined areas of the gingiva, lips, chin and tongue, as all terminal branches of the N. infraorbitalis and N. alveolaris inferior are also anaesthetised.

Abbreviations: ASA = anterior superior alveolar block, B = buccal block, GP = greater palatine block, IA = inferior alveolar block, IN = incisivus block, IO = infraorbital block, MSA = middle superior alveolar block, NP = nasopalatine block, PSA = posterior superior alveolar block

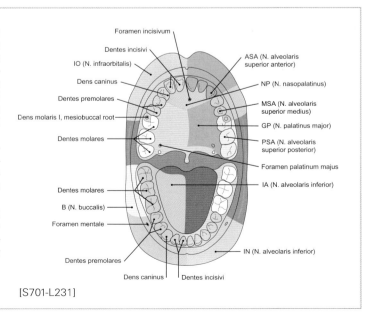

Foramen incisivum
Dentes incisivi
IO (N. infraorbitalis)
Dens caninus
Dentes premolares
Dens molaris I, mesiobuccal root
Dentes molares
Dentes molares
B (N. buccalis)
Foramen mentale
Dentes premolares
Dens caninus | Dentes incisivi
ASA (N. alveolaris superior anterior)
NP (N. nasopalatinus)
MSA (N. alveolaris superior medius)
GP (N. palatinus major)
PSA (N. alveolaris superior posterior)
Foramen palatinum majus
IA (N. alveolaris inferior)
IN (N. alveolaris inferior)

[S701-L231]

Fossa pterygopalatina and Ganglion pterygopalatinum

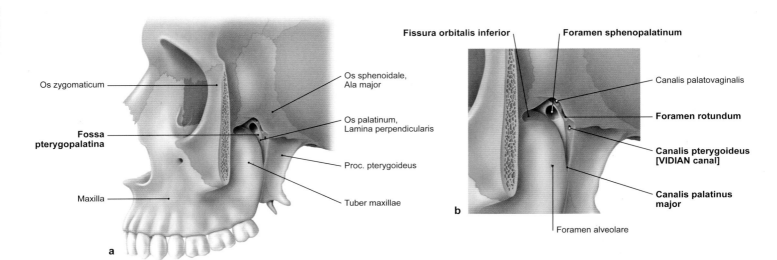

Os zygomaticum

Fossa pterygopalatina

Maxilla

Os sphenoidale, Ala major

Os palatinum, Lamina perpendicularis

Proc. pterygoideus

Tuber maxillae

a

Fissura orbitalis inferior

Foramen sphenopalatinum

Canalis palatovaginalis

Foramen rotundum

Canalis pterygoideus [VIDIAN canal]

Canalis palatinus major

b

Foramen alveolare

Fig. 8.156a and b   Fossa pterygopalatina, left side; lateral view; for colour chart, see p. XIII. [S700-L275]
a Overview.
b Detail in magnification.
The Fossa pterygopalatina is a neural switching area between the middle cranial fossa, the orbit and the nose. The maxilla, Os palatinum and Os sphenoidale also define the margins of this fossa. It is confined at

the front by the Tuber maxillae, at the back by the Proc. pterygoideus, medially by the Lamina perpendicularis of the Os palatinum and above by the Ala major of the Os sphenoidale. The fossa continues into the Fissura orbitalis inferior above. At the back, the fossa opens into the retropharyngeal space; laterally it opens widely into the Fossa infratemporalis.

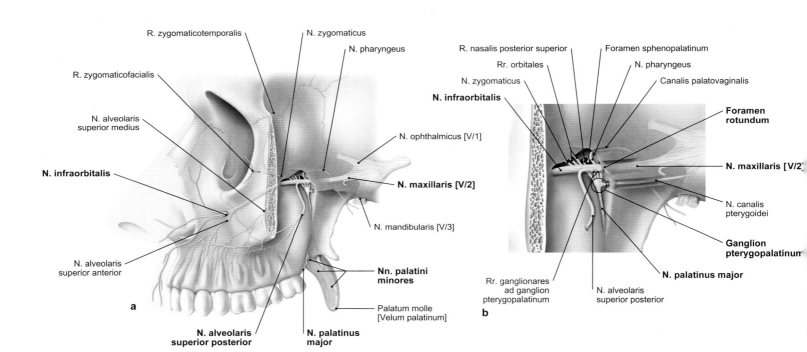

R. zygomaticotemporalis

N. zygomaticus

N. pharyngeus

R. zygomaticofacialis

N. alveolaris superior medius

N. infraorbitalis

N. ophthalmicus [V/1]

N. maxillaris [V/2]

N. mandibularis [V/3]

N. alveolaris superior anterior

Nn. palatini minores

Palatum molle [Velum palatinum]

a

N. alveolaris superior posterior

N. palatinus major

R. nasalis posterior superior

Rr. orbitales

N. zygomaticus

N. infraorbitalis

Foramen sphenopalatinum

N. pharyngeus

Canalis palatovaginalis

Foramen rotundum

N. maxillaris [V/2]

N. canalis pterygoidei

Ganglion pterygopalatinum

N. palatinus major

Rr. ganglionares ad ganglion pterygopalatinum

N. alveolaris superior posterior

b

Fig. 8.157a and b   N. maxillaris [V/2], left side; lateral view. [S700-L275]
a Terminal branches.
b Topographical relationship with the Ganglion pterygopalatinum.
The N. maxillaris [V/2] exits the base of the skull through the **Foramen rotundum** to enter the Fossa pterygopalatina, and exits this fossa through the **Fissura infraorbitalis.** In the Fossa pterygopalatina, the orbital branches, the N. zygomaticus, the N. alveolaris superior posterior and the Rr. ganglionares to the **Ganglion pterygopalatinum** branch off.

Sensory nerve fibres run within the Rr. ganglionares of the N. maxillaris [V/2] via the **Ganglion pterygopalatinum** to reach the soft and hard palate. Parasympathetic fibres from the Nucleus salivatorius superior reach the Ganglion pterygopalatinum via the N. facialis [VII] (N. intermedius), the N. petrosus major and the N. canalis pterygoidei, and are switched here from preganglionic to postganglionic. The postganglionic parasymphathetic fibres innervate the lacrimal, nasal and palatine glands. Postganglionic sympathetic fibres which originate from the N. caroticus internus (Plexus caroticus internus), assemble as the N. petrosus profundus and pass through the Ganglion pterygopalatinum to the lacrimal, nasal and palatine glands.

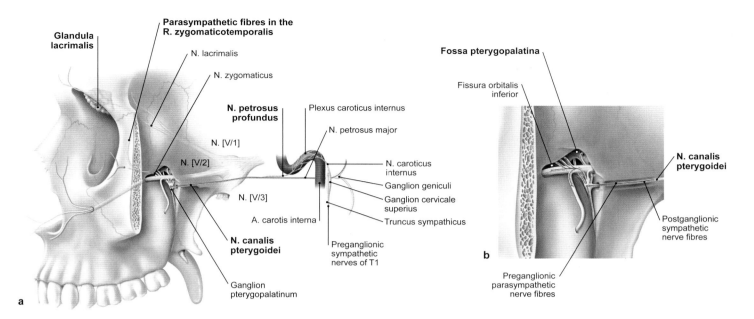

Fig. 8.158a and b **N. canalis pterygoidei, left side;** lateral view. [S700-L275]
a Overview.
b Nerves in the Fossa pterygopalatine.
Parasympathetic fibres of the N. facialis [VII], which form the N. petrosus major, reach the Ganglion pterygopalatinum and are switched here

from pre- to postganglionic fibres which then run downwards to the lacrimal, nasal and palatine glands. **Postganglionic sympathetic** fibres originating from the Plexus caroticus internus, assemble to the N. petrosus profundus and pass through the Ganglion pterygopalatinum without switching. They also reach the lacrimal, nasal and palatine glands.

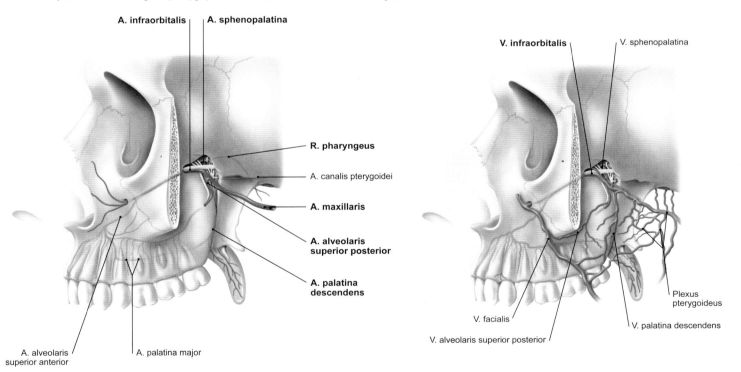

Fig. 8.159 **A. maxillaris in the Fossa pterygopalatina, left side;** lateral view. [S700-L275]
In the Fossa pterygopalatina, the A. maxillaris divides into its **terminal branches:** Aa. infraorbitalis, sphenopalatina, alveolaris superior posterior, palatina descendens and R. pharyngeus.

Fig. 8.160 **Veins in the Fossa pterygopalatina, left side;** lateral view. [S700-L275]
The Vv. infraorbitalis, sphenopalatina, alveolaris superior posterior and palatina descendens drain into the **Plexus pterygoideus,** which lies in the Fossa infratemporalis.

Clinical remarks

A lesion of the parasympathetic fibres exiting the brain in association with the N. facialis [VII], which finally reach the lacrimal gland via branches of the N. ophthalmicus [V/1] can result in a reduced production of lacrimal fluid by the lacrimal gland, leading to a **dry eye syndrome** ('SICCA' syndrome).

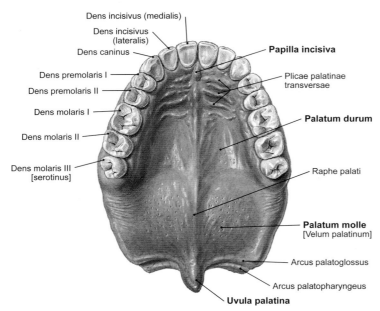

Dens incisivus (medialis)
Dens incisivus (lateralis)
Dens caninus
Dens premolaris I
Dens premolaris II
Dens molaris I
Dens molaris II
Dens molaris III [serotinus]

Papilla incisiva
Plicae palatinae transversae
Palatum durum
Raphe palati
Palatum molle [Velum palatinum]
Arcus palatoglossus
Arcus palatopharyngeus
Uvula palatina

Fig. 8.161 Hard palate, Palatum durum, and soft palate, Palatum molle; view from below. [S700]
The palate (Palatum) forms the roof of the oral cavity and the floor of the nasal cavity. It therefore forms a border between the oral and nasal cavities. At the front it consists of the hard palate (Palatum durum) and at the back the soft palate (Palatum molle).
The **hard palate** contributes to the phonation of consonants and serves as an abutment for the tongue when crushing food. Here, located on both sides of the midline, are several shallow, corrugated, mucosal ridges (Plicae palatinae transversae, Rugae palatinae). They serve to grind and hold ingested food.
The **soft palate** is flexible and blocks off the nasopharynx during swallowing by folding back onto the posterior pharyngeal wall.

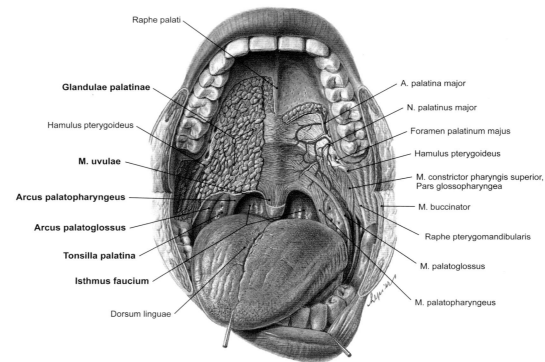

Raphe palati
Glandulae palatinae
Hamulus pterygoideus
M. uvulae
Arcus palatopharyngeus
Arcus palatoglossus
Tonsilla palatina
Isthmus faucium
Dorsum linguae

A. palatina major
N. palatinus major
Foramen palatinum majus
Hamulus pterygoideus
M. constrictor pharyngis superior, Pars glossopharyngea
M. buccinator
Raphe pterygomandibularis
M. palatoglossus
M. palatopharyngeus

Fig. 8.162 Oral cavity, Cavitas oris, and palatine muscles, Mm. palati; frontal view. [S700]
The palate is covered by a thick mucosal layer firmly attached to the periosteum. In its subepithelial layers, 'clusters' of small salivary glands (Glandulae palatinae) are found. The movable soft palate joins up towards the back and at its end, forms the uvula. The latter consists of a muscle (M. uvulae) and mucosal glands.

Laterally, the **palatine arches** (Arcus palatoglossus and Arcus palatopharyngeus), which at their base have muscles of the same name (Mm. palatoglossus and palatopharyngeus), insert into the soft palate and the uvula. The palatine arches frame the Tonsilla palatina on one side. They create the **pharyngeal isthmus** (Isthmus faucium), the muscle-controlled entrance to the pharynx.

→ T 4

Clinical remarks

Cleft formations of the palate, jaw and face can vary greatly. They are attributable to an insufficient mesenchymal proliferation, as a result of which the jaw and nasal crests fail to fuse. The uni- or bilateral clefting of the upper lip is commonly known as a 'harelip'. In severe forms, the clefting continues backwards into the palate as **lip-jaw-palate fissures** which occur in 1:2,500 births, and affect girls more

frequently than boys. An **isolated cleft palate** occurs when the two halves of the secondary palate do not fuse with each other or do not fuse with the primary palate. The mildest form is a cleft uvula (**Uvula bifida**). These clefts are not genetic malformations, but can be attributed to a folic acid deficiency in the mother's diet during pregnancy.

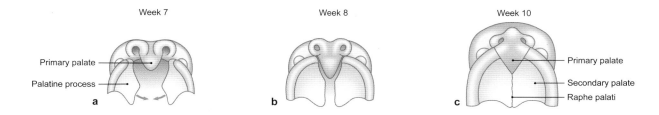

Week 7

Primary palate
Palatine process
a

Week 8

b

Week 10

Primary palate
Secondary palate
Raphe palati
c

Fig. 8.163a–c   Development of the palate, separation of the nasal and oropharyngeal cavities. [E838]
From the medial nasal prominences, the intermaxillary segment emerges from the depths, from which the philtrum of the upper lip, part of the maxilla (with the four incisors), and part of the palate (which forms the primary palate) develop. The primary palate extends into the anterior part of the oronasal cavity. The main part of the definitive bony palate is formed by the palatine processes which develop from the maxillary processes. In the seventh week, the tongue moves into a caudal position, the palatine processes are aligned horizontally and grow towards each other between the nasal cavity and the oral cavity, and merge in the midline to become the secondary palate. In the anterior part, these palatine processes fuse with the primary palate.

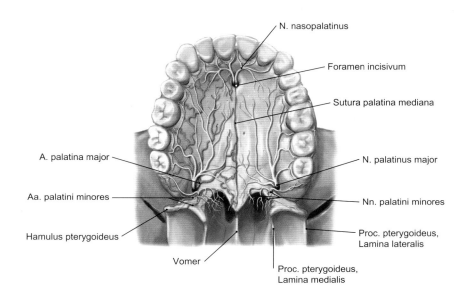

N. nasopalatinus
Foramen incisivum
Sutura palatina mediana
A. palatina major
N. palatinus major
Aa. palatini minores
Nn. palatini minores
Hamulus pterygoideus
Proc. pterygoideus, Lamina lateralis
Vomer
Proc. pterygoideus, Lamina medialis

Fig. 8.164   Arterial blood supply and nerves of the palate; view from below. [S702-L266]
Blood vessels and nerves reach the palate from cranially via the Foramen incisivum and the Foramina palatina majora and minora. The nerves are derived from the N. maxillaris [V/2].

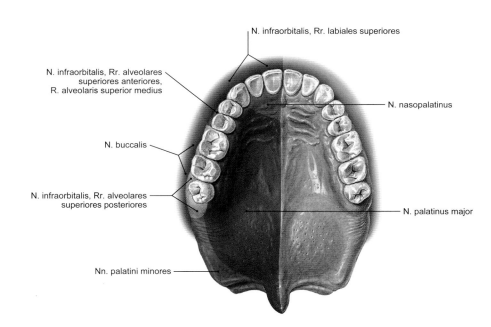

N. infraorbitalis, Rr. labiales superiores
N. infraorbitalis, Rr. alveolares superiores anteriores, R. alveolaris superior medius
N. nasopalatinus
N. buccalis
N. infraorbitalis, Rr. alveolares superiores posteriores
N. palatinus major
Nn. palatini minores

Fig. 8.165   Sensory innervation of the mucous membrane of the hard palate, Palatum durum, the soft palate, Palatum molle, as well as of the gingiva and the Vestibulum oris; view from below. [S700]
The sensory innervation of the palatine mucosa, upper lip, cheeks and gums is provided by various branches of the N. trigeminus [V]: N. maxillaris [V/3] and N. buccalis of the N. mandibularis [V/2].

Muscles of the palate

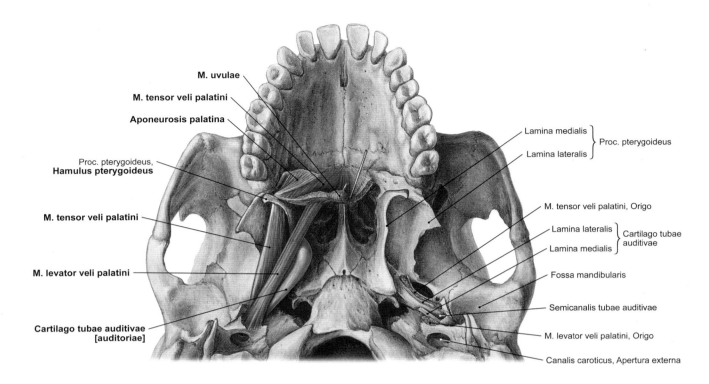

Fig. 8.166   M. levator veli palatini, M. tensor veli palatini and cartilage of the auditory tube, Cartilago tubae auditivae; view from below. [S700]

The M. tensor veli palatini and M. levator veli palatini provide tension to the **Aponeurosis palatina.** Both muscles are attached at the base of the skull. The Hamulus pterygoideus serves as a hypomochlion (centre of rotation of a joint) for the M. tensor veli palatini. The muscles pull the soft palate backwards and upwards upon contraction, which functions as a **closure between the nasopharynx and oropharynx** during the swallowing process. In addition, these muscles participate in the opening of the Tuba auditiva [auditoria] (→ Fig. 10.36).

→ T 4

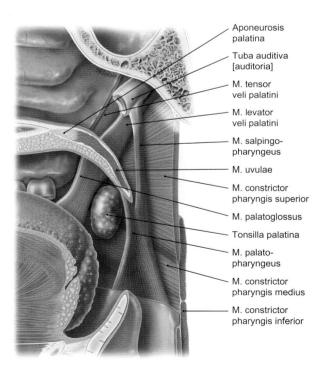

Fig. 8.167   Muscles of the soft palate, Palatum molle, right side; view from the left side. [S702-L238]/[E633-003]

In addition to the M. tensor veli palatini and M. levator veli palatini depicted in → Fig. 8.166 – which serve to raise the soft palate and open the Tuba auditiva – the M. uvulae of the M. palatoglossus and the M. palatopharyngeus radiate into the **Aponeurosis palatina,** serving to squeeze out the mucous glands of the uvula. The last two muscles pull the soft palate downwards upon contraction which reopens the passage **between the nasopharynx and oropharynx** after swallowing.

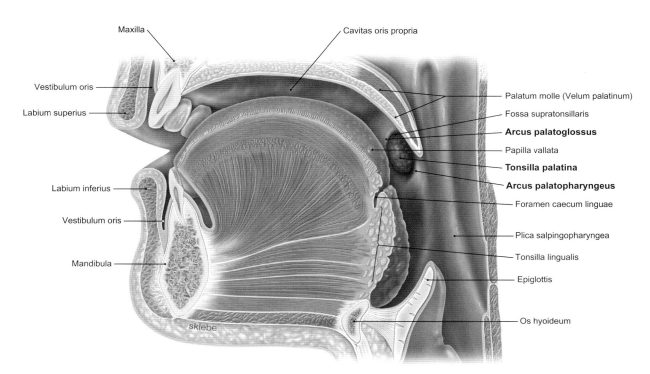

Fig. 8.168   Tongue, Lingua, in the oral cavity; medial view of a sagittal section of the oral cavity. [S700-L238]
Behind the Sulcus terminalis, the base of the tongue and the lingual tonsil (Tonsilla lingualis) are connected. The Tonsilla lingualis is part of the WALDEYER's tonsillar ring, which also includes the Tonsilla palatina which is located between the two palatine arches (Arcus palatoglossus and Arcus palatopharyngeus).

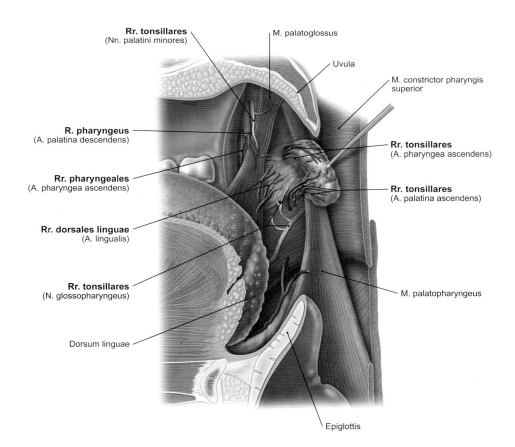

Fig. 8.169   Blood supply and innervation of the palatine tonsil, right side; medial view. [S702-L238]
Involved in the blood supply of the Tonsilla palatina are the **Rr. tonsillares** of the A. palatina ascendens, the R. pharyngeus of the A. palatina descendens and the Rr. pharyngeales of the A. pharyngea ascendens, as well as the Rr. dorsales linguae of the A. lingualis. The innervation of the tonsillar bed is provided by the **Rr. tonsillares** of the Nn. palatini minores and the N. glossopharyngeus [IX].

Palatine tonsil, blood supply

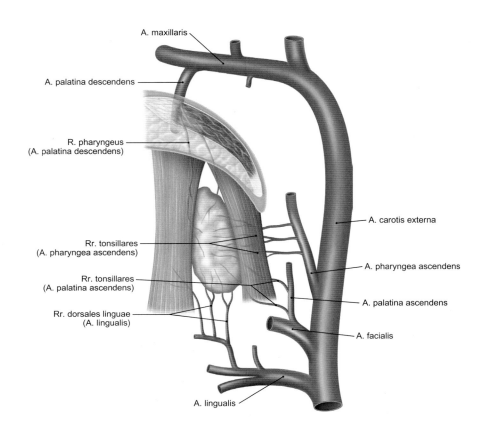

A. maxillaris

A. palatina descendens

R. pharyngeus
(A. palatina descendens)

A. carotis externa

Rr. tonsillares
(A. pharyngea ascendens)

A. pharyngea ascendens

Rr. tonsillares
(A. palatina ascendens)

A. palatina ascendens

Rr. dorsales linguae
(A. lingualis)

A. facialis

A. lingualis

Fig. 8.170   Blood supply of the palatine tonsil, Tonsilla palatina, right side; medial view, schematic diagram. [S700-L275]
The Tonsilla palatina receives blood from four different arteries:
- R. pharyngeus of the **A. palatina descendens** from the A. maxillaris
- Rr. pharyngeales of the **A. pharyngea ascendens** from the A. carotis externa
- Rr. tonsillares of the **A. palatina ascendens** from the A. facialis
- Rr. dorsales linguae of the **A. lingualis** from the A. carotis externa.

Pharyngeal lymphoid ring (WALDEYER's ring)	
Definition	**Components**
A group of lymphoepithelial tissues that is located at the transition from the oral cavity and the nasal cavity to the pharynx. As a whole, they form a ring. The pharyngeal lymphoid ring gives immune defence and is part of the mucosa-associated lymphoid tissue (MALT).	• pharyngeal tonsil (Tonsilla pharyngea) → Fig. 8.108, → Fig. 8.131 • tubal tonsils (Tonsillae tubariae) → Fig. 8.162 • palatine tonsils (Tonsillae palatinae) → Fig. 8.162 • lingual tonsil (Tonsilla lingualis) • bilateral parapharyngeal MALT aggregates

Clinical remarks

The fascia in the pharynx and neck form partially conjoined spaces or compartments, which allow the spread of infections within these compartments (→ figure). An infection of the palatine tonsils (**tonsillitis**) can lead to bacteria spreading into the pharyngeal space in the neck (→ Fig. 11.26) and from there into other spaces in the neck which can result in abscesses and sepsis.

Frequently recurrent infection of the palatine tonsils is an indication for their surgical removal **(tonsillectomy),** one of the most common surgical ENT procedures. Postoperative bleeding can occur for up to three weeks (in rare cases even longer) after the operation, and is feared as a serious complication.

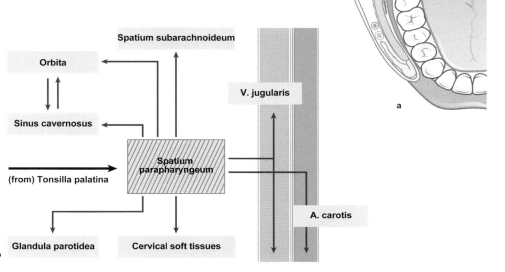

[S701-L126]/[G1060-003]

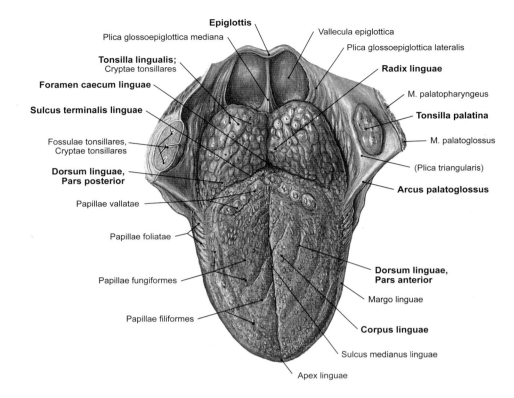

Fig. 8.171   Tongue, Lingua; view from above. [S700]
On the **dorsum of the tongue** (Dorsum linguae), the Sulcus medianus linguae divides the tongue into a right and a left half. The Sulcus terminalis linguae (a V-shaped furrow) forms the border between the Corpus linguae and the Radix linguae, and divides the tongue into a Pars anterior and a Pars posterior. At the tip of the Sulcus terminalis linguae, the surface epithelium sinks into the **Foramen caecum linguae.** This foramen is where the thyroid gland started its descent from the ectoderm of the floor of the mouth before reaching its final destination in front of the larynx (origin of the Ductus thyroglossalis).

The mucosa of the Pars anterior is rough since it contains multiple small, partially macroscopically visible papillae (Papillae linguales, filiformes, foliatae, fungiformes and vallatae), which play a role in the perception of touch and taste sensations.
The **root of the tongue** (Radix linguae) is covered by the lingual tonsil, which is framed laterally by the two palatine arches, Arcus palatoglossus and Arcus palatopharyngeus, and at the back by the epiglottis. From the root of the tongue, the unpaired Plica glossoepiglottica mediana and the paired Plicae glossoepiglotticae laterales extend to the epiglottis and delineate the Valleculae epiglotticae.

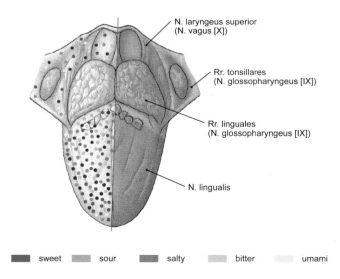

| sweet | sour | salty | bitter | umami |

Fig. 8.172   Innervation and sense of taste of the dorsum of the tongue. [S700-L238]
The N. lingualis, a branch of the N. mandibularis [V/3], provides the sensory innervation of the Pars anterior of the tongue, while the Rr. linguales of the N. glossopharyngeus [IX] supply the area of the Sulcus terminalis linguae, and the N. laryngeus superior, a branch of the N. vagus [X], innervates the base of the tongue.
Taste sensations from the **anterior two-thirds** of the tongue are conveyed by branches of the N. facialis [VII] (Chorda tympani, N. intermedius) to the upper part of the Tractus solitarius in the brainstem; the

perikarya of these sensory fibres are located in the Ganglion geniculi. Taste sensations from the **posterior third** of the tongue are projected to the lower part of the Tractus solitarius in the brainstem by sensory fibres of the N. glossopharyngeus [IX] and N. vagus [X]. The perikarya of these nerve fibres reside in the Ganglion inferius of the N. glossopharyngeus [IX] or the N. vagus [X].
All the areas in the anterior two-thirds of the tongue are capable of perceiving all five basic senses of taste, albeit with different intensity. One therefore perceives the taste of sweet things at the tip of the tongue and bitter things at the posterior one-third of the tongue.

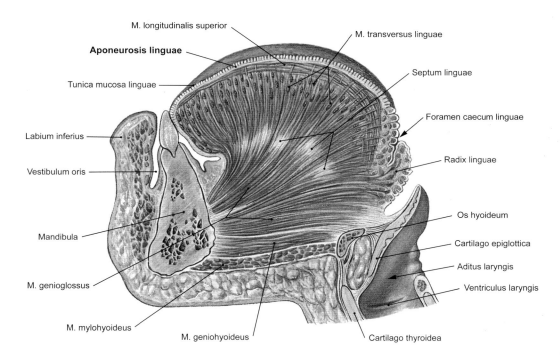

Fig. 8.173 labels: M. longitudinalis superior, Aponeurosis linguae, Tunica mucosa linguae, Labium inferius, Vestibulum oris, Mandibula, M. genioglossus, M. mylohyoideus, M. geniohyoideus, M. transversus linguae, Septum linguae, Foramen caecum linguae, Radix linguae, Os hyoideum, Cartilago epiglottica, Aditus laryngis, Ventriculus laryngis, Cartilago thyroidea

Fig. 8.173 Tongue, Lingua, and muscles of the tongue, Mm. linguae; median section. [S700]
The tongue is a highly flexible muscular body. It plays a significant role in chewing and swallowing and makes sucking and speaking possible. It is also an important instrument of taste and contains the taste organ. A distinction is made between internal and external muscles which originate from the skeleton and radiate into the body of the tongue. The external muscles change the position of the tongue, while the internal muscles of the tongue modify its shape. The majority of these muscles insert at the largest part of the **Aponeurosis linguae,** a tough plate of connective tissue beneath the mucosa of the dorsum of the tongue.

→ T 3.1

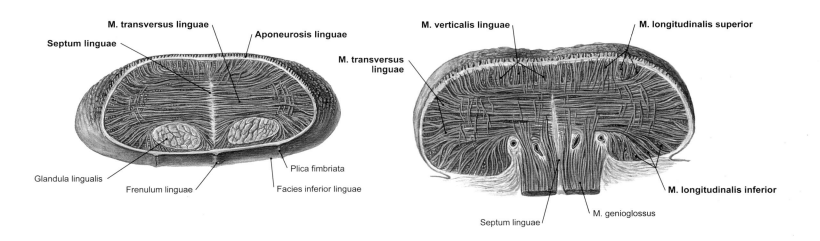

Fig. 8.174 labels: M. transversus linguae, Septum linguae, Aponeurosis linguae, Glandula lingualis, Frenulum linguae, Plica fimbriata, Facies inferior linguae

Fig. 8.175 labels: M. verticalis linguae, M. longitudinalis superior, M. transversus linguae, M. longitudinalis inferior, Septum linguae, M. genioglossus

Fig. 8.174 Tongue, Lingua, and internal muscles of the tongue, Mm. linguae interni; cross-section through the tip of the tongue. [S700]
The internal muscles of the tongue weave through the spatial planes like wickerwork. In the median plane, the Septum linguae intersects the tongue incompletely into two halves. Agonistic and antagonistic muscles facilitate the flexibility of the tongue. In the area of the tip of the tongue there is a salivary gland (Glandula lingualis, gland of BLANDIN-NUHN) on both sides.

→ T 3.1

Fig. 8.175 Tongue, Lingua, and internal muscles of the tongue, M. linguae interni; cross-section at the level of the middle part. [S700]
The internal muscles originate and insert in the tongue. A distinction is made between the Mm. longitudinales superior and inferior, transversus linguae and verticalis linguae. The muscles are perpendicular to each other in the three spatial planes and they interlace. The powerful malleability of the tongue makes functions such as chewing, sucking, singing, talking and whistling possible. The M. genioglossus belongs to the external muscles of the tongue.

→ T 3.1

Hyoid bone and hyoid bone musculature

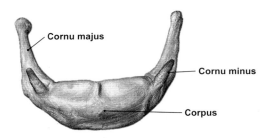

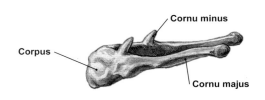

Fig. 8.176 Hyoid bone, Os hyoideum; frontal view from above. [S700]
The horseshoe-shaped hyoid consists of a body (Corpus) and the paired greater and lesser horns (Cornua majora and minora).

Fig. 8.177 Hyoid bone, Os hyoideum; lateral view. [S700]

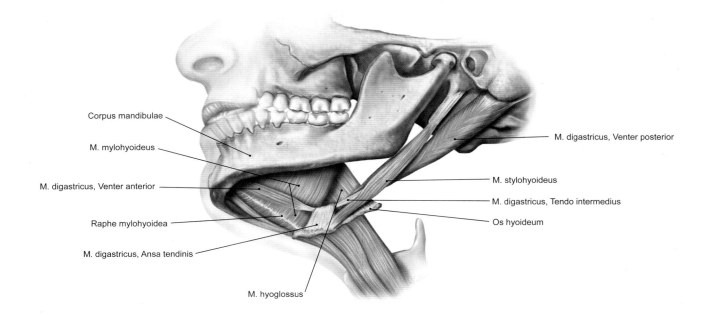

Fig. 8.178 Oral region; lateral view from below. [S700-L266]
The muscular oral diaphragm, **Diaphragma oris,** consists of the two Mm. mylohyoidei and forms the floor of the oral cavity. In addition, the Mm. geniohyoidei (not shown) and digastrici are part of the structure of the floor of the mouth. Since all muscles are directly or indirectly linked to the hyoid, they are treated together with the Mm. stylohyoidei as **Mm. suprahyoidei** (suprahyoid muscles). Functionally, the floor of the mouth represents an adjustable abutment for the tongue.

→ T 3.2, T 10

Clinical remarks

Touching the base of the tongue, the palatine arches or the posterior wall of the pharynx triggers a **swallowing** or **gag reflex.** The muscles of the tongue, pharynx, larynx and oesophagus are part of these reflexes.
Allergic reactions can result in a life-threatening swelling of the mucosal lining of the soft palate.
Inflammation of the palatine mucosa, in particular of the soft palate, typically leads to severe difficulty in swallowing.
Circulatory disorders of the brainstem are often associated with paralysis of the palatine muscles, resulting in difficulties swallowing and tube ventilation disorders. In affected patients, there may be a paralysis of the soft palate (lesion of the nuclear areas of the N. glossopharyngeus [IX] and N. vagus [X]). Due to paralysis of the M. levator veli palatini, the soft palate may hang down on the affected side. The uvula moves to the healthy side.
Often the tongue is the first site of injury during **chemical burns and scalding.** At the margin of the tongue, potential **precancerous** conditions may occur in the form of hyperkeratoses or leukoplakias.

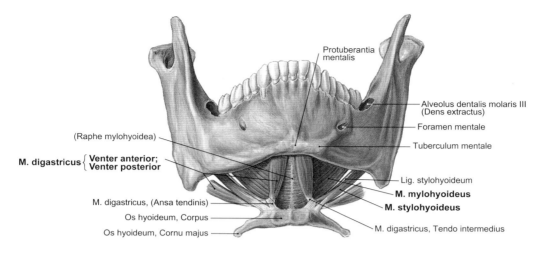

Protuberantia mentalis

Alveolus dentalis molaris III (Dens extractus)

Foramen mentale

Tuberculum mentale

(Raphe mylohyoidea)

M. digastricus { Venter anterior; Venter posterior

Lig. stylohyoideum

M. mylohyoideus

M. stylohyoideus

M. digastricus, (Ansa tendinis)

Os hyoideum, Corpus

Os hyoideum, Cornu majus

M. digastricus, Tendo intermedius

Fig. 8.179 Lower jaw, Mandibula, and muscles of the floor of the mouth, Mm. suprahyoidei; frontal view. [S700]
The oral diaphragm (Diaphragma oris) is formed by muscles that belong to the suprahyoid muscles. The central muscle of the floor of the mouth is the **M. mylohyoideus,** which extends between the two Rami mandibulae on both sides to the front; both parts of the muscle join in the midline at

the Raphe mylohyoidea. Underneath that is the paired Venter anterior of the **M. digastricus,** which is connected via an intermediate tendon to the Venter posterior of the M. digastricus. The intermediate tendon is fixed to the hyoid bone by means of a connective tissue loop. As the third suprahyoid muscle, the **M. stylohyoideus** can be seen coming from the hyoid.

→ T 10

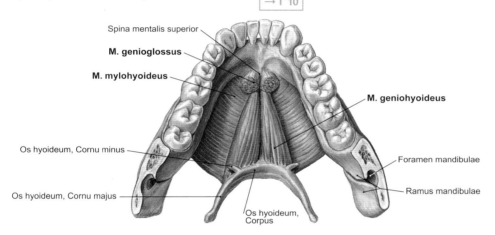

Spina mentalis superior

M. genioglossus

M. mylohyoideus

M. geniohyoideus

Os hyoideum, Cornu minus

Foramen mandibulae

Ramus mandibulae

Os hyoideum, Cornu majus

Os hyoideum, Corpus

Fig. 8.180 Lower jaw, Mandibula, muscles of the floor of the mouth, Mm. suprahyoidei, and hyoid bone, Os hyoideum; view from above. [S700]
The Diaphragma oris formed by both Mm. mylohyoidei can be seen, on which the paired **Mm. geniohyoidei,** belonging to the suprahyoid

muscles, run from the inner surface of the Mandibula to the hyoid bone. The overlying M. genioglossus, which is part of the external muscles of the tongue, has been severed just behind its origin at the Spina mentalis superior of the Mandibula.

→ T 10

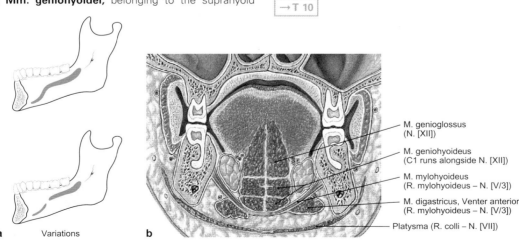

M. genioglossus (N. [XII])

M. geniohyoideus (C1 runs alongside N. [XII])

M. mylohyoideus (R. mylohyoideus – N. [V/3])

M. digastricus, Venter anterior (R. mylohyoideus – N. [V/3])

Platysma (R. colli – N. [VII])

a   Variations   b

Fig. 8.181a and b Linea mylohyoidea and structure of the floor of the oral cavity.
a Variants of the Linea mylohyoidea; medial view of a cross-section of the Mandibula. Schematic presentation of two variants of the Linea mylohyoidea on the insde of the Mandibula. [S700-L126]

b Structure of the floor of the oral cavity; frontal sectional view. The following structures lie on top of each other from exterior/inferior to interior/superior: (1) Platysma, (2) M. digastricus, Venter anterior; (3) M. mylohyoideus; (4) M. geniohyoideus; (5) M. genio-glossus. [S700-L238]/[G1080]

→ T 10

Muscles of the tongue

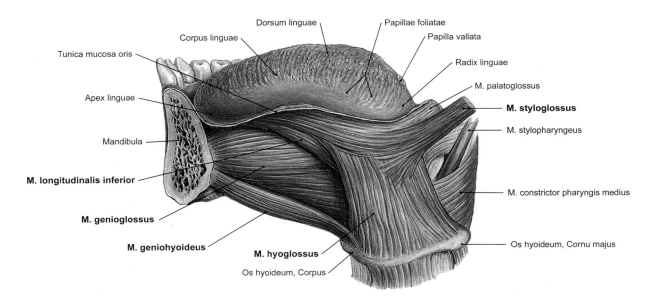

Fig. 8.182 Tongue, Lingua, and external muscles of the tongue, Mm. linguae externi; view from the left side. [S700]
The external muscles radiate into the tongue. They consist of the **Mm. genioglossus, hyoglossus and styloglossus.** The M. palatoglossus is also part of the external muscles of the tongue. The M. hyoglos-sus can receive functional support from the M. chondroglossus, which originates from the lesser horn of the Os hyoideum (→ Fig. 8.183 and → Fig. 8.184).

→ T 3.2

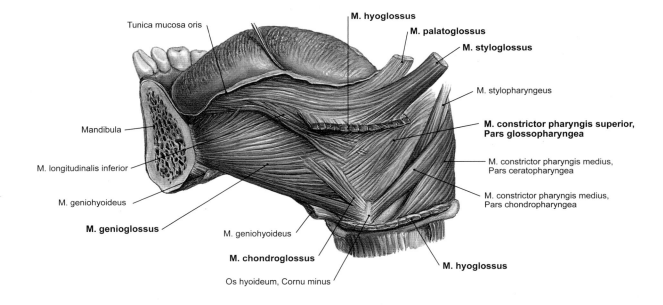

Fig. 8.183 Tongue, Lingua, and external muscles of the tongue, Mm. linguae externi; view from the left side. [S700]
With the M. hyoglossus removed, the small **M. chondroglossus** is vis-ible, which originates from the lesser horn of the Os hyoideum and functionally supports the M. hyoglossus. At the posterior aspect, in ad-dition to the external muscles of the tongue, the M. palatoglossus and the Pars glossopharyngea of the M. constrictor pharyngis superior ra-diate into the tongue.

→ T 3.2

Clinical remarks

The tongue can only be fully extended if the M. genioglossus is in-tact. In a state of **deep unconsciousness** the M. genioglossus goes slack. In the supine position, the tongue slips into the pharynx and can block the airway. This is why unconscious people must always be placed in a stable position on their side as a precaution.

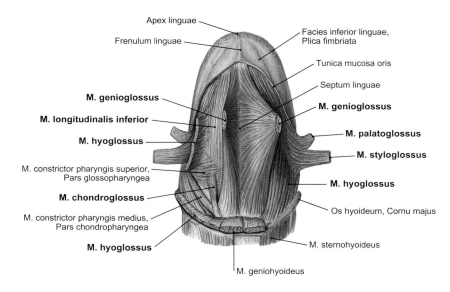

Apex linguae
Frenulum linguae
Facies inferior linguae, Plica fimbriata
Tunica mucosa oris
Septum linguae
M. genioglossus
M. genioglossus
M. longitudinalis inferior
M. palatoglossus
M. hyoglossus
M. styloglossus
M. constrictor pharyngis superior, Pars glossopharyngea
M. hyoglossus
M. chondroglossus
Os hyoideum, Cornu majus
M. constrictor pharyngis medius, Pars chondropharyngea
M. hyoglossus
M. sternohyoideus
M. geniohyoideus

Fig. 8.184   Muscles of the tongue, Mm. linguae; inferior view. [S700]
The M. genioglossus was removed at its mandibular origin. Also, the Mm. styloglossus and palatoglossus were removed. Laterally, the M. hyoglossus (severed at the right side of the tongue) and M. chon-droglossus are shown, which are also external muscles of the tongue. At the bottom of the tongue runs the M. longitudinalis inferior (internal muscle of the tongue).

→ T 3.2

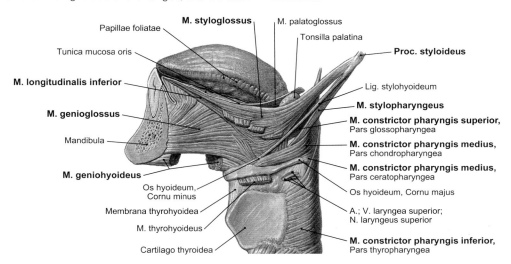

M. styloglossus
M. palatoglossus
Papillae foliatae
Tonsilla palatina
Tunica mucosa oris
Proc. styloideus
M. longitudinalis inferior
Lig. stylohyoideum
M. genioglossus
M. stylopharyngeus
Mandibula
M. constrictor pharyngis superior, Pars glossopharyngea
M. constrictor pharyngis medius, Pars chondropharyngea
M. geniohyoideus
M. constrictor pharyngis medius, Pars ceratopharyngea
Os hyoideum, Cornu minus
Os hyoideum, Cornu majus
Membrana thyrohyoidea
A.; V. laryngea superior; N. laryngeus superior
M. thyrohyoideus
Cartilago thyroidea
M. constrictor pharyngis inferior, Pars thyropharyngea

Fig. 8.185   External muscles of the tongue, Mm. linguae externi, and pharyngeal muscles, Mm. constrictores pharyngis; lateral view; mandibular arch removed. [S700]
The Lig. stylohyoideum extends between the M. styloglossus and M. stylopharyngeus. Located below this ligament are the pharyngeal muscles, the M. constrictor pharyngis superior with the Pars glosso-pharyngea, as well as the M. constrictor pharyngis medius with the Partes chondropharyngea and ceratopharyngea. Below the hyoid bone is the M. constrictor pharyngis inferior with the Pars thyropharyngea.

→ T 3.2, T 6

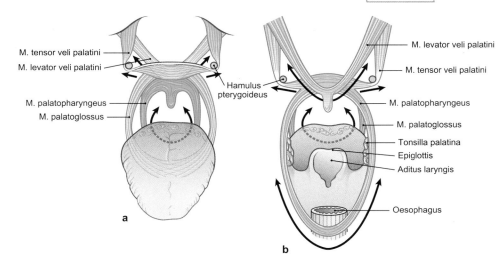

M. tensor veli palatini
M. levator veli palatini
M. levator veli palatini
M. tensor veli palatini
Hamulus pterygoideus
M. palatopharyngeus
M. palatopharyngeus
M. palatoglossus
M. palatoglossus
Tonsilla palatina
Epiglottis
Aditus laryngis
Oesophagus
a
b

Fig. 8.186a and b   Muscular loop system for the act of swallowing. [S700-L126]
a Anterior view.
b Posterior view.
Along with the M. palatopharyngeus and the palatine muscles (M. tensor veli palatini and the M. levator veli palatini), the M. palatoglossus forms a muscular loop structure which is critically impor-tant for narrowing the Isthmus faucium during swallowing (see also palate → Fig. 10.37, and act of swallowing → Fig. 11.20).

→ T 4

Compartments of the floor of the mouth, and vessels and nerves of the tongue

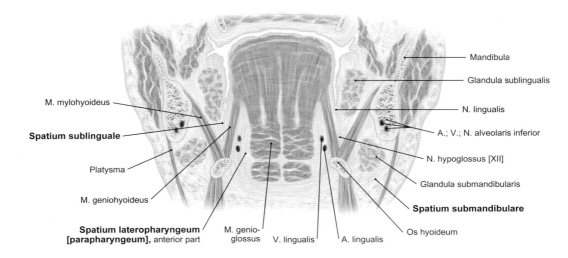

M. mylohyoideus

Spatium sublinguale

Platysma

M. geniohyoideus

Spatium lateropharyngeum [parapharyngeum], anterior part

M. genio-glossus

V. lingualis

A. lingualis

Mandibula

Glandula sublingualis

N. lingualis

A.; V.; N. alveolaris inferior

N. hypoglossus [XII]

Glandula submandibularis

Spatium submandibulare

Os hyoideum

Fig. 8.187 Compartments of the floor of the mouth, Diaphragma oris; horizontal section in the area of the Os hyoideum. [S702-L127] The muscles of the oral diaphragm are separated from each other by loose connective tissue spaces. These spaces, which are so-called compartments of the oral diaphragm, are the **Spatium parapharyn-** **geum,** in which the A. and V. lingualis run, the **Spatium sublinguale,** in which the N. lingualis runs, and the **Spatium submandibulare** with the Glandula submandibularis. All compartments of the oral diaphragm are posteriorly connected to the neurovascular structures of the neck.

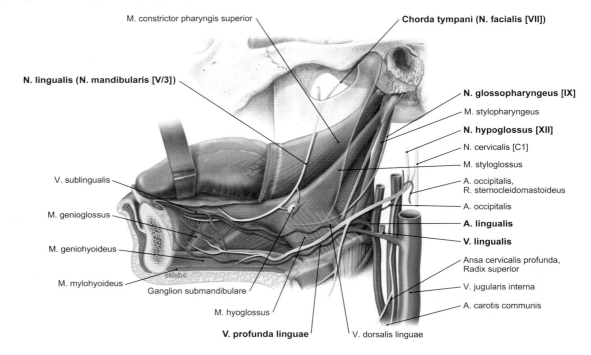

M. constrictor pharyngis superior

Chorda tympani (N. facialis [VII])

N. lingualis (N. mandibularis [V/3])

V. sublingualis

M. genioglossus

M. geniohyoideus

M. mylohyoideus

Ganglion submandibulare

M. hyoglossus

V. profunda linguae

V. dorsalis linguae

N. glossopharyngeus [IX]

M. stylopharyngeus

N. hypoglossus [XII]

N. cervicalis [C1]

M. styloglossus

A. occipitalis, R. sternocleidomastoideus

A. occipitalis

A. lingualis

V. lingualis

Ansa cervicalis profunda, Radix superior

V. jugularis interna

A. carotis communis

Fig. 8.188 Vessels and nerves of the tongue, Lingua; lateral view; mandibular arch removed. [S700-L238]

Clinical remarks

If **abscesses in the floor of the mouth** spread dorsally and caudally, and via the neurovascular structures of the neck into the mediastinum, this may give rise to life-threatening conditions. Inflammations in the soft tissue of the lower jaw are usually associated with a swelling of the submental and submandibular lymph nodes, which are palpable under the chin or in the submandibular triangle.

A unilateral **peripheral lesion of the N. hypoglossus [XII]** (in the example given in → figure on the right side) makes the outstretched tongue deviate to the affected side (in the example to the right side). Muscular atrophy can cause creasing of the mucosal surface on the paralysed side.

[G435]

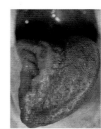

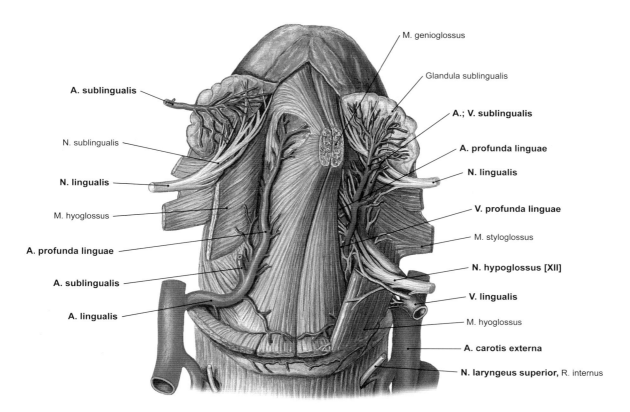

M. genioglossus

Glandula sublingualis

A. sublingualis

A.; V. sublingualis

N. sublingualis

A.; V. sublingualis

A. profunda linguae

N. lingualis

N. lingualis

M. hyoglossus

V. profunda linguae

A. profunda linguae

M. styloglossus

A. sublingualis

N. hypoglossus [XII]

A. lingualis

V. lingualis

M. hyoglossus

A. carotis externa

N. laryngeus superior, R. internus

Fig. 8.189 Vessels and nerves of the tongue, Lingua; frontal view from below. [S700]

The **arterial** supply of the tongue is provided by the A. lingualis from the A. carotis externa. Branches of the A. lingualis are the A. profunda linguae, which penetrates deep into the musculature of the tongue, mainly supplying the muscles of the middle and anterior parts of the tongue, and the A. sublingualis, which passes to the sublingual gland (Glandula sublingualis) and to the floor of the mouth. Projecting backwards, the Rr. dorsales linguae can communicate with each other, whereas all other branches are separated by the Septum linguae from each other and can therefore only provide arterial blood to one half of the tongue. The **venous** blood is drained via the V. lingualis. It is laterally adjacent to the M. hyoglossus and drains the blood of the tongue into the V. jugularis interna. The V. lingualis collects blood from the Vv. sublingualis, profunda linguae and dorsales linguae as well as from the V. comitans nervi hypoglossi.

With the exception of the M. palatoglossus which is innervated by the Plexus pharyngeus, the **motor** innervation of the tongue is via the N. hypoglossus [XII]. Sensory innervation in the anterior two-thirds of the tongue is provided by the N. lingualis, a branch of the N. mandibularis [V/3], in the region of the Sulcus terminalis by the N. glossopharyngeus [IX], and at the base of the tongue by the N. laryngeus superior (branch of the N. vagus [X]).

Branches of the A. lingualis:
- (R. hyoideus)
- Rr. dorsales linguae
- R. suprahyoideus
- A. sublingualis
- A. profunda linguae.

Innervation of the tongue

Nerve	Quality	Areas innervated
N. lingualis (branch of [V/3])	sensitive	anterior ⅔ of the tongue
N. glossopharyngeus [IX]	sensitive, sensory	posterior ⅓ of the tongue
N. vagus [X], N. laryngeus superior (branch of [X])	sensitive, sensory	transition to the epiglottis
Chorda tympani (branch of the N. intermedius as part of [VII])	sensory parasympathetic	• Papillae fungiformes • Glandula submandibularis, Glandula sublingualis, small salivary glands in the oral mucosa
N. hypoglossus [XII]	motor	all muscles of the tongue with the exception of the M. palatoglossus
Plexus pharyngeus (branches of [IX and X])	motor	M. palatoglossus

Clinical remarks

In the mucosa under the tongue is a **subepithelial venous plexus.** Therefore, medications administered sublingually are rapidly absorbed.

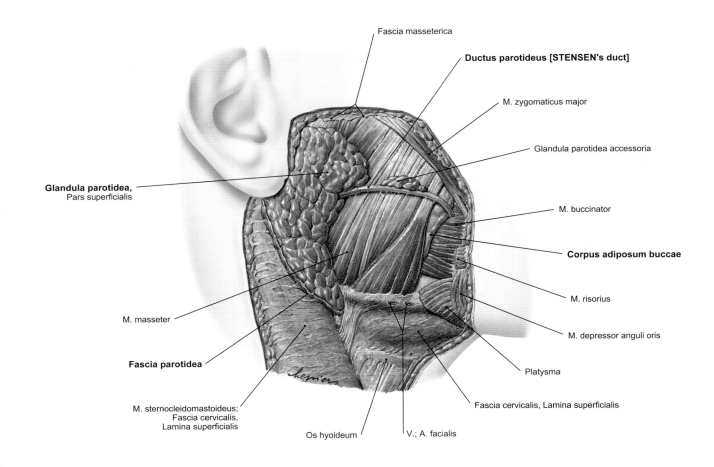

Fascia masseterica

Ductus parotideus [STENSEN's duct]

M. zygomaticus major

Glandula parotidea accessoria

M. buccinator

Corpus adiposum buccae

M. risorius

M. depressor anguli oris

Platysma

Fascia cervicalis, Lamina superficialis

V.; A. facialis

Os hyoideum

M. sternocleidomastoideus;
Fascia cervicalis,
Lamina superficialis

Fascia parotidea

M. masseter

Glandula parotidea,
Pars superficialis

Fig. 8.190   Parotid gland, Glandula parotidea, right side; lateral
view. [S700]
The purely serous Glandula parotidea is the largest oral salivary gland.
Its size and dimensions are quite variable. The Pars superficialis of the
gland is located immediately in front of the outer ear. It is surrounded by
a fascia of dense connective tissue (Fascia parotidea) (edges of the cut
shown).

The Fascia parotidea is the continuation of the Lamina superficialis of
the Fascia cervicalis. At the anterior margin of the gland, the Ductus
parotideus exits and runs horizontally across the upper half of the
M. masseter to the M. buccinator, piercing it, and, in the Papilla ductus
parotideus, opens into the Vestibulum oris opposite the second upper
molar tooth. Around the excretory duct, accessory glandular tissue
(Glandula parotidea accessoria) can often be found.

Clinical remarks

Surgical removal of tumours in the Glandula parotidea can result in
gustatory sweating (FREY's syndrome). During surgery, the sympathetic and parasympathetic nerve fibres innervating the glandular
parenchyma are severed. With postoperative regeneration, parasympathetic fibres may occasionally synapse with formerly sympathetically innervated sweat glands of the skin. Since the neurotransmitter
for the sympathetic innervation of the sweat glands is acetylcholine
(as with the parasympathetic nervous system), former sympathetically innervated sweat glands are now parasympathetically inner-

vated. In the case of parasympathetic activation (e. g. if a person is
hungry and sees something delicious to eat), the sweat glands are
also activated. Beads of sweat form on the cheek (gustatory sweating).
Parotitis epidemica, or mumps, is very painful, as the glandular tissue cannot expand when swelling occurs within the organ fascia.
Malignant **tumours of the Glandula parotidea** can lead to peripheral facial nerve lesions; in contrast, benign tumours of the Glandula
parotidea usually do not destroy the N. facialis [VII].

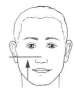

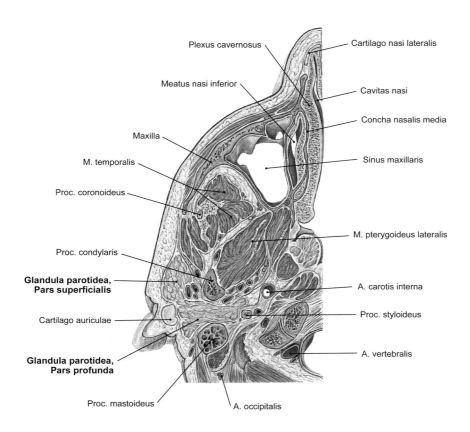

Plexus cavernosus

Meatus nasi inferior

Maxilla

M. temporalis

Proc. coronoideus

Proc. condylaris

Glandula parotidea, Pars superficialis

Cartilago auriculae

Glandula parotidea, Pars profunda

Proc. mastoideus

A. occipitalis

Cartilago nasi lateralis

Cavitas nasi

Concha nasalis media

Sinus maxillaris

M. pterygoideus lateralis

A. carotis interna

Proc. styloideus

A. vertebralis

Fig. 8.191 Parotid gland, Glandula parotidea, and masticatory muscles, Mm. masticatorii; horizontal section; view from below. [S700]
The Glandula parotidea consists of two parts. The upper **Pars superficialis** is located immediately in front of the outer ear. Projecting deep into the retromandibular fossa, the larger part of the gland **(Pars profunda)** is free of fascia. In this section, parts of the Mm. temporalis and pterygoideus lateralis can be seen between the Glandula parotidea and Sinus maxillaris.

Salivary glands of the oral cavity (Glandulae salivariae oris)	
In the oral cavity, there are three large salivary glands (Glandulae salivariae majores) and numerous small salivary glands (Glandulae salivariae minores).	
Large salivary glands	• parotid gland (Glandula parotidea) → Fig. 8.73, → Fig. 8.75, → Fig. 8.99, → Fig. 8.192, → Fig. 8.200 • submandibular gland (Glandula submandibularis) → Fig. 8.75, → Fig. 8.194 to → Fig. 8.200 • sublingual gland (Glandula sublingualis) → Fig. 8.115, → Fig. 8.195 to → Fig. 8.200
Small salivary glands	• labial glands (Glandulae labiales) → Fig. 8.126 • cheek (Glandulae buccales) → Fig. 8.126 • tongue (Glandulae linguales) → Fig. 8.174, → Fig. 8.198, → Fig. 8.199, → Fig. 8.200 • palatine glands (Glandulae palatinae) → Fig. 8.162 • molar glands (Glandulae molares)

8

Openings of the salivary glands

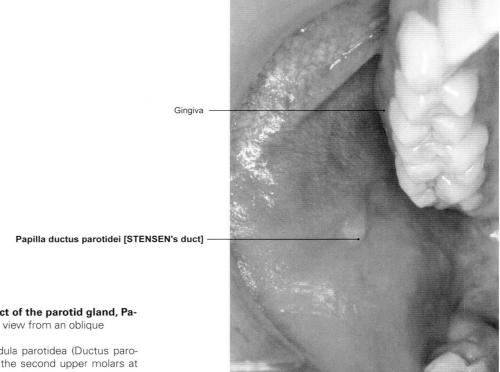

Fig. 8.192 Opening of the excretory duct of the parotid gland, Papilla ductus parotidei, right side; inferior view from an oblique angle. [S700-T910]
The excretory glandular duct of the Glandula parotidea (Ductus parotideus, STENSEN's duct) opens opposite the second upper molars at the Papilla ductus parotidei into the oral vestibule.

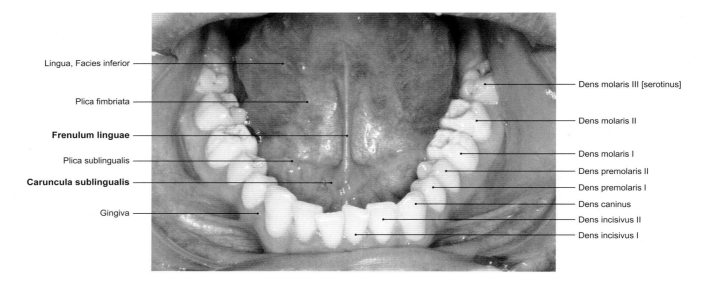

Fig. 8.193 Opening of the excretory duct of the submandibular gland, sublingual caruncle, Caruncula sublingualis; frontal superior view. [S700-T910]
The excretory duct of the Glandula submandibularis (Ductus submandibularis, WHARTON's duct) runs along the floor of the mouth (→ Fig. 8.196 and → Fig. 8.197), merges with the main excretory duct of the Glandula sublingualis (Ductus sublingualis major), and opens into the Cavitas oris propria at the Caruncula sublingualis on both sides of the Frenulum linguae and behind the incisors.

Clinical remarks

Malformations in the excretory duct system, especially of the Ductus submandibularis, can lead to the formation of a **ranula** (with saliva-filled retention cysts).
In kidney disease, increased levels of renally cleared substances can be detected in the saliva. Lime deposits from the saliva can lead to the formation of tartar, especially at the lingual side of the lower incisors, or to salivary stones **(sialoliths)** in the excretory ducts of the salivary glands with associated salivary colic, obstructions of the Ductus parotideus, and swelling of the gland, salivary gland tumours. Therapeutic radiation in the treatment of tumours of the head and neck or radioactive radiation can result in a **'dry mouth' syndrome** with swallowing and speech difficulties. **Inflammation** of the salivary glands can be acute or chronic.

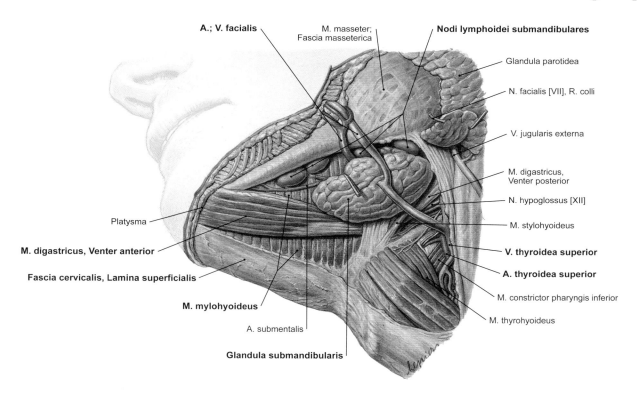

A.; V. facialis
M. masseter; Fascia masseterica
Nodi lymphoidei submandibulares
Glandula parotidea
N. facialis [VII], R. colli
V. jugularis externa
M. digastricus, Venter posterior
N. hypoglossus [XII]
M. stylohyoideus
V. thyroidea superior
A. thyroidea superior
M. constrictor pharyngis inferior
M. thyrohyoideus
Platysma
M. digastricus, Venter anterior
Fascia cervicalis, Lamina superficialis
M. mylohyoideus
A. submentalis
Glandula submandibularis

Fig. 8.194 Submandibular gland, Glandula submandibularis, left side; inferior view from a lateral oblique angle. [S700]
The Glandula submandibularis lies in the Trigonum submandibulare. The gland has its own fascia, enclosed in the compartment of the Lamina superficialis of the Fascia cervicalis (→ Fig. 11.9, → Fig. 11.10). The gland has a direct topographical relationship to the A. and V. facialis.

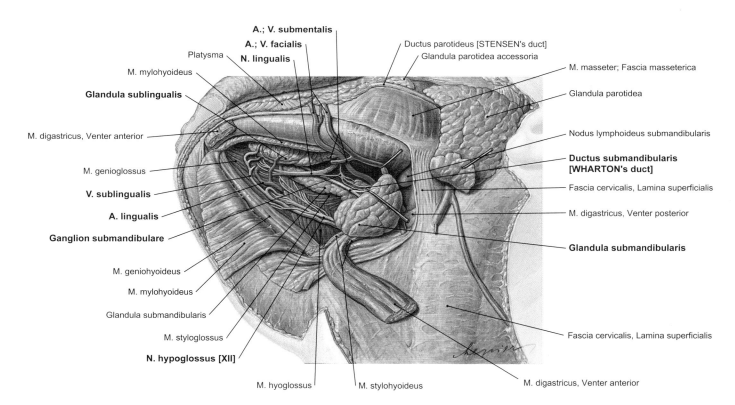

A.; V. submentalis
A.; V. facialis
Platysma
N. lingualis
M. mylohyoideus
Glandula sublingualis
M. digastricus, Venter anterior
M. genioglossus
V. sublingualis
A. lingualis
Ganglion submandibulare
M. geniohyoideus
M. mylohyoideus
Glandula submandibularis
M. styloglossus
N. hypoglossus [XII]
M. hyoglossus
M. stylohyoideus
Ductus parotideus [STENSEN's duct]
Glandula parotidea accessoria
M. masseter; Fascia masseterica
Glandula parotidea
Nodus lymphoideus submandibularis
Ductus submandibularis [WHARTON's duct]
Fascia cervicalis, Lamina superficialis
M. digastricus, Venter posterior
Glandula submandibularis
Fascia cervicalis, Lamina superficialis
M. digastricus, Venter anterior

Fig. 8.195 Submandibular gland, Glandula submandibularis, and sublingual gland, Glandula sublingualis, left side; lateral inferior view. [S700]
The superficial portion of the Glandula submandibularis has been moved back, the M. mylohyoideus is separated from the Mandibula and folded back medially. Below the removed muscle, the deep glandular portion of the Glandula submandibularis and the Glandula sublingualis, which lies parallel to the Corpus mandibulae, can be seen.
The **arterial** supply of the glands occurs via the Aa. facialis, submentalis and lingualis. The **venous** blood flows via the V. sublingualis and the V. submentalis into the V. facialis or directly into the V. jugularis interna. The Nodi lymphoidei submentales and submandibulares are the **regional lymph nodes.**

Salivary glands

Submandibular and sublingual gland

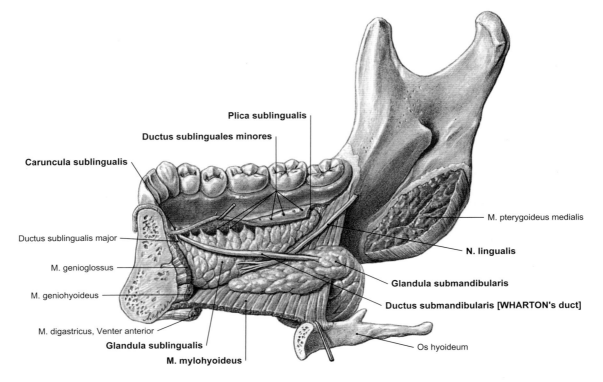

Plica sublingualis

Ductus sublinguales minores

Caruncula sublingualis

M. pterygoideus medialis

Ductus sublingualis major

N. lingualis

M. genioglossus

Glandula submandibularis

M. geniohyoideus

Ductus submandibularis [WHARTON's duct]

M. digastricus, Venter anterior

Os hyoideum

Glandula sublingualis

M. mylohyoideus

Fig. 8.196 Submandibular gland, Glandula submandibularis, and sublingual gland, Glandula sublingualis, right side; medial view. [S700]
The Glandula sublingualis lies on the M. mylohyoideus, lateral to the M. genioglossus. Sometimes it pierces the floor of the mouth. The glandular body makes the mucosa at the floor of the mouth bulge out as the Plica sublingualis, which contains multiple small excretory duct open-

ings (Ductus sublinguales minores) from the posterior part of the gland. The lower portion of the Glandula submandibularis embraces the posterior margin of the M. mylohyoideus in an uncinate manner, and continues above the muscle into the Ductus submandibularis. The N. lingualis runs between the Glandula submandibularis and the Glandula sublingualis below the Ductus submandibularis to the tongue.

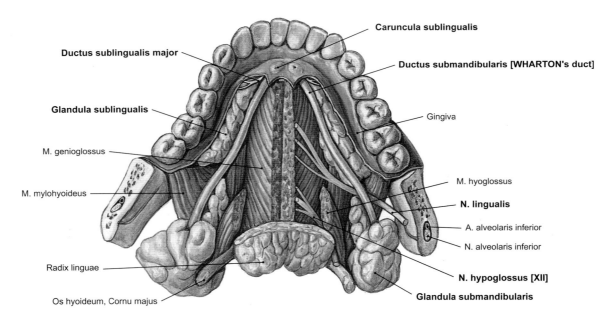

Ductus sublingualis major

Caruncula sublingualis

Ductus submandibularis [WHARTON's duct]

Glandula sublingualis

Gingiva

M. genioglossus

M. hyoglossus

M. mylohyoideus

N. lingualis

A. alveolaris inferior

N. alveolaris inferior

Radix linguae

N. hypoglossus [XII]

Os hyoideum, Cornu majus

Glandula submandibularis

Fig. 8.197 Sublingual gland, Glandula sublingualis, and submandibular gland, Glandula submandibularis; superior view. [S700]
The anterior portion of the Glandula sublingualis has a single greater excretory duct **(Ductus sublingualis major),** which joins the Ductus

submandibularis on the M. hyoglossus, where they open together on the Caruncula sublingualis. The N. hypoglossus [XII] reaches the tongue between the M. hyoglossus and the M. genioglossus.

Clinical remarks

The excretory duct system of the Glandula submandibularis is most commonly affected by salivary stones **(sialoliths).** Salts stored in the thickened saliva form crystalline structures, which can then be depo-

sited as sialoliths and block the excretory duct of the salivary gland. When eating, the gland swells rapidly and is painful (clinical remarks → Fig. 8.193).

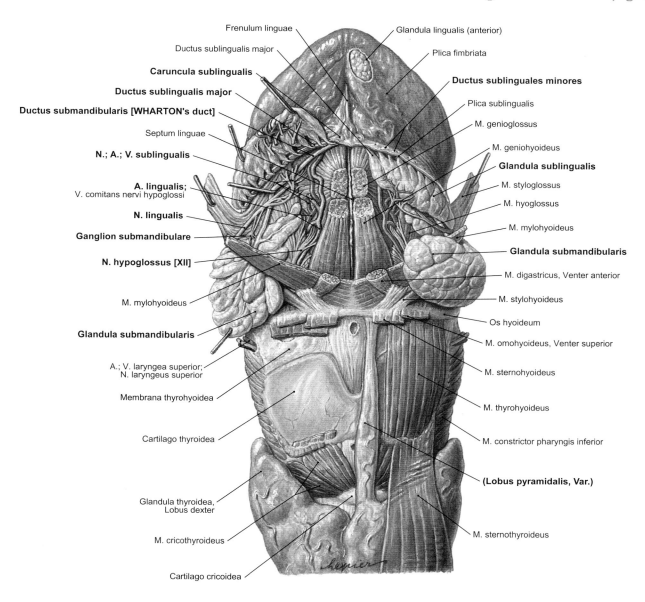

Frenulum linguae
Ductus sublingualis major
Caruncula sublingualis
Ductus sublingualis major
Ductus submandibularis [WHARTON's duct]
Septum linguae
N.; A.; V. sublingualis
A. lingualis;
V. comitans nervi hypoglossi
N. lingualis
Ganglion submandibulare
N. hypoglossus [XII]
M. mylohyoideus
Glandula submandibularis
A.; V. laryngea superior;
N. laryngeus superior
Membrana thyrohyoidea
Cartilago thyroidea
Glandula thyroidea,
Lobus dexter
M. cricothyroideus
Cartilago cricoidea

Glandula lingualis (anterior)
Plica fimbriata
Ductus sublinguales minores
Plica sublingualis
M. genioglossus
M. geniohyoideus
Glandula sublingualis
M. styloglossus
M. hyoglossus
M. mylohyoideus
Glandula submandibularis
M. digastricus, Venter anterior
M. stylohyoideus
Os hyoideum
M. omohyoideus, Venter superior
M. sternohyoideus
M. thyrohyoideus
M. constrictor pharyngis inferior
(Lobus pyramidalis, Var.)
M. sternothyroideus

Fig. 8.198 Vessels and nerves of the tongue, Lingua, and large salivary glands, Glandulae salivariae majores; frontal inferior view. [S700]
The frontal view of the elevated tongue shows a subepithelial venous plexus on the underside of the tongue. On the right, the Glandula sublingualis has been folded upwards, which gives a clear view of the un-

derlying N. lingualis and the Ductus submandibularis (WHARTON's duct). The N. hypoglossus [XII] penetrates the tongue slightly deeper. As a frequent remnant of the development of the thyroid, a Lobus pyramidalis can be seen in front of the larynx, which may extend up to the hyoid bone.

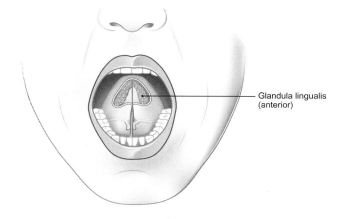

Glandula lingualis
(anterior)

Fig. 8.199 Lingual gland, Glandula lingualis (anterior), gland of BLANDIN-NUHN, anterior view from below. [S700-L126]
The Glandula lingualis (anterior) is a paired salivary gland in the area of the tip of the tongue. The gland produces a seromucous fluid which is secreted via short secretory ducts into the crypts of the epithelium on the underside of the tongue near the Frenulum linguae.

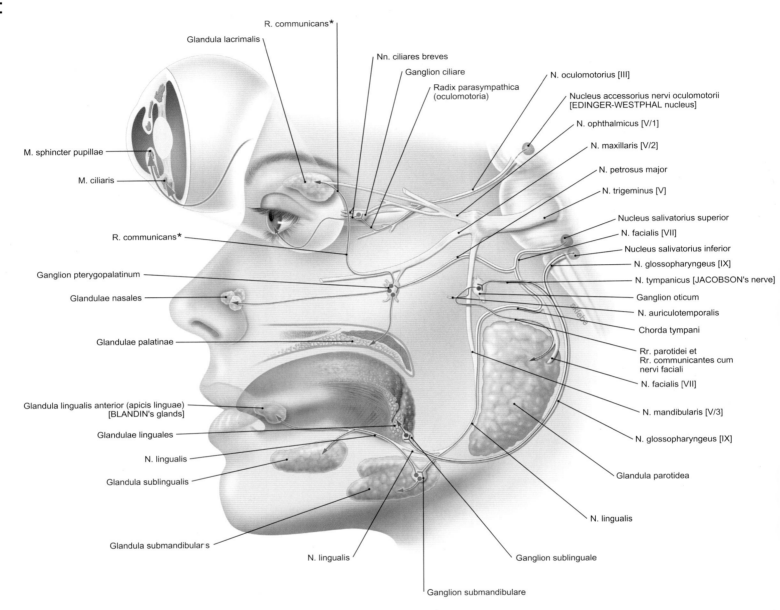

Fig. 8.200 Innervation of the glands of the head with autonomic ganglia; schematic drawing. [S700-L238]

Parasympathetic fibres originate from the lower and upper salivatory nuclei (Nucleus salivatorius superior and Nucleus salivatorius inferior). **Preganglionic parasympathetic** fibres run to the ganglia of the head (Ganglia oticum, submandibulare, sublinguale, pterygopalatinum, ciliare) with various nerves. Here, these fibres synapse and, as short postganglionic fibres, reach their target structures (glands). **Preganglionic**

sympathetic fibres for the head originate from the lateral horn of the spinal cord and are mostly switched in the Ganglion cervicale superius (upper ganglion of the sympathetic trunk) to postganglionic fibres. The **postganglionic** fibres form sympathetic plexuses around the arteries (e.g. A. carotis interna) and reach their target structures along with the blood vessels or by joining local nerves.

* anastomosis of the lacrimal gland

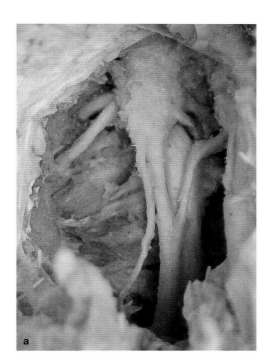

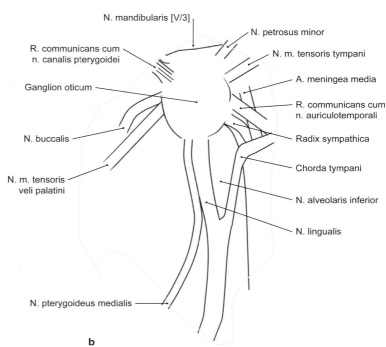

N. mandibularis [V/3]

R. communicans cum
n. canalis pterygoidei

Ganglion oticum

N. buccalis

N. m. tensoris
veli palatini

N. pterygoideus medialis

N. petrosus minor

N. m. tensoris tympani

A. meningea media

R. communicans cum
n. auriculotemporali

Radix sympathica

Chorda tympani

N. alveolaris inferior

N. lingualis

a

b

Fig. 8.201a and b   Ganglion oticum on the left with its branches;
view from the right. [F885]
a Photographic overview.
b Corresponding schematic drawing.
The parasympathetic Ganglion oticum is located immediately below the
Foramen ovale in the Fossa infratemporalis below the cranial base. It
has a close topographical relationship with the N. mandibularis [V/3], A.
meningea media, M. tensor veli palatini and Pars cartilaginea of the Tuba
auditiva. Passing through the ganglion are motor, sympathetic and parasympathetic fibres. The motor and sympathetic fibres run all the way
without switching, while the parasympathetic fibres are switched from
pre- to postganglionic. They reach the ganglion via the N. petrosus minor and leave it after switching via the R. communicans cum nervi auriculotemporali, a branch of the N. mandibularis [V/3]. After a short pas-

sage in the N. auriculotemporalis, the nerve fibres within the Glandula
parotidea join up with fibres of the N. facialis [VII] before leaving them
after a short distance and arriving at the glandular parenchyma (Rr. communicantes cum nervi faciali). The parasympathetic fibres are not only
responsible for the secretory innervation of the Glandula parotidea, but
also innervate the Glandulae buccales. The continuous motor fibres originate from the N. pterygoideus medialis (from [V/3]) and, after passing
through the Ganglion oticum, innervate the M. tensor tympani as the
N. musculi tensoris tympani, and also the M. tensor veli palatini as the
R. musculi tensoris veli palatini. The sympathetic fibres are postganglionic fibres, which have already been switched in the Ganglion cervicale superius and have reached the Ganglion oticum via the Plexus caroticus externus. After entering via the Ganglion oticum, they reach the
Glandula parotidea and the Glandulae buccales.

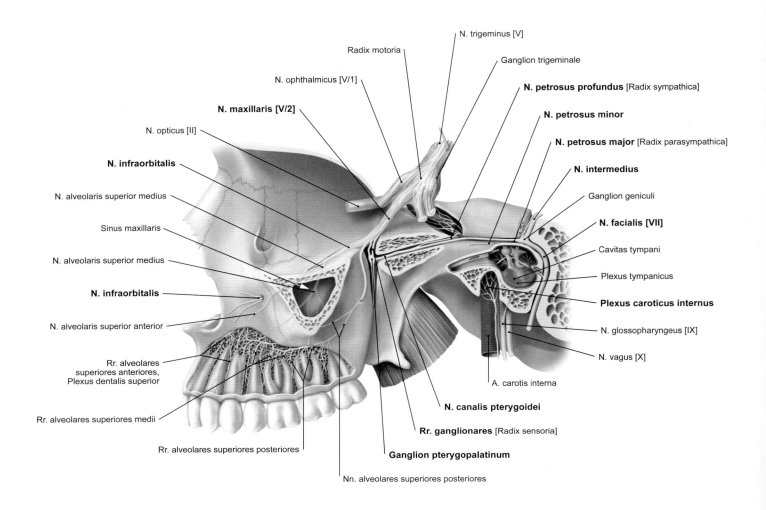

N. trigeminus [V]

Radix motoria

Ganglion trigeminale

N. ophthalmicus [V/1]

N. petrosus profundus [Radix sympathica]

N. maxillaris [V/2]

N. petrosus minor

N. opticus [II]

N. petrosus major [Radix parasympathica]

N. infraorbitalis

N. intermedius

N. alveolaris superior medius

Ganglion geniculi

Sinus maxillaris

N. facialis [VII]

N. alveolaris superior medius

Cavitas tympani

N. infraorbitalis

Plexus tympanicus

Plexus caroticus internus

N. alveolaris superior anterior

N. glossopharyngeus [IX]

Rr. alveolares
superiores anteriores,
Plexus dentalis superior

N. vagus [X]

A. carotis interna

Rr. alveolares superiores medii

N. canalis pterygoidei

Rr. ganglionares [Radix sensoria]

Rr. alveolares superiores posteriores

Ganglion pterygopalatinum

Nn. alveolares superiores posteriores

Fig. 8.202 Ganglion pterygopalatinum. [S700-L275]
Sensory nerve fibres run via the Rr. ganglionares of the N. maxillaris [V/2] through the Ganglion pterygopalatinum to reach the soft and hard palate. Parasympathetic fibres from the superior salivatory nucleus reach the Ganglion pterygopalatinum via the N. facialis [VII] (N. intermedius), the N. petrosus major and the N. canalis pterygoidei, and are switched here from preganglionic to postganglionic. The postganglionic parasympathetic fibres innervate the lacrimal, nasal and palatine glands. The postganglionic sympathetic fibres originate from the N. caroticus internus (Plexus caroticus internus), assemble to form the N. petrosus profundus and pass through the Ganglion pterygopalatinum to innervate the lacrimal, nasal and palatine glands.

Sample exam questions

To check that you are completely familiar with the content of this chapter, sample questions from an oral anatomy exam are listed here.

Explain the structure of the skull:

- Which bones border the orbit, which entry and exit points does the Orbita have, and what enters and exits?
- Which bones confine the nasal cavity?
- Which spaces hold air in the skull? How will these be ventilated?
- How are the cranial bones structured?
- What is meant by fontanelles, and when do they close?
- Explain the structure of the Articulatio temporomandibularis.
- How many and which teeth form part of the primary dentition?
- What are the special features of the Os temporale?

Describe the structure of the face:

- Which parts does the M. orbicularis oculi consist of? What are they used for?
- Which muscles in the face have a fascia, and which do not? Describe their functions.
- Describe the route of the N. facialis [VII] after exiting the Foramen stylomastoideum.
- Which masticatory muscles do you know, how are they supplied with blood and how are they innervated? Which muscles are innervated by the nerve which also innervates the masticatory muscles?
- Describe the inflow and outflow/anastomosis of the V. facialis.
- How is the Galea aponeurotica structured?
- Which structure is at risk of diseases of the Glandula parotidea?
- What is the juxtaoral organ, where is it, and how should it function?
- Into which lymph nodes does the lymph of the facial area drain?

Describe the structure of the nose:

- How are the bone and cartilage of the nose structured?
- How is the nose supplied with blood? How do arteries reach the nose?
- What is the Hiatus semilunaris, how is it confined and what usually drains or ends here?
- What is the KIESSELBACH's plexus?

Explain the structure of the oral cavity:

- Which structures open into the oral cavity?
- How is the oral cavity confined?

- Describe the innervation of the tongue.
- Which papillae occur on the tongue?
- Which muscles of the tongue do you know? How are they innervated?
- What is between the anterior and the posterior palatine arches?
- How is the Tonsilla palatina supplied arterially?
- How are the teeth innervated? Where should the dentist inject a local anaesthetic to numb the teeth of the maxilla and the Mandibula?
- What happens if the mandibular teeth are anaesthetised by a local injection before the Foramen mandibulae has been anaesthetised?
- How does the palate develop?
- Which muscles are involved in the movement of the soft palate?
- What is the problem with a cleft palate?

Explain the structure of the Fossa pterygopalatina:

- Which structures pass through the Fossa pterygopalatina?
- What is switched in the Ganglion pterygopalatinum?
- Which bones limit the Fossa pterygopalatina?
- Name the topographical relationships of the Fossa pterygopalatina.

Describe the structure of the floor of the mouth:

- Which muscles belong to the floor of the mouth?
- How are the muscles innervated?
- Which muscles of the floor of the mouth are involved in opening the jaw?

Explain the position and the structure of the salivary glands:

- What are the parts of the Glandula parotidea?
- To what does the Glandula parotidea have a topographical relationship?
- Describe the pathway of the Ductus parotideus.
- Where does it enter the Glandula sublingualis?
- Locate the orifice of the Ductus submandibularis.
- Where are the sympathetic and parasympathetic fibres for the innervation of the large salivary glands?
- Name the small salivary glands, describe their positions and say how many there are.
- How are the salivary glands supplied with blood?

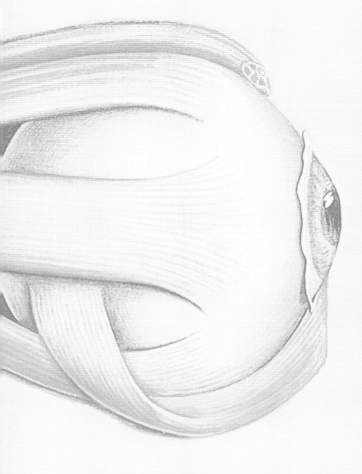

Eye

9

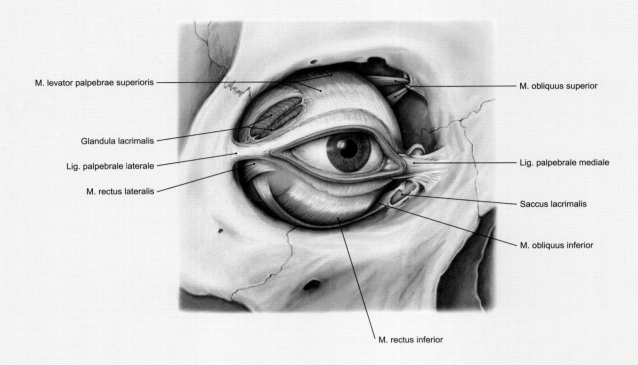

M. levator palpebrae superioris

Glandula lacrimalis

Lig. palpebrale laterale

M. rectus lateralis

M. obliquus superior

Lig. palpebrale mediale

Saccus lacrimalis

M. obliquus inferior

M. rectus inferior

Overview

The eye or organ of sight (Organum visus) is often referred to as the 'gateway to the soul' and is considered by many people to be the body's most important sensory organ. It includes the **eyeball** (Bulbus oculi), the optical apparatus and the auxiliary structures (Structurae oculi accessoriae), such as **extraocular muscles** (Mm. externi bulbi oculi), **eyelids** (Palpebrae), **conjunctiva** (Tunica conjunctiva) and the **lacrimal apparatus** (Apparatus lacrimalis). The Bulbus oculi has a diameter of approx. 24 mm and is encased in a **connective tissue capsule** (Vagina bulbi) and embedded in an **adipose body** (Corpus adiposum orbitae), together with the auxiliary structures (with the exception of the eyelids) in the bony **eye socket** (Orbita). The position of the Bulbus oculi can be adjusted to see in all directions with the help of six external (or extraocular) muscles; four rectus and two oblique. The Bulbus oculi itself consists of three layers. The outer layer is made up of the **outer (fi-**

brous) layer of the eyeball (Tunica fibrosa), the sclera and the cornea (Stratum corneum). The cornea is clear and forms the window to the outside world, through which anything to be seen enters the inner eye. Directly below the surface is the **middle (fibrous) layer of the eyeball** (Tunica vasculosa), consisting of the iris and the choroid (Corpus ciliare and Choroidea). Inside, the **inner layer of the eyeball** (Tunica interna) joins as the retina. This is where the receptors are situated which register the visual impression and then pass it on. The interior of the Bulbus oculi is separated in an **anterior** and a **posterior chamber** (Camera anterior and Camera posterior). The border between the two spaces forms the ocular lens (Lens oculi). The anterior chamber of the eye contains the intraocular fluid and the posterior chamber is filled with the **vitreous humour** (Corpus vitreum).

Main topics

After working through this chapter, you should be able to:

- understand the development of the eye from the three original tissue layers of the neuroectoderm of the diencephalon, the surface ectoderm of the head and the mesenchyme, and the resulting structure of the eye;
- name the structure of the Orbita and the structures involved in its development, as well as naming the structures which enter and exit;
- explain the content of the Orbita and differentiate between its different segments;
- describe the topographical relationships of the Orbita to its neighbouring structures;

- explain the structure of the auxiliary structures, such as eyelids, conjunctiva, lacrimal apparatus with lacrimal glands and the lacrimal drainage system in conjunction with the way they function;
- describe and distinguish between the structure and function of the extraocular muscles, how they are attached and anchored in the Orbita and the blood supply and innervation of the Bulbus oculi and the Orbita;
- explain the individual parts of the Bulbus oculi and describe their functions.

Clinical relevance

In order not to lose touch with prospective everyday clinical life with so many anatomical details, the following describes a typical case that shows why the content of this chapter is so important.

Orbital blow-out fracture

Case study

A 24-year-old student was playing squash on the first day of his semester vacation. During the game, he could not get out of the way quickly enough when the squash ball bounced back and hit him in the centre of his right eye (→ Fig. a). He clutched his right eye in pain. Using a mobile phone, his friend immediately called the emergency services and then obtained an ice pack from the squash court restaurant to hold against the eye.

Result of examination

During the initial examination, the emergency doctor noticed that the right Bulbus oculi seemed to be withdrawn into its socket (enophthalmos). The right eyelid structures were swollen, and there were also signs of bleeding into the soft tissue of the eye (monocular haematoma of the right side). Although the student could still see with this eye, he was almost completely unable to follow the doctor's finger moving in different directions. The student also complained of double vision and when the doctor brushed the skin below his right eye he felt no sensation.

Diagnostic procedure

The student was taken to the university eye hospital. A skull CT was performed which showed a fracture of the orbital floor with a shift or translocation of the eye socket content towards the right maxillary sinus (→ Fig. b). The N. infraorbitalis, the M. orbicularis inferior and the M. rectus inferior had shifted. The paranasal sinuses and the viscerocranium were otherwise intact. Other routine examinations of the eye revealed no evidence of retinal detachment or other damage within the Bulbus oculi. The patient had 100 % vision.

Diagnosis

A blow-out fracture to the right, with the participation of the N. infraorbitalis and entrapment of the lower extraocular muscles.

Treatment

The student was prepared for an operational orbital floor reconstruction procedure for the next morning. This is necessary, as all orbital floor fractures with symptoms such as double vision, sensory disturbances and enophthalmos, have to be operated on as soon as possible in order to prevent an ascending infection from the bacteria-populated maxillary sinus into the sterile Orbita. The pressure on the N. opticus could additionally lead to loss of vision or permanent double vision due to an atrophy of the eye muscles. As part of the operation, the soft tissue is first shifted back and the bone fragments replaced, as far as possible, in the correct position. This is followed by the orbital floor reconstruction with homologous material (e.g. lyophilised dura). Alternatively, the reconstruction can be performed using alloplastic materials (e.g. plastic or metallic osteosynthesis material).

Further developments

The postoperative recovery was satisfactory. After one week there were hardly any problems with double vision. The soft tissue shell of the external eye was only slightly swollen and had taken on a yellow-green colour.

Dissection lab

Isolated orbital floor fractures (blow-out fractures) are rare in relation to the total number of central facial fractures.

 Sports, traffic and workplace accidents, as well as violent crime are the most common causes of isolated orbital floor fractures.

It is far more common to encounter an orbital floor fracture in combination with other fractures. It is important to consider the complexity of the bony structures of the viscerocranium and the passage of the neurovascular pathways, particularly during the physical examination, in order to be able to determine the true extent of the damage. It is necessary to pay attention in particular to the bones and the surrounding bone structures involved in the composition of the eye socket in the dissection lab.

 Take note of the thin bony walls when dissecting the eye socket.

One must continually remind oneself of just how many structures there are in such close proximity.

Back in the clinic

Due to the impact of the squash ball, the Bulbus oculi was pushed back into the funnel-shaped Orbita. Generally speaking, injuries of the blood vessels in the soft tissue shell of the eye and the eyelids are more common than a nerve injury. Sometimes the N. opticus can also be compressed into its bony canal (Canalis nervi optici). The N. infraorbitalis is often affected because it extends into the cheek via the Fissura orbitalis inferior and the Foramen infraorbitale. That is why testing for sensitivity (lightly brushing against the skin), especially of the lower eyelid, cheeks and upper lip, is so important.

Three of the four orbital walls border on the sinuses. In the case of this student, the contusion of the Bulbus oculi broke the orbital floor.

 The orbital floor is also the roof of the maxillary sinus, inside which the N. infraorbitalis runs.

As a result, the M. rectus inferior and the M. orbitalis inferior are squeezed into the gap caused by the fracture. This explains the double vision in the initial examination. With a fracture of the Paries medialis, which is largely formed by the Lamina papyracea of

 The Lamina papyracea is aptly named as it is almost transparent.

the Os ethmoidale, the air from the ethmoidal cells can penetrate into the orbital adipose tissue or under the skin of the eyelid (subcutaneous emphysema). This results in a soft crackling sound in the palpation of the eyelid. Until such time as the injury is completely healed, the patient must not wipe his nose. Nose drops can be prescribed to ease inflammation or congestion. After any midfacial fracture, a check for a CSF leak must be made. In this event, a clear secretion (liquor) could be trickling out of the nose. Due to the risk of infection with an open connection between the Orbita and the paranasal sinuses, treatment with an antibiotic is imperative.

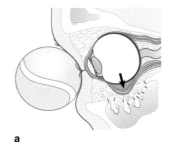 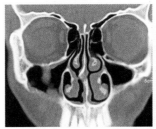

a   b

Fig. a Accidental cause: the ball hits the Bulbus oculi, which causes an orbital floor fracture, leading to a shift of the eye socket content into the maxillary sinus. [S700-L126]

Fig. b Coronary skull CT: fracture of the orbital floor on the left with a shift of the orbital structures into the maxillary sinus. [R349]

Development fourth to fifth week

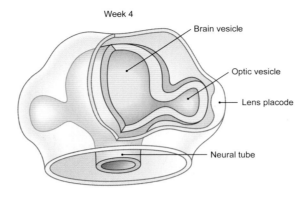

Week 4

Brain vesicle

Optic vesicle

Lens placode

Neural tube

Fig. 9.1 Eye development, fourth week. [E838]
In the fourth week, the optic vesicles (Vesicula optica) evert out of the diencephalon area of the prosencephalon. The optic vesicles make their way further towards the surface and induce the formation of a lens placode in the surrounding surface ectoderm.

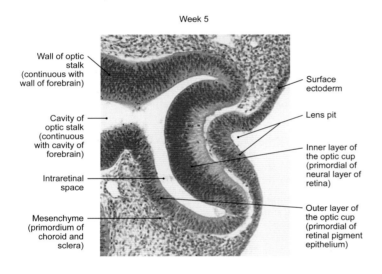

Week 5

Wall of optic stalk (continuous with wall of forebrain)

Cavity of optic stalk (continuous with cavity of forebrain)

Intraretinal space

Mesenchyme (primordium of choroid and sclera)

Surface ectoderm

Lens pit

Inner layer of the optic cup (primordial of neural layer of retina)

Outer layer of the optic cup (primordial of retinal pigment epithelium)

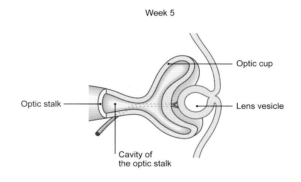

Week 5

Optic cup

Optic stalk

Lens vesicle

Cavity of the optic stalk

Fig. 9.2 Eye development, fifth week; photomicrograph of a sagittal section. [E347-09]
The image shows the optic vesicles which have everted out into the optic cup (or ophthalmic cup) and have already formed a close connection with the lens placode. Located between the two layers of the optic cup (primordium of the retina) and in the optic stalk (primordium of the N. opticus [II]), the intraretinal space is still relatively wide.

Fig. 9.3 Eye development, fifth week. [E838]
The spherical lens vesicle everts from the surface ectoderm and is surrounded on all sides by the optic vesicles, forming the optic cup. The optic cup is still connected with the diencephalon by a small optic stalk, the former Sulcus opticus.

Structure and function

Development of the eye
The development of the eye starts at the beginning of the fourth week when the optic vesicles evert out of the diencephalon area of the prosencephalon. Quite quickly, the anterior pole folds inwards to form a primitive optic cup. The retinal pigment epithelium is formed from the posterior section of the outer layer of the optic cup, whereas the epithelia of the Corpus ciliare and the iris are formed from its anterior section. The inner layer of the optic cup forms the retina. At the point of contact between the optic cup and the surface ectoderm, the lens vesicle separates and sinks below the surface. The epithelia of the cornea and conjunctiva are also formed by the ectoderm. Most of the other parts of the middle and external eye are of mesenchymal origin. In the beginning, the lens system is made up of a blood vessel network (which includes the A. hyaloidea), which regresses later. The proximal stump of the A. hyaloidea becomes the A. centralis retinae.

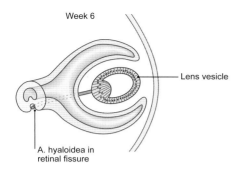

Week 6

Lens vesicle

A. hyaloidea in
retinal fissure

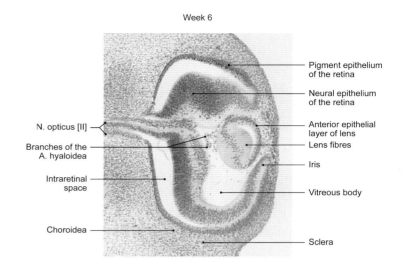

Week 6

Pigment epithelium
of the retina

Neural epithelium
of the retina

Anterior epithelial
layer of lens

Lens fibres

Iris

Vitreous body

Sclera

N. opticus [II]

Branches of the
A. hyaloidea

Intraretinal
space

Choroidea

Fig. 9.4   Eye development, sixth week. [E838]
At the deepest point of the optic cup – a longitudinal groove – the optic fissure becomes visible. This optic fissure contains blood vessels and the first nerve fibres of the later N. opticus [II]. During the development stage, the blood vessels supply the inside of the optic cup via the A. and V. hyaloidea. During the seventh month of pregnancy, the blood vessels in the optic cup disappear; in the N. opticus [II], the vessels remain as the A. and V. centralis retinae.

Fig. 9.5   Eye development, sixth week; photomicrograph of a sagittal section. [E347-09]
In the sixth week the epithelial cells in the posterior wall of the lens vesicle elongate and form the lens fibres.

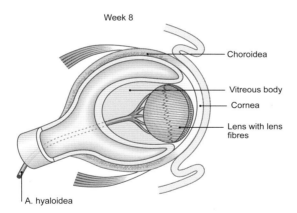

Week 8

Choroidea

Vitreous body

Cornea

Lens with lens
fibres

A. hyaloidea

Fig. 9.6   Eye development, eighth week. [E838]
Mesenchymal cells migrate into the optic cup and form the vitreous body (Corpus vitreum) which is composed of vitreous humour, a gelatinous substance embedded with tiny fibres. The vitreous body gives the eyeball its firm shape.

Clinical remarks

Developmental defects of the eye are relatively rare. Inherited blindness has an incidence of 20 per 100,000 live births and in most cases, coincides with other (mental) disabilities. In certain rare cases, remnants of the A. hyaloidea make their way from the N. opticus into the vitreous body or even into the lens and can cause a clouding of the lens. In most cases, the **persistence of the A. hyaloidea** is without clinical significance. The term **cyclopia** refers to the partial or complete merging of both eyes in the middle of the face (→ figure). It is a malformation of the face and eye. This congenital abnormality or absence of ocular tissue from the Orbita is known as **anophthalmia.**

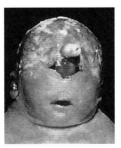

Male newborn with cyclopia. Cyclopia is a malformation of the face and eye associated with a proboscis-shaped nasal process above a single merged eye. [E347-09]

Bony eye socket

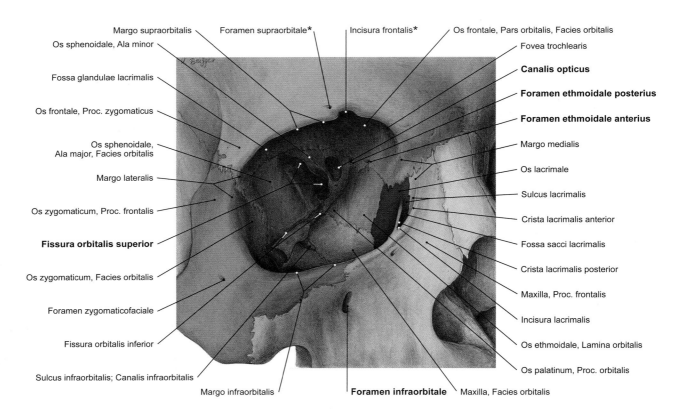

Margo supraorbitalis — Foramen supraorbitale* — Incisura frontalis* — Os frontale, Pars orbitalis, Facies orbitalis

Os sphenoidale, Ala minor — Fovea trochlearis

Fossa glandulae lacrimalis — **Canalis opticus**

Foramen ethmoidale posterius

Os frontale, Proc. zygomaticus — **Foramen ethmoidale anterius**

Os sphenoidale, Ala major, Facies orbitalis — Margo medialis

Margo lateralis — Os lacrimale

Os zygomaticum, Proc. frontalis — Sulcus lacrimalis

Crista lacrimalis anterior

Fissura orbitalis superior — Fossa sacci lacrimalis

Crista lacrimalis posterior

Os zygomaticum, Facies orbitalis — Maxilla, Proc. frontalis

Foramen zygomaticofaciale — Incisura lacrimalis

Fissura orbitalis inferior — Os ethmoidale, Lamina orbitalis

Os palatinum, Proc. orbitalis

Sulcus infraorbitalis; Canalis infraorbitalis — Maxilla, Facies orbitalis

Margo infraorbitalis — **Foramen infraorbitale**

Fig. 9.7   Eye socket, Orbita, right side; frontal view from an oblique angle; for a colour chart, see p. XIII. [S700]
The orbital walls are formed from seven bones (Os frontale, Os ethmoidale, Os lacrimale, Os palatinum, maxilla, Os sphenoidale and Os zygomaticum). The Paries lateralis borders on the Fossa temporalis, and the Paries medialis is located close to the ethmoidal cells and the nasal cavity. In the posterior aspect there are close topographical relationships to the middle cranial fossa, Canalis opticus and the Fossa pterygopalatina.

* These structures can be formed as foramina or Incisurae.

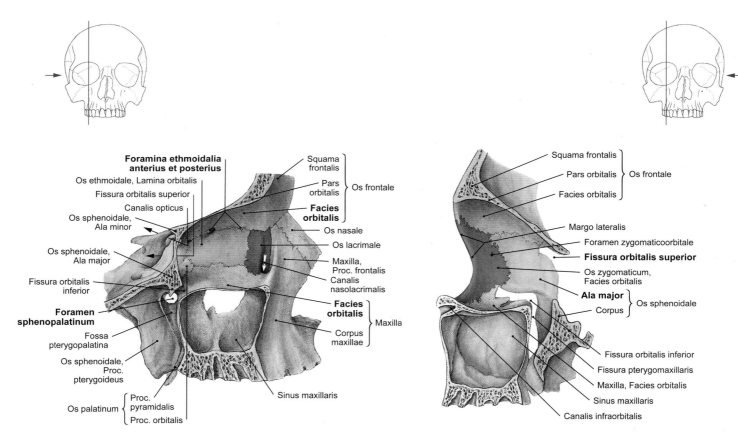

Foramina ethmoidalia anterius et posterius — Squama frontalis

Os ethmoidale, Lamina orbitalis — Pars orbitalis — } Os frontale

Fissura orbitalis superior — **Facies orbitalis**

Canalis opticus — Os nasale

Os sphenoidale, Ala minor — Os lacrimale

Os sphenoidale, Ala major — Maxilla, Proc. frontalis

Canalis nasolacrimalis

Fissura orbitalis inferior — **Facies orbitalis**

Foramen sphenopalatinum — Maxilla

Fossa pterygopalatina — Corpus maxillae

Os sphenoidale, Proc. pterygoideus

Os palatinum { Proc. pyramidalis / Proc. orbitalis } — Sinus maxillaris

Squama frontalis — }
Pars orbitalis — } Os frontale
Facies orbitalis — }

Margo lateralis

Foramen zygomaticoorbitale

Fissura orbitalis superior

Os zygomaticum, Facies orbitalis

Ala major — } Os sphenoidale
Corpus — }

Fissura orbitalis inferior

Fissura pterygomaxillaris

Maxilla, Facies orbitalis

Sinus maxillaris

Canalis infraorbitalis

Fig. 9.8   Medial wall of the eye socket, Paries medialis orbitae, right side; lateral view; for a colour chart, see p. XIII. [S700]

Fig. 9.9   Lateral wall of the eye socket, Paries lateralis orbitae, right side; medial view; for a colour chart, see p. XIII. [S700]

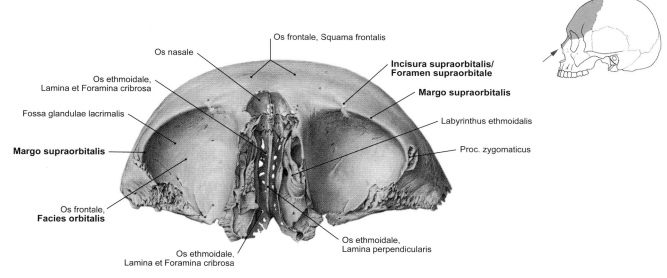

Fig. 9.10 **Roof of the eye socket, Paries superior orbitae;** inferior view; for a colour chart, see p. XIII. [S700]

The roof of the Orbita is also the floor of both the anterior cranial fossa and parts of the Sinus frontalis. All bones of the Labyrinthus ethmoidalis are extremely thin and can be easily fractured during surgical procedures.

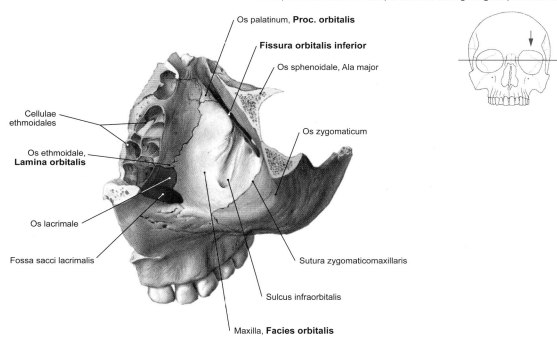

Fig. 9.11 **Floor of the eye socket, Paries inferior orbitae, left side;** superior view; for a colour chart, see p. XIII. [S700]
The floor of the Orbita is also the roof of the Sinus maxillaris. In its posterior aspect is the Sulcus infraorbitalis, the anterior aspect of which

continues in a bony canal through the maxilla and comes out as a Foramen infraorbitale (not visible) below the Orbita.

Clinical remarks

Although the medial bony wall is paper thin (hence the name Lamina papyracea), in the event of a blunt trauma against the Bulbus oculi (e.g. if a tennis ball hits the centre of the eye), the result is usually a fracture of the orbital floor (a so-called **blow-out fracture,** → figure). As a result, intraorbital structures (M. rectus inferior and M. obliquus inferior) can be trapped in the fracture gap or be translocated into the Sinus maxillaris **(orbital hernia).** Reduced mobility of the eyeball can cause double vision, an enophthalmos or a vertical gaze palsy. Involvement of the N. infraorbitalis, which runs along the orbital floor, is likely if **sensory dysfunction** in the dermal area of the upper jaw occurs.

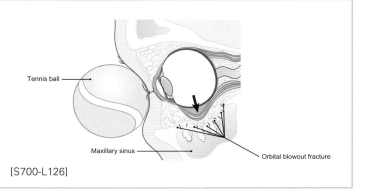

[S700-L126]

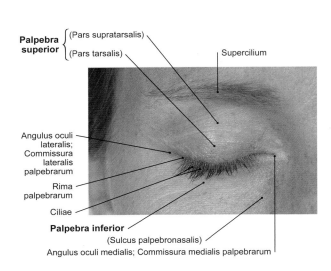

Palpebra superior (Pars supratarsalis) (Pars tarsalis)

Supercilium

Angulus oculi lateralis; Commissura lateralis palpebrarum

Rima palpebrarum

Ciliae

Palpebra inferior

(Sulcus palpebronasalis)

Angulus oculi medialis; Commissura medialis palpebrarum

Fig. 9.12 Eye, Oculus, right side, with eyelids closed. [S700]
On average, a human eye blinks 20–30 times per minute. Each eyelid movement distributes a tear film across the surface of the eye. Blinking involves a consecutive contraction of the M. orbicularis oculi from temporal to nasal and results in a wiping motion in the direction of the medial angle of the eye. Mechanical irritations (e.g. a sudden draft, dust particles, flies) activate the blink reflex (also known as the corneal reflex) which serves to protect the surface of the eye.

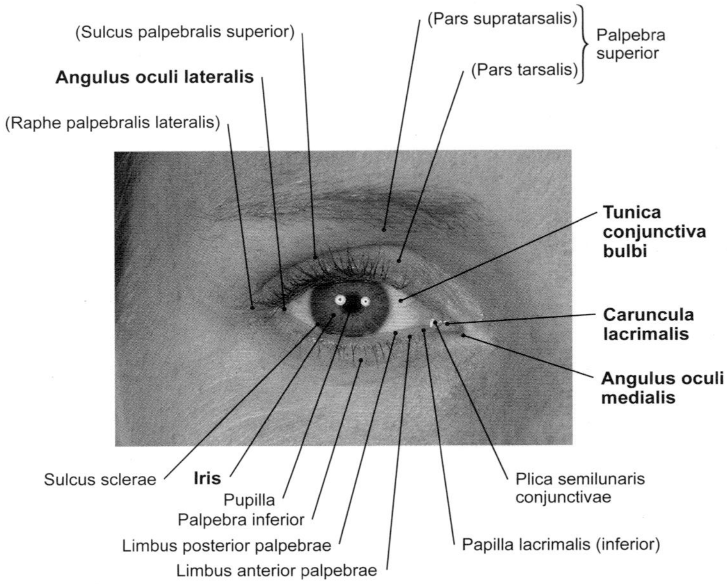

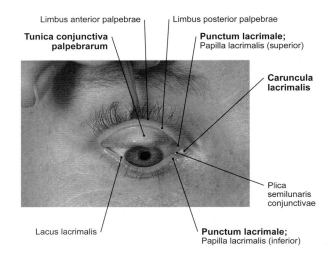

(Sulcus palpebralis superior) (Pars supratarsalis)

Angulus oculi lateralis

(Pars tarsalis)

Palpebra superior

(Raphe palpebralis lateralis)

Tunica conjunctiva bulbi

Caruncula lacrimalis

Angulus oculi medialis

Sulcus sclerae   **Iris**

Pupilla

Palpebra inferior

Limbus posterior palpebrae

Limbus anterior palpebrae

Plica semilunaris conjunctivae

Papilla lacrimalis (inferior)

Fig. 9.13 Eye, Oculus, right side, with eyelids open. [S700]
The normal width between the upper and lower eyelids in an adult ranges between 6 and 10 mm, and the distance between the temporal and medial angle of the eye is 28–30 mm.

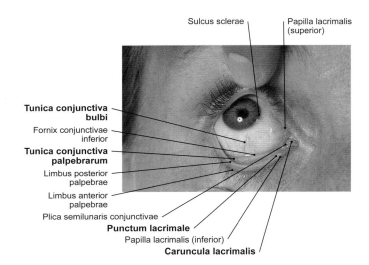

Sulcus sclerae

Papilla lacrimalis (superior)

Tunica conjunctiva bulbi

Fornix conjunctivae inferior

Tunica conjunctiva palpebrarum

Limbus posterior palpebrae

Limbus anterior palpebrae

Plica semilunaris conjunctivae

Punctum lacrimale

Papilla lacrimalis (inferior)

Caruncula lacrimalis

Fig. 9.14 Eye, Oculus, right side, with upper and lower eyelids pulled back. [S700]
With the exception of the cornea, the conjunctiva (a translucent thin mucous layer with blood vessels), covers the part of the eyeball near the eye surface and the side of the eyelids directed towards the eyeball.

Limbus anterior palpebrae   Limbus posterior palpebrae

Tunica conjunctiva palpebrarum

Punctum lacrimale; Papilla lacrimalis (superior)

Caruncula lacrimalis

Lacus lacrimalis

Plica semilunaris conjunctivae

Punctum lacrimale; Papilla lacrimalis (inferior)

Fig. 9.15 Eye, Oculus, right side, with upper eyelid ectropion. [S700]
The Conjunctiva palpebrae and the Conjunctiva bulbi cover the rear side of the eyelid and the eyeball, respectively. Both conjunctival parts merge at the upper and lower Conjunctiva fornicis. The latter is also referred to as the conjunctival sac. It is possible to apply eyedrop medication here.

Clinical remarks

A number of diseases involve the **tightening** or **widening of the eyelids.** Damage to the sympathetic fibres leads to a paralysis of the M. tarsalis superior and thus to a narrowing of the eyelids. Paralysis of the N. oculomotorius causes ptosis of the upper eyelid (which hangs down) due to the paralysis of the elevating muscle of the upper eyelid (M. levator palpebrae superioris). In contrast, a facial nerve palsy due to the paralysis of the muscle that closes the eyelids (M. orbicularis oculi) leads to a widening of the eyelids. An **inflam-**mation of the conjunctiva (conjunctivitis) is encountered frequently in individuals wearing contact lenses. In patients with anaemia, the conjunctiva appears to be off-white and pale, because the normal blood vessel pattern is missing due to the lack of erythrocytes. This condition can be diagnosed using a simple method. The examining physician pushes the lower eyelid down and examines the conjunctival sac.

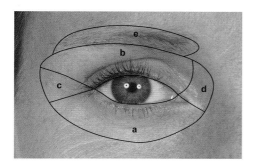

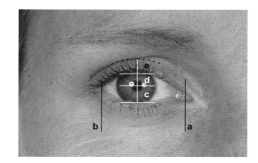

Fig. 9.16   Skin area around the eye, Oculus, right side. [S700]/[E1043]

The eye and eyelid area are central elements of the face. They characterise the appearance of a person to a great extent. Loss of elasticity of the thin eyelid skin in old age and increased life expectancy in the industrialised nations result in more and more people seeking corrective eyelid surgery (blepharoplasty). This surgery differs according to the structural peculiarities of different eye areas:

a Lower eyelid area.
b Upper eyelid area.
c Temporal canthal area.
d Nasal canthal area.
e Eyebrow area.

Fig. 9.17   Palpebral fissure and eyelid width of the eye, Oculus, right side. [S700]/[E1043]

The palpebral fissure is the distance between the two vertical lines through the nasal (**a**) and temporal (**b**) canthus areas. On average, it is between 28 and 30 mm. The distances of the bottom (**c**) and top margins (**e**) of the eyelids from the centre of the pupil (**d**) are referred to as 'upper (MRD1) and lower (MRD2) margin-to-reflex distances'. The result given by these two distances gives the palpebral fissure height or 'eyelid opening width', which is normally between 10 and 12 mm. The distance between the dotted line and (**e**) defines the lid fold. The distance between the upper eyelid border and the upper eyelid fold is on average 9–12 mm (women) and 7–9 mm (men), but can vary greatly and is often covered by the eyebrows.

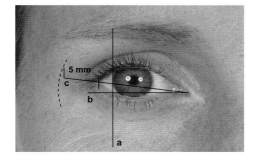

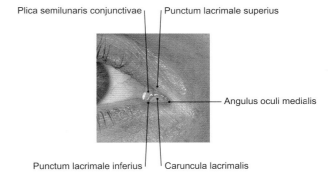

Plica semilunaris conjunctivae — Punctum lacrimale superius

Angulus oculi medialis

Punctum lacrimale inferius — Caruncula lacrimalis

Fig. 9.18   Proportions of the eye, Oculus, right side. [S700]/[E1043]

The nasal canthus is slightly lower than the temporal canthus. This is indicated by the angle between a horizontal (**b**) and the connection line (**c**) between the nasal canthus and the temporal canthus. The distance between the temporal canthus and outer border of the Orbita is approx. 5 mm. The highest point of the eyebrow curve is normally in the lateral third of the eye and is shown by the vertical line (**a**).

Fig. 9.19   Medial angle (corner) of the eye, Angulus oculi medialis, right side. [S700]/[E1043]

At the nasal canthus, Angulus oculi medialis (Epicanthus medialis, Commissura medialis palpebrarum), there is a small, crescent-shaped fold of skin (Plica semilunaris conjunctivae), which is known as the third eyelid. In humans, and in the majority of primates, vestigial remnants of the nictitating membrane (Membrana nicitans) still remain in the corner of the eye (nasal canthus). Animals with an intact nictitating membrane can draw a transparent or translucent third eyelid across the eye for protection and to moisten it while maintaining vision. In addition, the lacrimal caruncle (Caruncula lacrimalis), is the small, pink, globular nodule at the inner corner (nasal canthus) of the eye. This is also regarded as a modified part of the conjunctiva which is sometimes present in adipose tissue. In the mucous membrane which covers it are goblet cells and intraepithelial mucosal glands. A few millimeters away from the medial canthus are the openings to the upper (Punctum lacrimale superius) and the lower (Punctum lacrimale inferius) lacrimal points. They are the entrance to the lacrimal drainage system (→ Fig. 9.40ff.). The Punctum lacrimale inferius in adults is approx. 6.5 mm away from the nasal angle, while the Punctum lacrimale superius is only approx. 6 mm away. When the eyelid is closed, the two lacrimal points do not come into contact with each other. The opening of the lacrimal point is directed slightly towards the rear.

Eyelids

Structure

Fig. 9.20 Upper eyelid, Palpebra superior; image of a microscopic specimen; azan stain; sagittal section, magnified. [S700]
The eyelid can be divided into an outer and inner lamina. The outer lamina is composed of the striated M. orbicularis oculi with its Pars palpebralis. The inner lamina consists of the palpebral conjunctiva (Tunica conjunctiva palpebrarum), the tarsal plate (Tarsus) with the integrated MEIBOM's glands (Glandulae tarsales, modified sebaceous glands) and, close to the rim of the eyelid, muscle fibres of the Pars palpebralis of the M. orbicularis oculi (muscle of RIOLAN, Fasciculi ciliares) radiating into the tarsal plate.

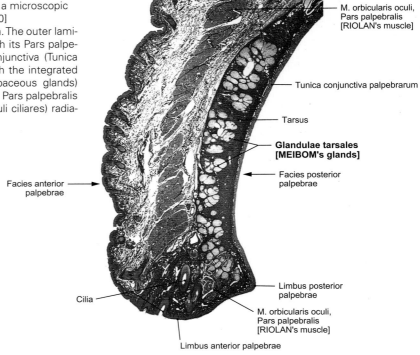

M. orbicularis oculi, Pars palpebralis [RIOLAN's muscle]

Tunica conjunctiva palpebrarum

Tarsus

Glandulae tarsales [MEIBOM's glands]

Facies posterior palpebrae

Facies anterior palpebrae

Limbus posterior palpebrae

M. orbicularis oculi, Pars palpebralis [RIOLAN's muscle]

Cilia

Limbus anterior palpebrae

Fig. 9.21 M. orbicularis oculi, right side; frontal view, showing only the medial half of the muscle. [S700-L285]/[E1043]
The orbital opening and the Septum orbitale are surrounded by the circular Pars orbitalis of the M. orbicularis oculi. The Pars palpebralis of this muscle extends into the eyelids. Hereby, the muscle forms the muscular foundation of the upper and lower eyelids and facilitates the closing of the eyes. Its innermost part in the rim area of the upper and lower eyelid forms the muscle of RIOLAN (→ Fig. 9.20).

→ T 1.3

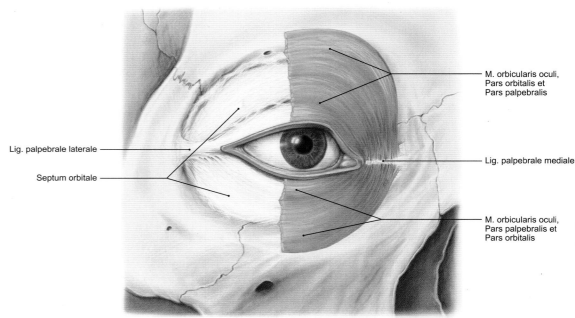

M. orbicularis oculi, Pars orbitalis et Pars palpebralis

Lig. palpebrale mediale

M. orbicularis oculi, Pars palpebralis et Pars orbitalis

Lig. palpebrale laterale

Septum orbitale

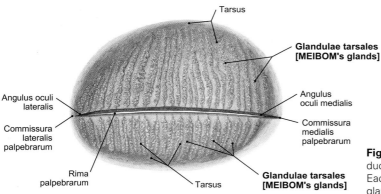

Tarsus

Glandulae tarsales [MEIBOM's glands]

Angulus oculi medialis

Commissura medialis palpebrarum

Angulus oculi lateralis

Commissura lateralis palpebrarum

Rima palpebrarum

Tarsus

Glandulae tarsales [MEIBOM's glands]

Fig. 9.22 Eyelids, Palpebrae, right side; posterior view; glandular ducts of the Glandulae tarsales in a translucent specimen. [S700]
Each eyelid contains approx. 25–30 individual glands, each with its own glandular duct opening into the rim of the eyelid (Rima palpebrarum).

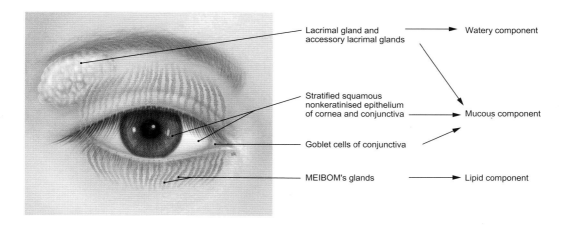

Lacrimal gland and accessory lacrimal glands → Watery component

Stratified squamous nonkeratinised epithelium of cornea and conjunctiva → Mucous component

Goblet cells of conjunctiva → Mucous component

MEIBOM's glands → Lipid component

Fig. 9.23 **Structures of the eye surface** involved in the formation of the three components of the tear film; schematic illustration. [S700-L238]

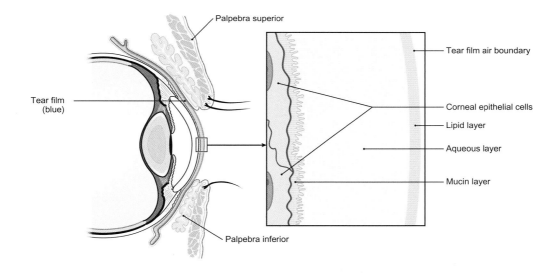

Palpebra superior

Tear film air boundary

Tear film (blue)

Corneal epithelial cells

Lipid layer

Aqueous layer

Mucin layer

Palpebra inferior

Fig. 9.24 **Tear film;** schematic model. [S700-L126]/[T419/P310]
The tear film consists mostly of water (> 99 %). It lubricates the epithelia of the cornea and the conjunctiva as a thin fluid layer up to 40 µm thick and forms a refractive surface. The tear film presents an isotonic electrolyte solution in which water and electrolytes as well as lipids and numerous peptides and proteins (> 1.500) are present, forming a barrier against pathogenic microorganisms. It can be subdivided into three layers: a superficial lipid layer, which counteracts the evaporation of the underlying aqueous layer. As part of the mucin layer and via membrane-bound mucins, the lipid layer is fixed to the epithelial cells of the cornea and the conjunctiva.

Eye

Tear film and M. orbicularis oculi

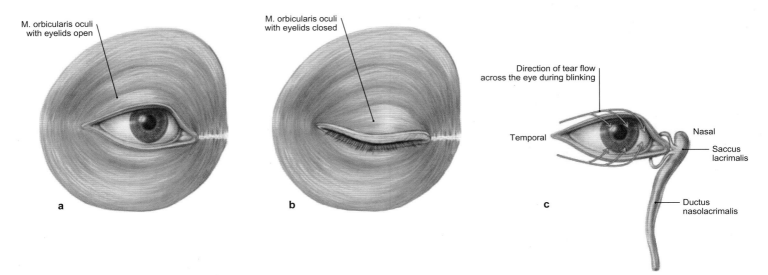

M. orbicularis oculi
with eyelids open

M. orbicularis oculi
with eyelids closed

Direction of tear flow
across the eye during blinking

Temporal

Nasal

Saccus
lacrimalis

Ductus
nasolacrimalis

a

b

c

Fig. 9.25a–c Dynamics of the tear film. [S700-L285]/[T419/P310]
a The tear film lubricates the epithelia of the cornea and the conjunctiva and protects the surface of the eye.
b Constant renewal of the thin tear film through the blinking movement of the eye ensures the lubrication and protection of the eye. Hereby the tear film is functionally slightly delayed in being transported by the

muscle fibres of the M. orbicularis oculi from the temporal to the nasal area.
c The 'used-up' lacrimal fluid (tears) is ultimately 'wiped' in the direction of the medial canthus. Here a lacrimal lake (Lacus lacrimalis) is formed, which is collected and drained via the upper and lower lacrimal points into the efferent tear ducts each time the eyelid blinks.

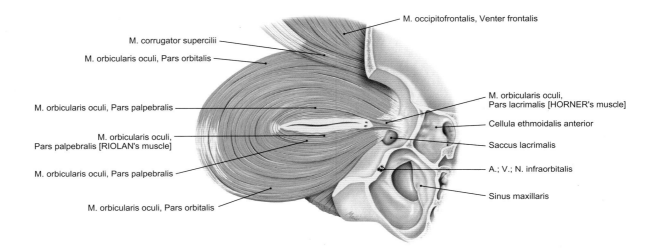

M. corrugator supercilii

M. orbicularis oculi, Pars orbitalis

M. orbicularis oculi, Pars palpebralis

M. orbicularis oculi,
Pars palpebralis [RIOLAN's muscle]

M. orbicularis oculi, Pars palpebralis

M. orbicularis oculi, Pars orbitalis

M. occipitofrontalis, Venter frontalis

M. orbicularis oculi,
Pars lacrimalis [HORNER's muscle]

Cellula ethmoidalis anterior

Saccus lacrimalis

A.; V.; N. infraorbitalis

Sinus maxillaris

Fig. 9.26 M. orbicularis oculi, left side; posterior view. [S700-L127]/[E633-003]
At the nasal canthus, the Pars lacrimalis of this muscle (HORNER's muscle) can be seen, which is important for the drainage of the lacrimal fluid (tears).
The M. orbicularis oculi consists of three parts:
• The **Pars orbitalis** is responsible for the voluntary firm occlusion of the eyelids.
• A contraction of the **Pars palpebralis** triggers the eyelid movement (blinking), which can be carried out randomly, but usually involuntarily.
The **Pars lacrimalis** (HORNER's muscle) is situated around the lacrimal canal and is important for the drainage of lacrimal fluid (tears). When the

eye is closed, the two **lacrimal points** (Puncta lacrimalia: Punctum lacrimale superius and Punctum lacrimale inferius) are immersed in the lacrimal lake (Lacus lacrimalis) in the nasal third of the medial canthus. It is assumed that the contraction of the Pars lacrimalis results in a suction effect (pressure-suction pump mechanism). The tear fluid is sucked via the lacrimal points through the upper and lower lacrimal canaliculus (Canaliculi lacrimales superior and inferior) into the lacrimal sac (Saccus lacrimalis). The lower lacrimal canaliculus transports most of the tear fluid.

→ T 1.3

Clinical remarks

Injuries to the N. facialis can result in the paralysis of the M. orbicularis oculi with the inability to close the eye **(lagophthalmos).** If the patient closes the eye, the Bulbus oculi rolls upward in the normal manner (the external eye muscles are intact), so that one only sees the white of the eye (sclera) **(BELL's phenomenon;** → Fig. 12.152).

If the eye cannot close, the film of lacrimal fluid can no longer keep the eye moist. The cornea dries out after a short time and takes on a milky appearance. The patient is unable to see with this eye. In the case of a facial paralysis, not being able to close the eyes presents the greatest challenge in the treatment of patients.

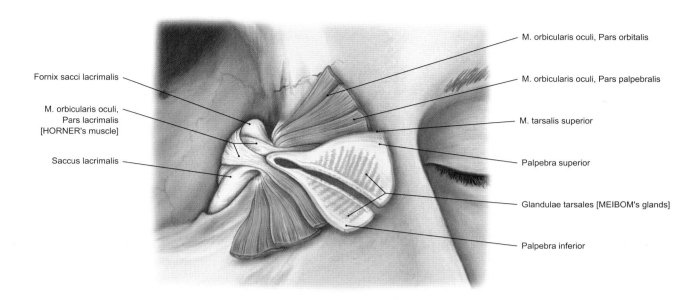

M. orbicularis oculi, Pars orbitalis

M. orbicularis oculi, Pars palpebralis

M. tarsalis superior

Palpebra superior

Glandulae tarsales [MEIBOM's glands]

Palpebra inferior

Fornix sacci lacrimalis

M. orbicularis oculi, Pars lacrimalis [HORNER's muscle]

Saccus lacrimalis

Fig. 9.27   M. orbicularis oculi and eyelids, Palpebrae; detached and folded over to the outside, right side. [S700-L285]/[E1043]
The Pars lacrimalis (HORNER's muscle) of the M. orbicularis oculi encloses the Canaliculi lacrimales (not visible because they are surrounded by the muscle, → Fig. 9.28) from behind and runs to the back of the lacrimal sac (Saccus lacrimalis; → Fig. 9.26 and → Fig. 9.43). The fibres of the Pars lacrimalis in the upper eyelid, Palpebra superior, are interlaced with those of the lower eyelid, Palpebra inferior. The Pars lacrimalis of the M. orbicularis oculi (HORNER's muscle) is essential for the

drainage of the lacrimal fluid (tears) through the lacrimal canaliculi. This so-called 'tear pump' function is not yet fully understood. It is thought that the lacrimal muscle fibres surrounding the canaliculi create a 'pressure-suction effect'. The muscle fibres influence the Septum lacrimale of the posterior lacrimal sac wall via small tendons so that their contractions expand the lumen of the lacrimal sac. On the back of the eyelids we can see the shimmer of the Glandulae tarsales (also called MEIBOM's glands).

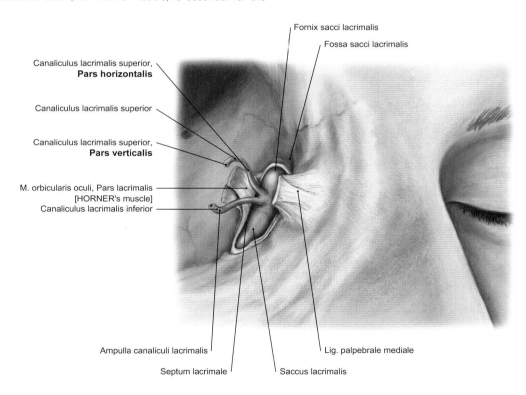

Fornix sacci lacrimalis

Fossa sacci lacrimalis

Canaliculus lacrimalis superior, **Pars horizontalis**

Canaliculus lacrimalis superior

Canaliculus lacrimalis superior, **Pars verticalis**

M. orbicularis oculi, Pars lacrimalis [HORNER's muscle]

Canaliculus lacrimalis inferior

Ampulla canaliculi lacrimalis

Septum lacrimale

Saccus lacrimalis

Lig. palpebrale mediale

Fig. 9.28   M. orbicularis oculi, Pars lacrimalis, lacrimal canaliculi, Canaliculi lacrimales, lacrimal sac, Saccus lacrimalis, and medial palpebral ligament, Lig. palpebrale mediale, right side. [S700-L285]/[E1043]
In the nasal canthus, one can see the detached Pars lacrimalis of the M. orbicularis oculi (HORNER's muscle), which is important for the drainage of lacrimal fluid (tears). It surrounds the upper (Canaliculus

lacrimalis superior) and lower lacrimal canaliculi (Canaliculus lacrimalis inferior) but it has been shortened so that we can see how the Pars lacrimalis runs behind the lacrimal sac (Saccus lacrimalis) and inserts here. At the posterior aspect of the lacrimal sac is the Lig. palpebrale mediale, which is attached to the bone shortly before the front margin of the Fossa lacrimalis (→ Fig. 9.43).

Orbital opening with blood supply and innervation

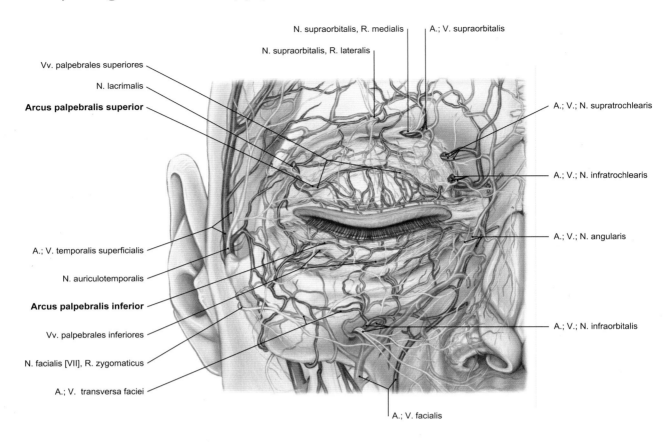

N. supraorbitalis, R. medialis

N. supraorbitalis, R. lateralis

A.; V. supraorbitalis

Vv. palpebrales superiores

N. lacrimalis

Arcus palpebralis superior

A.; V.; N. supratrochlearis

A.; V.; N. infratrochlearis

A.; V.; N. angularis

A.; V. temporalis superficialis

N. auriculotemporalis

Arcus palpebralis inferior

Vv. palpebrales inferiores

N. facialis [VII], R. zygomaticus

A.; V. transversa faciei

A.; V.; N. infraorbitalis

A.; V. facialis

Fig. 9.29 Arteries, veins, and nerves at the orbital opening, Aditus orbitalis, and in the periorbital area, right side; frontal view. [S700-L285]/[E1043]
The Arcus palpebrales superior and inferior create an arterial circle located above the Septum orbitale and surrounding the Orbita. The arterial circle is supplied by numerous arteries derived from the **supply area of the A. carotis interna** (A. supraorbitalis, Aa. palpebrales laterales of the A. lacrimalis, Aa. palpebrales mediales) and the **A. carotis externa**

(A. facialis, A. angularis, A. infraorbitalis, A. temporalis superficialis, A. zygomaticoorbitalis. The Nn. supra- and infraorbitalis are branches of the N. ophthalmicus [V/1] and N. maxillaris [V/2], respectively, and exit the Orbita through the eponymously named foramina (the N. supraorbitalis may exit the Orbita through the Incisura supraorbitalis). The sensory perception of the N. ophthalmicus [V/1] and N. maxillaris [V/2] can be tested at both nerve exit points.

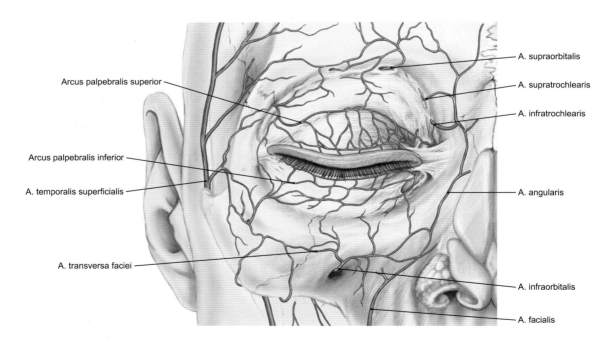

A. supraorbitalis

Arcus palpebralis superior

A. supratrochlearis

A. infratrochlearis

Arcus palpebralis inferior

A. temporalis superficialis

A. angularis

A. transversa faciei

A. infraorbitalis

A. facialis

Fig. 9.30 Arteries of the orbital opening, Aditus orbitalis, and the periorbital area, right side; frontal view. [S700-L285]/[E1043]
Above the Septum orbitale, the Orbita is surrounded by a circular network of communicating arteries, formed by the Arcus palpebrales superior and inferior. The vascular circle is fed by numerous arteries **derived**

from the A. carotis interna (A. supraorbitalis, Aa. palpebrales laterales of the A. lacrimalis, Aa. palpebrales mediales) and the **A. carotis externa** (A. facialis, A. angularis, A. infraorbitalis, A. temporalis superficialis, A. zygomaticoorbitalis).

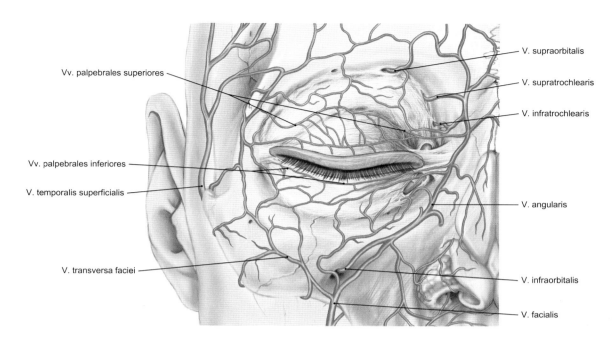

Fig. 9.31 **Veins of the orbital opening, Aditus orbitalis, and the periorbital area, right side**; frontal view. [S700-L285]/[E1043]
The venous blood is drained from the eyelid area via the Vv. palpebrales superiores and inferiores to the V. temporalis superficialis, the V. trans- versa faciei and the **V. facialis.** Due to the absence of venous valves, the blood drains nasally into the Vv. angularis, infra- and supratrochlearis and supraorbitalis and thereby **via the Orbita to the Sinus caverno-sus.**

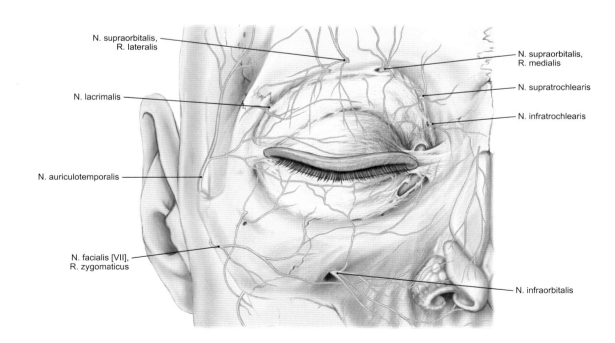

Fig. 9.32 **Nerves of the orbital opening, Aditus orbitalis, and the periorbital area, right side;** frontal view. [S700-L285]/[E1043]
The Nn. supra- and infraorbitalis, branches of the N. ophthalmicus [V/1] and N. maxillaris [V/2], leave the Orbita via the eponymously named foramina (the N. supraorbitalis can also leave the Orbita via an Incisura supraorbitalis]. At these **nerve exit points,** the sensitivity of the N. ophthalmicus [V/1] and the N. maxillaris [V/2] are tested (trigeminal pressure points).

Clinical remarks

A granulomatous inflammation, usually caused by an occlusion of the excretory duct of the MEIBOM's gland, is referred to as a **chalazion.** An immovable, painless protrusion, with a size between that of a grape seed and a hazelnut, it can be palpated just underneath the rim of the eyelid (→ Fig. a).

A stye (**hordeolum)** is a painful, mostly purulent inflammation of individual glands of the eyelids (usually caused by bacteria). Inflammation of the rim of the eyelid often results in **blepharitis** with the typical symptoms for dry eyes, such as a burning sensation, the feeling of having sand in one's eye, a mild form of photophobia and redness of the eyelid rims (→ Fig. b).

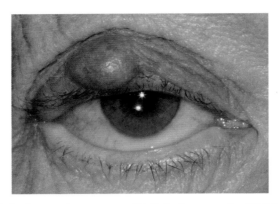

a Chalazion on the upper eyelid, Palpebra superior. [S700-T867]

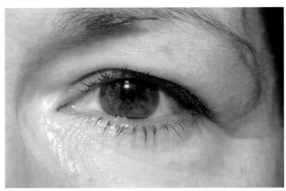

b Inflammation of the rims of the eyelids, seborrhoeic blepharitis. [S700-T867]

When the eyelid droops or turns outwards, this condition is called an **ectropion.** In most cases, the lower eyelid is affected. The most common form is a **senile ectropion** (Ectropium atonicum) which is caused by weakening of the muscles and a change in the conjunctive tissue in the elderly (→ Fig. c). This means that the eye can no longer be fully closed (lagophthalmos); or that there is a constant slow flow of tears (epiphora) with lacrimal fluid flowing over the rims of the eyelids, because the lacrimal points are no longer in contact with the Bulbus oculi. Additionally, a dry eye is vulnerable to chronic conjunctivitis or corneal ulceration. First-line treatment is surgical correction.

When dysfunction of a lacrimal gland is suspected, e. g. in the context of a facial paralysis, a **SCHIRMER's test** is carried out. For this purpose, a standardised long filter paper strip is applied to the conjunctival sac to absorb the tear fluid and it changes colour (→ Fig. d). At a normal rate of tear production, more than two-thirds of the paper strip should be coloured within five minutes. If only a small part of the paper strip changes colour, a reduced amount of lacrimal fluid (tears) is being produced. Another test for the tear film is the measurement of the **tear break-up time** (tearscope test), which helps to determine if the tear ducts can maintain a continuous protective film across the entire surface of the eye. A normal break-up time is 20–30 seconds. A break-up time of under 10 seconds is an indication of a dysfunction.

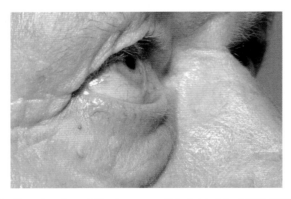

c Senile ectropion of the lower eyelid, right side. [S700-T867]

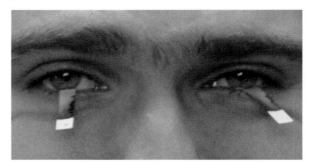

d SCHIRMER's test is performed on a healthy person. [S700-T912]

After just two minutes, the two yellow SCHIRMER's paper strips display a clear purple coloration. Within five minutes, the paper strips are completely purple.

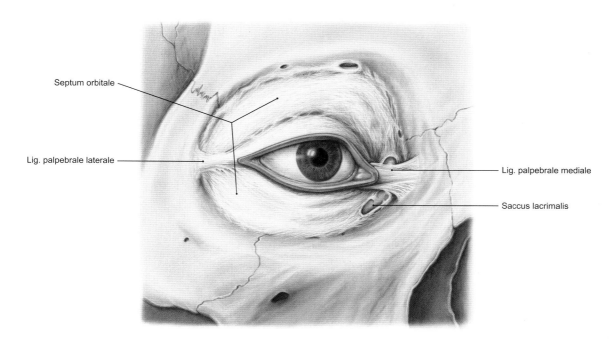

Septum orbitale

Lig. palpebrale laterale

Lig. palpebrale mediale

Saccus lacrimalis

Fig. 9.33 Orbital opening, Aditus orbitalis, right side, with Septum orbitale, eyelid lamina and palpebral ligaments; frontal view on the side. [S700-L285]/[E1043]
The Septum orbitale is a lamina of connective tissue that partially closes the orbital opening (Aditus orbitalis). It is attached to the walls of the

Orbita on the periorbita (periost). The Septum orbitale extends to the eyelid lamina, Tarsus superior and Tarsus inferior, and is laterally strengthened by the Ligg. palpebralia laterale and mediale.

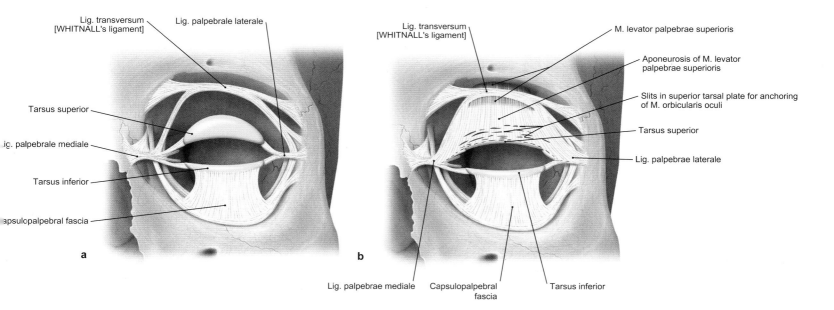

Lig. transversum [WHITNALL's ligament]

Lig. palpebrale laterale

Tarsus superior

Lig. palpebrale mediale

Tarsus inferior

Capsulopalpebral fascia

a

Lig. transversum [WHITNALL's ligament]

M. levator palpebrae superioris

Aponeurosis of M. levator palpebrae superioris

Slits in superior tarsal plate for anchoring of M. orbicularis oculi

Tarsus superior

Lig. palpebrae laterale

b

Lig. palpebrae mediale

Capsulopalpebral fascia

Tarsus inferior

Fig. 9.34a and b Orbital opening, Aditus orbitalis, right side, with Septum orbitale, tarsal plates and eyelid ligaments; frontal view. [S700-L127]
a Illustration of the connective tissue structures without the Levator aponeurosis.
b Illustration of the connective tissue structures with the Levator aponeurosis.
The Septum orbitale is a connective tissue membrane, respectively connecting the tarsal plate of the upper and lower eyelids to the rims of

the Orbita via ligaments. The connective tissue structures at the orbital margin merge with the periorbita (periosteum of the orbital opening) and form a support structure for the fatty tissue in the Orbita. The Ligg. palpebralia mediale and laterale and the Lig. transversum, known as WHITNALL's ligaments, are the strongest of the supporting ligaments in the upper section of the Orbita.

Eyelids and lacrimal gland

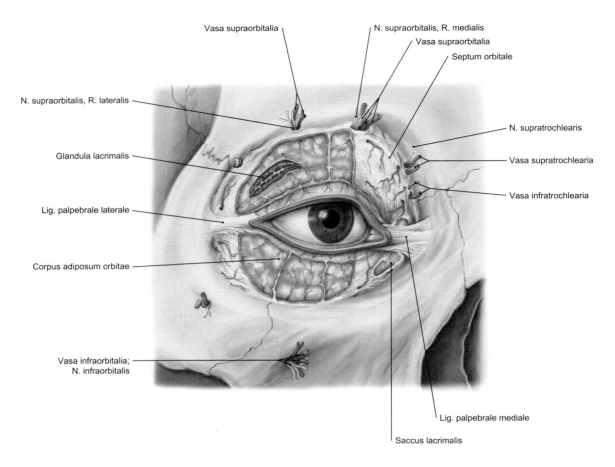

Fig. 9.35 Orbital cavity, Aditus orbitalis, Septum orbitale (partially removed), eyelid lamina and eyelid ligaments, right side; frontal view from the side. [S700-L285]/[E1043]
The orbital fatty tissue below the Septum orbitale is here known as post-septal, preaponeurotic fat (situated in front of the attachment site

of the tendon of the M. levator palpebrae superioris). In the outer upper quadrant is the anterior part of the lacrimal gland (Glandula lacrimalis), directly behind the Septum orbitale.

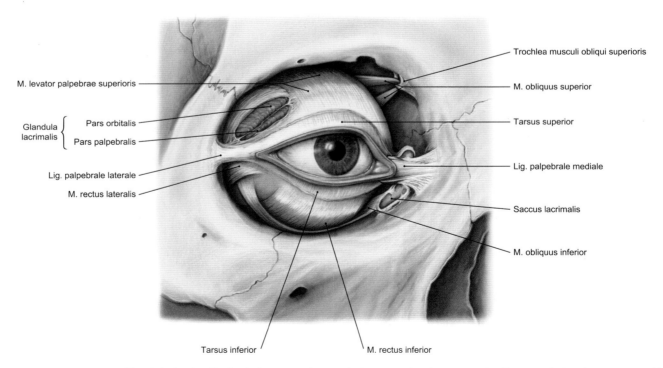

Fig. 9.36 Lacrimal glands, Glandula lacrimalis, in their connective tissue capsules on the eyeball, Bulbus oculi, right side; frontal view from the side. [S700-L285]/[E1043]
After removal of the postseptal fat (Corpus adiposum orbitae), and the Septum orbitale, the lacrimal glands (Glandula lacrimalis) can be seen in

their connective tissue capsule. The capsule has been removed in the front section. The lacrimal gland is divided by the tendon of the M. levator palpebrae superioris into a larger upper part (Pars orbitalis), and a smaller lower palpebral part (Pars palpebralis).

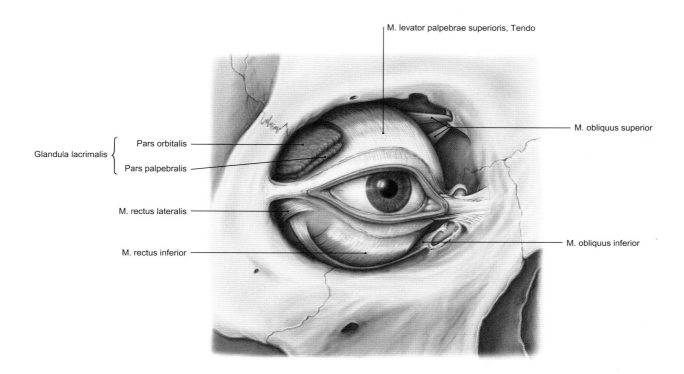

M. levator palpebrae superioris, Tendo

Glandula lacrimalis {
Pars orbitalis
Pars palpebralis

M. rectus lateralis

M. rectus inferior

M. obliquus superior

M. obliquus inferior

Fig. 9.37 Lacrimal gland, Glandula lacrimalis, on the eyeball, Bulbus oculi, right side; frontal view on the side. [S700-L285]/[E1043] After removal of the connective tissue capsules of the lacrimal gland (Glandula lacrimalis), their expansion in the upper lateral quadrant on the Bulbus oculi in relation to the course of the tendon of the M. levator palpebrae superioris is visible.

Clinical remarks

Inflammation of the lacrimal gland, Glandula lacrimalis (dacryoadenitis; → figure) causes protrusion of the Septum orbitale and a narrowing of the palpebral fissure.

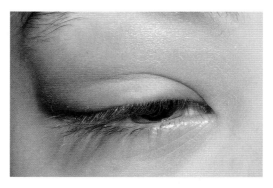

Swelling of the eyelid in acute dacryoadenitis (inflammation of the lacrimal gland); right side. [S700-T867]

Lacrimal gland, innervation

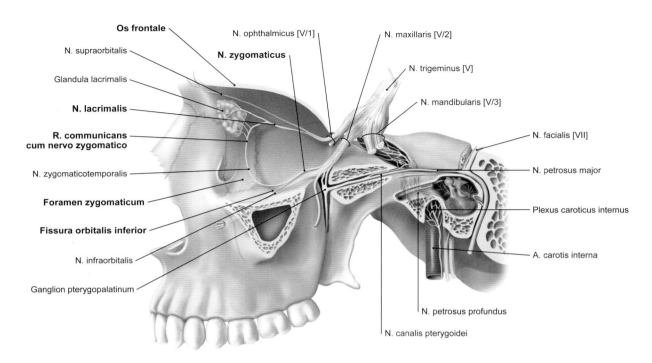

Fig. 9.38 Innervation of the lacrimal gland, Glandula lacrimalis, right side; medial view on the lateral wall of the Orbita. [S700-L275]

The lacrimal gland and the N. lacrimalis are both visible, as well as the connection between the N. zygomaticus and the N. lacrimalis via the R. communicans cum nervo zygomatico.

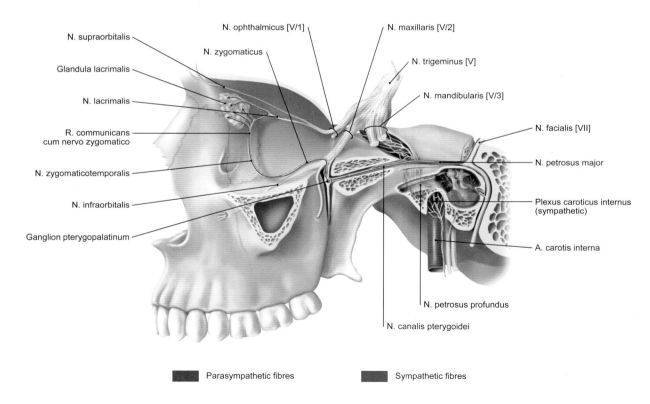

Parasympathetic fibres   Sympathetic fibres

Fig. 9.39 Sympathetic and parasympathetic innervation of the lacrimal gland, Glandula lacrimalis; schematic drawing. [S700-L275] In the Ganglion cervicale superius, preganglionic sympathetic nerve fibres are synapsed to postganglionic nerve fibres, which reach the lacrimal gland by accompanying the A. carotis interna, A. ophthalmica and A. lacrimalis, or by parting already from the A. carotis interna at the Foramen lacerum and running from here along with the parasympathe-

tic nerve fibres to the lacrimal gland. Preganglionic parasympathetic nerve fibres run via the intermedius portion of the N. facialis without synapsing through the geniculate ganglion (Ganglion geniculi) via the N. petrosus major and N. canalis pterygoidei to the Ganglion pterygopalatinum. Here, they synapse onto postganglionic nerve fibres, and via the R. communicans cum nervo zygomatico, along with the N. zygomaticus, reach the N. lacrimalis and hereby the lacrimal gland.

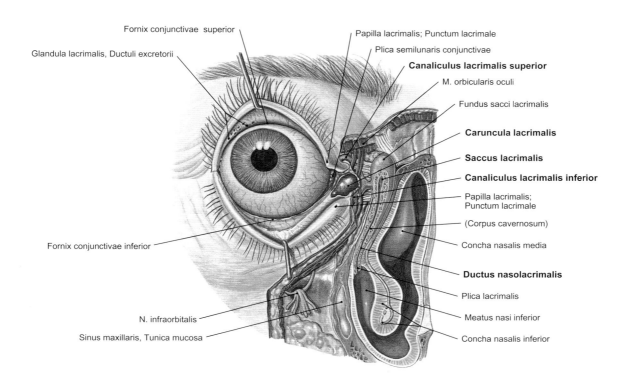

Fornix conjunctivae superior
Glandula lacrimalis, Ductuli excretorii
Fornix conjunctivae inferior
N. infraorbitalis
Sinus maxillaris, Tunica mucosa

Papilla lacrimalis; Punctum lacrimale
Plica semilunaris conjunctivae
Canaliculus lacrimalis superior
M. orbicularis oculi
Fundus sacci lacrimalis
Caruncula lacrimalis
Saccus lacrimalis
Canaliculus lacrimalis inferior
Papilla lacrimalis; Punctum lacrimale
(Corpus cavernosum)
Concha nasalis media
Ductus nasolacrimalis
Plica lacrimalis
Meatus nasi inferior
Concha nasalis inferior

Fig. 9.40 Lacrimal apparatus, Apparatus lacrimalis, right side; frontal view; the eyelids have been pulled away from the Bulbus oculi, thereby making it possible to see into the upper and lower conjunctival sac; the nasolacrimal duct has been opened up to the Meatus nasi inferior. [S700]
The draining nasolacrimal duct is composed of the upper and lower lacrimal canaliculi (Canaliculi lacrimales superior and inferior), the lacrimal sac (Saccus lacrimalis) and the nasolacrimal duct (Ductus nasolacrimalis). The Ductus nasolacrimalis exits into the lower nasal meatus (Meatus nasi inferior) beneath the lower nasal concha (Concha nasalis inferior).

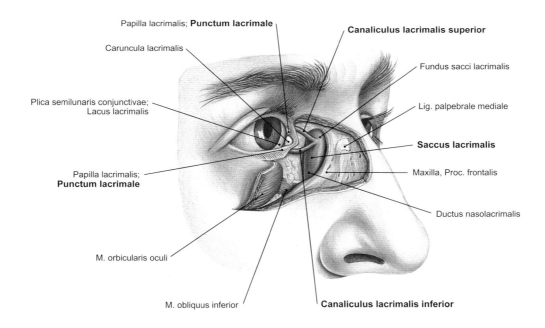

Papilla lacrimalis; **Punctum lacrimale**
Caruncula lacrimalis
Plica semilunaris conjunctivae; Lacus lacrimalis
Papilla lacrimalis; **Punctum lacrimale**
M. orbicularis oculi
M. obliquus inferior

Canaliculus lacrimalis superior
Fundus sacci lacrimalis
Lig. palpebrale mediale
Saccus lacrimalis
Maxilla, Proc. frontalis
Ductus nasolacrimalis
Canaliculus lacrimalis inferior

Fig. 9.41 Lacrimal apparatus, Apparatus lacrimalis, right side; frontolateral view; after removal of skin, muscles and the Septum orbitale in the medial canthus. [S700]
The lacrimal sac (Saccus lacrimalis) is located in the Fossa sacci lacrimalis and continues caudally as the Ductus nasolacrimalis in a bony enclosure, bordered at the front by the maxilla and posteriorly by the Os lacrimale. Each Canaliculus lacrimalis originates as a 0.25 mm (upper) to 0.3 mm (lower) wide, round, oval or slit-shaped Punctum lacrimale which continues as an approx. 2 mm long vertical tube which then bends almost at a right angle and proceeds as an approx. 8 mm horizontal segment. In the majority of cases (65–70 %), both canaliculi merge to form a common tube approx. 1–2 mm long that opens into the lacrimal sac about 2–3 mm below the Fornix sacci lacrimalis.

Lacrimal gland and lacrimal apparatus

Lacrimal apparatus

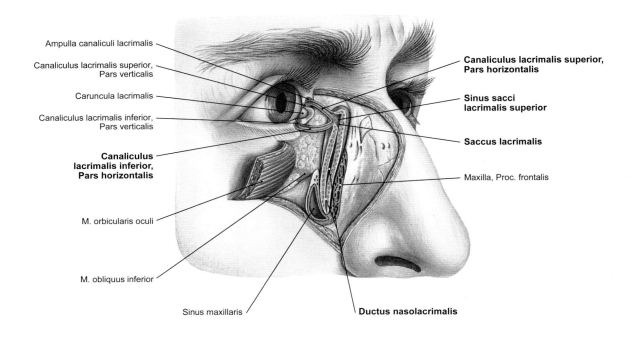

Ampulla canaliculi lacrimalis

Canaliculus lacrimalis superior, Pars verticalis

Caruncula lacrimalis

Canaliculus lacrimalis inferior, Pars verticalis

Canaliculus lacrimalis inferior, Pars horizontalis

M. orbicularis oculi

M. obliquus inferior

Sinus maxillaris

Canaliculus lacrimalis superior, Pars horizontalis

Sinus sacci lacrimalis superior

Saccus lacrimalis

Maxilla, Proc. frontalis

Ductus nasolacrimalis

Fig. 9.42 Lacrimal apparatus, Apparatus lacrimalis, right side; horizontal section at the level of the lacrimal sac. [S700]
The Canaliculi lacrimales consist of a short Pars verticalis and then bend almost at a right angle into the Pars horizontalis which is about four times as long. This right-angled bend becomes more rounded with increasing age. At the juncture between the Pars verticalis and Pars horizontalis, each canaliculus enlarges to form the Ampulla canaliculi lacrimalis. The Pars horizontalis is located close to the rim of the eyelid and projects towards the bony Fossa sacci lacrimalis of the orbita which contains the Saccus lacrimalis. The Partes horizontales have a diameter of 0.3–0.6 mm, but can easily expand up to 1.5 mm.
In more than 95 % of cases, the Partes horizontales of the upper and lower Canaliculus lacrimalis merge to form a single duct. After passing

through the Septum lacrimale which covers the Fossa sacci lacrimalis (→ Fig. 9.43), the duct penetrates the wall of the lacrimal sac approx. 2.5–4 mm below the Fundus sacci lacrimalis and opens into the lumen of the lacrimal sac (Sinus sacci lacrimalis superior, MAIER's sinus).
A cavernous body of tissue, functionally supporting the transport of the lacrimal fluid, surrounds the lumen of the lacrimal sac. Swelling of this cavernous tissue reduces or blocks the transport of lacrimal fluid and the tears (lacrimal fluid) run down the cheek (crying). The blood vessels of the cavernous tissue dilate when a foreign particle enters the conjunctival sac or when experiencing strong emotions (e. g. intense happiness or sadness).

Dimensions of the tear ducts			
Structure			**Dimensions**
Punctum lacrimale	superius		Ø 0.25 mm
	inferius		Ø 0.3 mm
Canaliculus lacrimalis	superior	Pars verticalis	Length: 1.8–2.25 mm, Ø 0.08–0.1 mm
		Pars horizontalis	Length: 7–9 mm, always approx. 0.5 mm shorter than the Canaliculus inferior, Ø 0.3–0.6 mm
	inferior	Pars verticalis	Length: 1.8–2.25 mm, Ø 0.08–0.1 mm
		Pars horizontalis	Length: 7–9 mm, always approx. 0.5 mm shorter than the Canaliculus superior, Ø 0.3–0.6 mm
Saccus lacrimalis	vertically		Ø 12 mm
	sagittally		Ø 5–6 mm
	transversely		Ø 4–5 mm
Ductus nasolacrimalis	total		Length: 12.4 mm
	bony cavity		Length: 10 mm
			Ø 4.6 mm

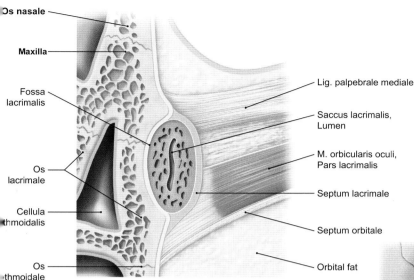

Os nasale
Maxilla
Fossa lacrimalis
Os lacrimale
Cellula ethmoidalis
Os ethmoidale

Lig. palpebrale mediale
Saccus lacrimalis, Lumen
M. orbicularis oculi, Pars lacrimalis
Septum lacrimale
Septum orbitale
Orbital fat

Fig. 9.43 Lacrimal apparatus, Apparatus lacrimalis, right side; horizontal section at the level of the lacrimal sac, Saccus lacrimalis. [S700-L275]
The Lig. palpebrale mediale inserts on the anterior margin of the Fossa lacrimalis. The Pars lacrimalis of the M. orbicularis oculi passes laterally of the Septum orbitale and at the posterior aspect of the lacrimal sac. The close proximity to the ethmoidal cells (Cellulae ethmoidales) is clear to see in this illustration.

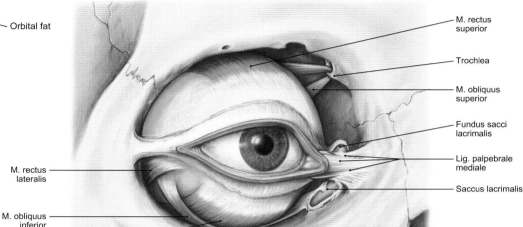

M. rectus superior
Trochlea
M. obliquus superior
Fundus sacci lacrimalis
Lig. palpebrale mediale
Saccus lacrimalis
M. rectus lateralis
M. obliquus inferior
M. rectus inferior

Fig. 9.44 Lacrimal apparatus, Apparatus lacrimalis, in the Orbita, right side; frontal view from the side. [S700-L285]/[E1043]
The tear sac lies directly behind the Lig. palpebrale mediale, with its fundus protruding from behind it. Below the Lig. palpebrale mediale, the tear sac passes into the Fossa lacrimalis; compare → Fig. 9.28.

→ T 2

Clinical remarks

The most common diseases of the lacrimal drainage system are inflammation (**dacryocystitis;** Fig. a), narrowing **(dacryostenosis)** and stone formation **(dacryolithiasis).** This mainly leads to excessive watering of the eye **(epiphora).** Dacryostenosis can also be hereditary. In most cases a congenital stenosis is based on a persistent membrane of HASNER, a thin connective tissue membrane at the transition to the lower nasal passage, which ruptures shortly after birth in most cases. However, if persistent, it must be pierced by the doctor.
The **development of the efferent tear ducts** is a complex process, particularly associated with congenital narrowing or closure of the Ductus nasolacrimalis in the area of the lower nasal passage. In up to 6 % of newborns, the Ductus nasolacrimalis does not correctly meet up with the Meatus nasi. There are various causes:

• The Ductus nasolacrimalis does not make a connection with the lower nasal passage and terminates blindly over the bony nasal floor (→ Fig. b).
• The Ductus nasolacrimalis terminates in the bony wall of the Sinus maxillaris (→ Fig. c).
• The lumen of the nasolacrimal canal does not connect to the lower nasal passage and is covered by a mucosal fold (→ Fig. d), which is the most common malformation.
• The opening of the Ductus nasolacrimalis is displaced by a bony lamella of the lower nasalis muscle which has folded over laterally (→ Fig. e).

These infants suffer from epiphora (watery eyes) and/or chronic inflammations of the efferent tear ducts. Mostly the membranes open by themselves in the first nine months of life, but if not, an ophthalmic surgical intervention is advisable.

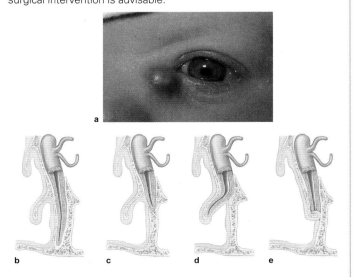

a

b   c   d   e

Inflammation of the lacrimal sac (dacryocystitis) in an infant (a) and congenital narrowing or closure of the Ductus lacrimalis (b–e). a [S700-T867], b–e [S700-L285]

Extraocular muscles

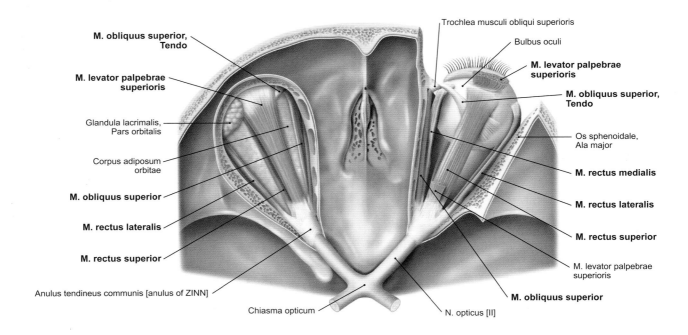

Fig. 9.45 Extraocular muscles, Mm. bulbi; superior view; after removal of the roof of the Orbita on both sides and removal of most of the M. levator palpebrae superioris, as well as the orbital fat body on the right side. [S700-L275]

→ T 2

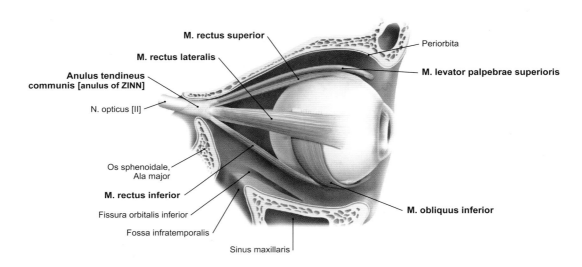

Fig. 9.46 Extraocular muscles, Mm. bulbi, right side; lateral view; after removal of the lateral wall of the Orbita. [S700-L275]
The Bulbus oculi is controlled by six extraocular muscles (four rectus muscles: Mm. recti superior, inferior, medialis and lateralis; two oblique muscles: Mm. obliqui superior and inferior). With the exception of the M. obliquus inferior (origin at the Facies orbitalis of the lateral maxilla of the Incisura lacrimalis in the anterior medial area of the Orbita) and the M. obliquus superior (origin at the Corpus ossis sphenoidalis medial of the Anulus tendineus communis and the dural sheath of the N. opticus), all other extraocular muscles originate from the **anulus of ZINN (Anulus tendineus communis).**

All six muscles insert at the sclera. The four extra ocular rectus muscles insert anterior to the equator of the Bulbus oculi, while the two oblique muscles insert posterior to the equator. A tendinous pulley-like structure (trochlea), which attaches to the anterior upper area of the Os frontale and acts as a hypomochlion for the M. obliquus superior, redirects this muscle back to its insertion area at the top of the eyeball, posterior to its equator. The anulus of ZINN is also the origin of the elevating muscle of the upper eyelid (M. levator palpebrae superioris) which projects into the upper eyelid (Palpebra superior).

→ T 2

Clinical remarks

A **paralysis of the M. levator palpebrae superioris** (resulting from damage to the N. oculomotorius [III]) leads to **ptosis** (drooping of the eyelid). The patient does not usually suffer from double vision (diplopia), since the affected eyelid is above the pupil. Raising the drooping eyelid, however, causes double vision, because the Mm. recti superior, inferior and medialis are also paralysed. Even in the case of damage to the N. abducens [VI] and the N. trochlearis [IV] there will be a paralytic squint, resulting in diplopia.

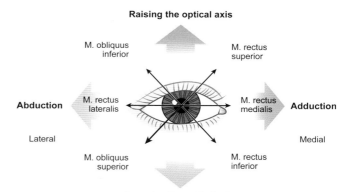

Fig. 9.47 Function of the extraocular muscles, Mm. bulbi. [S700-L126]

The clinical evaluation of ocular motility is carried out by **testing the nine main viewing directions (straight ahead, right, left, top, bottom, top left, top right, bottom left, bottom right).** The muscles activated for each direction are shown for both eyes. The synchronised movement of both eyeballs is a very complex issue as the innervated muscle of the different cranial nerves (Nn. oculomotorius, trochlearis and abducens) must be coordinated synergistically. The extraocular muscles are very finely innervated and their fine structure distinguish them from the normal striated muscles.

Muscle	Function	Innervation
M. rectus superior	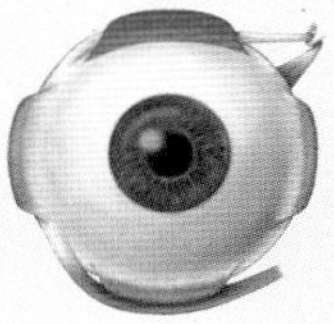 Raising the optical axis Adduction of the eyeball and turning it inwards	N. oculomotorius [III], R. superior
M. rectus inferior	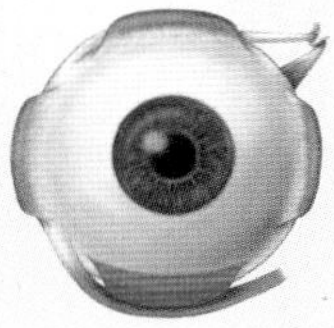 Lowering the optical axis Adduction of the eyeball and turning it outwards	N. oculomotorius [III], R. inferior
M. rectus lateralis	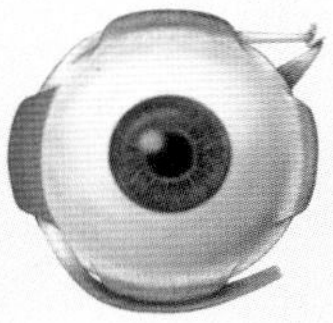 Abduction of the eyeball	N. abducens [VI]
M. rectus medialis	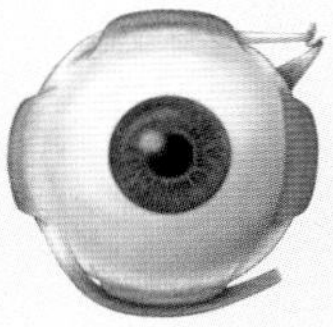 Adduction of the eyeball	N. oculomotorius [III], R. inferior
M. obliquus inferior	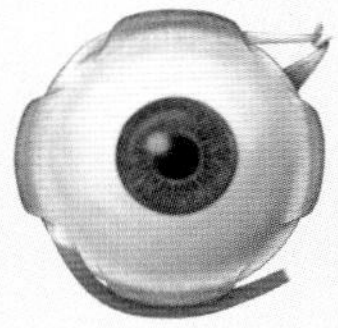 Raising the optical axis Abduction of the eyeball and turning it outwards	N. oculomotorius [III], R. inferior
M. obliquus superior	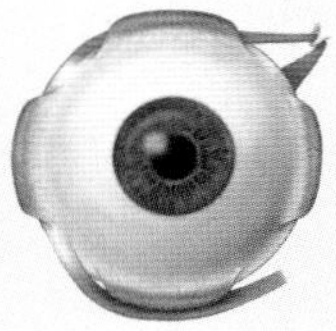 Lowering of the optical axis Abduction of the eyeball and turning it inwards	N. trochlearis [IV]

Fig. 9.48 Function and innervation of the extraocular muscles entering at the Bulbus oculi. [S700-L285]

The muscle is shown in dark red each time.

→ T 2

─ **Clinical remarks** ──────────────────────────────

In the case of **oculomotor nerve palsy,** with the exception of the M. rectus lateralis (N. abducens) and the M. obliquus superior (N. trochlearis [IV]), all extraocular muscles cease to function. Because the two unaffected muscles predominate, the gaze of the eye is directed downwards and outwards (down and out). Since the M. levator palpebrae superioris has failed, the patient has a ptosis. The patient cannot see with the affected eye and therefore does not experience double vision. Only when the drooping eyelid is manually raised does the patient complain of diplopia.

Extraocular muscles

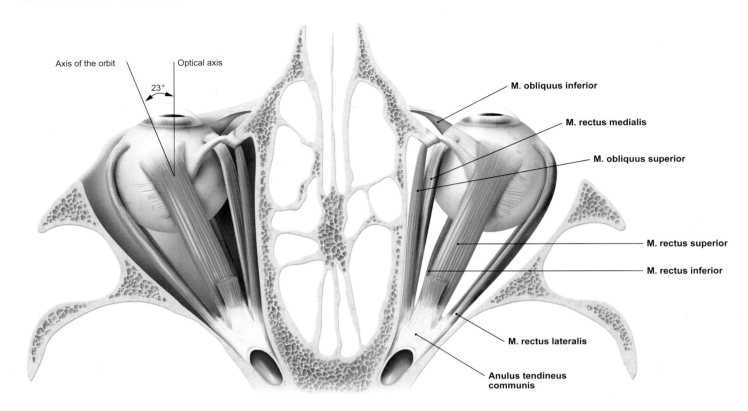

Fig. 9.49 Extraocular muscles, Mm. bulbi; superior view. [S700-L275] Shown are the anulus of ZINN (Anulus tendineus communis) and the insertion sites of the muscles at the Bulbus oculi.

The optical axis and the axis of the Orbita differ by an angle of 23°. This is the reason why the Fovea centralis (the area of most acute vision) is located lateral to the Papilla nervi optici (blind spot).

→ T 2

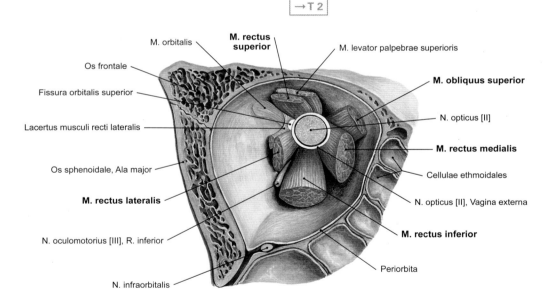

Fig. 9.50 Extraocular muscles, Mm. bulbi, right side; frontal view onto the posterior wall of the Orbita. [S700]

The periorbital space near the Fissura orbitalis superior contains smooth muscle fibres innervated by the Sympathicus; collectively, these form the M. orbitalis.

→ T 2

Clinical remarks

Damage to the N. trochlearis [IV] can cause **palsy of the trochlear nerve.** Paralysis of the M. obliquus superior causes the visual axis to point medially (nasal) and upward because the normal abduction and downward movement of the eyeball by the superior oblique muscle is absent. **Abducens nerve palsies** are the most frequent palsies of the extraocular muscles (in part, because the N. abducens [VI] [→ Fig. 9.51] runs through the centre of the Sinus cavernosus and can be damaged more easily here than in the peripheral zone of the sinus where the N. oculomotorius [III] and N. trochlearis [IV] are located). Paralysis of the M. rectus lateralis shifts the visual axis medially (nasally).

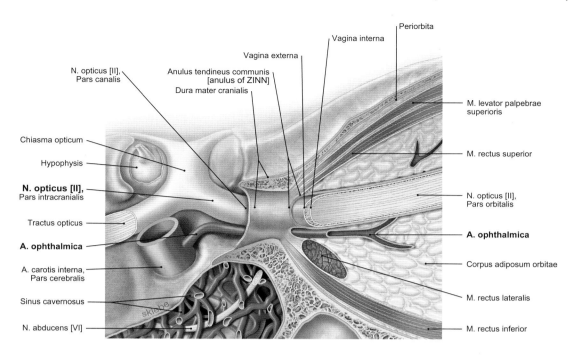

Fig. 9.51 Optic nerve, N. opticus [II], right side; lateral view; after the opening of the Canalis opticus. [S700-L238]

The N. opticus [II] runs along the A. ophthalmica (branch of the A. carotis interna) through the Canalis opticus and the Anulus tendineus communis (anulus of ZINN) into the Orbita.

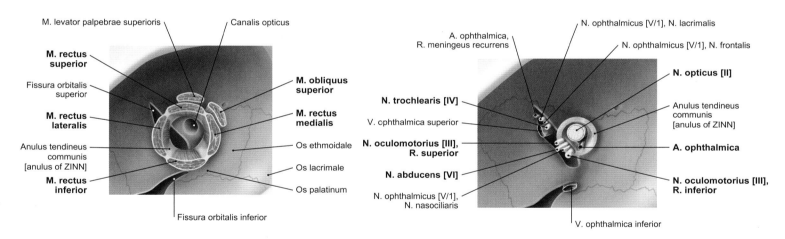

Fig. 9.52 Muscular origins at the Anulus tendineus communis (anulus of ZINN), right side; frontal view. [S700-L275]
The Mm. rectus superior, rectus medialis, rectus inferior and rectus lateralis originate from the Anulus tendineus communis. The neurovascular bundle passing through the anulus of Zinn is not shown in this illustration (→ Fig. 9.53). The M. levator palpebrae superioris, which is shown here, originates from the Ala minor ossis sphenoidalis at the tip of the Orbita and outside of the Anulus tendineus communis. The M. obliquus superior comes from the Corpus ossis sphenoidalis, medial of the Anulus tendineus communis, at the dural sheath. Connective tissue fibres of its fascia radiate into the Anulus tendineus communis.

→ T 2

Fig. 9.53 Neurovascular pathways passing through the Canalis opticus and the Fissura orbitalis superior, right side; frontal view. [S700-L275]
The N. oculomotorius [III], N. nasociliaris, N. abducens [VI] and Radix sympathica ganglii ciliaris run via the Fissura orbitalis superior and through the Anulus tendineus communis (anulus of ZINN). The V. ophthalmica superior, the N. lacrimalis, the N. frontalis and the N. trochlearis [IV] also run via the Fissura orbitalis superior in the Orbita. But these neurovascular structures run outside of the Anulus tendineus communis (anulus of ZINN). Not shown are the V. ophthalmica inferior, A. infraorbitalis, N. infraorbitalis and N. zygomaticus which enter the Orbita through the Fissura orbitalis inferior. The A. centralis retinae runs centrally within the N. opticus [II] as the first branch of the A. ophthalmica.

Clinical remarks

The **orbital apex syndrome** may cause incomplete or complete paralysis of one or more extraocular muscles (ophthalmoplegia). The causes are usually chronic inflammation or tumours in the area of the tip of the Orbita. An **embolic occlusion of the A. centralis retinae** is a frequent vascular cause of acute blindness.

Arteries and nerves of the eye socket

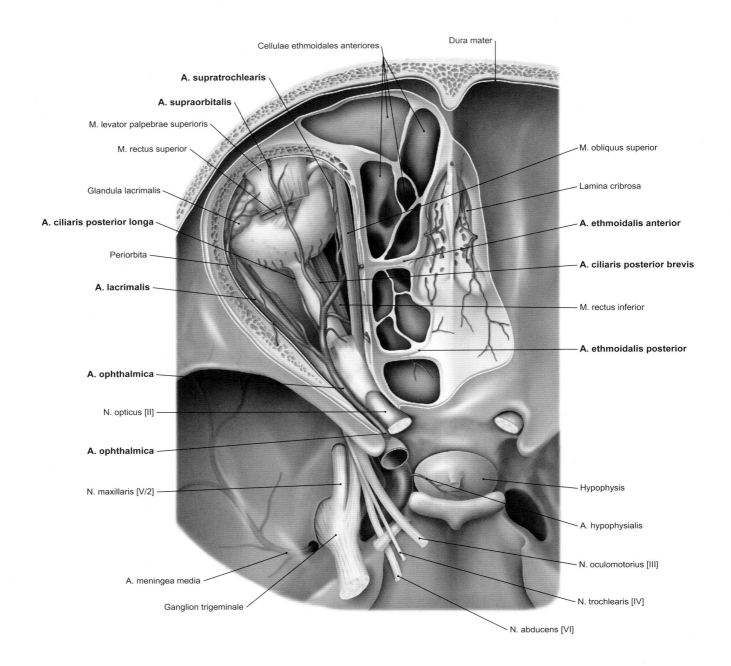

Cellulae ethmoidales anteriores

Dura mater

A. supratrochlearis

A. supraorbitalis

M. levator palpebrae superioris

M. rectus superior

Glandula lacrimalis

A. ciliaris posterior longa

Periorbita

A. lacrimalis

A. ophthalmica

N. opticus [II]

A. ophthalmica

N. maxillaris [V/2]

A. meningea media

Ganglion trigeminale

M. obliquus superior

Lamina cribrosa

A. ethmoidalis anterior

A. ciliaris posterior brevis

M. rectus inferior

A. ethmoidalis posterior

Hypophysis

A. hypophysialis

N. oculomotorius [III]

N. trochlearis [IV]

N. abducens [VI]

Fig. 9.54 Arteries of the eye, Oculus, and the eye socket, Orbita;
superior view of the opened orbitas on the left; orbital contents with
extraocular muscles. [S700-L275]
The A. ophthalmica is the main artery of the Orbita. It originates from
the Pars cerebralis of the A. carotis interna and normally runs slightly
below the N. opticus [II] through the Canalis opticus into the Orbita.
Here, the artery divides into many branches which supply the Bulbus

oculi and the structures of the Orbita with blood. Anastomoses exist via
a R. orbitalis to the A. meningea media (not shown), via the Aa. ethmoidales anterior and posterior to the blood vessels in the nose and via
blood vessels penetrating the Septum orbitale or the bone to the facial
arteries (Aa. supraorbitalis, supratrochlearis, palpebralis medialis and
lateralis, dorsalis nasi).

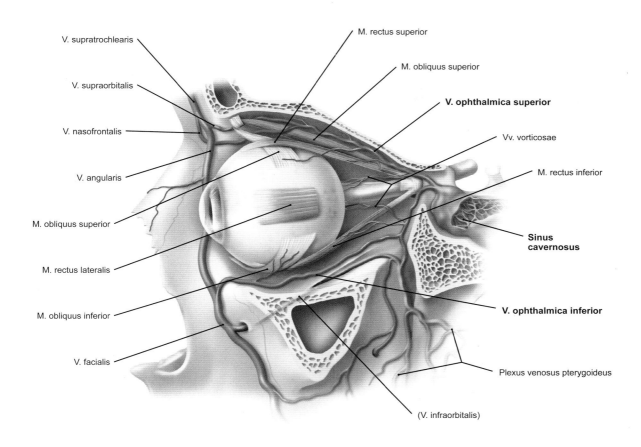

V. supratrochlearis
V. supraorbitalis
V. nasofrontalis
V. angularis
M. obliquus superior
M. rectus lateralis
M. obliquus inferior
V. facialis

M. rectus superior
M. obliquus superior
V. ophthalmica superior
Vv. vorticosae
M. rectus inferior
Sinus cavernosus
V. ophthalmica inferior
Plexus venosus pterygoideus
(V. infraorbitalis)

Fig. 9.55 Veins of the eye, Oculus, and the eye socket, Orbita, right side; lateral view into the Orbita; after removal of the lateral wall of the Orbita. [S700-L275]

The venous drainage occurs via the Vv. ophthalmicae superior and inferior. The latter is usually smaller than the A. ophthalmica superior. Venous anastomoses are present on the superficial and deep facial areas (Plexus pterygoideus) and the Sinus cavernosus.

Clinical remarks

Via the V. angularis running in the medial canthus and the intraorbitally running V. ophthalmica, there is a connection between the face (V. facialis) and the Sinus cavernosus. In the case of infections of the outer face areas (e.g. after squeezing out a pimple on the cheek)

there could be a **spread of germs** into the Sinus cavernosus with a subsequent **thrombosis** of the Sinus cavernosus (Clinical remarks → Fig. 12.70). At the first sign of an infection, the V. angularis must be ligated in order to prevent a sinus thrombosis.

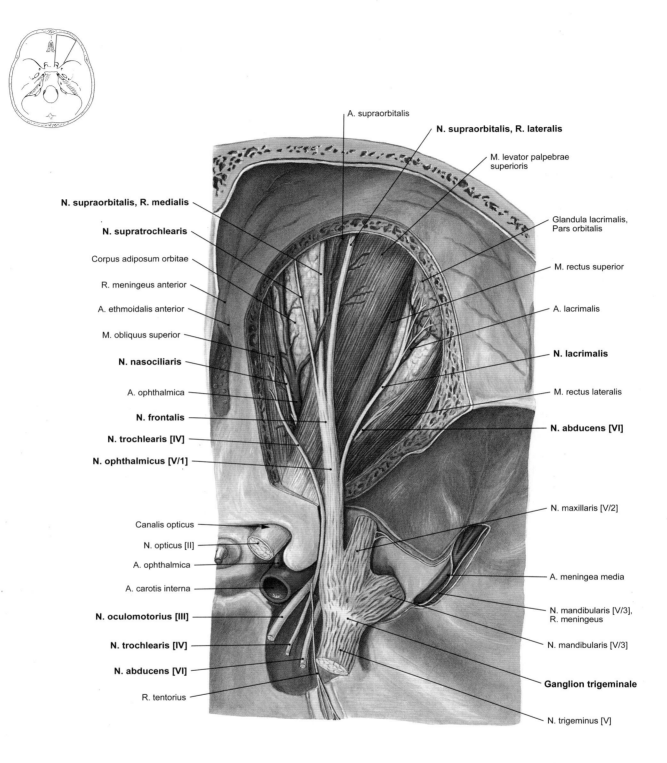

A. supraorbitalis

N. supraorbitalis, R. lateralis

M. levator palpebrae superioris

N. supraorbitalis, R. medialis

Glandula lacrimalis, Pars orbitalis

N. supratrochlearis

Corpus adiposum orbitae

M. rectus superior

R. meningeus anterior

A. ethmoidalis anterior

A. lacrimalis

M. obliquus superior

N. nasociliaris

N. lacrimalis

A. ophthalmica

M. rectus lateralis

N. frontalis

N. trochlearis [IV]

N. abducens [VI]

N. ophthalmicus [V/1]

N. maxillaris [V/2]

Canalis opticus

N. opticus [II]

A. ophthalmica

A. meningea media

A. carotis interna

N. oculomotorius [III]

N. mandibularis [V/3], R. meningeus

N. trochlearis [IV]

N. mandibularis [V/3]

N. abducens [VI]

Ganglion trigeminale

R. tentorius

N. trigeminus [V]

Fig. 9.56   Arteries and nerves of the eye socket, Orbita, right side; superior view on the opened Orbita (upper level of the Orbita); illustration of the Ganglion trigeminale (Ganglion semilunare, Ganglion GASSERI); bony roof of the Orbita, Periorbita and Corpus adiposum orbitae partially removed. [S700]
Depicted are the **pathway of the N. ophthalmicus [V/1],** superior view of the opened Fissura orbitalis superior and further branching into the Nn. lacrimalis and frontalis (including consecutive branching) as well as the more deeply running N. nasociliaris. It is also possible to see the gracile N. trochlearis [IV] which supplies the motor innervation of the M. obliquus superior, and the more deeply located N. abducens [VI] which innervates the M. rectus lateralis.

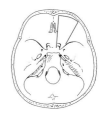

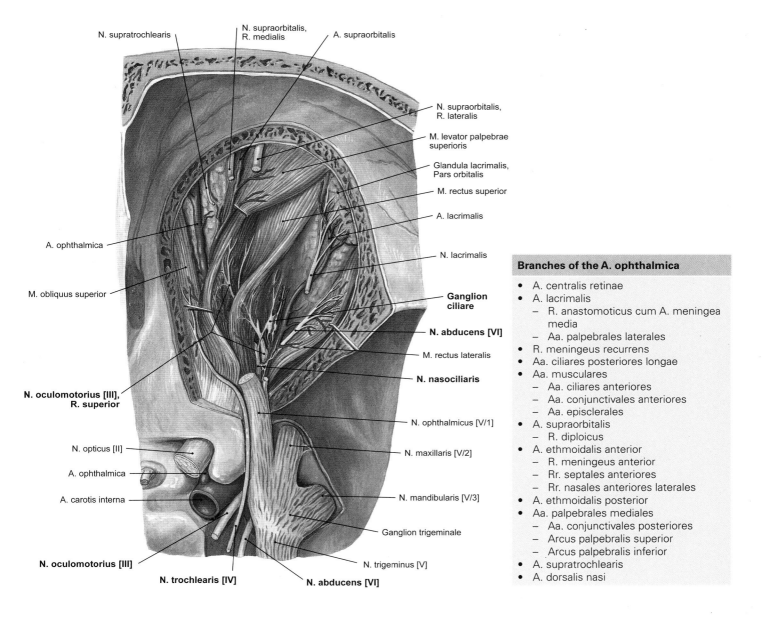

N. supratrochlearis

N. supraorbitalis, R. medialis

A. supraorbitalis

N. supraorbitalis, R. lateralis

M. levator palpebrae superioris

Glandula lacrimalis, Pars orbitalis

M. rectus superior

A. lacrimalis

N. lacrimalis

Ganglion ciliare

N. abducens [VI]

M. rectus lateralis

N. nasociliaris

N. ophthalmicus [V/1]

N. maxillaris [V/2]

N. mandibularis [V/3]

Ganglion trigeminale

N. trigeminus [V]

A. ophthalmica

M. obliquus superior

N. oculomotorius [III], R. superior

N. opticus [II]

A. ophthalmica

A. carotis interna

N. oculomotorius [III]

N. trochlearis [IV]

N. abducens [VI]

Branches of the A. ophthalmica

- A. centralis retinae
- A. lacrimalis
  - R. anastomoticus cum A. meningea media
  - Aa. palpebrales laterales
- R. meningeus recurrens
- Aa. ciliares posteriores longae
- Aa. musculares
  - Aa. ciliares anteriores
  - Aa. conjunctivales anteriores
  - Aa. episclerales
- A. supraorbitalis
  - R. diploicus
- A. ethmoidalis anterior
  - R. meningeus anterior
  - Rr. septales anteriores
  - Rr. nasales anteriores laterales
- A. ethmoidalis posterior
- Aa. palpebrales mediales
  - Aa. conjunctivales posteriores
  - Arcus palpebralis superior
  - Arcus palpebralis inferior
- A. supratrochlearis
- A. dorsalis nasi

Fig. 9.57 Arteries and nerves of the eye socket, Orbita, right side; superior view; after removal of the roof of the Orbita; illustration of the Ganglion ciliare; the M. levator palpebrae superioris and the M. rectus superior have been folded back. [S700]
Depicted are the nerve branches of the N. oculomotorius [III] entering beneath the muscles. After removal of the fat body beneath the muscles, the **Ganglion ciliare,** which is approx. 2 mm in size, becomes visible. Positioned lateral of the N. opticus [II], approx. 1 cm posterior to the Bulbus oculi, the Ganglion ciliare is embedded in the Corpus adi-

posum orbitae. The Ganglion ciliare contains perikarya of the postganglionic parasympathetic neurons, which synapse with the axons of preganglionic parasympathetic neurons located in the Nucleus oculomotorius accessorius (autonomicus, EDINGER-WESTPHAL nucleus). These parasympathetic fibres innervate the inner muscles of the eye (M. ciliaris and M. sphincter pupillae, → Fig. 8.132). Postganglionic sympathetic neurons for the M. dilatator pupillae pass through the Ganglion ciliare without switching. They were already switched from preganglionic to postganglionic in the Ganglion cervicale superius.

Arteries and nerves of the eye socket

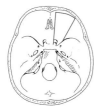

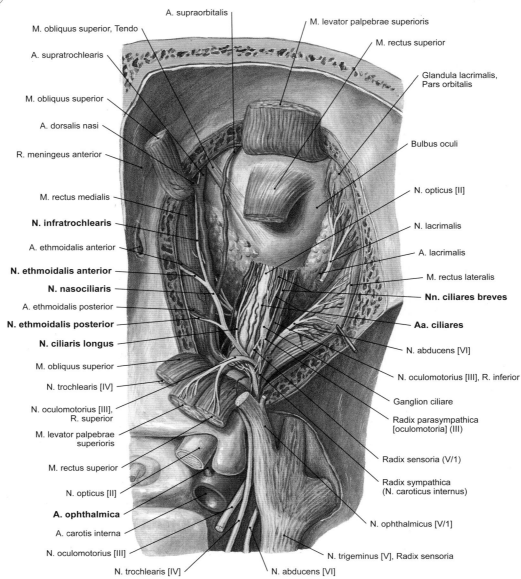

A. supraorbitalis

M. obliquus superior, Tendo

A. supratrochlearis

M. obliquus superior

A. dorsalis nasi

R. meningeus anterior

M. rectus medialis

N. infratrochlearis

A. ethmoidalis anterior

N. ethmoidalis anterior

N. nasociliaris

A. ethmoidalis posterior

N. ethmoidalis posterior

N. ciliaris longus

M. obliquus superior

N. trochlearis [IV]

N. oculomotorius [III], R. superior

M. levator palpebrae superioris

M. rectus superior

N. opticus [II]

A. ophthalmica

A. carotis interna

N. oculomotorius [III]

N. trochlearis [IV]

N. abducens [VI]

M. levator palpebrae superioris

M. rectus superior

Glandula lacrimalis, Pars orbitalis

Bulbus oculi

N. opticus [II]

N. lacrimalis

A. lacrimalis

M. rectus lateralis

Nn. ciliares breves

Aa. ciliares

N. abducens [VI]

N. oculomotorius [III], R. inferior

Ganglion ciliare

Radix parasympathica [oculomotoria] (III)

Radix sensoria (V/1)

Radix sympathica (N. caroticus internus)

N. ophthalmicus [V/1]

N. trigeminus [V], Radix sensoria

Fig. 9.58 Arteries and nerves of the eye socket, Orbita, right side; superior view; after partial removal of the Mm. levator palpebrae superioris, rectus superior and obliquus superior. [S700]
The illustration shows the content of the **middle level of the Orbita.** One can recognise the network of arteries (Aa. ciliares) that supply the

N. opticus [II] branching off the A. ophthalmica which runs through the Orbita, as well as the Nn. ciliares longi and breves, the Ganglion ciliare and the branching out of the N. nasociliaris.

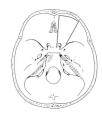

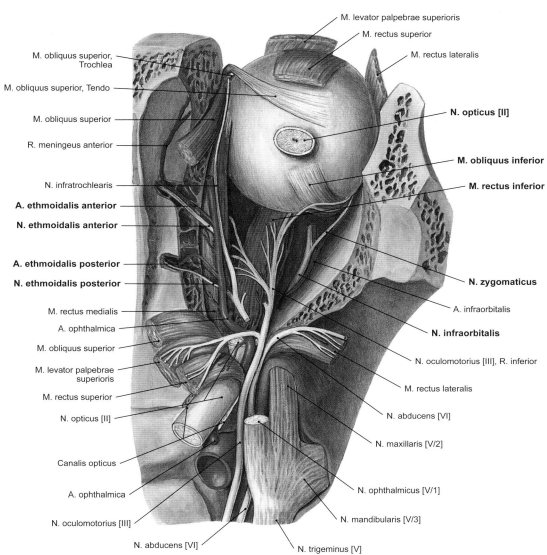

M. levator palpebrae superioris

M. rectus superior

M. rectus lateralis

M. obliquus superior, Trochlea

M. obliquus superior, Tendo

M. obliquus superior

R. meningeus anterior

N. infratrochlearis

A. ethmoidalis anterior

N. ethmoidalis anterior

A. ethmoidalis posterior

N. ethmoidalis posterior

M. rectus medialis

A. ophthalmica

M. obliquus superior

M. levator palpebrae superioris

M. rectus superior

N. opticus [II]

Canalis opticus

A. ophthalmica

N. oculomotorius [III]

N. abducens [VI]

N. opticus [II]

M. obliquus inferior

M. rectus inferior

N. zygomaticus

A. infraorbitalis

N. infraorbitalis

N. oculomotorius [III], R. inferior

M. rectus lateralis

N. abducens [VI]

N. maxillaris [V/2]

N. ophthalmicus [V/1]

N. mandibularis [V/3]

N. trigeminus [V]

Fig. 9.59 Arteries and nerves of the eye socket, Orbita, right side; superior view; the N. opticus [II] has been cut. [S700]
After removal of additional structures and the entire orbital fat body, the M. inferior rectus and the **lower level of the Orbita** are visible. The Bulbus oculi is rotated in such a way that the insertion site of the M. obliquus inferior, close to the entry site of the cut N. opticus [II], can be seen. On the medial side, the ethmoidal cells (Cellulae ethmoidales) are

opened up in order to show the pathway of the Nn. ethmoidales anterior and posterior as well as the Aa. ethmoidales anterior and posterior from the Orbita into the ethmoid bone. At the lower level, the lateral A. and N. infraorbitalis are visible. The N. zygomaticus, which contains sensory fibres, branches off from the N. infraorbitalis and innervates the lacrimal gland via postganglionic parasympathetic fibres.

Clinical remarks

The N. opticus [II] has a topographical connection to the sphenoidal sinus (Sinus sphenoidalis), with the consequence that **disease processes within the Sinus sphenoidalis** (sinusitis, tumours) can affect the N. opticus [III] because the bony wall which separates it

from the sphenoidal sinus is so thin. Sometimes, this bony wall is missing. During operations in the sphenoidal sinus, great care is required not to damage the N. opticus.

Nerves of the eye socket

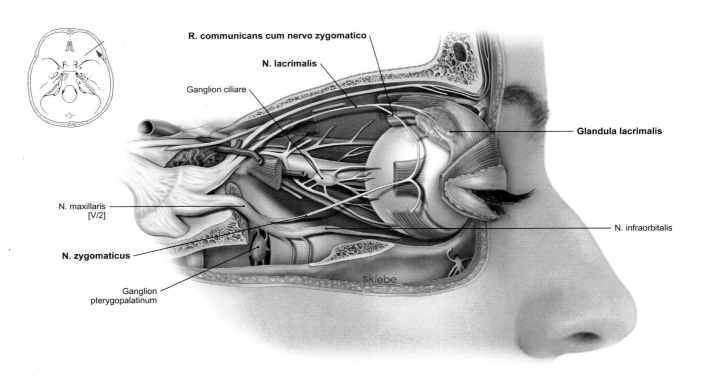

R. communicans cum nervo zygomatico

N. lacrimalis

Ganglion ciliare

Glandula lacrimalis

N. maxillaris
[V/2]

N. zygomaticus

N. infraorbitalis

Ganglion
pterygopalatinum

sklebe

Fig. 9.60 Nerves of the eye socket, Orbita, and the eye, Oculus, innervation of the lacrimal gland, Glandula lacrimalis, and illustration of the Ganglion ciliare, right side; lateral view; after removal of the temporal wall and the orbital fat body. [S700-L238]
The lacrimal gland is innervated via sympathetic, parasympathetic and somatosensory fibres. **Postganglionic parasympathetic fibres** originate from the Ganglion pterygopalatinum and stimulate glandular secretion. The fibres leave the Ganglion pterygopalatinum, travel alongside the N. zygomaticus (a branch of the N. maxillaris [V/2]), and anas-

tomose with the N. lacrimalis as R. communicans cum nervo zygomatico (→ Fig. 8.201 and → Fig. 9.38) to reach the lacrimal gland. The N. lacrimalis (a branch of the N. ophthalmicus [V/1]) provides the **sensory** innervation. The sympathetic fibres inhibit glandular secretion. **Postganglionic sympathetic fibres** originate from the Ganglion cervicale superius. Without synapsing, the fibres pass through the Ganglion pterygopalatinum and take the same route to the lacrimal gland as the parasympathetic fibres (→ Fig. 9.38).

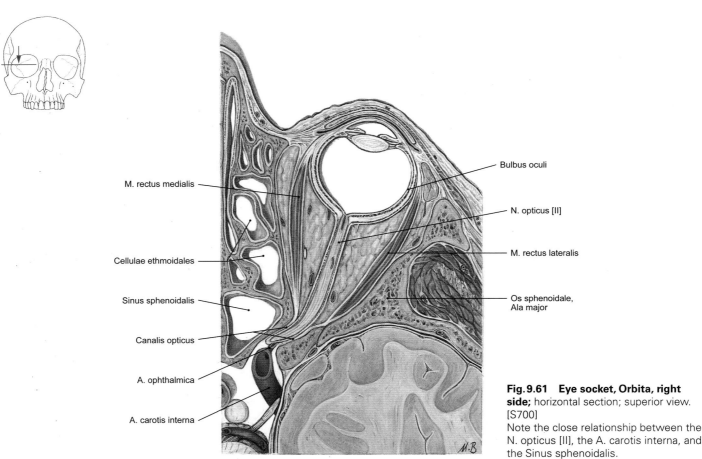

M. rectus medialis

Cellulae ethmoidales

Sinus sphenoidalis

Canalis opticus

A. ophthalmica

A. carotis interna

Bulbus oculi

N. opticus [II]

M. rectus lateralis

Os sphenoidale,
Ala major

Fig. 9.61 Eye socket, Orbita, right side; horizontal section; superior view. [S700]
Note the close relationship between the N. opticus [II], the A. carotis interna, and the Sinus sphenoidalis.

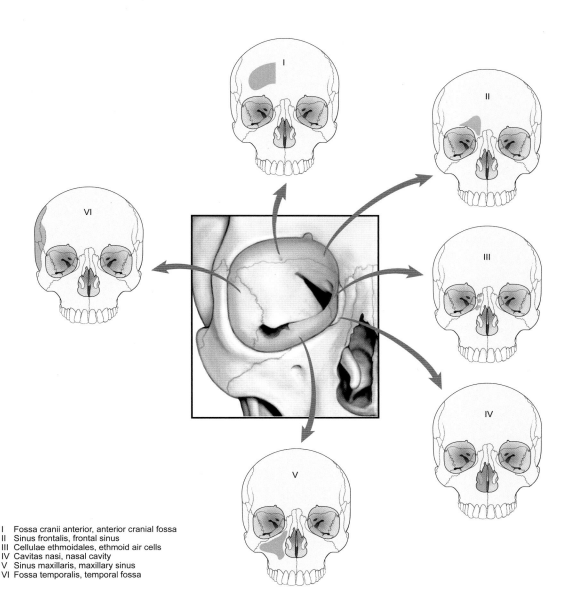

I   Fossa cranii anterior, anterior cranial fossa
II   Sinus frontalis, frontal sinus
III Cellulae ethmoidales, ethmoid air cells
IV   Cavitas nasi, nasal cavity
V   Sinus maxillaris, maxillary sinus
VI   Fossa temporalis, temporal fossa

Fig. 9.62   Topographical relationship between the eye socket, Orbita, and neighbouring areas, right side; frontal view. [S700-L126] The Orbita has a close topographical relationship with neighbouring areas. These areas include the anterior cranial fossa (Fossa cranii ante-rior), the frontal sinus (Sinus frontalis), the ethmoidal cells (Cellulae eth-moidales), the nasal cavity (Cavitas nasi), the maxillary sinus (Sinus ma-xillaris) and the temporal fossa (Fossa temporalis).

Clinical remarks

The treatment of diseases, particularly those affecting facial struc-tures, requires the interdisciplinary collaboration of numerous spe-cialist fields. Besides the ophthalmologist, the skills of otolaryngolo-gists, oromaxillofacial surgeons, neurosurgeons, radiologists and neurologists are involved in the treatment, as well as specialists of other disciplines (e.g. paediatricians, anaesthetists, nuclear medi-cine specialists, etc.). **Inflammation and tumours of the Orbita** can spread to the neighbouring areas (and vice versa) and require interdisciplinary therapy.

Eye socket, vertical section

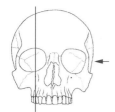

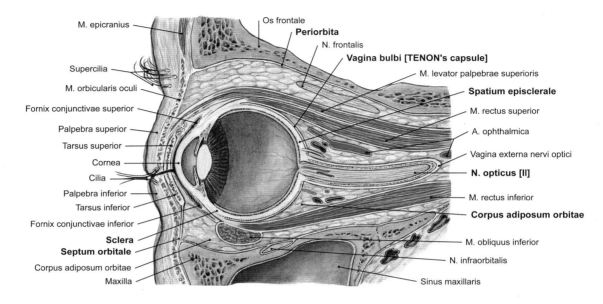

M. epicranius
Supercilia
M. orbicularis oculi
Fornix conjunctivae superior
Palpebra superior
Tarsus superior
Cornea
Cilia
Palpebra inferior
Tarsus inferior
Fornix conjunctivae inferior
Sclera
Septum orbitale
Corpus adiposum orbitae
Maxilla

Os frontale
Periorbita
N. frontalis
Vagina bulbi [TENON's capsule]
M. levator palpebrae superioris
Spatium episclerale
M. rectus superior
A. ophthalmica
Vagina externa nervi optici
N. opticus [II]
M. rectus inferior
Corpus adiposum orbitae
M. obliquus inferior
N. infraorbitalis
Sinus maxillaris

Fig. 9.63 Eye socket, Orbita, right side; medial view; vertical midline section. [S700]
The inside of the eye socket is coated with periosteum. All structures of the Orbita are embedded in adipose tissue (Corpus adiposum orbitae).

The entrance to the Orbita is restricted by the Septum orbitale. A thin layer or sheath of connective tissue fascia (Vagina bulbi, TENON's capsule) surrounds the eyeball. Between the Vagina bulbi and the sclera of the Bulbus oculi is a narrow gap called the Spatium episclerale.

Clinical remarks

Endocrine orbitopathy is an inflammation of the orbita-forming part of GRAVES' disease. This is an autoimmune disease, whereby it is assumed that the immune system erroneously produces antibodies which attack the tissues of the patient's own thyroid gland and eye sockets (e.g. extraocular muscle and the orbital fat body). The details of this disease mechanism are not yet fully understood. The disease phenotype is, however, a combination of a hyperfunction of the thyroid gland (hyperthyroidism) and exophthalmos (bulging of the eyes, → figure). Exophthalmos coincides with widening of the palpebral fissure, retraction of the eyelid, and distorted eye movements.
In order to choose an appropriate **surgical access route, the orbita** is divided into different parts according to clinical criteria:
• bulbar part – retrobulbar part
• central or intraconal (delineated by the cone-shaped arrangement of the extraocular rectus muscles) part – peripheral or extraconal part
• upper level – middle level – lower level of the Orbita:
  – The upper level is located between the roof of the Orbita and the M. levator palpebrae superioris. It contains: N. frontalis, N. trochlearis, N. lacrimalis, A. supraorbitalis, A. supratrochlearis, A. and V. lacrimalis and V. ophthalmica superior (→ Fig. 9.56).
  – The middle level is located between the extraocular rectus muscles and includes the intraconal space (→ Fig. 9.58). It contains:

N. oculomotorius, N. nasociliaris, N. abducens, N. zygomaticus, Ganglion ciliare, A. ophthalmica, V. ophthalmica superior, Aa. ciliares posteriores breves and longae.
– The lower level extends from the M. rectus inferior and the M. obliquus oculi inferior to the orbital floor (→ Fig. 9.59). It contains: N. infraorbitalis, A. infraorbitalis and V. ophthalmica inferior.

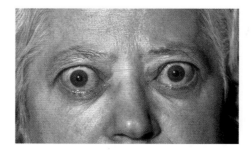

Patient with pronounced exophthalmos as part of GRAVES' ophthalmopathy. [S100]

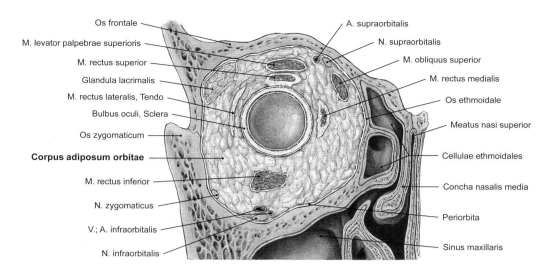

Os frontale
M. levator palpebrae superioris
M. rectus superior
Glandula lacrimalis
M. rectus lateralis, Tendo
Bulbus oculi, Sclera
Os zygomaticum
Corpus adiposum orbitae
M. rectus inferior
N. zygomaticus
V.; A. infraorbitalis
N. infraorbitalis

A. supraorbitalis
N. supraorbitalis
M. obliquus superior
M. rectus medialis
Os ethmoidale
Meatus nasi superior
Cellulae ethmoidales
Concha nasalis media
Periorbita
Sinus maxillaris

Fig. 9.64 **Eye socket, Orbita, right side;** frontal section through the Orbita at the level of the posterior aspect of the Bulbus oculi; frontal view. [S700]

All structures of the Orbita are embedded in the orbital fat body (Corpus adiposum orbitae); this structural fat forms a protective coating around the Orbita.

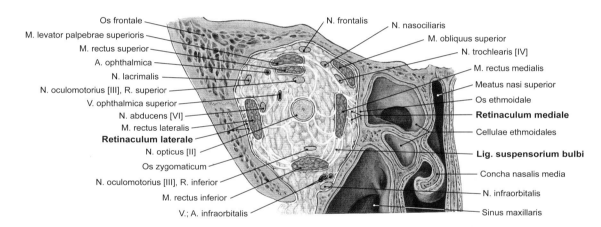

Os frontale
M. levator palpebrae superioris
M. rectus superior
A. ophthalmica
N. lacrimalis
N. oculomotorius [III], R. superior
V. ophthalmica superior
N. abducens [VI]
M. rectus lateralis
Retinaculum laterale
N. opticus [II]
Os zygomaticum
N. oculomotorius [III], R. inferior
M. rectus inferior
V.; A. infraorbitalis

N. frontalis
N. nasociliaris
M. obliquus superior
N. trochlearis [IV]
M. rectus medialis
Meatus nasi superior
Os ethmoidale
Retinaculum mediale
Cellulae ethmoidales
Lig. suspensorium bulbi
Concha nasalis media
N. infraorbitalis
Sinus maxillaris

Fig. 9.65 **Eye socket, Orbita, right side;** frontal section through the retrobulbar area of the Orbita; frontal view. [S700]
The Bulbus oculi and the structures of the retrobulbar space connect to the Periorbita and to each other via thin ligaments. The stronger ligaments are called Retinaculum mediale (between the M. rectus medialis

and Periorbita) and Retinaculum laterale (between the M. rectus lateralis and Periorbita) as well as a Lig. suspensorium bulbi (LOCKWOOD's ligament, between the M. rectus medialis and M. rectus inferior and Periorbita).

Clinical remarks

After **diabetic retinopathy,** retinal vein occlusions (in cases of diabetes mellitus) are the second most common vascular retinal diseases. Very often, the vein occlusions result from locally developing thrombi (thrombosis of the V. centralis retinae = **central venous thrombosis;** → figure). They are accompanied by significant loss of vision. Changes often occur in the retinal vessels of diabetic patients, which can lead to vitreous bleeding, resulting in a loss of vision. If the bleeding into the vitreous body does not resolve spontaneously after two to three months, a removal of the vitreous body (vitrectomy) is recommended in the case of poor vision.

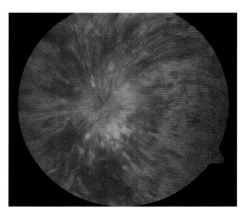

Central venous occlusion, left side. Bleeding is apparent in all quadrants of the retina. [S700-T867]

Eyeball, horizontal section

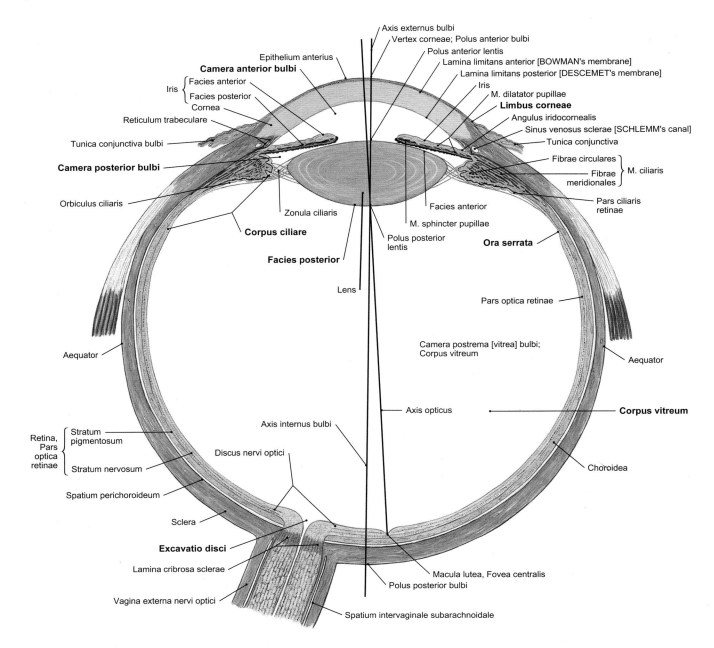

Axis externus bulbi
Vertex corneae; Polus anterior bulbi
Polus anterior lentis
Lamina limitans anterior [BOWMAN's membrane]
Lamina limitans posterior [DESCEMET's membrane]
Iris
M. dilatator pupillae
Limbus corneae
Angulus iridocornealis
Sinus venosus sclerae [SCHLEMM's canal]
Tunica conjunctiva
Fibrae circulares
Fibrae meridionales
M. ciliaris
Pars ciliaris retinae
Facies anterior
M. sphincter pupillae
Ora serrata
Pars optica retinae
Camera postrema [vitrea] bulbi; Corpus vitreum
Aequator
Corpus vitreum
Choroidea
Macula lutea, Fovea centralis
Polus posterior bulbi
Spatium intervaginale subarachnoidale

Epithelium anterius
Camera anterior bulbi
Iris
Facies anterior
Facies posterior
Cornea
Reticulum trabeculare
Tunica conjunctiva bulbi
Camera posterior bulbi
Orbiculus ciliaris
Zonula ciliaris
Corpus ciliare
Facies posterior
Polus posterior lentis
Lens
Aequator
Axis opticus
Axis internus bulbi
Discus nervi optici
Retina, Pars optica retinae
Stratum pigmentosum
Stratum nervosum
Spatium perichoroideum
Sclera
Excavatio disci
Lamina cribrosa sclerae
Vagina externa nervi optici

Fig. 9.66 Eyeball, Bulbus oculi, right side; schematic horizontal section at the level of the exit of the N. opticus [II]. [S700]

In the anterior part of the eye, the outer cover of the eyeball (Tunica fibrosa bulbi) is made up of the sclera and the **cornea.** Shaped like a convex disc, the cornea bulges out from the rest of the bulbus. At the Limbus corneae, the cornea merges into the less curved **sclera** which forms the Tunica fibrosa bulbi in the posterior part of the eye. The extraocular muscles insert from the outside onto the sclera. The Tunica vasculosa bulbi (vascular layer, uvea) lies beneath the sclera. Its anterior part consists of the **iris** and the ciliary body (Corpus ciliare), while the

choroid (Choroidea) forms the posterior part. At the Ora serrata, the ciliary body and the Choroidea meet. The Choroidea represents the most highly vascularised structure in the body. Its blood supply provides nutrients and oxygen to the adjacent retinal layer and is involved in thermoregulation of the eyeball. The **retina** is the innermost layer of the eyeball (Tunica interna bulbi). It contains the neural layer (Stratum nervosum; photoreceptive cells) and the pigmented layer (Stratum pigmentosum; pigment cells), and in the anterior part, the pigmented layer of the ciliary body and the epithelium of the iris. The inner space of the eyeball consists of the **vitreous body** (Corpus vitreum).

Clinical remarks

Various diseases (e.g. keratitis = corneal inflammation, keratoconus or chemical irritation) may require the surgical replacement of the cornea to restore proper vision **(corneal transplant).** Since the cornea is not vascularised, a transplant is significantly easier from an immunological point of view than the transplantation of a vascularised organ. Therefore, the corneal transplant (keratoplasty) is the world's most common type of human transplant surgery. **Retinal ablation** (Ablatio or Amotio retinae) describes the detachment of the inner parts of the retina (Stratum nervosum, neuroretina) from its supplying retinal pigment epithelium (Pars pigmentosa, RPE). Symp-

toms which include an increase in the number of coloured spots or flashes of light, may not be present, provided that the macula (point of central vision) is not affected. However, if the macula is detached from its supplying pigment epithelium for more than 48 hours, a permanent loss of function of the corresponding parts of the retina will occur. After a successful reattachment of the retina to the pigment epithelium, the functionality of the retina may improve, depending on the duration of the retinal ablation. If a complete retinal detachment is not corrected, the result will be loss of vision in the affected eye.

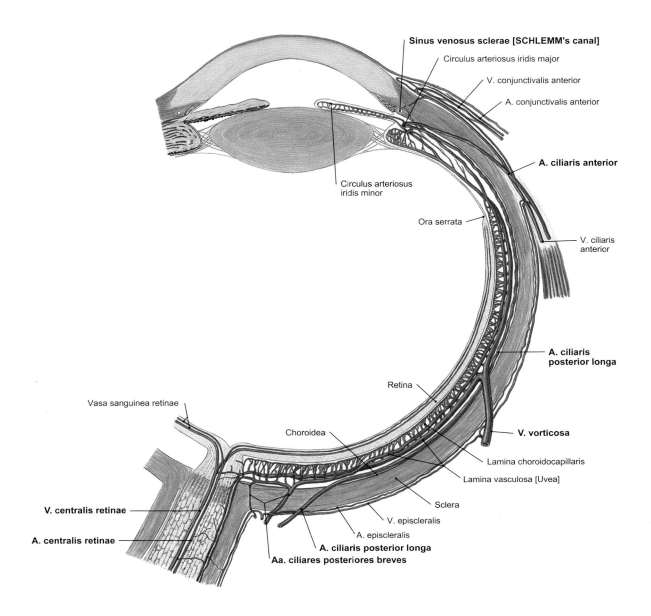

Fig. 9.67 Blood vessels of the eyeball, Bulbus oculi, right side; horizontal section at the level of the N. opticus [II]; view from above. [S700]

Arterial blood supply is shown in → Fig. 9.54. The venous drainage occurs via the V. centralis retinae, as well as via four to eight Vv. vorticosae (→ Fig. 9.55).
The latter pierce the sclera posterior to the equator of the eyeball and join the Vv. ophthalmica superior and inferior.

Dimensions of the eye ball (average values according to anatomical and ophthalmological literature)			
External bulbar diameter (Axis bulbi externus)	24.0 mm	Radius of curvature of the sclera	13.0 mm
Internal bulbar area (Axis bulbi internus)	22.5 mm	Radius of curvature of the cornea	7.8 mm
Thickness of the cornea	0.5 mm	Refractive index of the entire eye (distance vision)	59 dioptres
Depth of the anterior chamber	3.6 mm	Refractive index of the cornea	43 dioptres
Thickness of the lens	3.6 mm	Refractive index of the lens (distance vision)	19 dioptres
Distance between lens and retina	15.6 mm	Distance between the two pupils	61–69 mm
Thickness of the retina	0.3 mm		

Iridocorneal angle

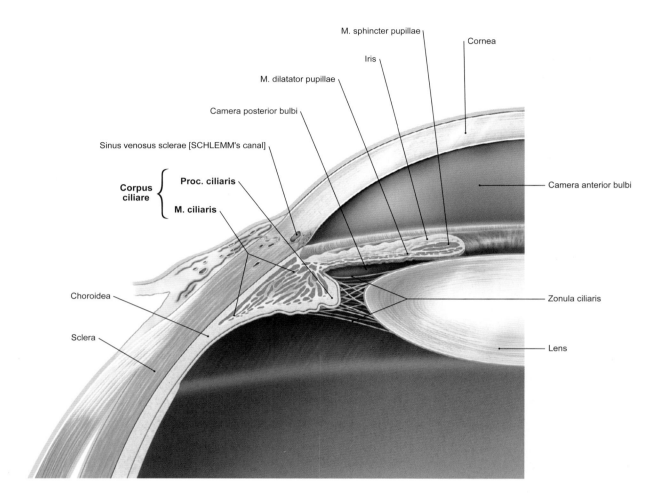

M. sphincter pupillae

Cornea

Iris

M. dilatator pupillae

Camera posterior bulbi

Sinus venosus sclerae [SCHLEMM's canal]

Camera anterior bulbi

Corpus ciliare { **Proc. ciliaris**

M. ciliaris

Choroidea

Zonula ciliaris

Sclera

Lens

Fig. 9.68 Iridocorneal angle, Angulus iridocornealis, and adjacent structures. [S700-L275]
The iridocorneal angle (Angulus iridocornealis) is bordered by the cornea, iris and sclera. The epithelium of the Corpus ciliare produces the aqueous humour which flows from the posterior chamber to the anterior chamber and through the trabecular meshwork in the Angulus iridocornealis into the SCHLEMM's canal where the fluid drains into the episcleral veins. The M. ciliaris is the major component of the ciliary body. It consists of meridional (longitudinal, BRÜCKE's muscle), radial, and circular (MÜLLER's muscle) muscle cells and is important for accommodation.

Clinical remarks

Glaucoma is caused by a malfunction of the intraocular fluid, often leading to a rise in the intraocular pressure (normally 15 mmHg). This mainly causes damage in the area of the optic nerve papilla with risk of blindness. Causes are, for example, a displacement of the iridocorneal angle, possibly through the iris and cornea moving closer together and blocking the canals (**acute or angle-closure glaucoma,** rare) or, in the case of an open angle, with impaired drainage through the trabecular mesh of the SCHLEMM's (**primary open-angle glaucoma,** common). Treatment is through medication which
closes the angle of the pupils (miotics). Thereby the intraocular fluid via the SCHLEMM's canal is increased and the intraocular pressure is reduced.
Genetically caused disorders affecting the connective tissue factor fibrillin 1 (**MARFAN syndrome**) lead to insufficiency of the zonular fibres with lens dislocation (lens luxation) as well as a permanent ball-shaped change to the lens of the eye (with impaired distance vision).

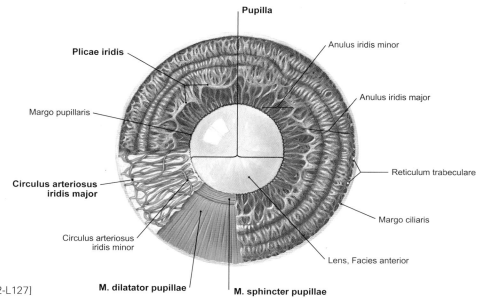

Fig. 9.69 **Iris and lens**; frontal view. [S702-L127]

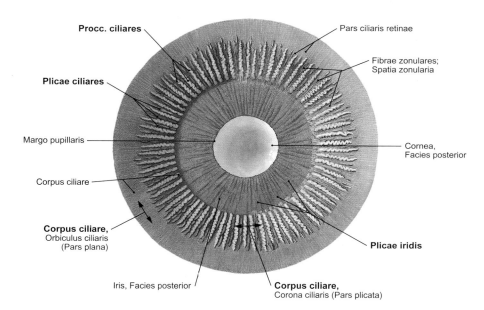

Fig. 9.70 **Iris and ciliary body, Corpus ciliare**; posterior view; after removal of the lens. [S700]

The Corpus ciliare is divided into a plane (Pars plana) and a raised part (Pars plicata). Approx. 70 ciliary processes (Procc. ciliares) originate from the latter. The Corpus ciliare is covered with ciliary epithelium, which, in the area of the Pars plicata, secretes the aqueous humour for the iridocorneal angle (Angulus iridocornealis). Zonular fibres (suspensory ligaments of the lens, Zonulae ciliares) traverse the distance between the ciliary epithelium and the lens capsule.

Clinical remarks

The **pupillary light reflex (PLR)** controls the intensity of the light reaching the retina. Bright light makes the pupil constrict (miosis) while dim light makes the pupil dilate (mydriasis). The retina and the optical nerve are the afferent (sensory) limb and the muscles of the pupil are the efferent (motor) limb of the pupillary light reflex (→ figure). The pupillary light reflex offers diagnostic information about the sensory (retina) and pupillomotor functions of the eye. [S700-L126]

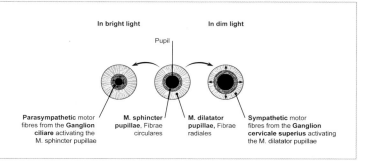

Lens

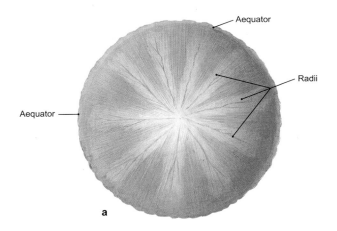

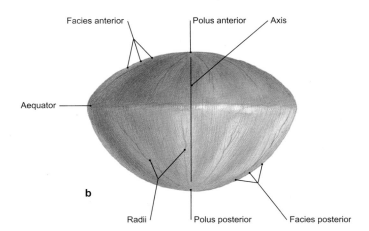

Fig. 9.71a and b Lens. [S700]
a Frontal view. Depending on its particular level of accommodation, the refractive index of the lens varies between 10–20 dioptres (for com-

parison, the refractive index of the cornea is 43 dioptres but cannot be modified).
b View from the equator.

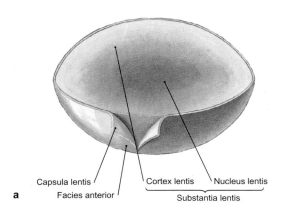

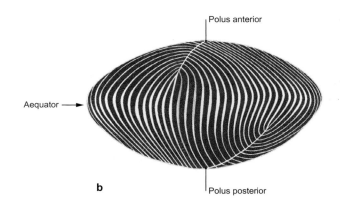

Fig. 9.72a and b Lens. [S700]
a Anterior oblique view; after meridional cut and partial detachment of the anterior lens capsule (Capsula lentis). The centres of the planes

are known as the anterior pole (Polus anterior) or posterior pole (Polus posterior).
b Lens fibres of a newborn infant; schematic drawing; view from the equator.

Clinical remarks

Accommodation of the eye depends on the lens increasing its diameter (becoming rounder) when the ciliary muscle which surrounds the lens, contracts. It bulges in the direction of the lens, thereby reducing its tension on the zonula fibres and the lens becomes rounder due to its inherent elasticity (→ Fig. a). With younger people, a change in the optical range of up to 15 dioptre is thereby possible. The continuous apposition of lens fibres reduces the elasticity of the lens (from the age of 40) to such an extent that the accommodation of the lens diminishes, i.e. the inability to properly focus on objects at various distances (age-related vision impairment, **presbyopia**).

Wearing an appropriate vision-correcting pair of glasses becomes necessary. A reduction in intracellular water content causes alterations in the proteins (crystallines) which are important for maintaining transparency of the lens. This leads to a cataract (grey senile cataract, **Cataracta senilis,** → Fig. b), which is the most common eye disease. A cataract can be diagnosed at an early stage by means of a slit-lamp examination. Cataract surgery is one of the most frequently performed surgical procedures in Western industrialised countries (approx. 10 % of all 80-year-old patients suffer from an advanced cataract).

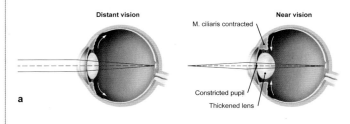

[S701-L275]

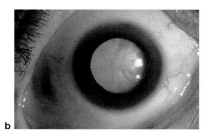

Senile cataracts, Cataracta senilis (a white opaque lens is evidence of an advanced cataract. [S700-T867]

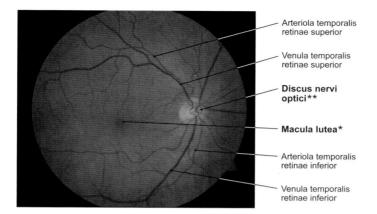

Arteriola temporalis
retinae superior

Venula temporalis
retinae superior

**Discus nervi
optici****

Macula lutea*

Arteriola temporalis
retinae inferior

Venula temporalis
retinae inferior

Fig. 9.73 Ocular fundus, Fundus oculi, right side; frontal view; ophthalmoscopic native imaging. [S700-T867]
The examination of the ocular fundus by direct ophthalmoscopy (fundoscopy) allows the clinical assessment of the condition of the retina, its blood vessels (in particular the A. and V. centralis retinae), the optic disc (Discus nervi optici), as well as the yellow spot (Macula lutea) and the point of central vision (Fovea centralis). The retinal vessels (A. and V. centralis retinae and their branches) may be assessed and, due to the vessel diameter (arteries – smaller diameter), differentiated from one

another. The papilla of the N. opticus [II] normally has a sharp margin, is yellow to orange in colour and contains a central depression (Excavatio disci). The Macula lutea (where most of the cone cells are located) sits 3–4 mm temporally of the N. opticus [II]. Numerous branches of the Vasa centralia retinae converge in a radial fashion onto the macula, but do not reach the centre (Fovea centralis). The latter is supplied via the Choroidea.
*   clin.: yellow spot
** clin.: blind spot (Discus = Papilla nervi optici)

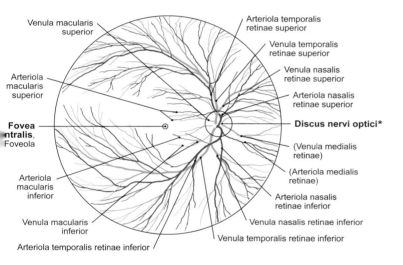

Venula macularis
superior

Arteriola
macularis
superior

**Fovea
ntralis,**
Foveola

Arteriola
macularis
inferior

Venula macularis
inferior

Arteriola temporalis retinae inferior

Arteriola temporalis
retinae superior

Venula temporalis
retinae superior

Venula nasalis
retinae superior

Arteriola nasalis
retinae superior

Discus nervi optici*

(Venula medialis
retinae)

(Arteriola medialis
retinae)

Arteriola nasalis
retinae inferior

Venula nasalis retinae inferior

Venula temporalis retinae inferior

**Fig. 9.74 Ocular fundus, Fundus oculi, and blood vessels of the
retina, Vasa sanguinea retinae, right side;** frontal view; schematic illustration of the pathway of the blood vessels. [S700-T899]
* Papilla nervi optici

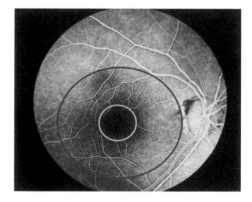

Fig. 9.75 Ocular fundus, Fundus oculi, right side; frontal view; fluorescence angiography during the arteriovenous phase with anatomic landmarks: macula (blue circle); fovea (yellow circle). [E282]

Clinical remarks

In case of a **retinal detachment** (Ablatio retinae), the retina takes on a whitish-yellow colour. Changes in blood vessels as in diabetic retinopathy or hypertension can be diagnosed at an early stage by fundoscopy. For advanced diagnostics, a fluorescence angiography may be performed (→ Fig. 9.75). With increased intracranial pressure (CSF), the papilla of the N. opticus [II] in the Bulbus oculi appears to be slightly protruding and its margins appear less well defined **(papilloedema).** Glaucoma also causes characteristic changes to the optic disc (papillary glaucoma; → figure). Pathological changes in the Macula lutea are frequently age-related. The most **frequent cause of blindness** in Western industrialised countries is age-related macular degeneration (AMD).

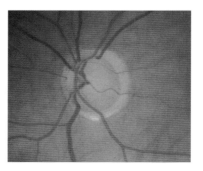

Concentric enlargement of the optic disc due to glaucoma.
[S700-T867]

Eyeball

Eye socket, MRI

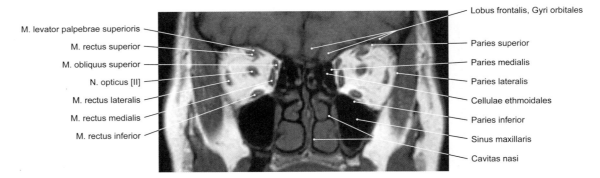

M. levator palpebrae superioris
M. rectus superior
M. obliquus superior
N. opticus [II]
M. rectus lateralis
M. rectus medialis
M. rectus inferior

Lobus frontalis, Gyri orbitales
Paries superior
Paries medialis
Paries lateralis
Cellulae ethmoidales
Paries inferior
Sinus maxillaris
Cavitas nasi

Fig. 9.76 Extraocular muscles, Mm. oculi; magnetic resonance image (MRI), frontal section of a healthy individual at the level of the orbital centre; frontal view. [S700-T916]

One can clearly see the close topographical relationship of the Orbita, Sinus maxillaris, Lobus frontalis, Cellulae ethmoidales and M. temporalis (not shown).

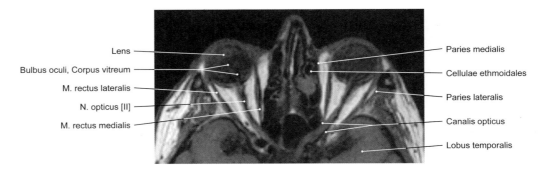

Lens
Bulbus oculi, Corpus vitreum
M. rectus lateralis
N. opticus [II]
M. rectus medialis

Paries medialis
Cellulae ethmoidales
Paries lateralis
Canalis opticus
Lobus temporalis

Fig. 9.77 Eyeball, Bulbus oculi, and extraocular muscles, Mm. bulbi; magnetic resonance image (MRI), cross-section of a healthy individual at the level of the N. opticus [II]; superior view. [S700-T916]

In this cross-section one can clearly see the slightly contorted pathway of the N. opticus [II], which is important as a reserve route for eye movement.

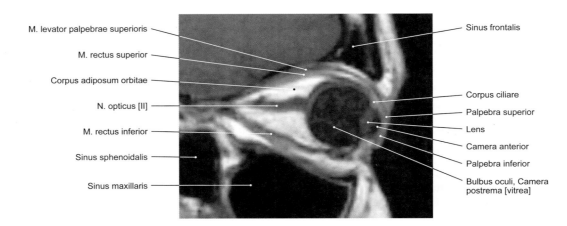

M. levator palpebrae superioris
M. rectus superior
Corpus adiposum orbitae
N. opticus [II]
M. rectus inferior
Sinus sphenoidalis
Sinus maxillaris

Sinus frontalis
Corpus ciliare
Palpebra superior
Lens
Camera anterior
Palpebra inferior
Bulbus oculi, Camera postrema [vitrea]

Fig. 9.78 Eyeball, Bulbus oculi, and extraocular muscles, Mm. bulbi; magnetic resonance image (MRI), sagittal section of a healthy individual at the level of the N. opticus [II]; lateral view. [S700]

On the MRI, the bulbar space and the retrobulbar space can easily be delimited due to the different layers of tissue.

→ T 2

Examination methods

Most visible structures of the eye can be examined in vivo using special optical instruments (e.g. magnifying glasses, ophthalmoscope, slit lamp) on the patient, e.g. cornea, aqueous humour, iridocorneal angle, iris, lens, vitreous body, retina with papilla of the N. opticus [II] and macula.

Imaging techniques can help in the diagnosis of chronic inflammation or of tumours which are located in areas of the Bulbus oculi that cannot be otherwise examined. Among the most frequently used imaging techniques for the examination of intraorbital structures and

their topographical relationships are **computed tomography** (CT) and **magnetic resonance imaging** (MRI). By intravenous administration of a contrast medium, these procedures can often reveal even more detailed information.

If the fundus of the eye cannot be assessed by an ophthalmoscopy (e.g. due to pathological changes, such as corneal opacity, cataract or bleeding into the vitreous humour), an **ultrasound examination** of the eye can be performed.

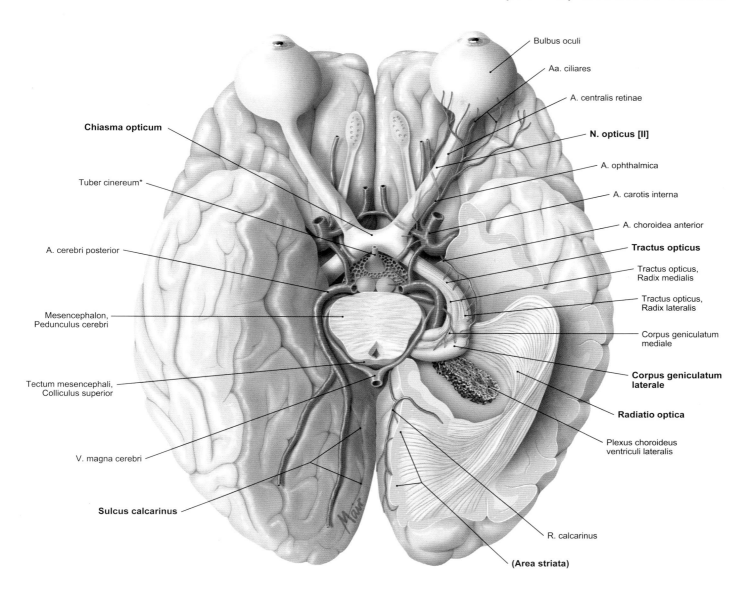

Bulbus oculi

Aa. ciliares

A. centralis retinae

N. opticus [II]

A. ophthalmica

A. carotis interna

A. choroidea anterior

Tractus opticus

Tractus opticus, Radix medialis

Tractus opticus, Radix lateralis

Corpus geniculatum mediale

Corpus geniculatum laterale

Radiatio optica

Plexus choroideus ventriculi lateralis

R. calcarinus

(Area striata)

Chiasma opticum

Tuber cinereum*

A. cerebri posterior

Mesencephalon, Pedunculus cerebri

Tectum mesencephali, Colliculus superior

V. magna cerebri

Sulcus calcarinus

Fig. 9.79 Brain, cerebrum, and blood supply of the visual pathway; inferior view. The pituitary gland has been removed at its infundibulum (*). It lies in close proximity to the Chiasma opticum. [S700-L127]

The visual pathway originates within the retina and contains the first three projection neurons and interneurons (horizontal cells, amacrine cells). Consecutively, from the outside to the inside, they are:

First neuron: photoreceptor cells of the retina (rods [approx. 120 million] and cones [approx. 6.5 million])

Second neuron: bipolar ganglion cells (perikarya in the Ganglion retinae), which receive the signals from the photoreceptor cells and transmit them to the multipolar ganglion cells (third neuron)

Third neuron: multipolar ganglion cells (approx. 10.5 million, perikarya in the Ganglion opticum).

This principle of the three neurons forming an intraretinal chain only applies to the cone cells. Up to 40 rod cells converge their signals onto one bipolar cell and this cell will then transmit these signals indirectly,

with the help of amacrine cells (20–50 different types of these cells have been described in the literature to date), to one multipolar ganglionic cell. The axons of the Ganglion opticum extend primarily to the Corpus geniculatum laterale (Radix lateralis), although several fibres also extend into the Area pretectalis and into the Colliculus superior (Radix medialis) as well as to the hypothalamus. The fibres run in the N. opticus [II] to the Chiasma opticum. Here they cross the nasal part of the retina to the opposite side. The fibres of the temporal part of the retina do not cross. In the Tractus opticus there are also fibres which transmit information from the contralateral half of the visual field.

Fourth neuron: Its axons travel primarily from the Corpus geniculatum laterale to the areas 17 and 18 of the cerebral cortex (Area striata, primary visual cortex with approx. 500 million neurons) in the area surrounding the Sulcus calcarinus.

A cortical enlargement takes place in the Area striata: approx. 50 % of the visual cortex processes the visual information in the central 3 % of the visual field.

Clinical remarks

Prior to activating the light-sensitive parts of the photoreceptors, light must penetrate through all the other layers of the retina (third neuron, second neuron); this is called the inversion of the retina. The photoreceptors (first neuron) are in close contact with the pigment epithelium, without developing actual adhesion structures between the pigment epithelium and photoreceptors. In this area, retinal detachment (**Ablatio** or **Amotio retinae**) can occur, which can lead to blindness if not treated.

Visual pathway

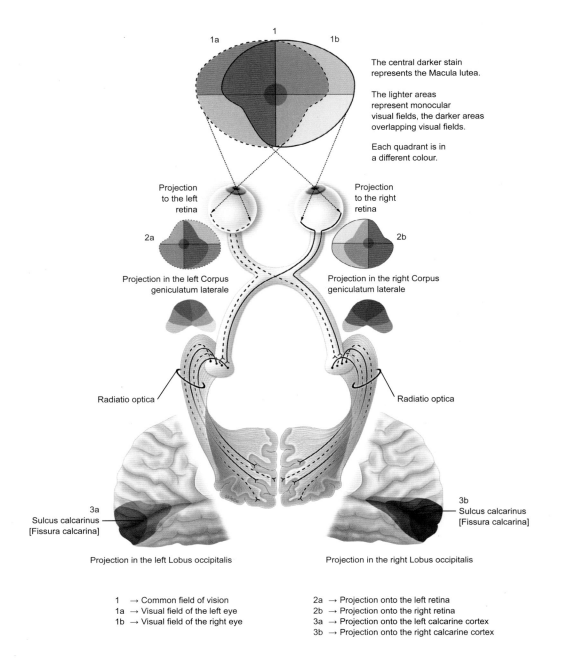

1a   1   1b

The central darker stain represents the Macula lutea.

The lighter areas represent monocular visual fields, the darker areas overlapping visual fields.

Each quadrant is in a different colour.

Projection to the left retina

Projection to the right retina

2a

2b

Projection in the left Corpus geniculatum laterale

Projection in the right Corpus geniculatum laterale

Radiatio optica

Radiatio optica

3a
Sulcus calcarinus
[Fissura calcarina]

3b
Sulcus calcarinus
[Fissura calcarina]

Projection in the left Lobus occipitalis

Projection in the right Lobus occipitalis

1 → Common field of vision	2a → Projection onto the left retina
1a → Visual field of the left eye	2b → Projection onto the right retina
1b → Visual field of the right eye	3a → Projection onto the left calcarine cortex
	3b → Projection onto the right calcarine cortex

Fig. 9.80 Visual pathway; schematic overview; superior view. The central visual field has a disproportionately large projection area. [S702-L238]

It is only at the level of the visual association cortices that the image is perceived as it actually appears. Until this point, it seems to be 'standing on its head'. Arranging the visual fields into four colours is used to show how information is transmitted and presented in the corresponding areas in the visual cortex and the various sections of the visual pathway.

⌐ Clinical remarks

Because of the close topographical relationship to the Chiasma opticum, if pituitary tumours increase in size, they can cause a **bitemporal hemianopsia**. Postchiasmatic or intracerebral lesions along the visual pathway can result in **homonymous hemianopsia.** Thus, for example, damage to the right Tractus opticus can lead to a left-sided homonymous hemianopsia. Damage to the left Radiatio optica (GRATIOLET's optic radiation) can cause a right-sided homonymous hemianopsia. Additional symptoms may include hemioptic pupillary rigidity, a degeneration of the pupil (after months) or optic papilla oedema. Underlying causes can be tumours, basal meningitis, aneurysm, ischaemia and bleeding. Loss of function in both visual cortices causes a **cortical amaurosis** (cortical blindness; → Fig. 12.129).

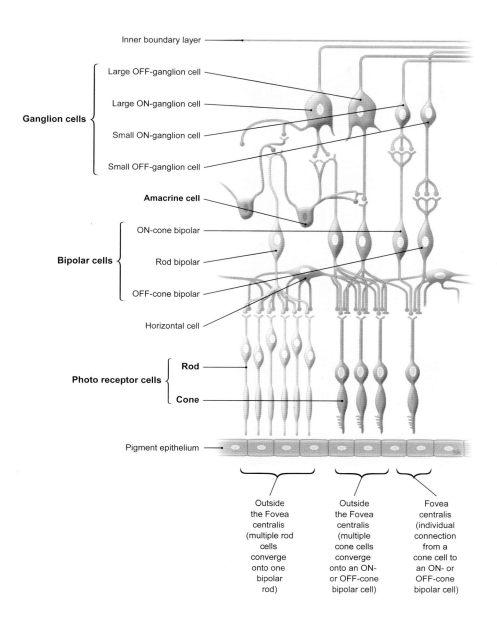

Inner boundary layer

Ganglion cells
- Large OFF-ganglion cell
- Large ON-ganglion cell
- Small ON-ganglion cell
- Small OFF-ganglion cell

Amacrine cell

Bipolar cells
- ON-cone bipolar
- Rod bipolar
- OFF-cone bipolar

Horizontal cell

Photo receptor cells
- **Rod**
- **Cone**

Pigment epithelium

Outside the Fovea centralis (multiple rod cells converge onto one bipolar rod)

Outside the Fovea centralis (multiple cone cells converge onto an ON- or OFF-cone bipolar cell)

Fovea centralis (individual connection from a cone cell to an ON- or OFF-cone bipolar cell)

Fig. 9.81 **Neuronal interconnections in the retina;** simplified diagram. [S702-L238]

The environment (visual field) is perceived with the stationary eye and is relayed to the retina. It contains the first three (cone cells) or four (rod cells) neurons of the visual tract. The first neurons are the photoreceptor cells (cone and rod cells); the second neurons are the bipolar ON- or OFF-cone cells which follow the bipolar rods. The third neurons are large or small ganglion cells that occur as ON- or OFF-ganglion cells for the cones; the third/fourth neuron of the retinal bipolar rod cells are amacrine cells and ganglion cells. Both rod and cone cells can project together onto a large ganglion cell. The area of the retina, of which the light leads to a response in a particular ganglion cell and the corresponding nerve fibres of the N. opticus [II], is referred to as the receptive field. If the receptive field is large, the resolution is only low; if it is small, the resolution is high. The ON- and OFF-ganglion cells, with their preliminary ON- and OFF-cone-bipolar cells thereby play a decisive role in the contrast enhancement (stimulating centre and inhibiting environment). These mechanisms are further reinforced by the horizontal cells as interneurons. However, the mechanisms are not yet fully understood.

Pupillary and accommodation reflex

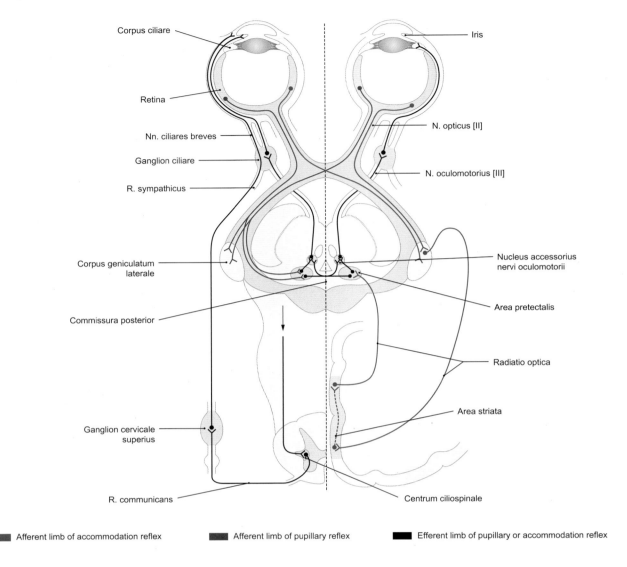

Corpus ciliare

Retina

Nn. ciliares breves

Ganglion ciliare

R. sympathicus

Corpus geniculatum laterale

Commissura posterior

Ganglion cervicale superius

R. communicans

Iris

N. opticus [II]

N. oculomotorius [III]

Nucleus accessorius nervi oculomotorii

Area pretectalis

Radiatio optica

Area striata

Centrum ciliospinale

■ Afferent limb of accommodation reflex　　　■ Afferent limb of pupillary reflex　　　■ Efferent limb of pupillary or accommodation reflex

Fig. 9.82 Pupillary, left side, and accommodation reflex, right side. [S702-L126]/[B500~T1191]/[G1088]
For an intact visualising process, it is not only conveying impressions to the awareness that is of great importance, but also the light-dark setting, the near-far setting, and the setting of the visual sight lines. These functions are coordinated by the pupillary reflex, the accommodation-convergence equipment of the eye and the convergence apparatus.
Pupillary reflex: multi-synaptically mediated reflectory adjustment of the width of the pupil to different lighting conditions. Activation of the photoreceptor cells of the retina, leading to the transmission of the signal into the Area pretectalis, from where the information is first interconnected and then routed to the parasympathetic Nucleus accessorius nervi oculomotorii (EDINGER-WESTPHAL nucleus) and the ciliospinal centre of the spinal cord. **Pupil constriction:** from the Nucleus accessorius nervi oculomotorii, the information reaches the Ganglion ciliare. After switching over, innervation of the M. sphincter pupillae (myosis) occurs. **Pupil dilatation:** after switching in the Centrum ciliospinale of the spinal cord and further switching in the Ganglion cervicale superius, the postganglionic sympathetic fibres with their arteries reach the M. dilatator pupillae (mydriasis).
Accommodation reflex and convergence reaction: in order to see close objects clearly, the refractive index of the lens must be increased

(through the accommodation reflex) and the object must be aligned with the centre of sight (through the convergence reaction). In addition, the depth of field must be increased by narrowing of the pupil (aperture). In the entire visual tract, the afferent reflex limbs of each side are identical (up to the visual cortex) and therefore contain the information of both eyes. **Accommodation:** in the efferent reflex limbs, neurons of the visual cortex project into the pretectal area via the tectum (Brachium colliculi superioris) and are configured in the same manner as for the light reflex (crossed and uncrossed). The increase in the refractive power of the lens is carried out by contraction of the general efferent fibres of the N. oculomotorius [III] innervated M. ciliaris, which induce miosis by contraction of the same fibres as for the innervated M. sphincter pupillae. **Convergence reaction:** caused by the somatic efferent fibres of the N. oculomotorius [III] to the eye muscles, because of the stimulation of the neurons of the Nucleus nervi oculomotorii by nerve fibres from the Area pretectalis. This is to activate the M. rectus medialis to move the respective bulb to the centre. At the same time, fibres from the Area pretectalis along the Fasciculus longitudinalis medialis to the Nucleus abducentis cause a slackening of the M. rectus lateralis.

Clinical remarks

Lesions of the retina and N. opticus [II] not only lead to blindness, but also to elimination of the pupillary reflex **(amaurotic pupillary rigidity)**. The direct light reaction of the eye is thereby terminated. Lesions of the efferent limb (e. g. damage to the N. oculomotorius[III]) result

in the elimination of direct and indirect light reaction **(complete pupillary rigidity)**. A loss of any light reaction in both eyes (e. g. in the case of damage to the mesencephalon) would be called a **reflective pupillary rigidity.**

Sample exam questions

To check that you are completely familiar with the content of this chapter, sample questions from an oral anatomy exam are listed here.

Explain the structure of the Orbita:

- Which bone borders the Orbita, which entry and exit points does the Orbita have, and what enters and exits?
- Which structures and cavities border the Orbita?
- What passes through the Canalis nervi optici?
- What runs along the floor of the Orbita?
- What lines the Orbita?
- How can the Orbita be divided?
- What are the weak points in the bony structure of the Orbita?
- Why is the middle wall of the Orbita called the Lamina papyracea?

Describe the entrance to the Orbita:

- Which structures close the opening of the Orbita? How are they structured?
- What is the Septum orbitale? Where is it?
- How is the skin around the opening of the Orbita innervated?
- Are there any vascular connections between the face and the Orbita? If so, which are they?
- Which muscles are involved in the opening and closing movements of the eyelid?
- What is the Conjunctiva bulbi and what is the Conjunctiva palpebrae? Where is the conjunctival sac?
- Where is the lacrimal gland? How is it innervated and how is it provided with blood? Where does it deposit its secretion? What is the function of this secretion?

Describe the structure of the efferent lacrimal ducts:

- Where is the lacrimal sac?
- Where does the nasolacrimal duct enter?
- What happens to used lacrimal fluid?
- How does lacrimal drainage work?
- Which muscle is essential for the drainage of the lacrimal fluid?

Explain the content of the Orbita:

- Which extraocular muscles do you know?
- How are the extraocular muscles innervated and supplied with blood?
- Where do the extraocular muscles have their insertion and their origin?
- In which direction does the Bulbus oculi move in the event of an isolated contraction of the M. obliquus superior?
- What is the trochlea, and what is its function?
- Which limbs go out from the N. ophthalmicus [V/1], and what innervates them?
- What is the anulus of ZINN? Which structures go through it?
- How is the Bulbus oculi fixed in the Orbita?
- Which different vascular connections are there between the Orbita and the nose?

Explain the innervation of the eye:

- Where is the Ganglion ciliare? What function does it have?
- What are the names of the inner eye muscles? How are they innervated?
- What is meant by HORNER's triad?
- What is switched in the Ganglion ciliare?

Describe the structure of the Bulbus oculi:

- Where is aqueous humour formed, and how is it circulated?
- How is the cornea structured?
- What is the Corpus ciliare? What is its function?
- How is the ocular lens structured, and how does it work?
- Which different layers participate in the structure of the Bulbus oculi?
- Explain the arrangement of the neurons in the retina.
- Which blood vessels supply the choroid?

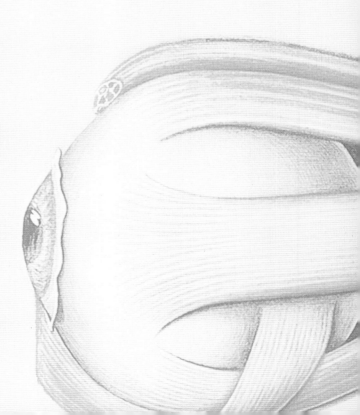

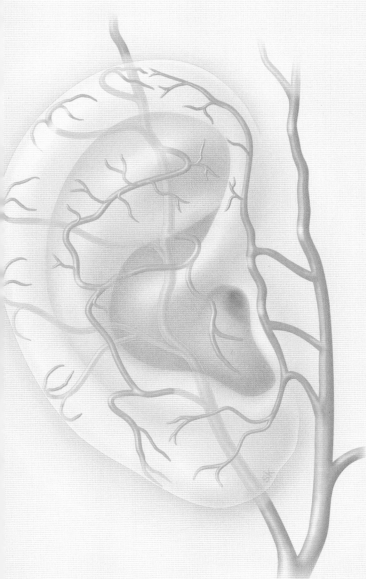

Ear

10

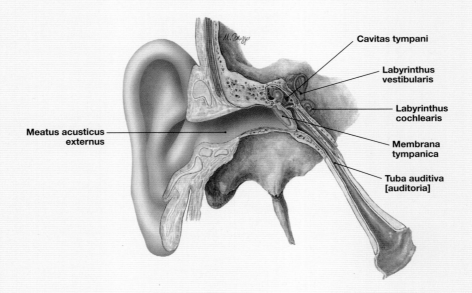

Cavitas tympani

Labyrinthus vestibularis

Labyrinthus cochlearis

Membrana tympanica

Tuba auditiva [auditoria]

Meatus acusticus externus

Overview

The ear is divided into the **outer ear, middle ear** and **inner ear.** Forming part of the outer ear are the **auricula** (Auricula pinna), the **outer ear canal** (Meatus acusticus externus) and the **eardrum** (Membrana tympanica). Behind the eardrum, located in the petrous part of the temporal bone (Pars petrosa ossis temporalis) and belonging to the middle ear, is the **tympanic cavity** (Cavitas tympani) with its **auditory ossicles: malleus, incus** and **stapes.** The tympanic cavity is connected via the **EUSTACHIAN tube** (auditory tube, Tuba auditiva, Tuba auditoria) to the nasopharynx and continues in adults via the mastoid antrum (Antrum mastoideum) into the ventilated areas of the mastoid process **(Cellulae mastoideae).** The auditory ossicles form a flexible chain for the transmission of sound waves conducted by the eardrum to the perilymph in the inner ear. The inner ear, which is also called the **labyrinth** and which, like the middle ear, is located in the petrous part of the temporal

bone, contains the **organ for hearing and equilibrium** (Organum vestibulocochleare). The **cochlea** is the organ for hearing. It contains ducts filled with perilymph and endolymph and records the vibrations of the lymphs, carried there by the sound-conducting apparatus of the ear. The vestibular organ is made up of three **bony semicircular canals** (Canales semicirculares ossei), two antechamber vesicles (**utriculus** and **sacculus**) and the endolymphatic duct **(Ductus endolymphaticus).** The vestibular cells, situated in the utriculus and the sacculus, register changes in the head or body position in vertical or horizontal positions (linear acceleration). The sensory cells in the semicircular canals register rotational acceleration. The action potentials arising in the perception areas of the vestibular organ responsible for hearing and equilibrium are relayed via the VIIIth cranial nerve (N. vestibulocochlearis).

Main topics

After working through this chapter, you should be able to:

- explain the anatomy of the outer ear, middle ear and inner ear and describe their content structures;
- clearly define the borders of the three regions, explain their proximity to neighbouring structures and put them in context with clinically relevant aspects;
- correctly describe the path and structure of the EUSTACHIAN tube, the muscles involved in the tube's function and the relationship to the middle ear;

- outline the functional context between tube ventilation, the tympanic cavity and the mastoid process cells;
- explain the neurovascular pathways in the Pars petrosa, including their route as well as the areas they supply and innervate;
- explain the development of the outer ear, middle ear and inner ear, including functional interrelations, and use those to make conclusions on developmental disorders.

Clinical relevance

In order not to lose touch with prospective everyday clinical life with so many anatomical details, the following describes a typical case that shows why the content of this chapter is so important.

Otitis media acuta

Case study
The three-year-old Maximilian has to be picked up from nursery school again soon after drop-off, because he has developed a fever and is touching his ear constantly. As the mother arrives, Maxi runs to her in tears. The nursery school teachers tell the mother that Maxi did not eat breakfast, kept asking to be hugged, started crying spontaneously and constantly touched his ear. The mother is already familiar with this pattern of behaviour and suspects a middle ear infection, which Maxi has already had quite often. She therefore takes him directly from the nursery school to the clinic.

Results of examination
The nurse ascertains that Maxi has a temperature of 38.7 °C. The paediatrician asks how Maxi slept the night before, whether he has been snoring lately, breathing through his mouth or been hard of hearing. The mother states that Maxi slept well the previous night, but had indeed snored. She could not say whether his hearing was worse. The mother points out that Maxi currently has a cold, with a thick yellow nasal discharge, but considers that normal at his age. Looking into his mouth, the paediatrician notices a fissured, slightly red and enlarged pharyngeal tonsil; the oral cavity is otherwise normal. Examination of the right ear using the otoscope reveals a dark red tympanic membrane bulging into the external auditory canal (→ Fig. a).

 Characteristic of an Otitis media acuta is a bulging and dark red tympanic membrane, as well as severe ear ache.

The left ear is without symptoms. When touching the cervical lymph nodes, the paediatrician can feel enlarged retroauricular lymph nodes. Pressure on Maxi's mastoid process does not elicit a pain response.

Diagnosis
Acute middle ear inflammation (Otitis media acuta)

Treatment
The paediatrician prescribes decongestant nasal drops and liquid ibuprofen for Maxi for pain relief and to lower the fever. The mother is to administer the nasal drops liberally and to apply them several times a day on both sides. Using an image of an ear, the paediatrician explains to the mother the connection between the nasopharynx, the EUSTACHIAN tube and the middle ear to clarify why it is essential that Maxi must be given the nasal drops, and will need it for several days. If the situation does not improve over the next two days or if it deteriorates, the mother is to bring Maxi back to the doctor's immediately or take him to A & E at the hospital. But the paediatrician expects that the condition will improve rapidly.

Further developments
The liquid ibuprofen is effective as expected. Shortly after taking it, Maxi already appears significantly improved, the fever lessens, he begins to interact and play again, and is almost back to his usual self. In the evening, Maxi once again develops a high fever, and the mother once again gives him ibuprofen. She also administers the nasal drops regularly. Maxi is restless during the night, but has no fever. To be on the safe side, the mother gives him liquid ibuprofen again the next morning. The following day, and on subsequent days, the child is symptom-free. On the third day, the mother takes him back to the nursery school and asks the nursery teachers to administer the nasal drops to Maxi before he takes a nap at midday. At the nursery school, Maxi shows no symptoms either.

Dissection lab
In the dissection lab, one should look at the entrance to the EUSTACHIAN tube behind the choanae in the nasopharynx, and, if possible, the opened middle ear with the auditory ossicles.

 Malleus, incus and stapes

In addition, the connection from the nasopharynx via the EUSTACHIAN tube to the middle ear can be seen clearly using anatomical models.

Back at the clinic
The paediatrician diagnoses Maxi with Otitis media acuta. She explains to the mother that this is a common condition in early childhood, since the middle ear structures are still small, and there is a risk of ventilation disorders in the ear, especially in the context of infections, which can then lead to an acute inflammation.

 The EUSTACHIAN tube is still small and short in children. Hence a tube ventilation disorder can happen easily in the context of infections.

Such acute inflammations are to be differentiated from a chronic ventilation disorder in the middle ear, caused by an enlargement of the pharyngeal tonsil (Tonsilla pharyngea). Enlarged tonsils are also colloquially referred to as polyps, while Ear, Nose and Throat (ENT) specialists refer to them as adenoids or adenoid vegetation. In the worst case scenario, the enlarged pharyngeal tonsil obstructs the entrance of the EUSTACHIAN tube on both sides. The pharyngeal tonsil enlarges to the extent that the child can no longer breathe through the nose, only through the mouth. Since skull growth has not yet been completed, the child also develops the 'facial expression of a mouth breather' (Facies adenoidea). Because the ventilation of the EUSTACHIAN tube is disrupted, the child cannot hear very well and has difficulty learning to speak as a result. They have difficulty concentrating and – if already of school age – fall behind at school. In these children, the hyperplastic pharyngeal tonsil has to be surgically removed in order to improve the situation. In addition, a tympanostomy tube is placed into a lower quadrant of the tympanic membrane, which ensures ventilation via the external auditory canal in the short term. The tympanostomy tube, provided it does not fall out of its own accord, has to be removed after some time.

Middle ear infections are always fraught with risk due to the topographical proximity to neighbouring structures.

 The middle ear has six walls, through which a middle ear inflammation may spread to adjacent regions.

It can result in perforation of the tympanic membrane, inflammation of the mastoid process (mastoiditis), meningitis, brain abscess, thrombosis of the Sinus sigmoideus, spreading of germs into the A. carotis interna with subsequent sepsis, inflammation of the inner ear (labyrinthitis) or other complications.

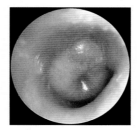

Fig. a Right tympanic membrane in Otitis media acuta; viewed through the otoscope from the outside via the external ear canal to the tympanic membrane, which is dark red and bulging. [G548]

Overview

Development

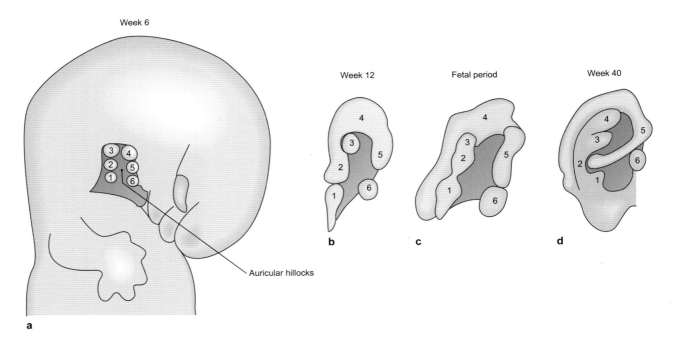

Week 6

Week 12

Fetal period

Week 40

Auricular hillocks

a

b

c

d

Fig. 10.1a–d   Development of the auricle from the six auricular hillocks, right side. [S700-L231]
Merging of the auricular hillocks (1–6) is a complicated process and disorders in this development are therefore not rare. The primordial auricle originates in the lower region of the neck. As the lower jaw develops, there is a cranial shift so that the outer ears are ultimately positioned at the same level as the eyes. Auricles at a lower position are very commonly associated

with other (often chromosomal) deformities. The external auditory canal develops from the posterior part of the first pharyngeal groove, which extends inwards as a cone-shaped tube, reaching the entodermal epithelial lining of the tympanic cavity (Recessus tubotympanicus). At the beginning of the ninth week, the epithelial cells of the acoustic floor proliferate and form an ear canal plate. This dissolves in the seventh month. A persistent plate in the external acoustic meatus results in congenital deafness.

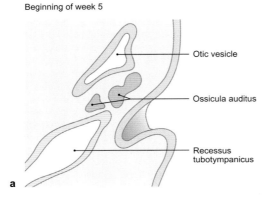

Beginning of week 5

Otic vesicle

Ossicula auditus

Recessus tubotympanicus

a

End of week 5

Auris interna

Incus

Malleus

Stapes

Meatus acusticus externs

b

Fig. 10.2a and b   Differentiation of the auditory ossicles, Ossicula auditus. [E838]
a Beginning of the fifth week.
b End of the fifth week.
At the beginning of the fifth week, in the mesenchyme of the first and second pharyngeal arch, the auditory ossicles begin to emerge. The

malleus and incus emerge from the first pharyngeal arch as derivatives of MECKEL's cartilage, as well as the M. tensor tympani, which is innervated by the first pharyngeal arch nerve, the N. mandibularis [V/3]. The stapes emerges from the second pharyngeal arch as a derivative of REICHERT's cartilage. It can be moved by the M. stapedius, which is innervated by the second pharyngeal arch nerve, the N. facialis [VII].

Structure and function

Development of the ear
On approx. the 22nd day, the **surface ectoderm** on both sides of the rhombencephalon will thicken. This cellular condensation, called an **otic placode,** subsequently folds inward, forming an **otic pit** and thereafter the **otic vesicle** (otocyst). Each vesicle is divided into a **ventral (rostral) section,** from which the saccule (sacculus) as well as the Ductus cochlearis emerge, and a **dorsal (occipital) section,** from which the utricle (utriculus), semicircular canals and Ductus endolymphaticus emerge. The rostral and occipital parts remain connected via a small duct. The resulting structures are in their entirety referred to as a **membranous labyrinth.**
The first pharyngeal groove and the first pharyngeal pouch grow towards each other. The external acoustic meatus is formed by the ectoderm of the first pharyngeal groove; the entoderm of the first

pharyngeal pouch forms the **middle ear.** Proximally, the latter narrows to form the **EUSTACHIAN tube** (auditory tube). The latter has a very narrow connection with the part of the foregut which will become the nasopharynx. Distally, the first pharyngeal pouch widens to form the **tympanic cavity.**
The Recessus tubotympanicus, which grows towards the advancing pharyngeal groove, forms on the lateral tympanic cavity wall. At the point of contact, only a thin membrane remains – the **tympanic membrane.** The **auditory ossicles** develop in the mesenchyme from the first and second pharyngeal arch at the beginning of the fifth week. On the outer edge of the first pharyngeal groove, six **auricular hillocks** form at the beginning of the sixth week, which merge in a complex way until birth to form the adult auricle.

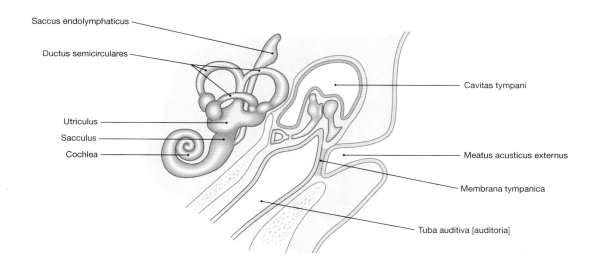

Saccus endolymphaticus
Ductus semicirculares
Utriculus
Sacculus
Cochlea

Cavitas tympani
Meatus acusticus externus
Membrana tympanica
Tuba auditiva [auditoria]

Fig. 10.3 Structures of the inner, middle and outer ear at birth.
[E838]
Up to the eighth month of pregnancy, the initially cartilaginous auditory ossicles are embedded in the mesenchyme. This gradually recedes and

is replaced by an entodermal mucosal lining that covers the entire tympanic cavity.

Clinical remarks

Congenital deafness occurs in two out of every 1,000 newborns. In approx. one third, a genetic defect is the cause. Other causes include infections during pregnancy, chronic diseases in the mother, medication, alcohol and nicotine. An inability to hear severely limits language-learning as well as structured thinking and communication. Early detection and subsequent therapy early on in life are therefore of enormous importance.

Auricular malformations are common. They are divided into three grades of dysplasia from mild (I) to severe (III) (→ figures). A severe dysplasia, for example, tends to include the genetically dominant FRANCESCHETTI syndrome (Dysostosis mandibulofacialis), which is characterised by malformation of the first pharyngeal arch and first pharyngeal groove, resulting in malformed outer ears and zygomatic bone, a receding chin and cleft palate.

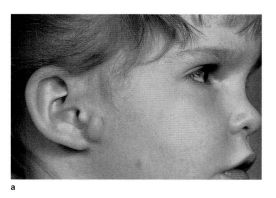

a

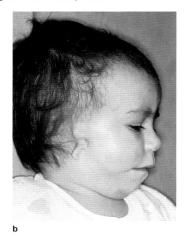

b

Child with preauricular skin adnexa, mild (grade I) auricular dysplasia. [E347-09]

Child with small, rudimentary auricle (microtia), and moderate (grade II) auricular dysplasia. The auricle is small and severely malformed. Often this also affects the external acoustic meatus. [E347-09]

Overview

Outer, middle and inner ear

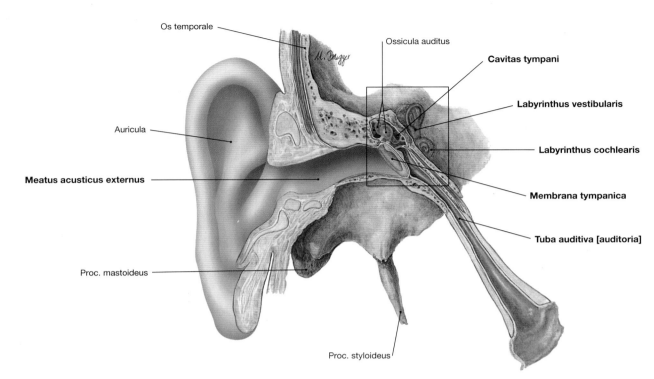

Fig. 10.4 Parts of the ear, auris, right side; longitudinal section through the external acoustic meatus, middle ear and EUSTACHIAN tube; frontal view. [S700]
Presentation of the auricle (Auricula), external auditory canal (Meatus acusticus externus), tympanic membrane (Membrana tympanica), tympanic cavity (Cavitas tympani), auditory ossicles (Ossicula auditus), auditory organ (Labyrinthus cochlearis) and vestibular organ (Labyrinthus vestibularis). Sound waves cause the tympanic membrane to vibrate **(aerotympanal conduction).** The vibrations are carried up to the oval window of the inner ear by the auditory ossicles (→ Fig. 10.24). Thereby the low acoustic imped-

ance (→ Fig. 10.16) in the air is adapted to the high impedance of the fluid-filled inner ear. Moreover, the inner ear can also utilise vibrations via the skull bones **(bone conduction).** Within the inner ear, sound energy continues to travel as a wave (migrating wave). The sensory cells of the inner ear transform the sound energy into an **electrical impulse** that is passed on to the brain via the N. cochlearis. The vestibular organ serves in the perception of rotational and linear accelerations. Movements of the endolymph in the vestibular organ result in a deflection of the cilia of the sensory cells which are synaptically linked to afferent fibres of the N. vestibularis.

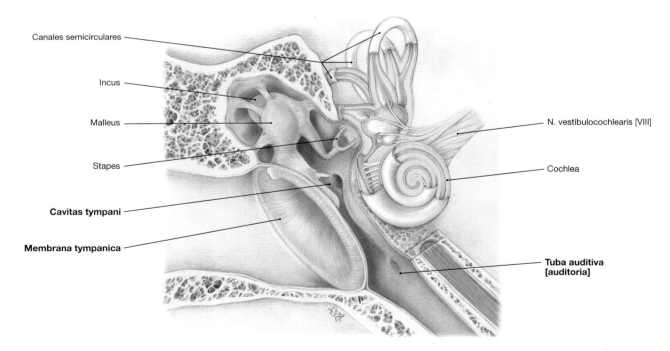

Fig. 10.5 Middle and inner ear, Auris media and interna, right side; section of → Fig. 10.4 frontal view. [S700-L285]
Apart from the tympanic membrane, the three auditory ossicles are visible in the tympanic cavity (Cavitas tympani): hammer-shaped malleus, anvil-shaped incus and stirrup-like stapes, as well as parts of the membranous labyrinth (Labyrinthus membranaceus, blue).

Clinical remarks

It is not rare for mechanical manipulation (e.g. cleaning the external auditory canal with a cotton swab) or injuries to result in an inflammation in the auricle area and the external acoustic meatus **(Otitis externa).**

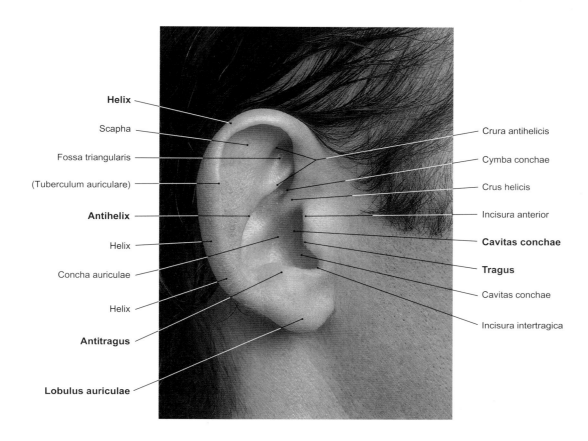

Helix

Scapha

Fossa triangularis

(Tuberculum auriculare)

Antihelix

Helix

Concha auriculae

Helix

Antitragus

Lobulus auriculae

Crura antihelicis

Cymba conchae

Crus helicis

Incisura anterior

Cavitas conchae

Tragus

Cavitas conchae

Incisura intertragica

Fig. 10.6   Auricle, Auricula, right side; lateral view. [S700]
The basic framework of the auricle is made up of elastic cartilage. The skin across the lateral surface is attached to the perichondrium and cannot be moved; the skin on the back of the auricle is movable. There is no subcutaneous fat tissue. The earlobe (Lobulus auriculae) is non-cartilaginous.

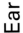

Auricle, blood vessels and innervation

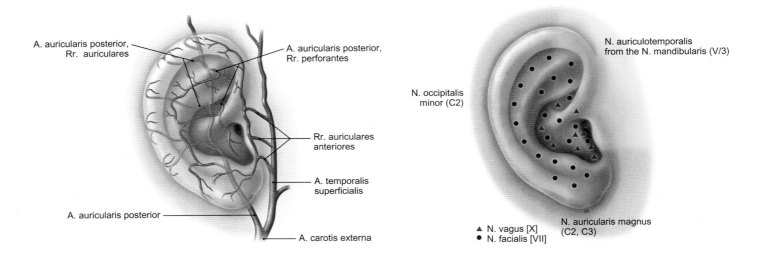

A. auricularis posterior, Rr. auriculares

A. auricularis posterior, Rr. perforantes

Rr. auriculares anteriores

A. temporalis superficialis

A. auricularis posterior

A. carotis externa

N. auriculotemporalis from the N. mandibularis (V/3)

N. occipitalis minor (C2)

▲ N. vagus [X]
● N. facialis [VII]

N. auricularis magnus (C2, C3)

Fig. 10.7   Arteries of the auricle, Auricula, right side; lateral view. [S700-L238]
Due to its exposed position, the auricle is highly vascularised (protection against freezing and heat loss). The vessels are **branches of the A. carotis externa** (A. auricularis posterior, A. temporalis superficialis).

Fig. 10.8   Sensory innervation of the auricle, Auricula, right side; lateral view. [S700-L238]/[E402-004]
Innervation at the front of the auricle is supplied by the **N. auriculotemporalis** (from the N. mandibularis [V/3]), behind and below the ear by the **Plexus cervicalis** (N. auricularis magnus, N. occipitalis minor), at the auricle itself by the **N. facialis [VII]** (it is not entirely clear which part exactly it supplies), and at the entrance to the external acoustic meatus by the **N. vagus [X]**.

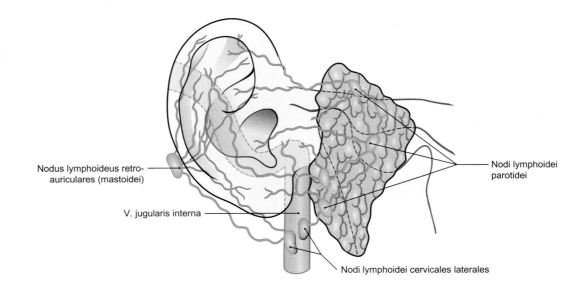

Nodus lymphoideus retro-auriculares (mastoidei)

V. jugularis interna

Nodi lymphoidei parotidei

Nodi lymphoidei cervicales laterales

Fig. 10.9   Lymphatic drainage from the auricle, Auricula, right side; lateral view. [S700-L126]
The lymph of the auricle is drained via the parotid (Nodi lymphoidei parotidei superficiales et profundi) and retroauricular (Nodi lymphoidei re-

troauriculares, Nodi lymphoidei mastoidei) lymph nodes into the lateral cervical lymph nodes (Nodi lymphoidei cervicales laterales) along the V. jugularis interna.

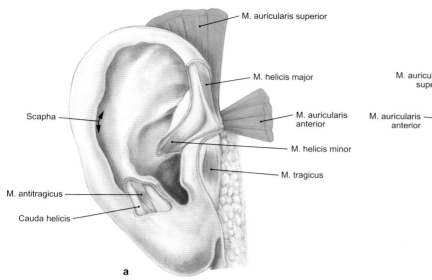

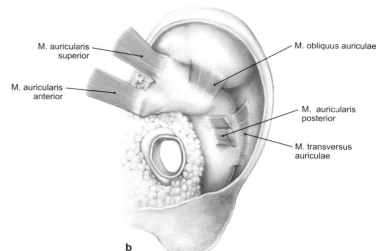

Fig. 10.10 a and b Mm. auriculares and cartilage of the auricle, Auricula, right side. [S700-L285]
a Lateral view.
b Dorsal view.
Quite often, rudimentary muscles are still attached to the auricle (some people can move their ears). This mimic musculature (innervated by the

N. auricularis posterior, a branch of the N. facialis [VII]), forms part of a rudimentary sphincter system, which is still very well developed in many animals. Horses, for example, turn their auricles towards the direction of sound. Hedgehogs and bears close off their external acoustic meatus so as not to be disturbed by noise during hibernation.

→ T 1.2

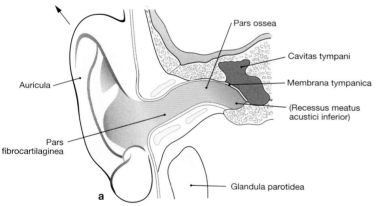

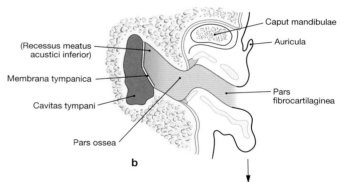

Fig. 10.11a and b External acoustic meatus, Meatus acusticus externus, right side; schematic drawing. [S700-L126]
a Frontal section.
b Horizontal section.
The external acoustic meatus is S-shaped and is formed by the Pars tympanica of the Os temporale. In order to be able to inspect the tympanic membrane with an otoscopic mirror or a microscope (otoscopy), the auricle has to be pulled upwards and to the back. This stretches the cartilaginous part of the external acoustic meatus and the tympanic

membrane can be seen (at least partially). **Innervation** of the external acoustic meatus (not shown) occurs via the N. meatus acustici externi of the N. auriculotemporalis (anterior and superior wall), the R. auricularis of the N. vagus [X] (posterior wall and part of inferior wall) and via the Rr. auriculares of the N. facialis [VII] and the N. glossopharyngeus [IX] (posterior wall and tympanic membrane).
Arrows: Direction in which the examiner pulled the auricle, to stretch the external acoustic meatus and to gain a view of the tympanic membrane.

Clinical remarks

- An inflammation of the elastic cartilage **(auricular perichondritis)** may occur as a result of injuries or insect stings to the auricle. Treatment includes topical application of disinfecting agents as well as local and systemic application of glucocorticoids and antibiotics.
- Since the earlobe is well supplied with blood, is very easily accessible and has no elastic cartilage, it is often used to take a blood sample, e.g. in diabetic patients, to measure blood glucose levels.

- Abnormalities of the auricle often require plastic-reconstructive surgery.
- Due to the sensory innervation of the external acoustic meatus by the N. vagus [X], manipulations in the external acoustic meatus (e.g. the removal of cerumen or foreign objects) almost always initiates a cough reflex. In severe cases the manipulation can cause vomiting or a collapse.

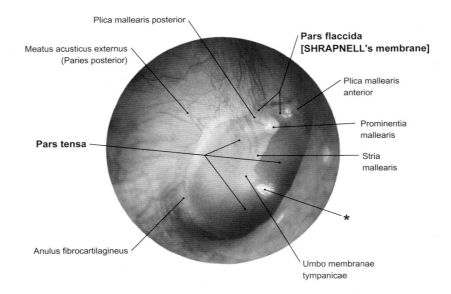

Plica mallearis posterior

Meatus acusticus externus
(Paries posterior)

**Pars flaccida
[SHRAPNELL's membrane]**

Plica mallearis
anterior

Prominentia
mallearis

Stria
mallearis

Pars tensa

*

Anulus fibrocartilagineus

Umbo membranae
tympanicae

**Fig. 10.12   Tympanic membrane, Membrana tympanica, right
side;** lateral view; otoscopic image. [S700]
The Pars tympanica of the Os temporale separates the anterior, inferior
and posterior aspects of the Meatus acusticus externus. In its superior
aspect, the bony ring is interrupted by the Incisura tympanica (attachment site of the Pars flaccida of the tympanic membrane). With the

exception of the Incisura tympanica, the otherwise circular Sulcus tympanicus is located within the Pars tympanica (the Pars tensa of the tympanic membrane is attached here by an Anulus fibrocartilagineus).

* typically positioned light reflex

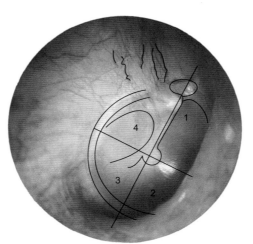

1 Anterior superior (AS) quadrant
2 Anterior inferior (AI) quadrant
3 Posterior superior (PS) quadrant
4 Posterior inferior (PI) quadrant

**Fig. 10.13   Tympanic membrane, Membrana tympanica, right
side, divided into four quadrants;** lateral view. [S700]

When illuminating the tympanic membrane with its shiny, pearly appearance, a triangular light reflex in the anterior lower quadrant is usually
produced, which allows for conclusions to be made about its tension.

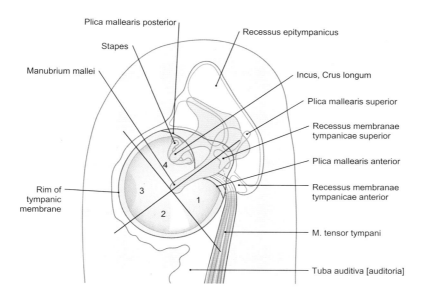

Plica mallearis posterior
Recessus epitympanicus
Stapes
Manubrium mallei
Incus, Crus longum
Plica mallearis superior
Recessus membranae tympanicae superior
Plica mallearis anterior
Recessus membranae tympanicae anterior
Rim of tympanic membrane
M. tensor tympani
Tuba auditiva [auditoria]

Fig. 10.14 Tympanic membrane, Membrana tympanica and the recessus of the tympanic cavity, Cavitas tympani, right side, divided into four quadrants; lateral view; schematic diagram. [S700-L126]

Dividing into four quadrants is of practical clinical relevance. The auditory ossicles are located in the upper quadrants. In addition, the Chorda tympani and the attaching tendon of the M. tensor tympani are positioned here (→ Fig. 12.148).

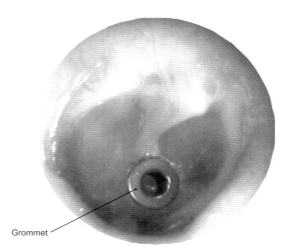

Grommet

Fig. 10.15 Tympanostomy tube in the anterior lower quadrant. [S700-T720]
To avoid injury to the structures of the middle ear, a paracentesis (small surgical incision of the tympanic membrane) is performed in the ante-

rior lower or posterior lower quadrant. The incision is used to insert a tympanostomy tube (grommet) for long-term ventilation.

Clinical remarks

The Pars flaccida of the tympanic membrane is thinner than the Pars tensa and therefore the most likely location with a **purulent middle ear infection** (Otitis media) (→ Fig. a) for a spontaneous perforation. Tympanic cavity effluent can be seen and drained through the tympanic membrane. To do this, a paracentesis is carried out in the anterior and posterior lower quadrants (→ Fig. b) and the draining inflammatory secretion is suctioned off. For long-term drainage and ventilation, a tympanostomy tube (grommet, myringotomy tube) is inserted

at the location of the tympanic membrane incision (→ Figs. c and d; → Fig. 10.15). Excessive production of cerumen (earwax) often results in a ceruminal plug that may close the external acoustic meatus **(Cerumen obturans)** and lead to conductive hearing loss. The bitter substances in the cerumen normally serve to keep microorganisms and insects (flies, small beetles, etc.) away.
[E625]

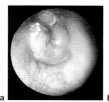
a

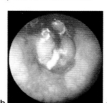
b

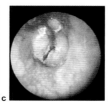
c

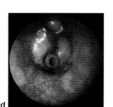
d

Middle ear

Auditory ossicles

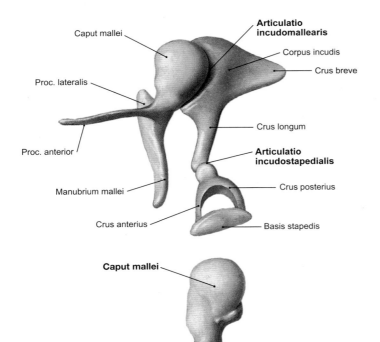

Fig. 10.16 Auditory ossicles, Ossicula auditus, right side; medial view from above. [S700]

The auditory bones of the auditory ossicular chain are connected consecutively and linked by true joints (Articulatio incudomallearis – a saddle joint – and Articulatio incudostapedialis – a spheroidal joint). The auditory ossicles form a flexible chain for the transmission of sound waves conducted by the tympanic membrane to the perilymph of the inner ear. Low air impedance has to be transferred to the significantly higher inner ear air impedance. This requires an amplification of the sound waves (impedance matching), which is achieved by the difference in size of the area of the tympanic membrane (55 mm²) to the area of the oval window (3.2 mm²; 17-fold) and the lever action of the auditory ossicle chain (1.3-fold). Thus, the acoustic pressure amplifies by 22-fold.

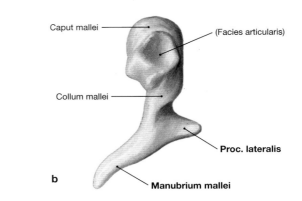

Fig. 10.17a and b Malleus, right side. [S700]
a Frontal view.
b Posterior view.

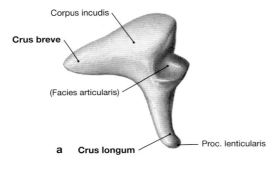

Fig. 10.18a and b Incus, right side. [S700]
a Lateral view.
b Medial view.

Fig. 10.19 Stapes, right side; superior view. [S700]

Clinical remarks

Defects in the chain of transmission (tympanic membrane, auditory ossicles) result in **conductive hearing loss.** In the event of a complete loss of acoustic pressure transmission, a hearing loss of approx. 20 dB sets in. A typical disorder that leads to such a hearing loss is **otosclerosis.** This is a localised disorder of the petrous part of the temporal bone. The base of the stapes progressively attaches to the oval window through ossification of the Lig. anulare stapediale (→ figure), causing a gradual worsening of conductive hearing. Inflammatory foci in the area of the cochlea may also cause inner ear hearing loss. Women aged 20–40 years are affected twice as often as men. In 70 % of cases, otosclerosis affects both ears.

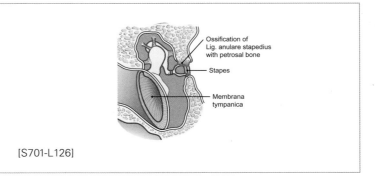

[S701-L126]

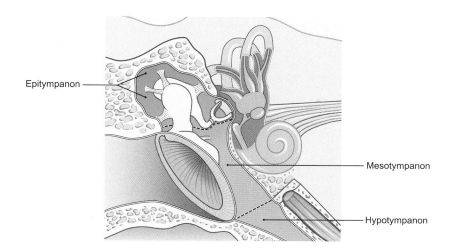

Epitympanon

Mesotympanon

Hypotympanon

Fig. 10.20 Levels of the tympanic cavity, Cavitas tympani, right side; frontal view. [S702-L126]

From a clinical perspective, the tympanic cavity is divided into three sections according to their positioning in relation to the tympanic membrane:

*   The **epitympanum** (Recessus epitympanicus, epitympanic recess, attic) contains the suspension apparatus and the majority of the au-

ditory ossicles, and is connected to the Antrum mastoideum via the mastoid cells.
*   The **mesotympanum** contains the Manubrium mallei, the Proc. lenticularis of the incus, and the tendon of the M. tensor tympani.
*   The **hypotympanum** leads into the Tuba auditiva [auditoria] via the Recessus hypotympanicus.

The boundaries between the three sections are defined by dashed lines.

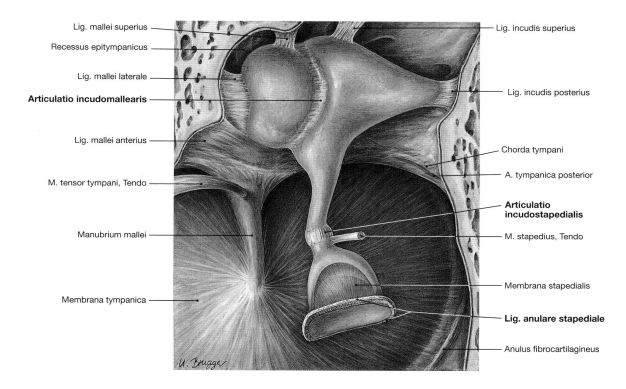

Lig. mallei superius

Recessus epitympanicus

Lig. mallei laterale

Articulatio incudomallearis

Lig. mallei anterius

M. tensor tympani, Tendo

Manubrium mallei

Membrana tympanica

Lig. incudis superius

Lig. incudis posterius

Chorda tympani

A. tympanica posterior

Articulatio incudostapedialis

M. stapedius, Tendo

Membrana stapedialis

Lig. anulare stapediale

Anulus fibrocartilagineus

Fig. 10.21 Joints and ligaments of the auditory ossicles, Articulationes and Ligg. ossiculorum auditus, right side; medial view from above. [S700]

The malleus and incus are secured via ligaments in the epitympanum and are flexibly interconnected via the saddle joint (Articulatio incudo-

mallearis). The stapes is in contact with the incus via the spheroidal joint (Articulatio incudostapedialis). Its base (Basis stapedis) is attached in the oval window (syndesmosis) by the Lig. anulare stapediale. All structures in the tympanic cavity, including the Chorda tympani, are lined with middle ear mucosa.

Clinical remarks

In childhood, one of the most common causes of conductive hearing loss is an occlusion of the Tuba auditiva (tubal occlusion) due to an inflammation of the tube **(EUSTACHIAN catarrh)** or in cases of restricted nasal breathing due to **enlarged pharyngeal tonsils (ade-**

noids). If the tubal function disorder persists over a longer period of time, restructuring of the mucosa of the middle ear takes place. As a result, an actively secreting epithelium develops, with fluid retention formation in the tympanic cavity (seromucous tympanum).

191

Tympanic cavity

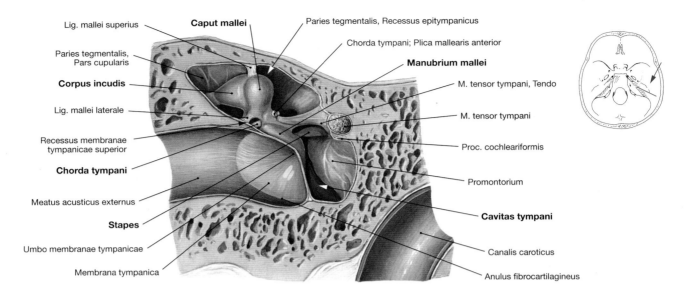

Fig. 10.22 Tympanic cavity, Cavitas tympani, right side; frontal section; frontal view. [S700]
The tympanic cavity is an air-filled hollow space inside the middle ear containing the auditory ossicles. It is located directly behind the tympanic membrane and is ventilated via the EUSTACHIAN tube [Tuba auditiva/auditoria], aiding pressure equalisation. The distance between the epitympanum and the hypotympanum is 12–15 mm at a depth of 3–7 mm. The inner volume is only about 1 cm³.

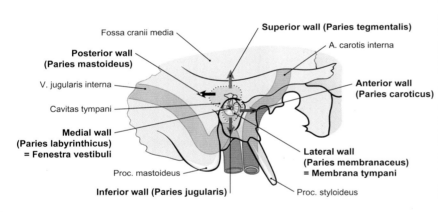

Topographical connections of the tympanic cavity (Cavitas tympani)		
Mastoid process (Paries mastoideus)	Posterior wall (Proc. mastoideus)	→
V. jugularis (Paries jugularis)	Inferior wall (Fossa jugularis)	↓
A. carotis interna (Paries caroticus)	Anterior wall (carotid canal)	←
Middle cranial fossa (Paries tegmentalis)	Superior wall (middle cranial fossa)	↑
Oval window (Paries labyrinthicus)	Medial wall (labyrinth)	⬭
Tympanic membrane (Paries membranaceus)	Lateral wall (tympanic membrane)	◎

Fig. 10.23 Topographical relationships between the tympanic cavity, Cavitas tympani, to adjacent structures, right side; lateral view; schematic drawing. [S702-L126]
A thin bony plate (Tegmen tympani, **Paries tegmentalis**) separates the epitympanum from the middle cranial fossa. The anterior wall of the mesotympanum (**Paries caroticus**) is in close proximity to the A. carotis interna. The lateral wall (**Paries membranaceus**) is formed almost exclusively by the tympanic membrane. The EUSTACHIAN tube [Tuba auditiva/auditoria] opens into the tympanic cavity in the inferior wall section. The posterior wall (**Paries mastoideus**) is adjacent to the mastoid process (Proc. mastoideus). In the upper posterior section, a direct connection exists to the pneumatised areas of the mastoid (Aditus ad antrum). The medial wall (**Paries labyrinthicus;** → Fig. 10.24 and → Fig. 10.26) separates the cochlea from the tympanic cavity. The inferior wall of the tympanic cavity (**Paries jugularis**) forms part of the hypotympanum. It separates the tympanic cavity from the V. jugularis interna. The bone is very thin at that point and partially pneumatised.

Clinical remarks

An acute middle ear infection (**Otitis media**) is one of the most common illnesses in childhood. It is commonly caused by bacteria and viruses entering the middle ear through the EUSTACHIAN tube during or after an infection of the nasopharynx. The inflammation is characterised by a reddening of the mucous membrane, mucosal oedema, granulocytic infiltration and a formation of pus. Since the suppuration cannot exit via the inflamed and therefore blocked tubes, the inflammation can spread to the surrounding area and cause severe **complications,** such as:

- rupturing of the tympanic membrane (most common; via the Paries membranaceus)
- mastoiditis (via the Paries mastoideus, Antrum mastoideum)
- thrombophlebitis and thrombosis of the V. jugularis (via the Paries jugularis)
- sepsis (bacteria spreading into the blood via the Paries caroticus)
- brain abscess and/or meningitis (via the Paries tegmentalis)
- labyrinthitis (with vertigo and hearing impairment via the Paries labyrinthicus).

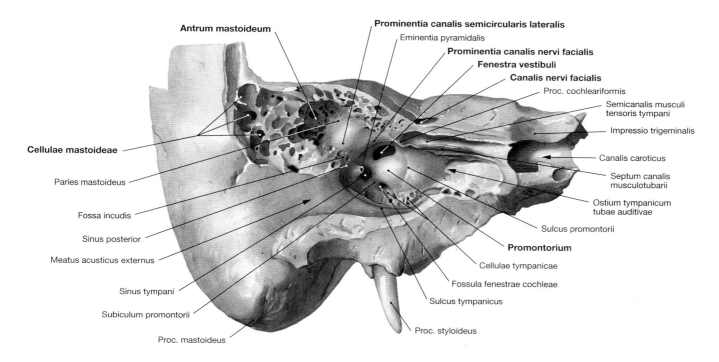

Antrum mastoideum

Prominentia canalis semicircularis lateralis

Eminentia pyramidalis

Prominentia canalis nervi facialis

Fenestra vestibuli

Canalis nervi facialis

Proc. cochleariformis

Semicanalis musculi tensoris tympani

Impressio trigeminalis

Canalis caroticus

Septum canalis musculotubarii

Ostium tympanicum tubae auditivae

Sulcus promontorii

Promontorium

Cellulae mastoideae

Paries mastoideus

Fossa incudis

Sinus posterior

Meatus acusticus externus

Sinus tympani

Subiculum promontorii

Proc. mastoideus

Cellulae tympanicae

Fossula fenestrae cochleae

Sulcus tympanicus

Proc. styloideus

Fig. 10.24 Medial wall, Paries labyrinthicus, of the tympanic cavity, Cavitas tympani, right side; vertical section through the longitudinal axis of the petrous part of the temporal bone; anterolateral view. [S700]
Above the oval window, the lateral semicircular canal makes the wall of the tympanic cavity bulge out from the Prominentia canalis semicircularis lateralis. The N. facialis [VII] passes through the medial wall in the

Canalis nervi facialis. The canal makes the horizontal Prominentia canalis nervi facialis bulge towards the medial wall. The Tuba auditiva [auditoria] starts at the Ostium tympanicum tubae auditivae and is demarcated at the top by the Septum canalis musculotubarii from the Semicanalis musculi tensoris tympani. The mastoid process (Proc. mastoideus) is typically pneumatised (Cellulae mastoideae) and is connected to the tympanic cavity via the Antrum mastoideum.

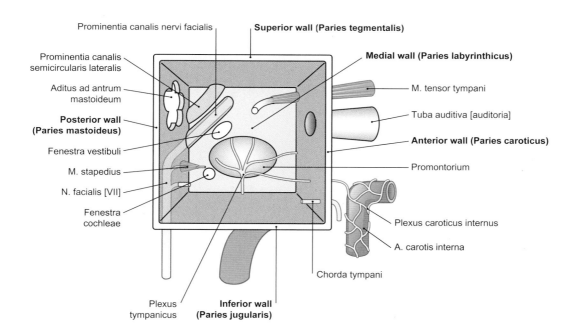

Prominentia canalis nervi facialis

Superior wall (Paries tegmentalis)

Prominentia canalis semicircularis lateralis

Aditus ad antrum mastoideum

Posterior wall (Paries mastoideus)

Fenestra vestibuli

M. stapedius

N. facialis [VII]

Fenestra cochleae

Plexus tympanicus

Inferior wall (Paries jugularis)

Medial wall (Paries labyrinthicus)

M. tensor tympani

Tuba auditiva [auditoria]

Anterior wall (Paries caroticus)

Promontorium

Plexus caroticus internus

A. carotis interna

Chorda tympani

Fig. 10.25 Medial wall, Paries labyrinthicus, of the tympanic cavity, Cavitas tympani, right side; anterolateral view, schematic drawing. [S702-L126]/[E402-004]
The illustration presents the tympanic cavity as a rectangular box with six walls, whereby the lateral wall in which the tympanic membrane

would be positioned has been omitted. The illustration serves as a basic orientation, facilitating navigation of the anatomical images (→ Fig. 10.24 and → Fig. 10.26) as well as the structures positioned in or passing through the bone.

Middle ear

Tympanic cavity

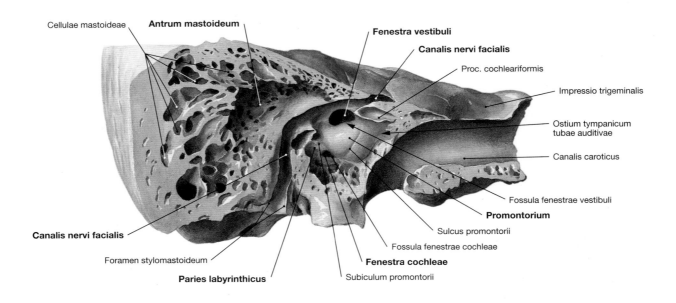

Cellulae mastoideae
Antrum mastoideum
Fenestra vestibuli
Canalis nervi facialis
Proc. cochleariformis
Impressio trigeminalis
Ostium tympanicum tubae auditivae
Canalis caroticus
Fossula fenestrae vestibuli
Promontorium
Sulcus promontorii
Fossula fenestrae cochleae
Fenestra cochleae
Subiculum promontorii
Paries labyrinthicus
Foramen stylomastoideum
Canalis nervi facialis

**Fig. 10.26   Medial wall, Paries labyrinthicus, of the tympanic cavi-
ty, Cavitas tympani, right side;** anterolateral view; after removal of
the lateral wall and the adjacent parts of the anterior and superior
wall; Canalis nervi facialis and Canalis caroticus opened. [S700]
The medial wall of the tympanic cavity forms the boundary to the inner
ear (labyrinth). It has two openings:

* the **oval window** (Fenestra vestibuli), in which the base of the
  stapes (Basis stapedis) is attached to the Lig. anulare stapediale
* the **round window** (Fenestra cochleae), located more inferiorly, occluded by the Membrana tympanica secundaria.

Between the oval and the round window, the basal cochlear turn
creates a prominent bulge in the medial wall of the tympanic cavity
towards the promontorium.

Clinical remarks

An inflammation of the Cellulae mastoideae **(mastoiditis)** is often an
inflammatory process in the tympanic cavity. It is one of the most
frequent complications of a middle ear inflammation (Otitis media).
The inflammation can spread from the mastoid to the soft tissue

parts behind and in front of the outer ear, the M. sternocleidomastoideus, the inner ear, the Sinus sigmoideus, the meninges, and the
N. facialis [VII].

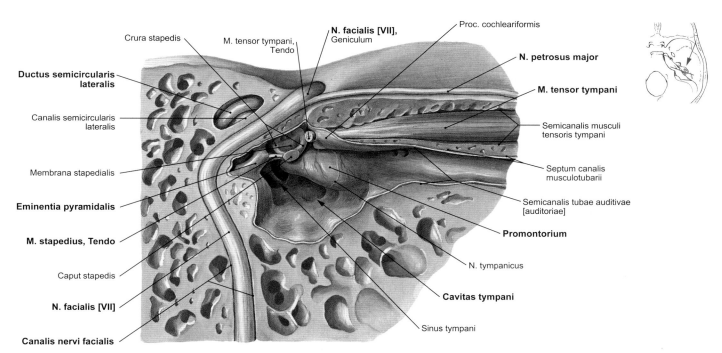

Ductus semicircularis lateralis

Canalis semicircularis lateralis

Membrana stapedialis

Eminentia pyramidalis

M. stapedius, Tendo

Caput stapedis

N. facialis [VII]

Canalis nervi facialis

Crura stapedis

M. tensor tympani, Tendo

N. facialis [VII], Geniculum

Proc. cochleariformis

N. petrosus major

M. tensor tympani

Semicanalis musculi tensoris tympani

Septum canalis musculotubarii

Semicanalis tubae auditivae [auditoriae]

Promontorium

N. tympanicus

Cavitas tympani

Sinus tympani

Fig. 10.27 N. facialis [VII], tympanic cavity, Cavitas tympani and EUSTACHIAN tube [Tuba auditiva [auditoria], right side; vertical section of the longitudinal axis of the petrous part of the temporal bone; frontal view; facial canal opened. [S700]
The N. facialis [VII] is composed of two branches, the actual N. facialis and the N. intermedius. Both branches merge deep inside the facial canal (Canalis nervi facialis) to form the N. intermediofacialis (generally referred to as N. facialis [VII]). It arches around the tympanic cavity and

generates the Prominentia canalis nervi facialis in the medial wall of the tympanic cavity. The Eminentia pyramidalis protrudes underneath. Located inside is the N. facialis [VII] which innervates the M. stapedius (→ Fig. 12.153). Its tendon exits from the Eminentia pyramidalis and inserts inferolaterally at the small stapedial head.
Function of the M. stapedius: attenuation of vibrations at the oval window by tilting of the stapes, decreasing of acoustic transmission, protection against excessive noise.

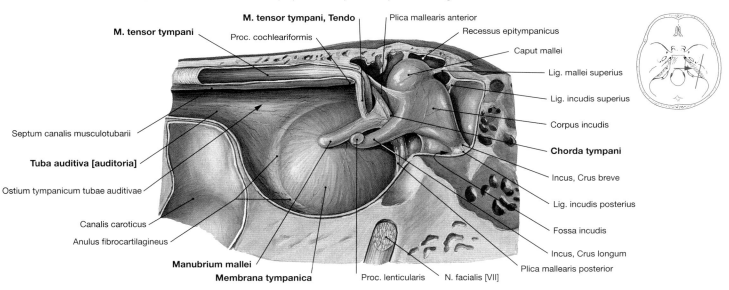

M. tensor tympani

Septum canalis musculotubarii

Tuba auditiva [auditoria]

Ostium tympanicum tubae auditivae

Canalis caroticus

Anulus fibrocartilagineus

Manubrium mallei

Membrana tympanica

M. tensor tympani, Tendo

Proc. cochleariformis

Plica mallearis anterior

Recessus epitympanicus

Caput mallei

Lig. mallei superius

Lig. incudis superius

Corpus incudis

Chorda tympani

Incus, Crus breve

Lig. incudis posterius

Fossa incudis

Incus, Crus longum

Plica mallearis posterior

Proc. lenticularis

N. facialis [VII]

Fig. 10.28 Lateral wall, Paries membranaceus, of the tympanic cavity, Cavitas tympani, right side; medial view. [S700]
The Canalis musculotubarius enters the tympanic cavity from the front. It contains two bony semicanals (Semicanales) that are separated by a bony septum. The M. tensor tympani and the EUSTACHIAN tube run inside it. The tendon of the M. tensor tympani makes a right angle at the Pro. cochleariformis and proceeds towards the Manubrium mallei.

Function of the M. tensor tympani: increasing the tension of the tympanic membrane by pulling on the Manubrium mallei. This results in stiffening the chain of auditory ossicles for improved transfer of high frequency sound waves.
Shortly before the end of the Canalis nervi facialis, the **Chorda tympani** leaves the N. facialis [VII], runs backwards through its own bony canal, ending up in the tympanic cavity once again, runs through its centre embedded in mucosa, and between the malleus and the Crus longum of the incus. The Chorda tympani exits the cranial base via the Fissura sphenopetrosa (or the Fissura petrotympanica).

Clinical remarks

In the case of facial paralysis with involvement of the N. stapedius leading to paralysis of the N. stapedius, hearing on the affected side is altered. Loud noises are perceived as uncomfortably loud **(hyper-**

acusis), because of an insufficient damping action of the M. stapedius (through the tilting of the base of the stapes in the oval window).

Middle ear

Tympanic cavity

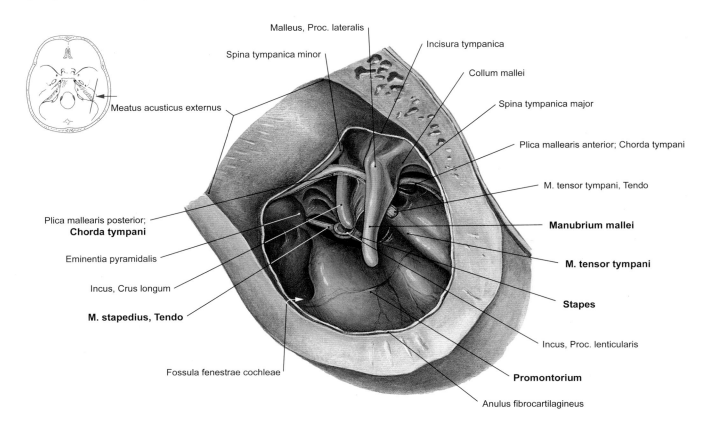

Malleus, Proc. lateralis

Spina tympanica minor

Incisura tympanica

Collum mallei

Meatus acusticus externus

Spina tympanica major

Plica mallearis anterior; Chorda tympani

M. tensor tympani, Tendo

Manubrium mallei

Plica mallearis posterior;
Chorda tympani

Eminentia pyramidalis

M. tensor tympani

Incus, Crus longum

Stapes

M. stapedius, Tendo

Incus, Proc. lenticularis

Fossula fenestrae cochleae

Promontorium

Anulus fibrocartilagineus

Fig. 10.29 Tympanic cavity, Cavitas tympani, right side; lateral view; after removal of the tympanic membrane and the mucous layer around the Chorda tympani. [S700]
View of the mucous-covered structures in the tympanic cavity.
The three auditory ossicles, covered by a mucous membrane, lie behind the eardrum in the main compartment (mesotympanum) and are (from lateral to medial): the malleus (hammer), incus (anvil) and stapes (stirrup). A mucous membrane lines the tympanic cavity, including the inner surface of the eardrum, the bony part of the EUSTACHIAN tube and the Cellulae mastoideae. Sometimes, mucous membrane layers extend outwards from the auditory ossicles, dividing the tympanic cavity into sections. Of the malleus, the handle (Manubrium mallei) and the short process (Proc. lateralis) as well as the neck (Collum mallei) can be seen in the figure. Medially, the incus is visible, of which the Crus longum and the Proc. lenticularis are recognisable. In the depths of the figure, the joint surface of the Caput stapedis can be seen articulating with the Proc. lenticularis of the incus. The Chorda tympani passes through the Crus longum incudis and the Manubrium mallei. Also visible in the figure are the tendon roots of the M. tensor tympani and of the M. stapedius.

─ Structure and function ─

With newborns, the tympanic cavity and the Antrum mastoideum are already formed; at this point, the mastoid does not yet contain any air cells (pneumatisation). Only in the first years of life, concluding around the sixth year of life, pneumatisation of the mastoid by the Antrum mastoideum takes place. The pneumatisation process and the extent of pneumatisation happens very variably. In this way, the zygomatic arch and the petrous portion of the temporal bone are also pneumatised, which is called extended pneumatisation. The pneumatisation can however also be much less (limited pneumatisation) or it can be absent and the mastoid process stays compact (compact bone). It is assumed that a patent and well-functioning EUSTACHIAN tube plays an important role in the degree of pneumatisation. Chronic middle ear infections are often associated with limited pneumatisation.

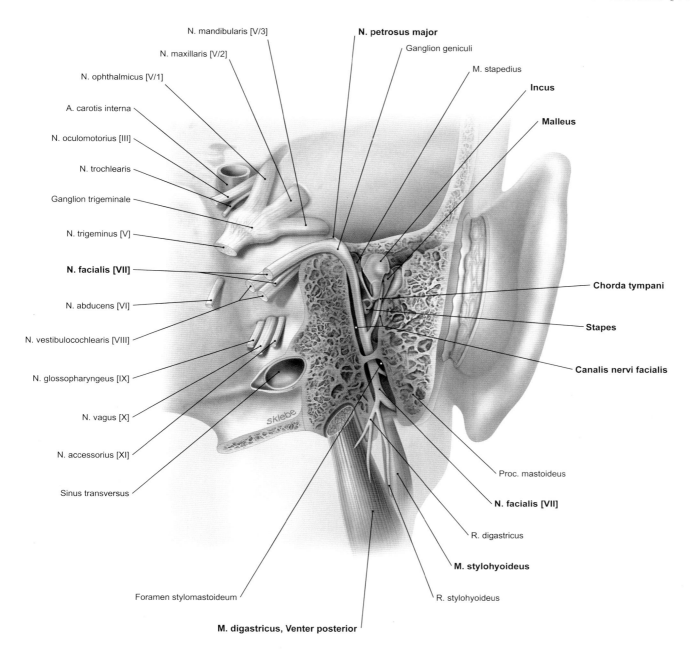

N. mandibularis [V/3]
N. maxillaris [V/2]
N. ophthalmicus [V/1]
A. carotis interna
N. oculomotorius [III]
N. trochlearis
Ganglion trigeminale
N. trigeminus [V]
N. facialis [VII]
N. abducens [VI]
N. vestibulocochlearis [VIII]
N. glossopharyngeus [IX]
N. vagus [X]
N. accessorius [XI]
Sinus transversus
Foramen stylomastoideum
M. digastricus, Venter posterior

N. petrosus major
Ganglion geniculi
M. stapedius
Incus
Malleus
Chorda tympani
Stapes
Canalis nervi facialis
Proc. mastoideus
N. facialis [VII]
R. digastricus
M. stylohyoideus
R. stylohyoideus

sklebe

Fig. 10.30   N. facialis [VII] in the petrous part of the temporal bone, Os temporale, Pars petrosa, right side; posterior view; petrous bone partially removed; facial canal and tympanic cavity opened. [S700-L238]

After removal of the Proc. mastoideus and opening of the facial canal and the tympanic cavity, the entire route of the N. facialis [VII] becomes visible with its exiting branches in the bony canal (→ Fig. 12.148).

Clinical remarks

Damage to the N. facialis [VII] can be associated with fractures of the petrous bone and inflammations of the middle ear or mastoid process, as well as with surgical interventions because of these conditions. Various testing methods are used in **facial nerve diagnostics** (e.g. at what level is the injury?) and in follow-up monitoring of facial paralysis: SCHIRMER test (lacrimal gland function), stapedius reflex test, taste perception test and sometimes also sialometry (measurement of salivary gland function) to check the Chorda tympani, as well as electromyography (EMG) and electroneurography (ENoG) to test facial muscle function.

N. facialis [VII], topography

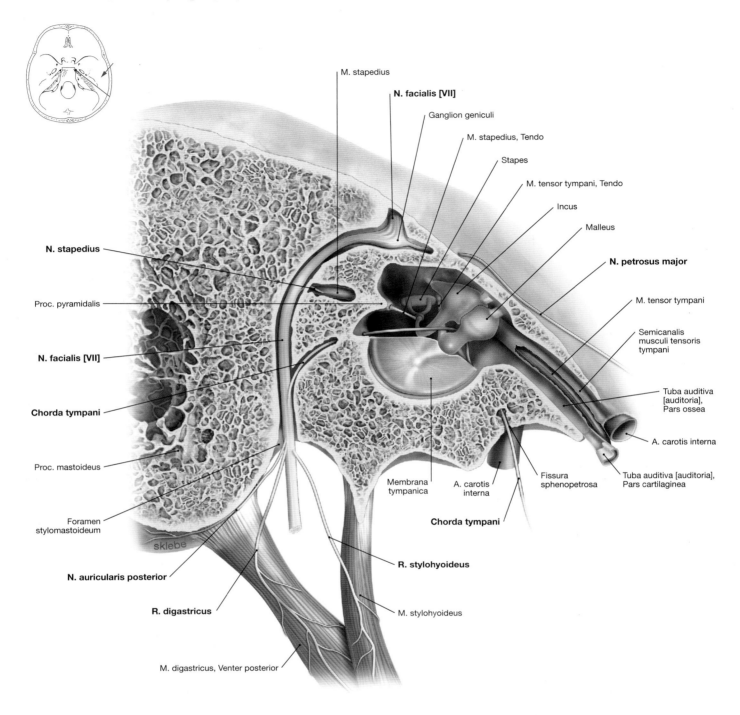

M. stapedius

N. facialis [VII]

Ganglion geniculi

M. stapedius, Tendo

Stapes

M. tensor tympani, Tendo

Incus

Malleus

N. petrosus major

M. tensor tympani

Semicanalis
musculi tensoris
tympani

Tuba auditiva
[auditoria],
Pars ossea

A. carotis interna

Tuba auditiva [auditoria],
Pars cartilaginea

Fissura
sphenopetrosa

A. carotis
interna

Membrana
tympanica

Chorda tympani

R. stylohyoideus

M. stylohyoideus

R. digastricus

N. auricularis posterior

M. digastricus, Venter posterior

Foramen
stylomastoideum

Proc. mastoideus

Chorda tympani

N. facialis [VII]

Proc. pyramidalis

N. stapedius

sklebe

Fig. 10.31 N. facialis [VII], right side; lateral view. [S700-L238]
Presentation of the N. facialis [VII] passing through the petrous bone,
up to shortly after exiting the Foramen stylomastoideum (cut off after
that). Within the bony facial canal, the **N. stapedius** diverges to innervate the M. stapedius, and the **Chorda tympani,** which regresses into
the tympanic cavity and passes almost 'free' within a mucosal fold between the malleus and the incus through the tympanic cavity to the
Fissura sphenopetrosa, where it exits the tympanic cavity again.

Clinical remarks

The pathway of the Chorda tympani renders it susceptible to injury in
surgery conducted on the middle ear. Isolated functional **loss of the**
Chorda tympani, with associated dry mouth and loss of taste sensation on the affected side, is common in middle ear inflammations.

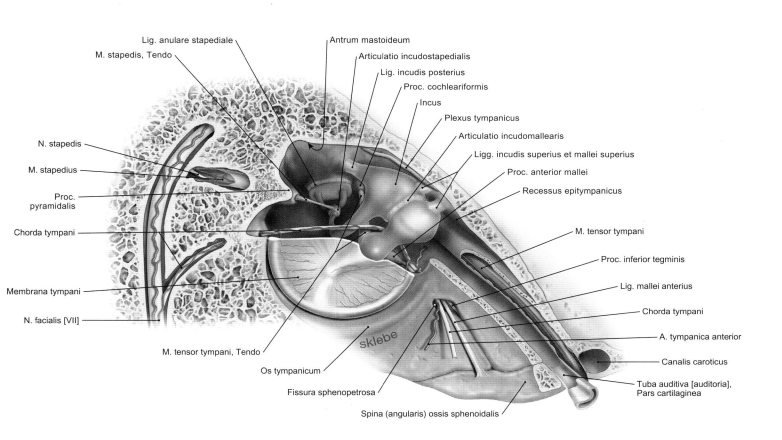

Lig. anulare stapediale
M. stapedis, Tendo
Antrum mastoideum
Articulatio incudostapedialis
Lig. incudis posterius
Proc. cochleariformis
Incus
Plexus tympanicus
Articulatio incudomallearis
Ligg. incudis superius et mallei superius
Proc. anterior mallei
Recessus epitympanicus

N. stapedis
M. stapedius
Proc. pyramidalis
Chorda tympani

M. tensor tympani
Proc. inferior tegminis
Lig. mallei anterius
Chorda tympani
A. tympanica anterior
Canalis caroticus
Tuba auditiva [auditoria], Pars cartilaginea

Membrana tympani
N. facialis [VII]
M. tensor tympani, Tendo
Os tympanicum
Fissura sphenopetrosa
Spina (angularis) ossis sphenoidalis

sklebe

Fig. 10.32 N. facialis [VII], and joints, ligaments and muscles of the auditory ossicles, Ossicula auditus, left side; lateral view, petrous bone partly removed. [S700-L238]

The Plexus tympanicus serve the sensory innervation of the middle ear mucosa, including the mucosa of the auditory or EUSTACHIAN tube [Tuba auditiva/auditoria] and the mastoid. In addition, it receives preganglionic, parasympathetic fibres from the N. tympanicus of the N. glossopharyngeus [IX], as well as the sympathetic fibres of the Nn. caroticotympanici from the Plexus caroticus internus. The N. petro-

sus minor, which is not visible, is formed by the Plexus tympanicus. The tympanic cavity is divided into the epi-, meso- and hypotympanum. The epitympanum contains the auditory ossicles except for the manubrium and the Proc. lenticularis incudis, the Recessus epitympanicus and the connection to the mastoid; the manubrium, the Proc. lenticularis incudis and the M. tensor tympani tendon lie in the mesotympanum. The Chorda tympani runs along the border between the epi- and mesotympanum. The EUSTACHIAN tube extends to the middle ear in the hypotympanum.

N. facialis [VII], topography

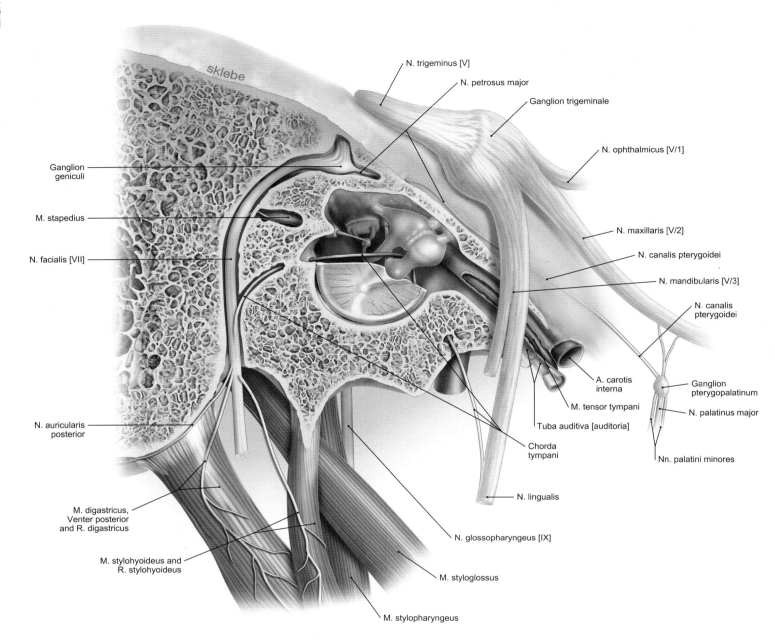

Ganglion trigeminale

N. trigeminus [V]

N. petrosus major

N. ophthalmicus [V/1]

N. maxillaris [V/2]

N. canalis pterygoidei

N. mandibularis [V/3]

N. canalis pterygoidei

Ganglion pterygopalatinum

N. palatinus major

Nn. palatini minores

A. carotis interna

M. tensor tympani

Tuba auditiva [auditoria]

Chorda tympani

N. lingualis

N. glossopharyngeus [IX]

M. styloglossus

M. stylopharyngeus

Ganglion geniculi

M. stapedius

N. facialis [VII]

sklebe

N. auricularis posterior

M. digastricus, Venter posterior and R. digastricus

M. stylohyoideus and R. stylohyoideus

Fig. 10.33 N. facialis [VII] in the petrous bone with connections to the N. trigeminus [V], cut through a right temporal bone in the area of the middle ear; with the N. petrosus major below the dura and the N. canalis pterygoidei shown transparently. [S700-L238]

At the Ganglion geniculi, the N. facialis provides the N. petrosus major as its first branch. It runs in the Os temporale medially to the front and emerges at the Hiatus nervi petrosi majoris on the Facies anterior of the Pars petrosa ossis temporalis below the dura. Here it runs in the Sulcus nervi petrosi majoris to the Foramen lacerum where it leaves from the middle cranial fossa. After passing through, its fibres run alongside the fibres of the N. petrosus profundus as the N. canalis pterygoidei [VIDI-ANUS] through the sphenoidal bone to the Fossa pterygopalatina,

thereby reaching the Ganglion pterygopalatinum. In the illustration, the pathway of the N. petrosus major through the Foramen lacerum is hidden by the N. mandibularis [V/3], while its pathway as the N. canalis pterygoidei is shown transparently within the bone, and the last part up to the Ganglion pterygopalatinum is only shown schematically. The nerve carries preganglionic parasympathetic fibres to the Ganglion pterygopalatinum for the innervation of the nasolacrimal glands. Shortly after the N. facialis [VII] passes through the Foramen stylomastoideum, the N. auricularis posterior branches off for the innervation of the auricles. Also shown is the connection of the N. facialis [VII] to the N. mandibularis [V/3] via the Chorda tympani, which carries preganglionic parasympathetic fibres and sensory taste fibres.

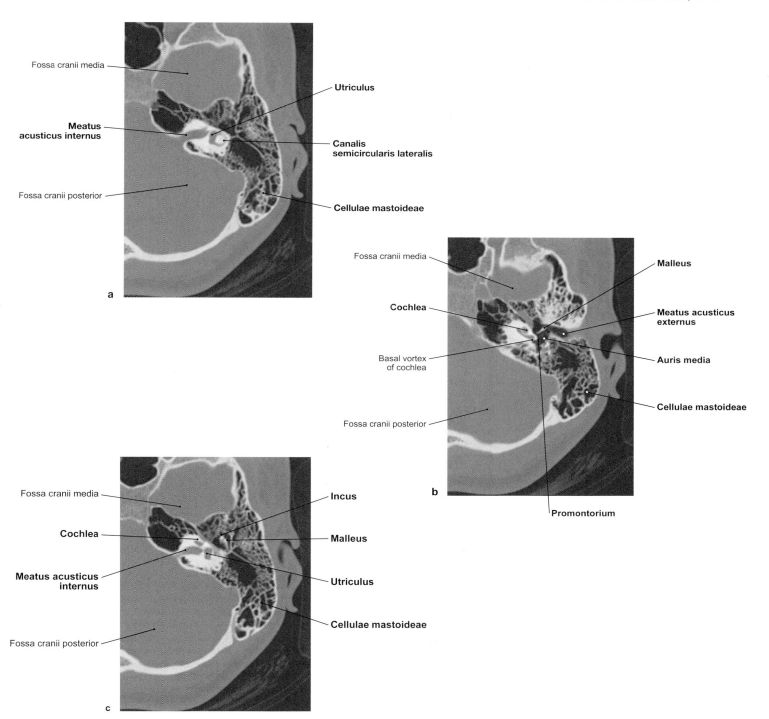

Fossa cranii media

Utriculus

Meatus acusticus internus

Canalis semicircularis lateralis

Fossa cranii posterior

Cellulae mastoideae

a

Fossa cranii media

Malleus

Cochlea

Meatus acusticus externus

Basal vortex of cochlea

Auris media

Fossa cranii posterior

Cellulae mastoideae

b

Promontorium

Fossa cranii media

Incus

Cochlea

Malleus

Meatus acusticus internus

Utriculus

Fossa cranii posterior

Cellulae mastoideae

c

Fig. 10.34a–c   Temporal bone, Os temporale, with middle and inner ear, left ear; computed tomography (CT) scan; inferior view. [E460]

A high-resolution CT scan is able to visualise in detail all middle ear and inner ear structures. Thus, for example, the internal acoustic meatus, the pneumatisation of the mastoid process, the positioning of the auditory ossicles, as well as the labyrinth, can be assessed.

Clinical remarks

The N. facialis [VII] can be accessed surgically via the Proc. mastoideus, for example, to provide relief in the context of an inflammatory swelling of the nerve. Upon careful removal of the mastoid bone, the posterior section of the bony canal is exposed.

Auditory tube

Auditory tube

Fig. 10.35 Cartilage of the EUSTACHIAN (auditory) tube, Cartilago tubae auditivae, right side; inferior view, exposed at the base of skull. [S700]

The approx. 4 cm long EUSTACHIAN tube (auditory tube, Tuba auditiva [auditoria]) projects at an oblique angle from a cranial posterolateral to an anteromedial caudal position and connects the tympanic cavity with the nasopharynx. Its function is pressure equalisation. For optimal transmission of sound waves, pneumatic pressure in the tympanic cavity (the tympanic membrane is airtight) has to be the same as in the external acoustic meatus. If this is not the case, e.g. during ascent or descent in a plane, some hearing is lost.

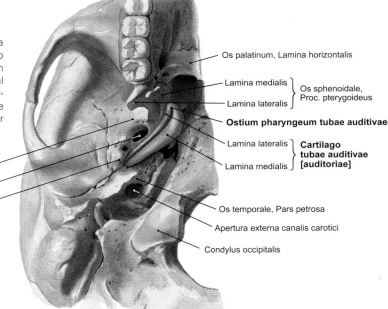

Os palatinum, Lamina horizontalis

Lamina medialis ⎱ Os sphenoidale,
Lamina lateralis ⎰ Proc. pterygoideus

Ostium pharyngeum tubae auditivae

Lamina lateralis ⎱ **Cartilago**
 tubae auditivae
Lamina medialis ⎰ **[auditoriae]**

Os temporale, Pars petrosa

Apertura externa canalis carotici

Condylus occipitalis

Os sphenoidale, Ala major, Facies temporalis

Foramen ovale

Spina ossis sphenoidalis

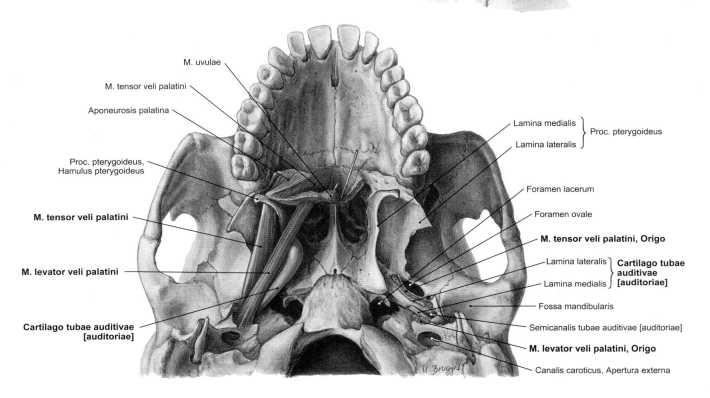

M. uvulae

M. tensor veli palatini

Aponeurosis palatina

Proc. pterygoideus,
Hamulus pterygoideus

M. tensor veli palatini

M. levator veli palatini

**Cartilago tubae auditivae
[auditoriae]**

Lamina medialis ⎱ Proc. pterygoideus
Lamina lateralis ⎰

Foramen lacerum

Foramen ovale

M. tensor veli palatini, Origo

Lamina lateralis ⎱ **Cartilago tubae**
 auditivae
Lamina medialis ⎰ **[auditoriae]**

Fossa mandibularis

Semicanalis tubae auditivae [auditoriae]

M. levator veli palatini, Origo

Canalis caroticus, Apertura externa

Fig. 10.36 M. levator veli palatini, M. tensor veli palatini and cartilage of the EUSTACHIAN tube, Cartilago tubae auditivae; inferior view. [S700]

The EUSTACHIAN tube ([Tuba auditiva/auditoria]; bony portion not visible) starts at the anterior wall of the tympanic cavity (Paries caroticus) along with the Ostium tympanicum tubae auditivae and leads to the pharyngeal opening (Ostium pharyngeum tubae auditivae), which protrudes posterolaterally into the nasopharynx. A distinction is made be-

tween a bony section (Pars ossea) and a cartilaginous section (Pars cartilaginea) which is about twice as long. The latter consists of a groove made of elastic cartilage (Cartilago tubae auditivae). The upside-down cartilage groove is medially enclosed by connective tissue (Lamina membranacea) to form a slit-shaped canal. The EUSTACHIAN tube is opened by the contraction of the Mm. tensor and levator veli palatini as part of the swallowing motion.

→ T 4

Clinical remarks

The EUSTACHIAN tube is lined by respiratory ciliated epithelium with goblet cells. The ciliary beat is in the direction of the nasopharynx. Failure of the protective mechanism in the tube can lead to an aggravated inflammation, such as the formation of a **EUSTACHIAN ca-**

tarrh or a middle ear inflammation. By air injection via the nose, adhesions and closures inside the tubes can be dissolved (e.g. swallowing to compensate for ambient pressure changes).

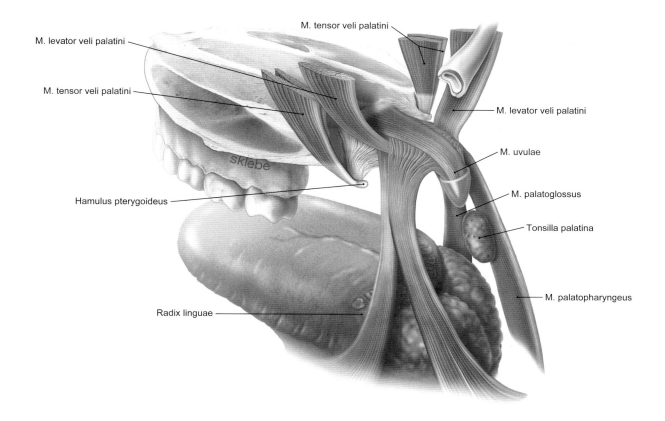

M. tensor veli palatini

M. levator veli palatini

M. tensor veli palatini

M. levator veli palatini

M. uvulae

M. palatoglossus

Hamulus pterygoideus

Tonsilla palatina

M. palatopharyngeus

Radix linguae

Fig. 10.37 Muscles of the soft palate, Palatum molle; left side; posterior view from the left. [S700-L238]

The basis of the soft palate is a plate of connective tissue (Aponeurosis palatina) into which four paired muscles and the unpaired **M. uvulae,** which forms the uvula, radiate.

The two lower paired muscles are the:

* **M. palatoglossus,** which forms the basis of the anterior palatoglossal archway (Arcus palatoglossus)
* **M. palatopharyngeus,** which forms the basis of the posterior palatopharyngeal archway (Arcus palatopharyngeus).

Between the two palatine archways is the Tonsilla palatina. During a contraction, the two paired muscles pull the soft palate down and thus reduce the Isthmus faucium.

The two upper paired muscles are the:

* **M. levator veli palatini,** which lifts the velum
* **M. tensor veli palatini,** which tenses the velum.

The contraction of the upper pairs of muscles, together with the contraction of the M. uvulae, causes the elevation and tension of the soft palate, which is drawn back to the wall of the pharynx, thereby separating the nasopharynx from the oropharynx (important for swallowing). In addition, the two upper muscles at the opening of the EUSTACHIAN tube (→ Fig. 10.36 and → Fig. 10.38) are also involved.

→ T 4

Clinical remarks

A **cleft palate** is associated with a loss of function of the Mm. tensor and levator veli palatini, because the Punctum fixum of the muscles is missing and they contract into a void (→ figure). Thereby the tube function is suspended. If left untreated, an **adhesive process** occurs in the middle ear due to the absence of middle ear ventilation. Affected children are very hard of hearing and often do not learn to speak. [S700-L238]

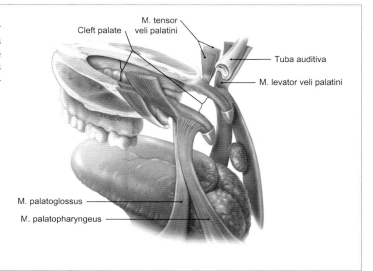

Cleft palate

M. tensor veli palatini

Tuba auditiva

M. levator veli palatini

M. palatoglossus

M. palatopharyngeus

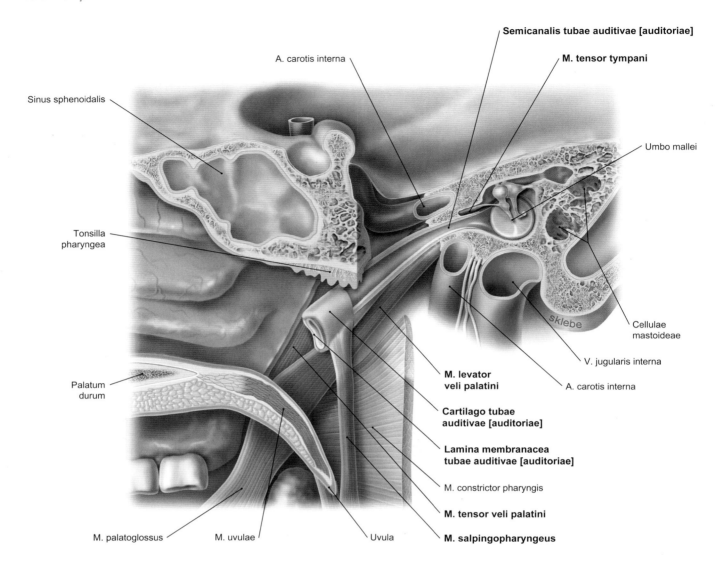

Sinus sphenoidalis

A. carotis interna

Semicanalis tubae auditivae [auditoriae]

M. tensor tympani

Umbo mallei

Tonsilla pharyngea

Cellulae mastoideae

Palatum durum

V. jugularis interna

M. levator veli palatini

A. carotis interna

Cartilago tubae auditivae [auditoriae]

Lamina membranacea tubae auditivae [auditoriae]

M. constrictor pharyngis

M. tensor veli palatini

M. palatoglossus

M. uvulae

Uvula

M. salpingopharyngeus

sklebe

Fig. 10.38 EUSTACHIAN tube (auditory tube, Tuba auditiva [auditoria]), right side; medial view. [S702-L238]
Presentation of the connection between the nasopharynx and the tympanic cavity as well as the position of the muscles. The **M. salpingo-** **pharyngeus** originates in the lower section of the cartilage of the tube of the nasopharynx. Its contraction causes the tube to close. At the same time, it lifts the pharynx.

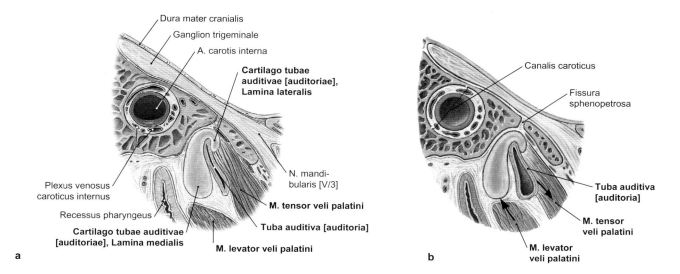

a

b

Fig. 10.39a and b   EUSTACHIAN tube (auditory tube, Tuba auditiva [auditoria]), right side; cross-sections at the level of the lateral section of the Pars cartilaginea; lateral view. [S700]
a Closed tube. The M. salpingopharyngeus (not shown) is involved in occluding the tube.
b Open tube. The effect of the muscles on the tube is illustrated by arrows.

The swallowing motion involves the contraction of the Mm. tensor and the levator veli palatini. The **contraction of the M. tensor veli palatini** causes the tubal lumen to expand by pulling on the Pars membranacea and on the upper edge of the cartilaginous part of the EUSTACHIAN tube. The **contraction of the M. levator veli palatini** causes the thickest part of the muscle to push against the tubal cartilage from below. In doing so, the groove is bent open and the tubal lumen expanded.

→ T 4, T 6.2

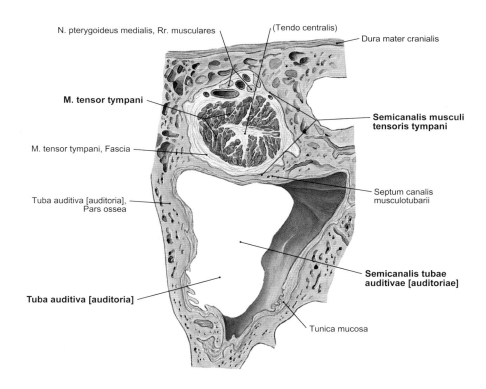

Fig. 10.40   EUSTACHIAN tube (auditory tube, Tuba auditiva [auditoria]), right side; cross-section at the level of the Pars ossea through the Canalis musculotubarius; lateral view. [S700]
The osseous part of the Tuba auditiva [auditoria] is inside a triangular bony canal (Semicanalis tubae auditivae of the Canalis musculotubarius)
of the Pars petrosa ossis temporalis. Separated by a thin bony wall, the M. tensor tympani proceeds inside the Semicanalis musculi tensoris tympani of the Canalis musculotubarius.

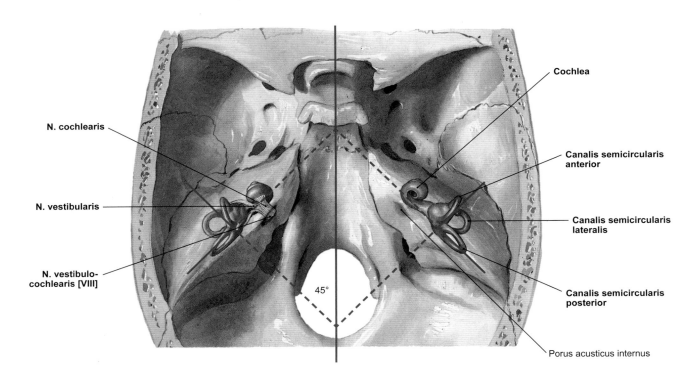

N. cochlearis

N. vestibularis

N. vestibulo-
cochlearis [VIII]

45°

Cochlea

Canalis semicircularis
anterior

Canalis semicircularis
lateralis

Canalis semicircularis
posterior

Porus acusticus internus

**Fig. 10.41   Inner ear, Auris interna and N. vestibulocochlearis
[VIII];** superior view; inner ear in its natural position projected onto the
petrous part of the temporal bone. [S702]

The tip of the cochlea is pointed anterolaterally. The semicircular canals
(Canales semicirculares) are positioned at a 45° angle in relation to the
main planes of the skull (frontal, sagittal and horizontal planes). This is
important in the assessment of CT scans of the skull.

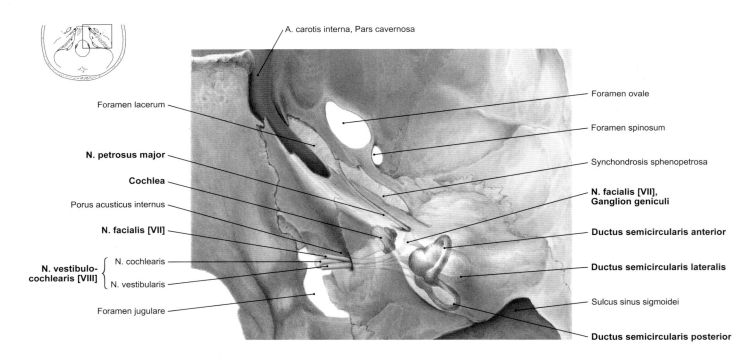

A. carotis interna, Pars cavernosa

Foramen lacerum

N. petrosus major

Cochlea

Porus acusticus internus

N. facialis [VII]

**N. vestibulo-
cochlearis [VIII]** { N. cochlearis
N. vestibularis

Foramen jugulare

Foramen ovale

Foramen spinosum

Synchondrosis sphenopetrosa

**N. facialis [VII],
Ganglion geniculi**

Ductus semicircularis anterior

Ductus semicircularis lateralis

Sulcus sinus sigmoidei

Ductus semicircularis posterior

**Fig. 10.42   Inner ear, Auris interna with N. facialis [VII] and N. ves-
tibulocochlearis [VIII], right side;** superior view of petrous part of the
temporal bone. [S700]
Upon entering the Porus acusticus internus, the N. facialis [VII] and its
intermedius part lie on top of the N. vestibulocochlearis [VIII] (in clinical
terms often also referred to as N. statoacusticus), which is composed
of the N. cochlearis and N. vestibularis. The nerves divide in the petrous
part of the temporal bone. The **N. cochlearis** follows a slightly arched
path anterior to the cochlea, and the **N. vestibularis** a slightly arched
posterior path. Shortly before reaching the labyrinth, it divides into a

Pars superior to the anterior and lateral semicircular canals as well as to
the sacculus, and into a Pars inferior to the utriculus and posterior semicircular canals. The perikarya of the neurons of both parts are combined
into the **Ganglion vestibulare.** The N. facialis [VII] proceeds above and
between the cochlea and the vestibular organ in the facial canal. The
main stem bends downward at a right angle at the outer knee of the
facial nerve. At the Ganglion geniculi, the **N. petrosus major** leaves the
N. facialis [VII]. It proceeds in a dural sac on the petrous bone in the direction of the Foramen lacerum and contains preganglionic parasympathetic fibres for the innervation of the lacrimal and nasal glands.

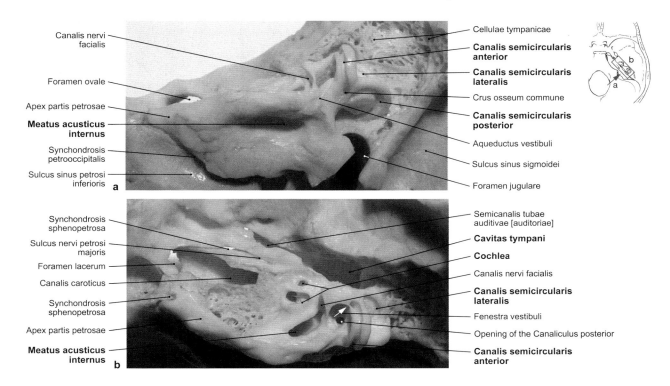

Canalis nervi facialis
Foramen ovale
Apex partis petrosae
Meatus acusticus internus
Synchondrosis petrooccipitalis
Sulcus sinus petrosi inferioris **a**

Cellulae tympanicae
Canalis semicircularis anterior
Canalis semicircularis lateralis
Crus osseum commune
Canalis semicircularis posterior
Aqueductus vestibuli
Sulcus sinus sigmoidei
Foramen jugulare

Synchondrosis sphenopetrosa
Sulcus nervi petrosi majoris
Foramen lacerum
Canalis caroticus
Synchondrosis sphenopetrosa
Apex partis petrosae
Meatus acusticus internus b

Semicanalis tubae auditivae [auditoriae]
Cavitas tympani
Cochlea
Canalis nervi facialis
Canalis semicircularis lateralis
Fenestra vestibuli
Opening of the Canaliculus posterior
Canalis semicircularis anterior

Fig. 10.43a and b   Bony labyrinth, Labyrinthus osseus, right side; hollowed out of the petrous part of the temporal bone. [S700]
a Posterior view from above.
b View from above.

The inner ear (Auris interna) is a complex network of bony canals and ampullary extensions in the Pars petrosa of the Os temporale (osseous labyrinth). Inside is a system of membranous tubes and sacs called the membranous labyrinth. It contains the vestibular and cochlear organ (Organum vestibulocochleare).

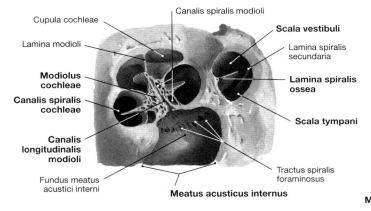

Cupula cochleae
Lamina modioli
Modiolus cochleae
Canalis spiralis cochleae
Canalis longitudinalis modioli
Fundus meatus acustici interni
Meatus acusticus internus

Canalis spiralis modioli
Scala vestibuli
Lamina spiralis secundaria
Lamina spiralis ossea
Scala tympani
Tractus spiralis foraminosus

Tractus spiralis foraminosus
Area nervi facialis
Area vestibularis superior
Crista transversa
Area vestibularis inferior
Foramen singulare
Area cochlearis
Meatus acusticus internus   Fundus meatus acustici interni

Fig. 10.44   Spiral canal of the cochlea, Canalis spiralis cochleae, right side; superior view; opened along the axis of the modiolus. [S700]
The cochlea consists of a spiral canal (Canalis spiralis cochleae), which is wound in 2½ turns around the cochlear modiolus (Modiolus cochleae). The Ganglion spirale cochleae is situated in the Canales spiralis and longitudinalis modioli and contains the perikarya of the bipolar nerve cells of the N. cochlearis. Originating from the modiolus, the Lamina spiralis ossea protudes into the cochlear canal.

Fig. 10.45   Internal acoustic meatus, Meatus acusticus internus and fundus of the internal acoustic meatus, Fundus meatus acustici interni, right side; medial view; after partial removal of the posterior wall. [S700]
The internal acoustic meatus starts at the Porus acusticus internus and projects laterally for about 1 cm. Here it ends in a perforated bony plate. The N. facialis [VII] and the N. vestibulocochlearis [VIII] run along the 1 cm long segment.

Clinical remarks

The **acoustic neuroma** (vestibular schwannoma) is a benign tumour of the SCHWANN cells which most frequently affects the N. vestibularis. It originates in the Meatus acusticus internus and grows extrusively into the posterior cranial fossa (cerebellopontine angle tumour, → arrow in figure), displacing adjacent structures. Early symptoms are impaired hearing and equilibrium.
[F276-006]

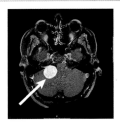

Bony labyrinth

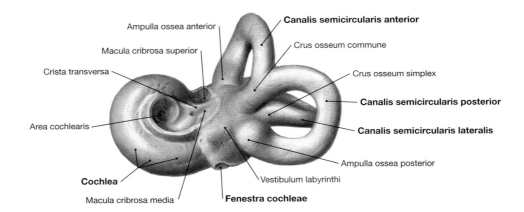

Ampulla ossea anterior
Macula cribrosa superior
Crista transversa
Area cochlearis
Cochlea
Macula cribrosa media
Canalis semicircularis anterior
Crus osseum commune
Crus osseum simplex
Canalis semicircularis posterior
Canalis semicircularis lateralis
Ampulla ossea posterior
Vestibulum labyrinthi
Fenestra cochleae

Fig. 10.46   Bony labyrinth, Labyrinthus osseus, right side; posterior oblique view, bony surroundings of the membranous labyrinth removed from the petrous part of the temporal bone. [S700]

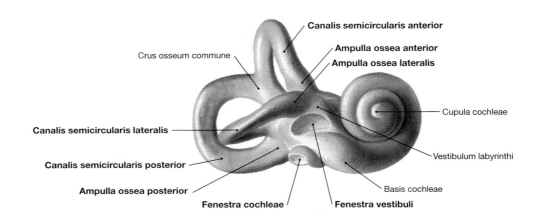

Crus osseum commune
Canalis semicircularis lateralis
Canalis semicircularis posterior
Ampulla ossea posterior
Fenestra cochleae
Canalis semicircularis anterior
Ampulla ossea anterior
Ampulla ossea lateralis
Cupula cochleae
Vestibulum labyrinthi
Basis cochleae
Fenestra vestibuli

Fig. 10.47   Bony labyrinth, Labyrinthus osseus, right side; lateral view; bony surroundings of the membranous labyrinth removed from the petrous part of the temporal bone. [S700]

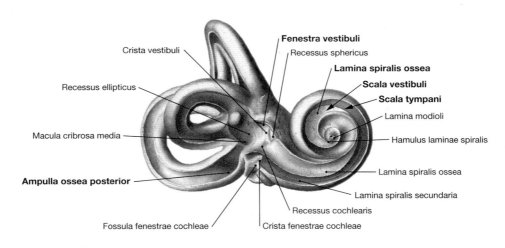

Crista vestibuli
Recessus ellipticus
Macula cribrosa media
Ampulla ossea posterior
Fossula fenestrae cochleae
Fenestra vestibuli
Recessus sphericus
Lamina spiralis ossea
Scala vestibuli
Scala tympani
Lamina modioli
Hamulus laminae spiralis
Lamina spiralis ossea
Lamina spiralis secundaria
Recessus cochlearis
Crista fenestrae cochleae

Fig. 10.48   Bony labyrinth, Labyrinthus osseus, right side; anterolateral view; hollowed out cavities. [S700]
The bony labyrinth consists of the vestibulum, three bony semicircular canals (Canales semicirculares ossei), the bony cochlea and the internal

accoustic meatus (Meatus acusticus internus). The cochlea and semicircular canals originate at the vestibulum. It is connected to the tympanic cavity via the oval window.

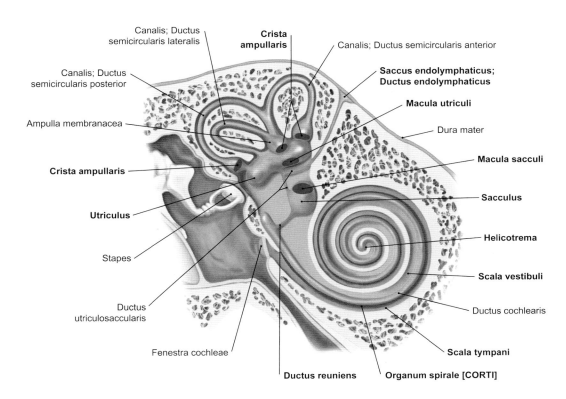

Canalis; Ductus semicircularis lateralis
Crista ampullaris
Canalis; Ductus semicircularis anterior
Canalis; Ductus semicircularis posterior
Saccus endolymphaticus; Ductus endolymphaticus
Ampulla membranacea
Macula utriculi
Dura mater
Crista ampullaris
Macula sacculi
Utriculus
Sacculus
Stapes
Helicotrema
Scala vestibuli
Ductus utriculosaccularis
Ductus cochlearis
Fenestra cochleae
Scala tympani
Ductus reuniens
Organum spirale [CORTI]

Fig. 10.49 Membranous labyrinth, Labyrinthus membranaceus, right side; longitudinal section through the petrous part of the temporal bone; frontal view, schematic drawing. [S700-L284]
The membranous labyrinth is filled with low-sodium and potassium-rich endolymph. It is not directly adjacent to the bony labyrinth, but separated from it by the perilymphatic space filled with perilymph. The membranous labyrinth is functionally divided into a vestibular and a cochlear compartment. The **vestibular labyrinth** includes the sacculus and utriculus located in the vestibulum, the Ductus utriculosaccularis, the three semicircular canals and the Ductus endolymphaticus, along with the Saccus endolymphaticus. The latter represents an epidural sac, located at the rear surface of the petrous bone, in which the endolymph is resorbed. The **cochlear labyrinth** is formed by the Ductus cochlearis. The Ductus reuniens connects the vestibular and cochlear labyrinth.

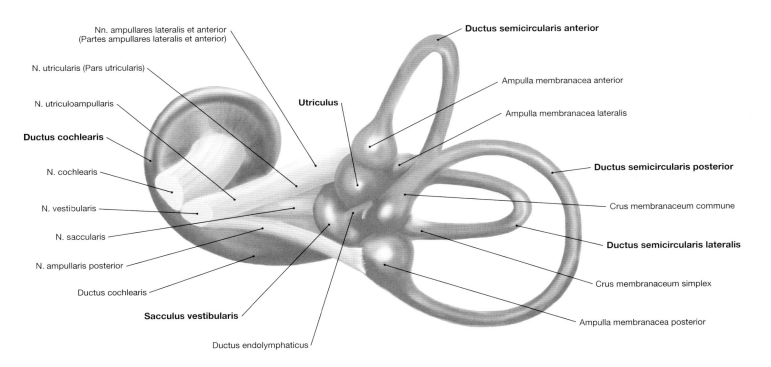

Nn. ampullares lateralis et anterior (Partes ampullares lateralis et anterior)
Ductus semicircularis anterior
N. utricularis (Pars utricularis)
Utriculus
Ampulla membranacea anterior
N. utriculoampullaris
Ampulla membranacea lateralis
Ductus cochlearis
N. cochlearis
Ductus semicircularis posterior
N. vestibularis
Crus membranaceum commune
N. saccularis
Ductus semicircularis lateralis
N. ampullaris posterior
Crus membranaceum simplex
Ductus cochlearis
Sacculus vestibularis
Ampulla membranacea posterior
Ductus endolymphaticus

Fig. 10.50 N. vestibulocochlearis [VIII] and membranous labyrinth, Labyrinthus membranaceus; semischematic overview, dorsal view. [S700-L284]
The membranous labyrinth includes the Ductus cochlearis, the sacculus, the utriculus, as well as the three membranous semicircular canals (Ductus semicirculares). The latter are in contact with the utriculus. Each semicircular canal forms an ampulla-shaped dilation (Ampulla membranacea) at the border to the utriculus. The superior and posterior semicircular canal unite to form a common canal (Crus commune). Each ampulla contains sensory epithelium (Crista ampullaris, not shown).

Blood supply and innervation of the membranous labyrinth

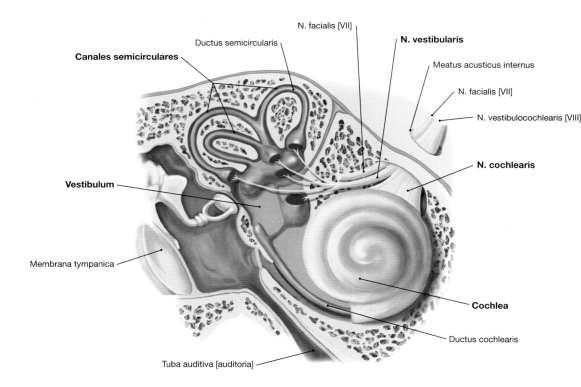

Fig. 10.51 **Innervation of the inner ear, Auris interna, right side;** longitudinal section through the petrous part of the temporal bone; frontal view, schematic drawing. [S700-L284]
The inner ear divides into the **bony labyrinth** (Labyrinthus osseus) which is surrounded by the compact bone of the petrous part of the temporal bone and includes a system of membranous tubes, the **membranous labyrinth** (Labyrinthus membranaceus).

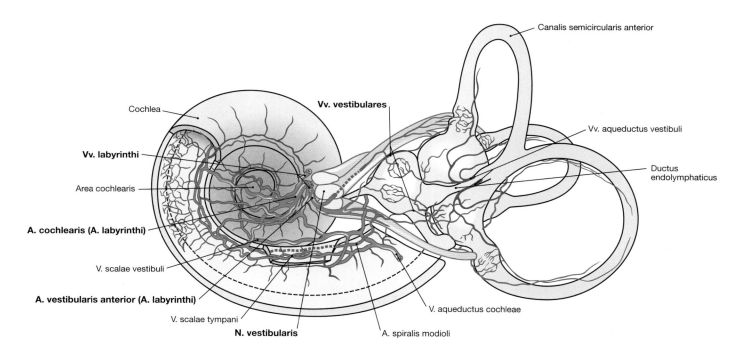

Fig. 10.52 **Blood supply and innervation of the inner ear, Auris interna, right side;** medial view. [S700-L126]/[B500~M282/L132]/[G1083]
The entire blood supply of the inner ear is via the branches of the **A. cochlearis (A. labyrinthi;** → Fig. 12.57), venous blood drainage is via the Vv. labyrinthi. The A. and V. inferior anterior cerebelli often project a few millimetres into the internal acoustic meatus (not shown) and branch into the A. and Vv. labyrinthi; supplying the labyrinth with blood (**caution:** the A. labyrinthi is a terminal artery).

Clinical remarks

Thrombotic occlusions of the A. labyrinthi or its afferent branches is associated with a loss of balance and hearing, because the A. labyrinthi is a terminal artery.
Attacks of vertigo, unilateral hearing loss and unilateral tinnitus are a triad of symptoms referred to as **MENIÈRE's disease.** Its etiology is not clear, but a hydropic swelling of the membranous labyrinth due to impaired resorption of endolymph (cochlear hydrops) is under discussion. The pressure imposed by the increased volume of endolymph damages the sensory cells of the vestibulocochlear system.

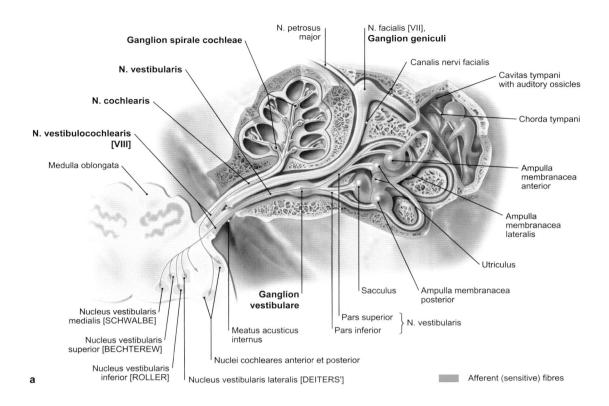

N. petrosus major

N. facialis [VII],
Ganglion geniculi

Ganglion spirale cochleae

Canalis nervi facialis

N. vestibularis

Cavitas tympani
with auditory ossicles

N. cochlearis

Chorda tympani

**N. vestibulocochlearis
[VIII]**

Medulla oblongata

Ampulla
membranacea
anterior

Ampulla
membranacea
lateralis

Utriculus

Nucleus vestibularis
medialis [SCHWALBE]

**Ganglion
vestibulare**

Sacculus

Ampulla membranacea
posterior

Nucleus vestibularis
superior [BECHTEREW]

Meatus acusticus
internus

Pars superior
Pars inferior } N. vestibularis

Nucleus vestibularis
inferior [ROLLER]

Nuclei cochleares anterior et posterior

Nucleus vestibularis lateralis [DEITERS']

■ Afferent (sensitive) fibres

a

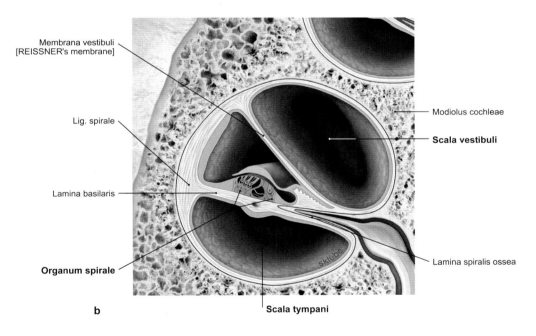

Membrana vestibuli
[REISSNER's membrane]

Modiolus cochleae

Scala vestibuli

Lig. spirale

Lamina basilaris

Lamina spiralis ossea

Organum spirale

Scala tympani

b

**Fig. 10.53a and b Cochlea, vestibular organ, Organum vestibula-
re, N. vestibulocochlearis [VIII] with nuclei and fibrous qualities,
N. facialis [VII] as well as the middle ear, Auris media;** view from
above, Pars petrosa opened. [S700-L238]

a After entry, the N. facialis [VII] proceeds via the Meatus acusticus internus between the cochlea and vestibular organ. At the Ganglion geniculi it bends forwards and downwards and is found in the topographical
proximity of the middle ear (→ Fig. 10.24, → Fig. 10.25, → Fig. 10.26).
The N. vestibulocochlearis [VIII] (syn.: N. statoacusticus) contains special somatic-afferent (SSA) fibres as well as efferent fibres that form the
olivocochlear bundle. Its **cochlear section** conducts hearing information to the anterior and posterior cochlear nuclei in the brainstem; its
vestibular section conducts body balance information to the Nuclei
vestibularis medialis, lateralis, superior and inferior in the brainstem.
The perikarya of the bipolar neurons for the cochlea are in the **Ganglion
spirale** and for the vestibular organ in the **Ganglion vestibulare.**

b The Membrana vestibuli (REISSNER's membrane) and the Membrana
basilaris (basilar membrane) divide the Canalis spiralis cochleae into
three areas:
- the **Scala vestibuli** (vestibular duct) filled with perilymph, which extends from the vestibulum to the helicotrema (opening between Scala vestibuli and Scala tympani in the uppermost turn of the cochlea)
- the **Ductus cochlearis** filled with endolymph
- the **Scala tympani** (tympanic duct) filled with perilymph, which extends from the helicotrema to the round window in the medial wall
of the tympanic cavity. The Scala vestibuli and the Scala tympani join
at the helicotrema.

The floor of the Ductus cochlearis is the basilar membrane (Lamina basilaris), which carries the cochlear organ (organ of CORTI). The endolymph
is formed by the Stria vascularis at the lateral bony wall of the cochlea.

Cochlea and sound conduction

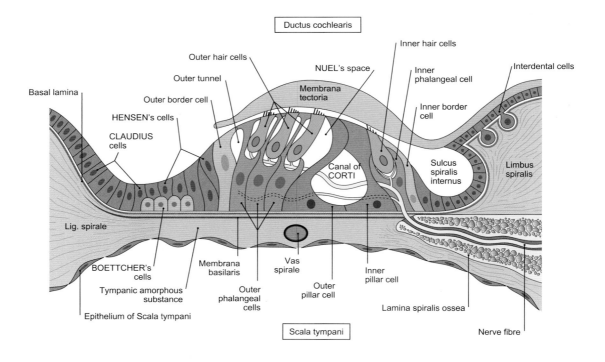

Fig. 10.54 Organum spirale, organ of CORTI; schematic drawing.
[R170-5-L107]
This is a very simplified presentation of the complex afferent and efferent innervation of the hair cells.

The organ of CORTI represents the actual cochlear organ. Here, cochlear sensory cells (hair cells) lie on the basilar membrane along with supporting cells and are covered by a gelatinous membrane (Membrana tectoria). The organ of CORTI extends over the whole length of the Ductus cochlearis.

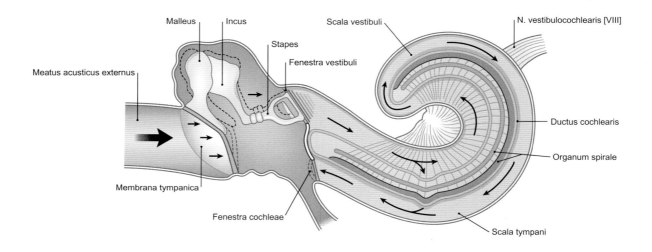

Fig. 10.55 Sound conduction. [S700-L126]
Sound conduction occurs via sound waves that enter via the external ear (auricle and external acoustic meatus) and are transmitted via the tympanic membrane and the auditory ossicular chain, which physically augments the amplitude of sound waves in the middle ear, via the base of the stapes to the perilymph. This produces wave movements (migrat-

ing waves) that migrate along the walls of the Ductus cochlearis (especially the basilar membrane). This results in a deflection of the organ of CORTI. The stereocilia of the inner hair cells are bent (deflection). These biomechanical events are converted by the sensory cells into receptor potentials (mechanical-electrical transduction).

Clinical remarks

Hair cell damage, e.g. after listening to very loud music or after an explosion (acoustic shock), is very commonly associated with **tinnitus.** In this, the term Tinnitus aurium ('ringing in the ears') or tinnitus

for short, refers to a symptom in which the affected person perceives sounds that are not perceptible to other people.

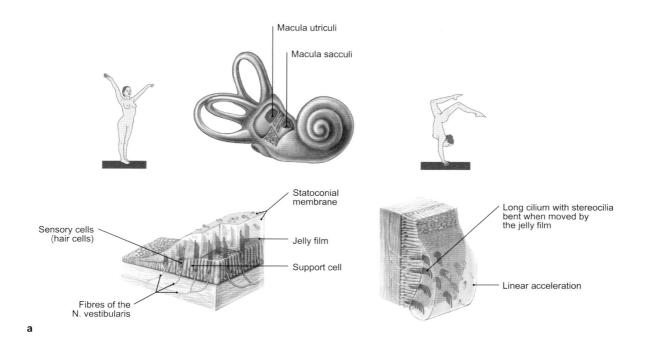

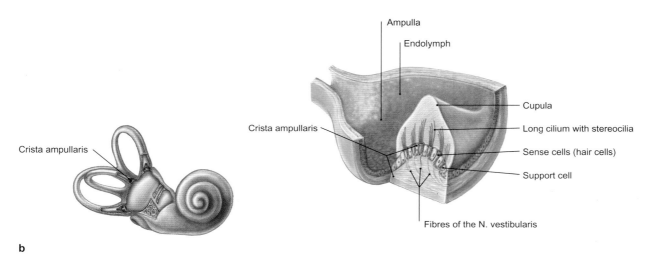

Fig. 10.56a and b Structure of the Maculae utriculi and sacculi and the Cristae ampullares. [S700-L285]

The vestibular labyrinth, filled with endolymph, is made up of the **saccule** (Macula sacculi – vertical linear accelerations), **utricle** (Macula utriculi – horizontal linear accelerations) and the **three semicircular canals** (Cristae ampullares with their Cupulae – horizontal linear accelerations).
a In both the saccule and the utricle, an oval epithelial segment (macula), 2 mm in length and equipped with sensory cells and support cells, projects above the remaining epithelium.

b In the ampullas, a transverse positioned segment made of sensory and support cells rises into the extended lumen (Cristae ampullaris). Above both of the maculae and the Cristae ampullares is a gelatinous mass called the statoconium membrane or otolithic membrane (maculae) or cupula (Cristae ampullares). The sensory cells, each of which has a long cilium of 60 μm in length and approx. 80 stereocilia, protrude into the gelatinous layer of the maculae and the Cristae ampullares and are activated by the fluid motion of the gelatinous layer (kinked, a) which results in the synaptic activation of afferent fibres of the N. vestibularis [VIII].

Clinical remarks

Labyrinthitis with dizziness, irritation or nystagmus, which can occur with cholesteatoma (syn.: peritoneal tuberosity of the ear made up of multilayered keratinising squamous epithelium; proliferating into the middle ear, with subsequent chronic purulent inflammation), Otitis media acuta, mastoiditis and after an injury to the skull. Infection routes are the round and oval window, gaps in the bony labyrinth (after trauma and bone erosion by infected pneumatic areas), or inflammation transmitted via nerves and vessels to the cochlear or vestibular ducts. The outcome is **sensorineural hearing loss** (perceptive deafness), or even hearing loss and destruction of the vestibular organ.

Hearing and equilibrium

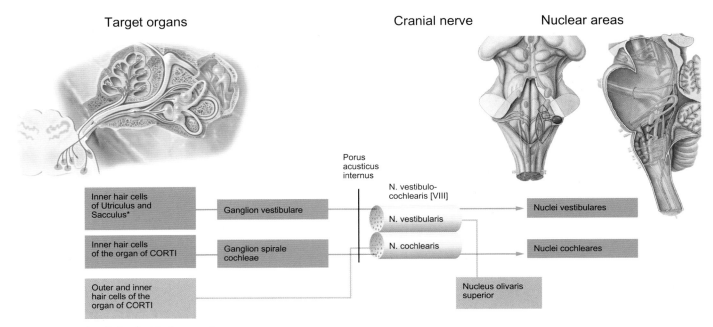

Target organs   Cranial nerve   Nuclear areas

Inner hair cells of Utriculus and Sacculus* → Ganglion vestibulare

Inner hair cells of the organ of CORTI → Ganglion spirale cochleae

Outer and inner hair cells of the organ of CORTI

Porus acusticus internus

N. vestibulo-cochlearis [VIII]

N. vestibularis

N. cochlearis

Nuclei vestibulares

Nuclei cochleares

Nucleus olivaris superior

* and hair cells of the three arcades

Fig. 10.57   Pathway, branches and fibrous qualities of the N. vestibulocochlearis [VIII]; schematic drawing. [S700-L127/L238]
Hearing and equilibrium perceptions are recorded by the outer and inner hair cells (sensory cells) of the organ of CORTI in the cochlea, or by the hair cells (sensory cells) of the utriculus and sacculus, as well as the three semicircular canals. The information is transmitted using the first neuron of the auditory and vestibular tract. The perikarya of the first neuron are positioned in the Ganglion spirale or in the Ganglion vestibulare. The axons of each first neuron form the N. cochlearis or the N. vestibularis, which combine to form the N. vestibulocochlearis [VIII]

(syn.: N. statoacusticus). The axons of the N. cochlearis project to the two Nuclei cochleares in the brainstem, and the axons of the N. vestibularis to the four Nuclei vestibulares. (For the proper names of nuclei → Fig. 10.53.)
Efferent axonal processes reach the hair cells of the inner ear (olivocochlear bundle) from the upper olivary complex. Initially the fibres accompany the N. vestibularis, and then within the Meatus acusticus internus pass over to the N. cochlearis (anastomosis of OORT), with which they reach the hair cells (→ Fig. 10.58).

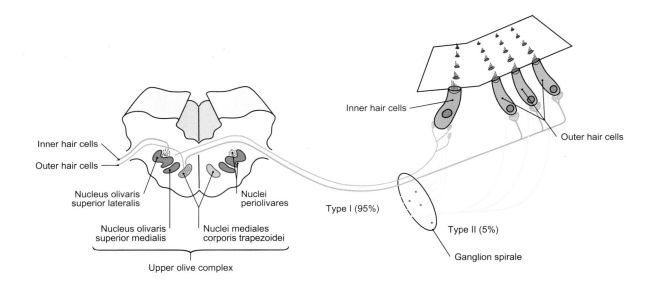

Inner hair cells

Outer hair cells

Inner hair cells

Outer hair cells

Nucleus olivaris superior lateralis

Nuclei periolivares

Nucleus olivaris superior medialis

Nuclei mediales corporis trapezoidei

Type I (95%)

Type II (5%)

Ganglion spirale

Upper olive complex

Fig. 10.58   Peripheral sections of the auditory pathway. Origins and terminal areas of the ganglion cells and of the olivocochlear efferent fibres; schematic drawing. [S702-L126]/[B500~M282/L132]/ [G1087]
In the organ of CORTI there are three to four rows of outer hair cells and a series of inner hair cells. The information registered by the outer hair cells in the bending of their stereocilia in the direction of the longest stereocilia (through contact with the tectorial membrane situated above the organ of CORTI) results in the activation of afferent pseudounipolar type II ganglion cells of which the perikarya are located in the Ganglion spirale (only 5 % of all ganglion cells of the Ganglion spirale). Most of their axons do not participate in the formation of the N. cochlearis, but

have intrinsic cochlear coordination functions. They serve as a cochlear augmentation mechanism, which is the prerequisite for a very low frequency hearing threshold and the ability to discriminate between frequencies. The inner hair cells activated by type I neurons are bipolar ganglion cells. A ganglia cell receives information from 10–20 inner hair cells. The axons of the bipolar ganglion cells of the perikarya, located in the Ganglion spirale, subsequently form the N. cochlearis and project to the Nuclei cochleares anterior and posterior. Efferent fibres reach the inner and outer hair cells (olivocochlear bundle) from the upper olivary complex. The efferent fibres synapse with the afferent fibres of the inner hair cells and the bases of the outer hair cells.

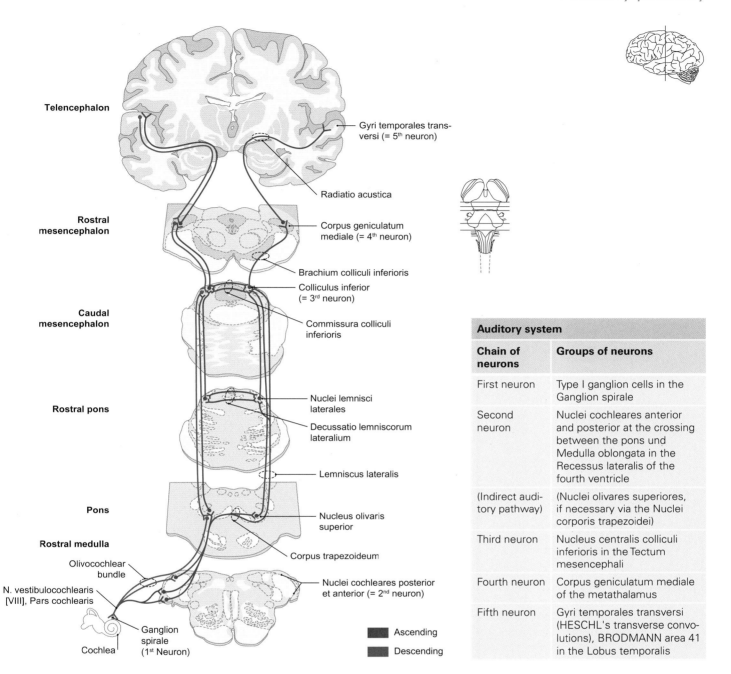

Telencephalon

Gyri temporales trans-
versi (= 5th neuron)

Radiatio acustica

**Rostral
mesencephalon**

Corpus geniculatum
mediale (= 4th neuron)

Brachium colliculi inferioris

Colliculus inferior
(= 3rd neuron)

**Caudal
mesencephalon**

Commissura colliculi
inferioris

Rostral pons

Nuclei lemnisci
laterales

Decussatio lemniscorum
lateralium

Lemniscus lateralis

Pons

Nucleus olivaris
superior

Rostral medulla

Corpus trapezoideum

Olivocochlear
bundle

N. vestibulocochlearis
[VIII], Pars cochlearis

Nuclei cochleares posterior
et anterior (= 2nd neuron)

Ganglion
spirale
(1st Neuron)

Cochlea

■ Ascending

■ Descending

Auditory system	
Chain of neurons	**Groups of neurons**
First neuron	Type I ganglion cells in the Ganglion spirale
Second neuron	Nuclei cochleares anterior and posterior at the crossing between the pons und Medulla oblongata in the Recessus lateralis of the fourth ventricle
(Indirect auditory pathway)	(Nuclei olivares superiores, if necessary via the Nuclei corporis trapezoidei)
Third neuron	Nucleus centralis colliculi inferioris in the Tectum mesencephali
Fourth neuron	Corpus geniculatum mediale of the metathalamus
Fifth neuron	Gyri temporales transversi (HESCHL's transverse convolutions), BRODMANN area 41 in the Lobus temporalis

Fig. 10.59 Auditory pathway. The most important neuronal stations and intersections of the central auditory pathway; schematic drawing. [S702-L127]/[G1081]

The function of the ascending auditory pathway is to transmit acoustic signals to the brain in order to process them and create an acoustic awareness. The auditory pathway is made up of a chain of five groups of neurons (→ table) and is organised tonotopically throughout. Tonotopy means the connections from the ear to the brain are constructed in such a way that the nerve endings in the brain reflect the neighbouring relationships of the cell bodies in the basilar membrane. In the cochlea,

the area proximal to the base is stimulated by high frequencies, the apical area by low frequencies. High frequencies tend to be represented laterally and low frequencies medially in the **primary auditory cortex** (Gyri temporales transversi, HESCHL's transverse convolutions), which is achieved via the axons of the fifth neuron as **Radiatio acustica.** The primary auditory cortex is involved in the perception of tones, sounds and simple acoustic patterns. Words, language or melodies are only processed once they reach the adjacent secondary auditory cortex (not shown).

Clinical remarks

To ascertain whether a hearing loss originates in the inner ear (sensory) or has neuronal (retrocochlear) causes, an **ABR (auditory brainstem response)** can be carried out, even before language development (when still an infant), to test the function of the inner ear and the central processing of impulses of the auditory pathway. For

this purpose, the **auditory evoked potential (AEP)** ascertained by standardised acoustic stimulation of the inner ear, using surface electrodes placed on the scalp, are assessed, including their latency and amplitude.

Vestibular tract

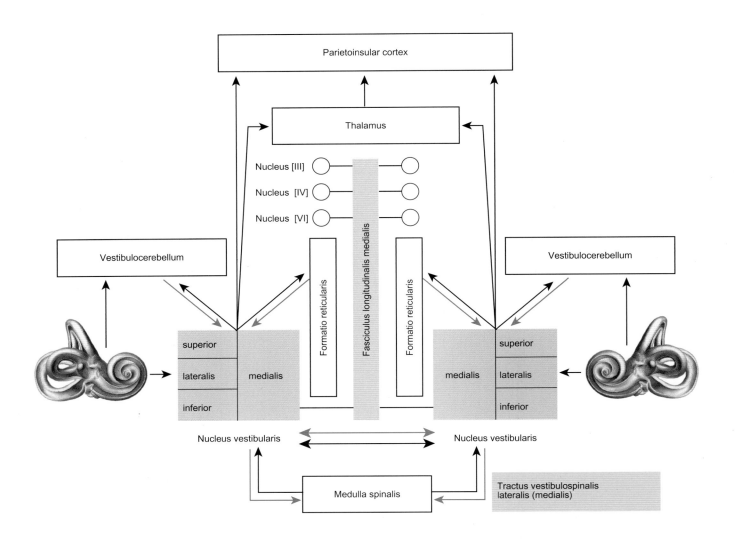

Fig. 10.60 Vestibular system, important afferences and efferences of the Nuclei vestibulares functioning as integration nuclei; schematic drawing. [S702-L127]/[G1081]

The vestibular system registers changes in the position and/or movement of the body, to maintain the body's balance (→ table). Thereby, the vestibular apparatus in the inner ear registers changes in position and movement. The registered impulses are forwarded not only to the vestibular nuclei in the Medulla oblongata, but also to the cerebellum (Lobus flocculonodularis as the main constituent of the vestibulocerebellum). Moreover, they are synchronised intensively with proprioceptive impulses generated by the GOLGI tendon organs and muscle spindles, which arrive via the spinal cord at the vestibular nuclei, as well as with information from the optical system (gaze stabilisation). The vestibular nuclei thus form an integration centre for quick adaptation to changes in body position or movement. This takes place subconsciously, without cortical interconnection. To activate awareness, an onward interconnection via the thalamus and cortex is necessary. Interestingly, to date no primary cortex area is known that can be assigned to the vestibular system alone. Instead, up to ten areas are under discussion as possibly being involved in impulse processing (e.g. the Sulcus intraparietalis, parietoinsular cortex, somatosensory cortex, hippocampus).

Vestibular system	
Chain of neurons	**Groups of neurons**
First neuron	Ganglion cells in the Ganglion vestibulare
Second neuron	Nuclei vestibulares superior, lateralis, inferior et medialis in the transition between the pons and Medulla oblongata
Third neuron	Thalamus (Nucleus posterior ventrolateralis)
Fourth neuron	Cortex: Sulcus intraparietalis, parietoinsular area, Gyrus postcentralis, BRODMANN area 7 and hippocampus

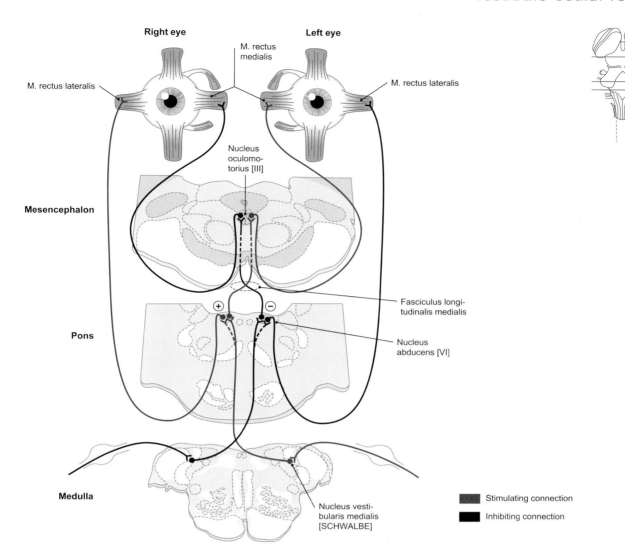

Right eye

Left eye

M. rectus medialis

M. rectus lateralis

M. rectus lateralis

Nucleus oculomotorius [III]

Mesencephalon

Fasciculus longitudinalis medialis

Pons

⊕ ⊖

Nucleus abducens [VI]

Medulla

Nucleus vestibularis medialis [SCHWALBE]

■ Stimulating connection

■ Inhibiting connection

Fig. 10.61 Vestibulo-ocular reflex with stimulation of the left lateral semicircular canal; schematic drawing. [S702-L127]/[G1081]
Of the visual cortex, 50 % processes the central 3 % of the visual field. For this reason, an important function of the vestibular organ is to enable positional adjustment of the eyes during head movements to ensure that the resulting image is projected simultaneously onto the Fovea centralis of the retina (area of sharpest vision) in both eyes. This reflexive coordinated adjustment process involves several nuclear and fibre systems within the vestibular system (→ Fig. 10.60). Activation of the sensory cells in the Cristae ampullares of the lateral semicircular canal when turning the head (to the left) results in an increased impulse frequency in the left N. vestibularis. Motor neurons of the contralateral Nucleus nervi abducentis are activated via the medial vestibular nucleus, causing the contraction of the M. rectus lateralis (right side). At the same time, interneurons activate the ipsilateral Nucleus nervi oculomotorii, which in turn causes the synchronous contraction of the M. rectus medialis (left side). Via the semicircular canal system of the opposite side, the two muscles acting as antagonists (M. rectus lateralis on the left and the M. rectus medialis on the right) receive opposing commands and thus act antagonistically (they relax). Movements of the head lead to such an eye movement in the opposite direction.

Clinical remarks

To objectify any **dizziness** perceived by the patient, and to locate a lesion, the vestibular organ has to be tested. Commonly used tests are the **ROMBERG test** (patient stands up with eyes closed and arms stretched forward) and the **UNTERBERGER step test** (patient marches on the spot with eyes closed) in order to rule out a tendency to fall over. Another method is the **nystagmus test** (nystagmus = ocular tremor) using magnifying glasses (FRENZEL glasses). Nystagmus means an uncontrollable, usually horizontal eye movement, characterised by a slow tracking movement and a quick return movement (comparable to eye movements when looking from a moving train). Shaking the patient's head rapidly back and forth helps the examiner test whether a provocation nystagmus can be triggered. The examiner performs this provocation nystagmus test in various positions. This would also reveal any latent nystagmus which may be present. The **thermal nystagmus test** is used in testing the labyrinth on either side. For this, the patient lies in a supine position with the head slightly elevated in a darkened room while each ear is irrigated with cold and warm water in turn. Cold water hereby physiologically triggers a nystagmus on the opposite side, warm water on the same side. A pathological level of under-excitability or unexcitability on one side suggests a peripheral function impairment.

Sample exam questions

To check that you are completely familiar with the content of this chapter, sample questions from an oral anatomy exam are listed here.

Explain the structure of the outer ear:

- Describe the development of the outer ear.
- What are auricular hillocks?
- Name some of the characteristic structures on the outer ear.
- What distinguishes the ear lobe from the rest of the outer ear?
- Where is the tragus located?
- Which sorts of things do you look at if you can trigger a tragus pressure pain in a patient?
- Insert your little finger into your ear and open and close your mouth several times. What do you notice?

Describe the external auditory canal:

- What is the pathway of the external auditory canal?
- What do you need to do in order to be able to look at the tympanic membrane with an otoscope?
- How is the external auditory canal constructed? Approximately how long is it?
- Which glands are located in the wall of the external auditory canal? What are their function?

Describe the structure of the tympanic membrane:

- How is the tympanic membrane constructed?
- Describe the development of the tympanic membrane.
- Why is the tympanic membrane clinically divided into quadrants? Which quadrants do you know?
- Why is the front lower quadrant often poorly visible?
- Which structures are located directly behind the tympanic membrane?
- What is the colour of a healthy tympanic membrane, and where is the light reflex?
- How is the tympanic membrane attached?
- Can air penetrate a healthy tympanic membrane?
- How can you test that your own tympanic membrane is intact?

Explain the structure of the tympanic cavity:

- With what does the tympanic cavity have a positional relationship?
- How big is the tympanic cavity?
- How far is the tympanic membrane from the medial tympanic cavity wall?
- How can the tympanic cavity be divided?

- Which structures are located in the tympanic cavity?
- How is the tympanic cavity ventilated?
- Are the auditory ossicles situated freely in the tympanic cavity?
- Are you aware of any other air-filled spaces in proximity to the tympanic cavity?

Describe the structure of the auditory ossicles.

- Which muscles are the auditory ossicles attached to?
- What is meant by a consensual reaction in relation to the M. stapedius?
- Why is the Chorda tympani at risk in surgery on the middle ear?
- What is the pathway of the N. facialis in relation to the tympanic cavity?

Explain the structure of the EUSTACHIAN tube:

- How is the EUSTACHIAN tube structured?
- Which muscles are involved in the tube's function, and how are they innervated?
- The bony part of the EUSTACHIAN tube is also referred to as the Semicanalis tubae auditivae. What is located in the other half (semicanal)?
- In cases of a cleft palate, what could be the cause of a tube function impairment?

Describe the structure of the inner ear:

- Where in the bony cochlea is the Pars petrosa?
- What is meant by the term 'labyrinth'?
- How is the inner ear supplied with blood?
- Describe sound conduction.
- What is the Ductus endolymphaticus?
- Where are the perikarya of the N. cochlearis located?
- What is the organ of CORTI?
- What are the membranous and the bony labyrinths?
- Where is the round window (Fenestra cochleae)?
- What is the helicotrema?

Explain the auditory pathway and control of the equilibrium:

- Describe the course of the auditory pathway.
- Which other nuclear areas is the vestibular organ in contact with?

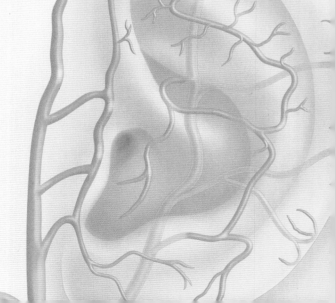

Neck

11

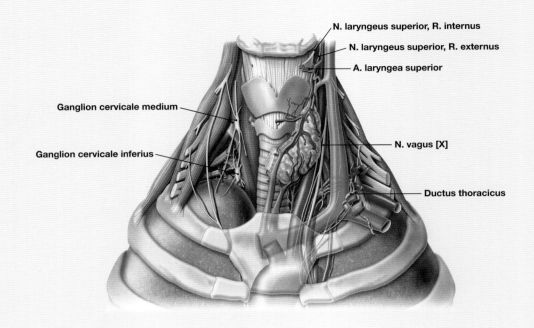

N. laryngeus superior, R. internus
N. laryngeus superior, R. externus
A. laryngea superior
Ganglion cervicale medium
N. vagus [X]
Ganglion cervicale inferius
Ductus thoracicus

Overview

The **neck** (collum, cervix) connects the head to the trunk. The respiratory and digestive tracts, the neurovascular pathways and the central nervous system are somatic connections using the neck as a transit route. An osseous base is provided by the cervical spine, on which the head rests and which allows free rotation relative to the trunk of up to almost 180°. The neck is the location of several specialised organs of the respiratory tract (thyroid gland, parathyroid glands, submandibular salivary glands and larynx). Externally, the neck area can be divided into the anterior, the lateral and posterior cervical regions; the latter is also called the nape (nucha). The upper boundary of the neck is formed by the lower rim of the Mandibula, the Proc. mastoideus and the Linea nuchalis superior up to the Protuberantia occipitalis externa. The neck area extends to the Manubrium sterni, the clavicula and a connecting line between the acromion, Spina scapulae and the spinous process of the seventh cervical vertebra. There are many different muscles governing the movement of the head, the skin of the neck and the hyoid bone in the neck, as well as the larynx and the cervical spine. Cervical fasciae divide the neck viscera into sections. The external appearance of the neck depends not only on the formative structure, the body type and age, but also in particular on the musculature of the neck and the amount and distribution of the subcutaneous fatty tissue.

Main topics

After working through this chapter, you should be able to:

- name the specific structures of the neck and describe the anatomical composition;
- know the boundaries of the neck and correctly name its topographical regions;
- functionally link the passive and active elements of the musculoskeletal system of the neck;
- specify the layers of the cervical fascia, their boundaries and the structures enclosed within;
- name the anatomical spaces of the neck and describe their boundaries;
- classify the neurovascular pathways of the neck and understand what particular areas they innervate or supply;
- name the skeletal elements and ligaments of the larynx;
- describe the laryngeal joints and muscles as well as their functions;

- explain significant functions of the larynx, its blood supply, lymphatic drainage and innervation;
- classify different sections of the larynx, with internal boundaries and spaces;
- explain terms such as arytenoid cartilages or phonation and respiration position;
- locate the blood vessels and nerves of the larynx in relation to the surrounding structures and name important landmarks;
- describe the principles of laryngeal development;
- explain how the thyroid and parathyroid glands developed from the pharynx;
- explain the functions of the thyroid and parathyroid glands;
- describe the upper oesophageal constriction and weak muscle triangles at the transition from the throat to the oesophagus.

Clinical relevance

In order not to lose touch with prospective everyday clinical life with so many anatomical details, the following describes a typical case that shows why the content of this chapter is so important.

Supraglottic squamous cell carcinoma

Case study
A 58-year-old bricklayer presents with hoarseness which has persisted for three months, a cough, a scratchy throat and a croaky voice at his general practitioner.

 For hoarseness lasting more than three weeks, an ENT specialist must always be consulted.

More recently, occasional pain in his neck is radiating to the right ear. He claims to be suffering from a cold and would like some medication to help him. The hoarseness does not particularly bother him, but he is also not in the best of health. The general practitioner barely knows the patient. He now learns that the patient has been a smoker for many years and likes to drink a beer with his colleagues at work, although this is not permitted. The bricklayer's voice sounds rough, deep and hoarse. He has no difficulty in swallowing, nor any shortness of breath. But he mentions that he has recently lost some weight because he has hardly any appetite. He doesn't mind this because he has to lose a little weight anyway.

 Secondary (accompanying) symptoms include fever, night sweats and weight loss, and their presence must be recorded in all patients with cancer.

The general practitioner refers the patient to an ENT specialist to ensure a rapid diagnosis.

Result of examination
The ENT specialist reads on the referral: hoarseness for three months, exclusion of a laryngeal tumour. After taking a thorough medical history, he examines the bricklayer carefully (examination of the ears, nose and throat), including the lymph nodes in the ENT area. A laryngoscopy shows an already advanced tumour of the supraglottis with partially ulcerated surface and raised exophytic edge (→ Fig. a). On the right side of the neck at the level of the larynx, the doctor palpates a slightly enlarged lymph node, not painful to the touch, in the area of the V. jugularis interna.

Having discussed the findings with the patient, he arranges an appointment at the clinic of the university hospital to take a sample biopsy which will determine any further steps to be taken in the coming week.

Diagnostic procedure
At the ENT clinic a microlaryngoscopy is performed under anaesthesia and numerous sample biopsies of the suspected tumour areas are taken, and an endoscopic examination of the other areas of the upper aerodigestive tract (panendoscopy) is performed to exclude a secondary tumour in another area. The microlaryngoscopy shows that the tumour is limited to the larynx, which is quite mobile; however, it has already infiltrated the postcricoid region, the right Cartilago arytenoidea and the medial wall of the Sinus piriformis. The pathological findings of the biopsies reveal a slightly horny squamous cell carcinoma. Therefore the patient is submitted to further staging. The X-ray image of the thorax and the ultrasound of the abdomen are normal. A CT (computed tomography) of the neck shows two enlarged and altered cervical lymph nodes on the right-hand side.

Diagnosis
Supraglottic squamous cell carcinoma right side, cT3 cN2b cM0 (→ Fig. a)

Treatment
The choice of treatment will be determined by the tumour size and location, and also the status of the local cervical lymph nodes. Due to the size of the tumour and evidence of lymph node metastases, the patient's larynx must be entirely removed. As part of the primary tumour treatment and to improve the prognosis, a neck dissection in the regional lymphatic drainage area is carried out. To achieve this, dissection of lymph node regions II, III and IV (lymphadenectomy) is performed (→ Fig. 11.92) on the right side of the neck.

Further developments
The complete resection of the larynx (laryngectomy) is a major operation. The larynx allows not only the articulation of sounds and voice, but also separates the respiratory tract from the digestive tract when swallowing. As part of a laryngectomy, a permanent laryngectomy stoma is created, meaning that the trachea opens to the outside in the area of the Fossa jugularis. This means that the respiratory and digestive tracts are completely separated from each other. The patient can no longer breathe through the nose.

Dissection lab
Malignant tumours of the larynx are the fifth most common malignant tumours worldwide and hence not a rare medical finding. In dissection classes, great importance should therefore be placed on understanding the regional lymph nodes in the neck, since they should be assessed during any physical examination.

 During a dissection, imagine that you are carrying out your first neck dissection. Pay attention to the topography of the blood vessels and nerves.

In addition, the division of the larynx into the supraglottis, glottis and subglottis is essential, especially for diagnostic imaging in the context of tumour-staging and so indispensable for any subsequent choice of treatment. Because of the location of tumours of the glottis, they are often identified at an early stage compared to, for example, carcinomas of the supraglottis (leading symptom: hoarseness).

Back in the clinic
A total laryngectomy causes the patient to lose his voice. For the bricklayer, this is actually 'the worst part of the whole operation', as he writes to the speech therapist on a piece of paper. Patients who have undergone a laryngectomy can follow various voice reconstruction and rehabilitation procedures. One method of voice reconstruction is the oesophageal speech method.

 Oesophageal speech sounds different because it is produced by the oesophagus instead of the vocal folds.

Through a variety of exercises in the area of the oesophageal entrance, a bulge of the mucous membrane develops, which takes over the function of the former vocal folds. Voice reconstruction can then be achieved by voluntarily controllable movements of air in the oesophagus and by the newly formed bulge of the Plica vocalis. Other methods favour voice prostheses for patients.

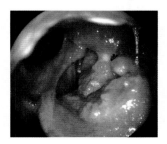

Fig. a Supraglottic carcinoma of the larynx, right side; easily recognisable on the epiglottis. [S700-T872]

11

Neck

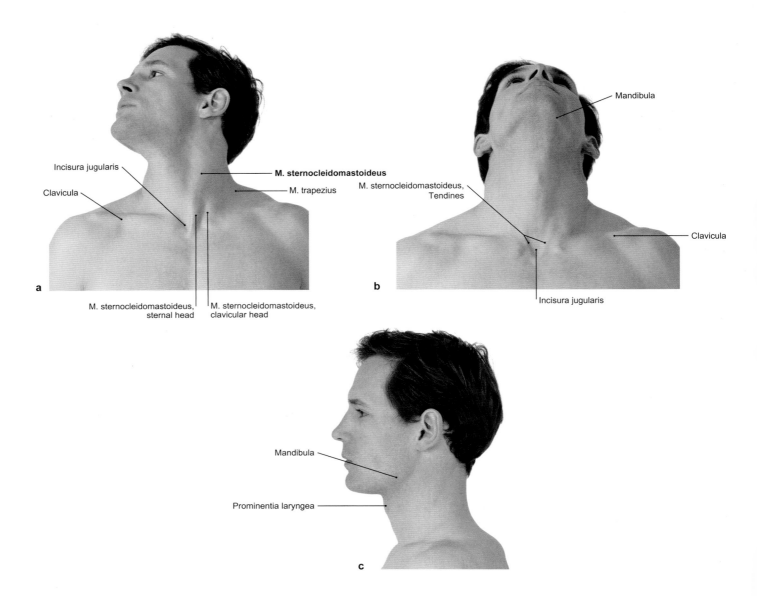

a

Incisura jugularis

Clavicula

M. sternocleidomastoideus

M. trapezius

M. sternocleidomastoideus, sternal head

M. sternocleidomastoideus, clavicular head

b

Mandibula

M. sternocleidomastoideus, Tendines

Clavicula

Incisura jugularis

c

Mandibula

Prominentia laryngea

Fig. 11.1a–c Surface anatomy of the anterior and lateral regions of the neck, Regiones cervicales anterior et lateralis. [S700-J803]

a Anterior view with head turned to the upper right.
b Anterior view with head turned upward.
c Lateral view from the left.

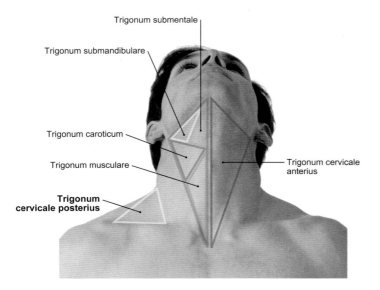

Trigonum submentale

Trigonum submandibulare

Trigonum caroticum

Trigonum musculare

Trigonum cervicale posterius

Trigonum cervicale anterius

Fig. 11.2   Position of the anterior and posterior triangle of the neck and subdivision of the Regio cervicalis anterior; anterior view [S701-J803/L126]
The anterior triangle of the neck (purple) is further subdivided into the Trigonum submentale (green), Trigonum submandibulare (yellow), Trigonum caroticum (red) and Trigonum musculare (blue).

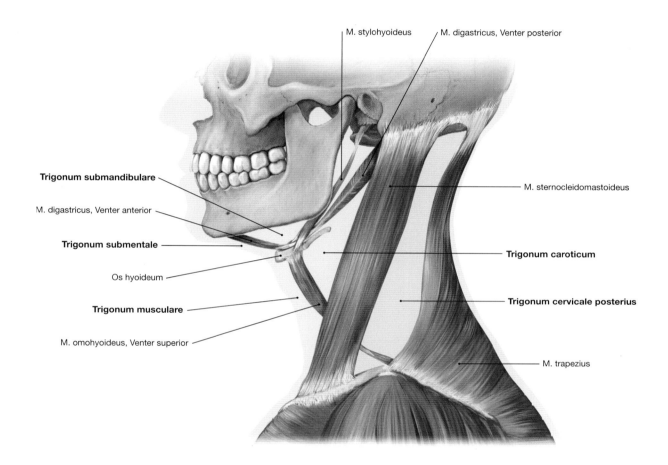

M. stylohyoideus

M. digastricus, Venter posterior

Trigonum submandibulare

M. digastricus, Venter anterior

Trigonum submentale

Os hyoideum

Trigonum musculare

M. omohyoideus, Venter superior

M. sternocleidomastoideus

Trigonum caroticum

Trigonum cervicale posterius

M. trapezius

Fig. 11.3 Anterior and lateral regions of the neck; Regiones cervicales anterior et lateralis, left side; lateral view. [S700-L266]
The boundaries of the **anterior triangle of the neck** (Regio cervicalis anterior [Trigonum cervicale anterius]) are the lower rim of the mandible, the anterior rim of the M. sternocleidomastoideus, and the Linea mediana cervicis. Located within the anterior triangle of the neck are the Trigonum submandibulare (margins: mandible, Venter anterior and Venter posterior of the M. digastricus), the Trigonum submentale (margins: Os hyoideum, Venter anterior of the M. digastricus, Linea mediana

cervicis), the Trigonum musculare (margins: Os hyoideum, Venter superior of the M. omohyoideus, M. sternocleidomastoideus, midline of the neck), and the Trigonum caroticum (margins: Venter superior of the M. omohyoideus, the lowest part of the M. stylohyoideus, Venter posterior of the M. digastricus, M. sternocleidomastoideus).
Boundaries of the **posterior triangle of the neck** (Regio cervicalis posterior [Trigonum cervicale posterius]) are the posterior rim of the M. sternocleidomastoideus, the anterior rim of the M. trapezius, the upper rim of the clavicula and the Os occipitale.

Neck muscles

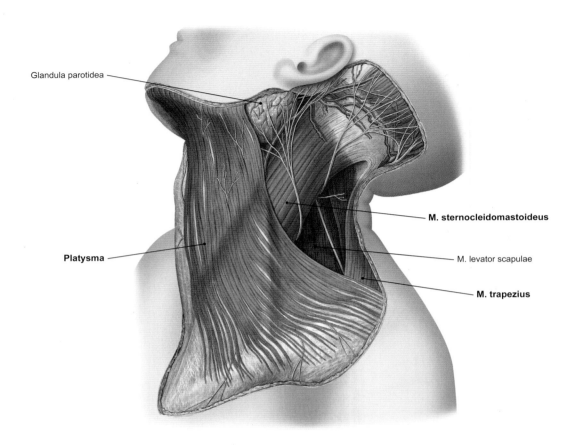

Glandula parotidea

M. sternocleidomastoideus

Platysma

M. levator scapulae

M. trapezius

Fig. 11.4 Muscles of the anterior and lateral neck regions, Regiones cervicales anterior et lateralis, superficial layer, left side; lateral view. [S700]
On the surface, the platysma (a mimetic muscle without fascia) forms a thin muscular layer located directly under the skin and extends from the Mandibula via the clavicula to the thorax. Lateral to the rear, the superficial cervical fascia has been removed. The upper part of the

M. sternocleidomastoideus, which serves as a reference structure in surgery, is visible, as well as the anterior rim of the M. trapezius below at the back. The lower pole of the Glandula parotidea, which lies between the platysma and the M. sternocleidomastoideus, can extend into the neck region to a variable degree. The M. levator scapulae can be identified deep in the posterior triangle of the neck.

→ T 1.6, T 9

Clinical remarks

There are several possible surgical access routes to the trachea:
* In the **coniotomy,** the Lig. cricothyroideum medianum (Lig. conicum, * in the → figure] is severed between the thyroid and cricoid cartilages. This gives access to the inner space of the larynx just below the vocal folds.
* For a **tracheostomy,** an upper access route above the isthmus of the thyroid gland (** in the → figure), a middle access route after severing the isthmus, and a lower access route below the isthmus of the thyroid gland (*** in the → figure) can be chosen (also → Fig. 11.64).

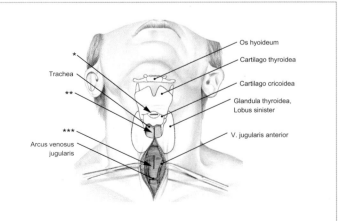

Trachea

*

**

***

Arcus venosus jugularis

Os hyoideum

Cartilago thyroidea

Cartilago cricoidea

Glandula thyroidea, Lobus sinister

V. jugularis anterior

Surgical access routes to open the trachea; ventral view; neck hyperextended dorsally. [S700]

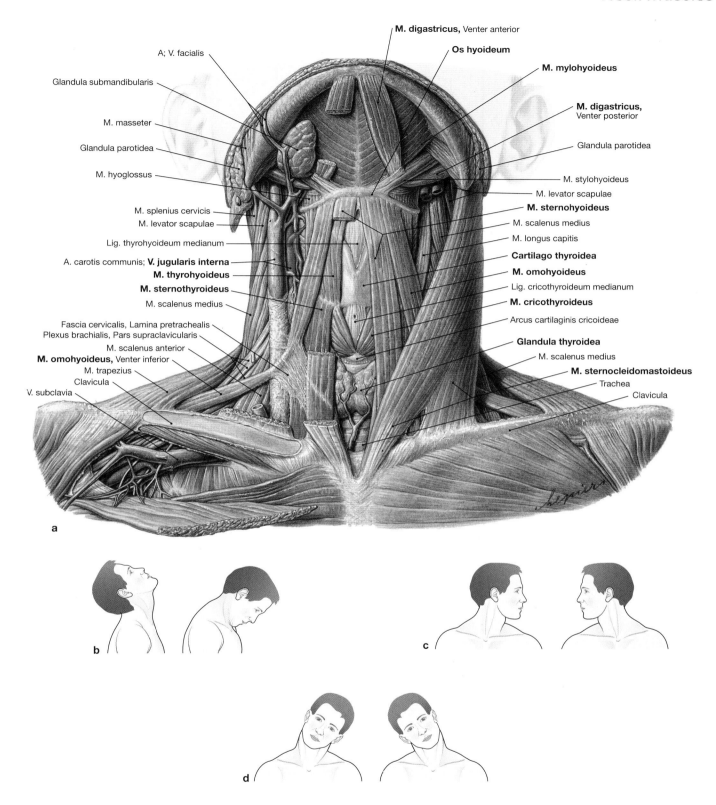

M. digastricus, Venter anterior

Os hyoideum

M. mylohyoideus

A; V. facialis

M. digastricus,
Venter posterior

Glandula submandibularis

Glandula parotidea

M. masseter

M. stylohyoideus

Glandula parotidea

M. levator scapulae

M. hyoglossus

M. sternohyoideus

M. scalenus medius

M. splenius cervicis

M. longus capitis

M. levator scapulae

Cartilago thyroidea

Lig. thyrohyoideum medianum

M. omohyoideus

A. carotis communis; **V. jugularis interna**

Lig. cricothyroideum medianum

M. thyrohyoideus

M. cricothyroideus

M. sternothyroideus

Arcus cartilaginis cricoideae

M. scalenus medius

Glandula thyroidea

Fascia cervicalis, Lamina pretrachealis
Plexus brachialis, Pars supraclavicularis

M. scalenus medius

M. scalenus anterior

M. sternocleidomastoideus

M. omohyoideus, Venter inferior

Trachea

M. trapezius

Clavicula

Clavicula

V. subclavia

a

b

c

d

Fig. 11.5a–d Neck muscles, Mm. colli and movements of the M. sternocleidomastoideus.

a Ventral view; chin elevated. **Superficially,** the M. sternocleidomastoideus runs from its two origins (Caput sternale and Caput claviculare) to the Proc. mastoideus. Its caudal part covers the origin of the **infrahyoid musculature** with the Mm. sternohyoideus, sternothyroideus, thyrohyoideus and omohyoideus, which stretch between the sternum, thyroid cartilage, hyoid bone, and scapula (M. omohyoideus). The M. omohyoideus is composed of two bellies separated by an intermediate tendon affixed to the connective tissue of the carotid sheath (Vagina carotica) and serves to keep the lumen of the V. jugularis interna

open. From bottom to top under the infrahyoid muscles can be seen the isthmus of the thyroid gland, the paired M. cricothyroideus (an outer laryngeal muscle), the thyroid cartilage and the hyoid bone. Above the hyoid bone, the floor of the mouth is formed by the M. mylohyoideus. [S700]

b–d Functionally, the **M. sternocleidomastoideus** raises the head with bilateral activity and bends the cervical spine dorsally **(b);** a one-sided activity leads to the head turning to the contralateral side **(c)** and to a lateral inclination on the ipsilateral side **(d).** [S700-L126]

→ T 9–T 12

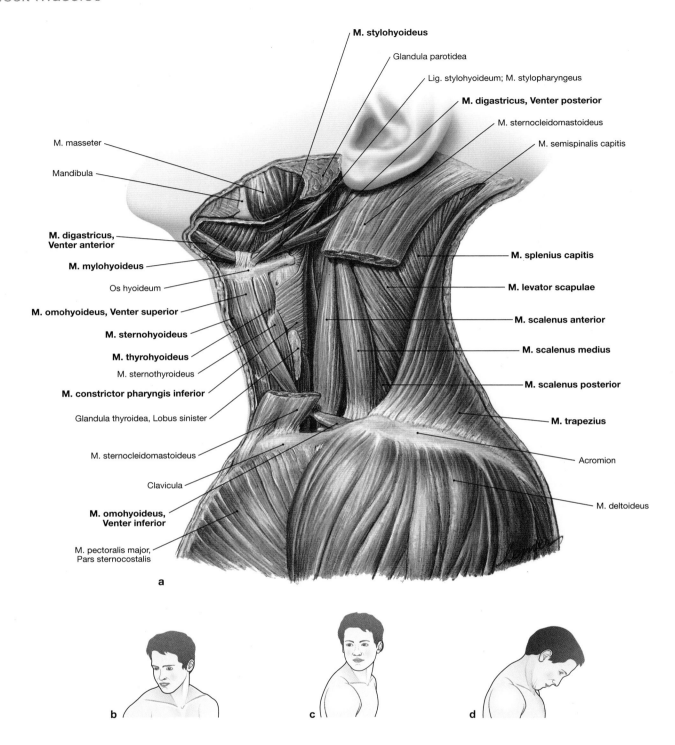

M. stylohyoideus

Glandula parotidea

Lig. stylohyoideum; M. stylopharyngeus

M. digastricus, Venter posterior

M. sternocleidomastoideus

M. semispinalis capitis

M. masseter

Mandibula

M. digastricus, Venter anterior

M. mylohyoideus

Os hyoideum

M. omohyoideus, Venter superior

M. sternohyoideus

M. thyrohyoideus

M. sternothyroideus

M. constrictor pharyngis inferior

Glandula thyroidea, Lobus sinister

M. sternocleidomastoideus

Clavicula

M. omohyoideus, Venter inferior

M. pectoralis major, Pars sternocostalis

M. splenius capitis

M. levator scapulae

M. scalenus anterior

M. scalenus medius

M. scalenus posterior

M. trapezius

Acromion

M. deltoideus

a

b   c   d

Fig. 11.6a–d   Neck muscles, Mm. colli, and movements.
a Lateral view. All muscle fasciae, the platysma and the middle portion of the M. sternocleidomastoideus have been removed. From anterior to posterior, the following structures can be seen: the **infrahyoid muscles** with the M. sternohyoideus, M. omohyoideus (Venter superior; the Venter inferior runs above the clavicula in the lateral triangle of the neck), Mm. thyrohyoideus and sternothyroideus, parts of the pharyngeal muscles (M. constrictor pharyngis inferior), the Mm. scaleni (anterior, medius and posterior), the M. levator scapulae, the M. splenius capitis, and the M. trapezius. Above the hyoid bone, three **suprahyoid**

muscles can be seen (M. digastricus with its Venter anterior and Venter posterior, M. mylohyoideus and M. stylohyoideus). [S700]
b–d Combined bilateral or one-sided muscle contractions of the superficial neck muscles facilitate complex movements of the head, such as dipping of the chin with simultaneous rotation to the side **(b)**, rotational movements for looking over the shoulder **(c),** or dropping the chin to the chest **(d).** [S700-L126]

→ T 9–T 12

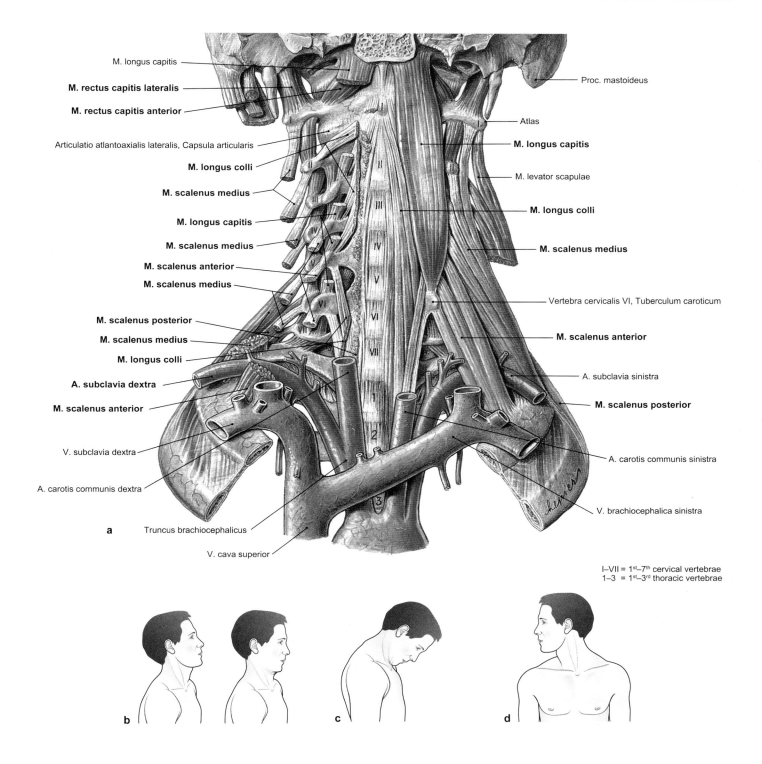

M. longus capitis

M. rectus capitis lateralis

M. rectus capitis anterior

Articulatio atlantoaxialis lateralis, Capsula articularis

M. longus colli

M. scalenus medius

M. longus capitis

M. scalenus medius

M. scalenus anterior

M. scalenus medius

M. scalenus posterior

M. scalenus medius

M. longus colli

A. subclavia dextra

M. scalenus anterior

V. subclavia dextra

A. carotis communis dextra

a Truncus brachiocephalicus

V. cava superior

Proc. mastoideus

Atlas

M. longus capitis

M. levator scapulae

M. longus colli

M. scalenus medius

Vertebra cervicalis VI, Tuberculum caroticum

M. scalenus anterior

A. subclavia sinistra

M. scalenus posterior

A. carotis communis sinistra

V. brachiocephalica sinistra

I–VII = 1st–7th cervical vertebrae
1–3 = 1st–3rd thoracic vertebrae

b **c** **d**

Fig. 11.7a–d   Prevertebral muscles and Mm. scaleni.

a Ventral view. The **prevertebral muscles** are located on both sides of the vertebral bodies of the cervical and upper thoracic spine and are covered by the Lamina prevertebralis of the Fascia cervicalis. The anterolateral parts of the atlas and axis are linked via the short M. rectus capitis anterior. In addition to this muscle, the M. longus capitis and the M. longus colli also form part of the prevertebral muscles. The M. rectus capitis lateralis belongs to the ventrolateral muscles, which have migrated to this region.

The **Mm. scaleni** anterior, medius and posterior run to the upper ribs and form a triangular-shaped muscle plate lateral to the cervical spine. The Mm. scalenus anterior and scalenus medius, together with the upper rim of the first rib, form the **scalene hiatus,** through which pass the A. subclavia and the Plexus brachialis (not shown).

Some authors distinguish between an anterior and a posterior scalene hiatus. The anterior scalene hiatus represents the pathway of the V. subclavia which runs in front of the M. scalenus anterior across the first rib, whereas the posterior scalene hiatus represents the passage of the A. subclavia and Plexus brachialis which runs between the Mm. scaleni anterior and medius across the first rib. Because the so-called 'anterior' scalene hiatus is not a real gap, one should only refer to the space between the M. scalenus anterior and M. scalenus medius as the scalene hiatus. [S700]

b–d The deep cervical muscles help to guide precise movements of the head and the cervical spine, such as stabilising the head and the cervical spine **(b)**, dropping the chin onto the chest **(c)**, and rotational movements for looking over the shoulder **(d)**. [S700-L126]

→ T 12, T 13

Cervical fasciae

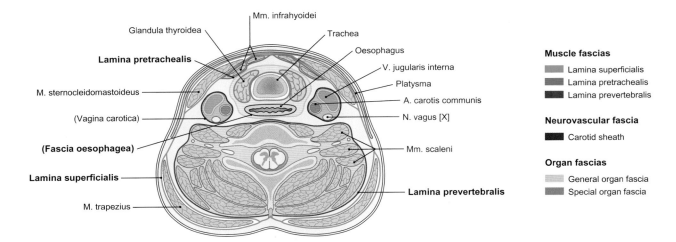

Muscle fascias
- Lamina superficialis
- Lamina pretrachealis
- Lamina prevertebralis

Neurovascular fascia
- Carotid sheath

Organ fascias
- General organ fascia
- Special organ fascia

Labels (clockwise): Mm. infrahyoidei · Trachea · Oesophagus · V. jugularis interna · Platysma · A. carotis communis · N. vagus [X] · Mm. scaleni · **Lamina prevertebralis** · M. trapezius · **Lamina superficialis** · **(Fascia oesophagea)** · (Vagina carotica) · M. sternocleidomastoideus · **Lamina pretrachealis** · Glandula thyroidea

Fig. 11.8 Cervical fasciae, Fasciae cervicales; cross-section through the neck. [S700-L126]
A distinction is made between a muscle fascia with three laminae, a neurovascular fascia, and an organ fascia which has two laminae.

Muscle fascias:
- Lamina superficialis (superficial lamina, encases the whole neck and ensheathes the M. sternocleidomastoideus as well as the Mm. levator scapulae and M. trapezius in the neck region)
- Lamina pretrachealis (middle lamina, surrounds infrahyoid muscles)
- Lamina prevertebralis (deep lamina, ensheathes the Mm. scaleni, prevertebral muscles and M. rectus capitis lateralis, and merges with the fascia of the autochthonous muscles of the back).

Neurovascular fascia:
- carotid sheath (ensheathes the Aa. carotides communis, interna and externa and V. jugularis interna, N. vagus [X]).

Organ fascias:
- general organ fascia (envelops all viscerae of the neck such as the pharynx, larynx, thyroid gland, parathyroid glands, upper part of the trachea, and oesophagus together with the Pars cervicalis)
- special organ fascia = organ capsule (encases all organs of the neck, e.g. Fascia oesophagea).

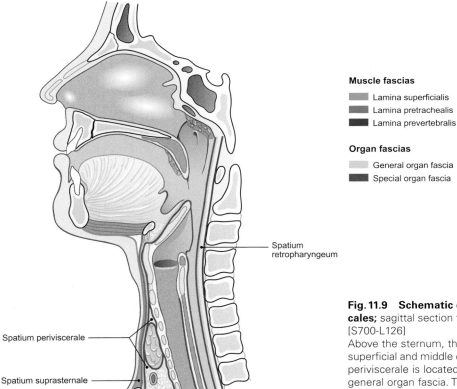

Muscle fascias
- Lamina superficialis
- Lamina pretrachealis
- Lamina prevertebralis

Organ fascias
- General organ fascia
- Special organ fascia

Labels: Spatium retropharyngeum · Spatium periviscerale · Spatium suprasternale

Fig. 11.9 Schematic drawing of the cervical fasciae, Fasciae cervicales; sagittal section through the neck at the level of the larynx. [S700-L126]
Above the sternum, the Spatium suprasternale is located between the superficial and middle cervical fascial lamina, and ventrally, the Spatium periviscerale is located between the middle cervical fascial lamina and general organ fascia. The Spatium retropharyngeum (→ Fig. 11.17) is located prevertebrally between the general organ fascia and the deep layer of the cervical fascial lamina.

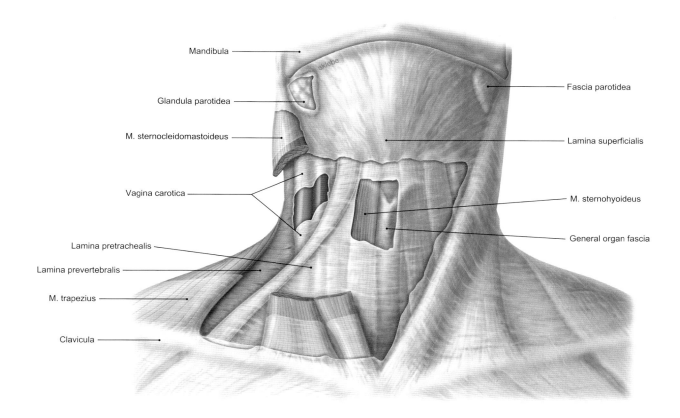

Mandibula

Glandula parotidea

M. sternocleidomastoideus

Vagina carotica

Lamina pretrachealis

Lamina prevertebralis

M. trapezius

Clavicula

Fascia parotidea

Lamina superficialis

M. sternohyoideus

General organ fascia

Fig. 11.10 Muscle fasciae of the neck, Fasciae cervicales; ventral view. [S700-L238]
The platysma was removed bilaterally. On the right side, the Lamina superficialis of the Fascia cervicalis is intact and forms a sheath around the M. sternocleidomastoideus. On the left side, the muscle and the Lamina superficialis of the Fascia cervicalis have mostly been removed.

Above the larynx, a small part of the middle cervical fascia has been removed to show the M. sternohyoideus, a muscle normally ensheathed by the middle cervical fascia, and the general organ fascia located below. At the posterior margin of the M. omohyoideus, the fenestrated carotid sheath as well as the deep lamina of the cervical fascia are visible.

Clinical remarks

Within the context of neck operations (e. g. neck dissections) the laminae of the cervical fascia and the areas of connective tissue delimited by them serve as reference structures. Between the cervical fascial laminae, bleeding and abscesses can spread within the connective tissue and caudally into the mediastinum **(descending abscess).** The weakness of the walls of the pharynx favours an invasion of microorganisms, most commonly into the parapharyngeal and retropharyngeal spaces **(parapharyngeal** [peripharyngeal], → figure, or **retropharyngeal abscess).**
Parapharyngeal abscess on the right, extending (black arrow tips) inside the anatomically defined area (Spatium lateropharyngeum); computed tomographical horizontal section. [R242]

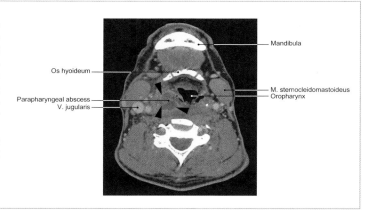

Os hyoideum

Parapharyngeal abscess
V. jugularis

Mandibula

M. sternocleidomastoideus
Oropharynx

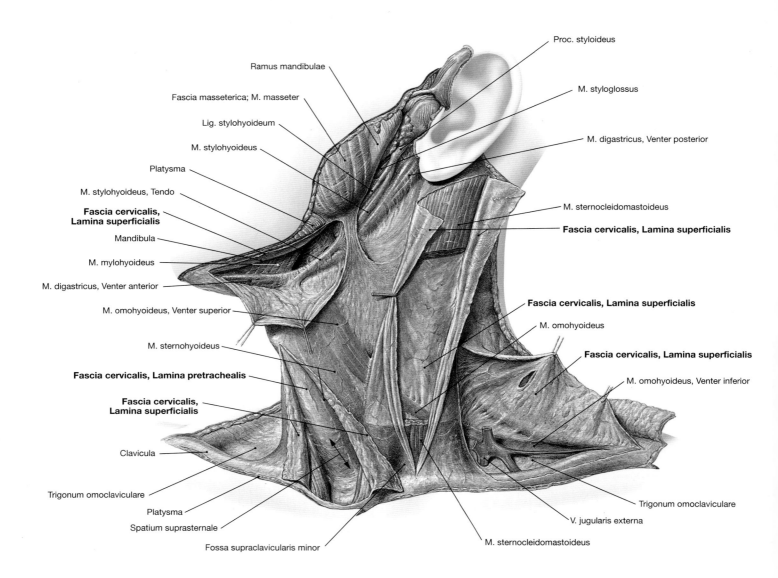

Proc. styloideus

Ramus mandibulae

M. styloglossus

Fascia masseterica; M. masseter

Lig. stylohyoideum

M. stylohyoideus

M. digastricus, Venter posterior

Platysma

M. stylohyoideus, Tendo

Fascia cervicalis, Lamina superficialis

M. sternocleidomastoideus

Mandibula

Fascia cervicalis, Lamina superficialis

M. mylohyoideus

M. digastricus, Venter anterior

M. omohyoideus, Venter superior

Fascia cervicalis, Lamina superficialis

M. omohyoideus

M. sternohyoideus

Fascia cervicalis, Lamina pretrachealis

Fascia cervicalis, Lamina superficialis

M. omohyoideus, Venter inferior

**Fascia cervicalis,
Lamina superficialis**

Clavicula

Trigonum omoclaviculare

Trigonum omoclaviculare

Platysma

V. jugularis externa

Spatium suprasternale

M. sternocleidomastoideus

Fossa supraclavicularis minor

Fig. 11.11   Cervical fascia, Fascia cervicalis, left side; ventral view. [S700]
The superficial lamina of the cervical fascia (Fascia cervicalis, Lamina superficialis) has been opened or removed in several places. The superficial lamina of the cervical fascia covering the M. sternocleidomastoideus has also been opened and the middle portion of the M. sternocleidomastoideus has been resected. Thus, the fascial sheath and the deep part of the superficial cervical fascia become visible. Above the Incisura jugularis of the sternum, the superficial fascia has been slit down to the Adam's apple of the larynx and has been folded back on both sides. Thereby the Spatium suprasternale is opened. Upon removal of the adipose tissue (the Arcus venosus jugularis can frequently be

found here, → Fig. 11.78), the middle lamina of the cervical fascia (Fascia cervicalis, Lamina pretrachealis) becomes visible, forming the posterior wall of the Spatium suprasternale. The superficial lamina of the cervical fascia is also removed down to the Mandibula and folded downward. Below this lamina, the tendon of the M. stylohyoideus, the M. mylohyoideus and the Venter anterior of the M. digastricus can be recognised. In the posterior triangle of the neck, the superficial cervical fascia has been removed from the clavicula and folded upward. Underneath, the V. jugularis externa can be seen, as well as an indication of the Venter inferior of the M. omohyoideus, which is ensheathed by the middle cervical fascia.

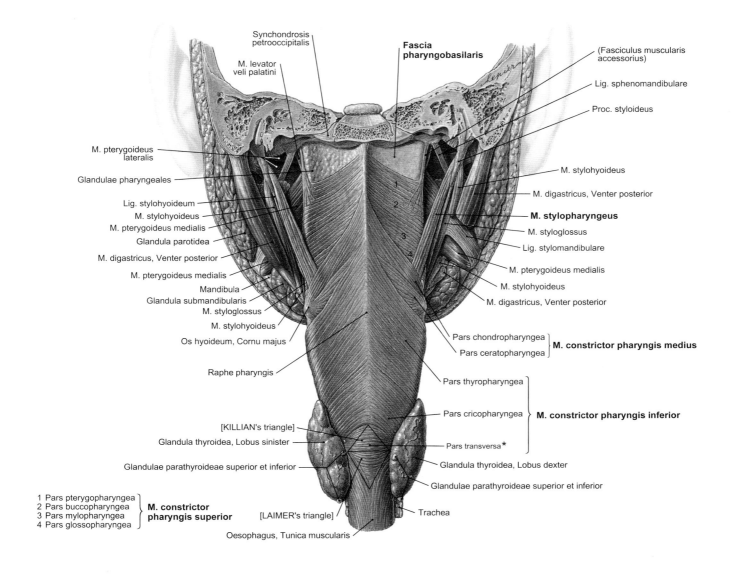

Fig. 11.12 **Pharyngeal muscles, Mm. pharyngis;** dorsal view. [S700]
The pharyngeal muscles (Tunica muscularis pharyngis) consist of the pharyngeal constrictors (Mm. constrictores pharyngis) and three pairs of pharyngeal levator muscles (Mm. levatores pharyngis). In the muscle-free upper part of the pharyngeal wall, the Tela submucosa and Tunica adventitia combine to form the Fascia pharyngobasilaris. The constricting and elevating pharyngeal muscles mainly act during swallowing, choking, as well as when speaking and singing.
The **Mm. constrictores pharyngis** superior, medius and inferior consist of different parts, enclosing the pharyngeal lumen in a horseshoe shape, and overlapping one another, with the inferior muscle slightly covering the lower margin of the superior muscle. The Pars cricopharyngea of the M. constrictor pharyngis inferior is composed of two muscle

parts which together form a triangle which is weak in muscle fibres (KILLIAN's dehiscence or KILLIAN's triangle). Dorsally, at the transition from the Pars fundiformis of the M. constrictor pharyngis inferior to the oesophagus there is also a muscle triangle (LAIMER's triangle), formed by radiating oesophageal muscle fibres. Standing on its head, the tip of the LAIMER's triangle touches the tip of the KILLIAN's triangle. The Pars fundiformis (of the Pars cricopharyngea of the M. constrictor pharyngis inferior) forms the basis for both triangles.
The muscles elevating the pharynx are the **Mm. palatopharyngeus, salpingopharyngeus** and **stylopharyngeus.**

* Pars fundiformis of the Pars cricopharyngea (KILLIAN's muscle)

→ T 6

Clinical remarks

KILLIAN's triangle can be a vulnerable point because of its muscle weakness, particularly in elderly men of advanced age. Due to increased intraluminal pressure, the pharyngeal wall bulges out through the muscular weak point as a **pharyngeal diverticulum** (ZENKER's diverticulum) into the retropharyngeal space. It can be filled with partly digested food, which leads to regurgitation (reflux) of undigested food into the oral cavity.
[S700-L127]

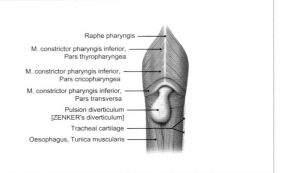

Attachment point and vascularisation of the pharynx

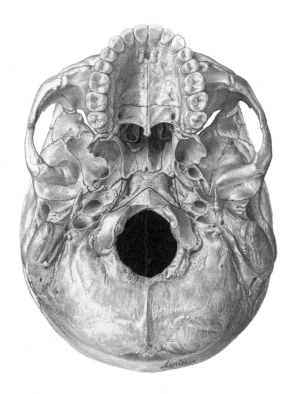

Fig. 11.13   Base of the skull, Basis cranii externa, with attachment point of the Fascia pharyngobasilaris and openings to the Spatium lateropharyngeum; caudal view. [S700]
The pharynx is suspended by the **Fascia pharyngobasilaris** (red line), located immediately in front of the cervical spine. The Fascia pharyngobasilaris is therefore located directly in front of the occipital condyles, and is laterally attached to the cranial base along the border between

the Os sphenoidale and Os occipitale. Lateral to these structures, the passageways of the A. carotis interna, V. jugularis, N. glossopharyngeus [IX], vagus [X], accessorius [XI] as well as the Truncus sympathicus are visible (as the Plexus caroticus internus), which cross over via the cranial base (→ Fig. 11.21, → Fig. 11.22 and → Fig. 11.24) on their way out of the Spatium lateropharyngeum (blue circles) or into it.

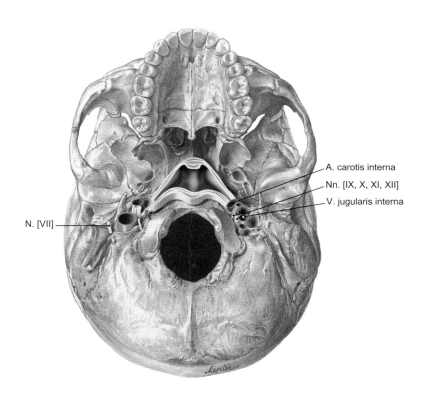

N. [VII]

A. carotis interna
Nn. [IX, X, XI, XII]
V. jugularis interna

Fig. 11.14   Passage of vessels and nerves of the pharynx and attachment point of the pharynx in the region of the base of the skull; caudal view. [S700-L127]

The attachment point of the pharynx at the base of the skull lies directly in front of the Foramen magnum. Laterally the vessels and nerves that accompany the pharynx pass through the base of the skull (see also → Fig. 11.18, → Fig. 11.19).

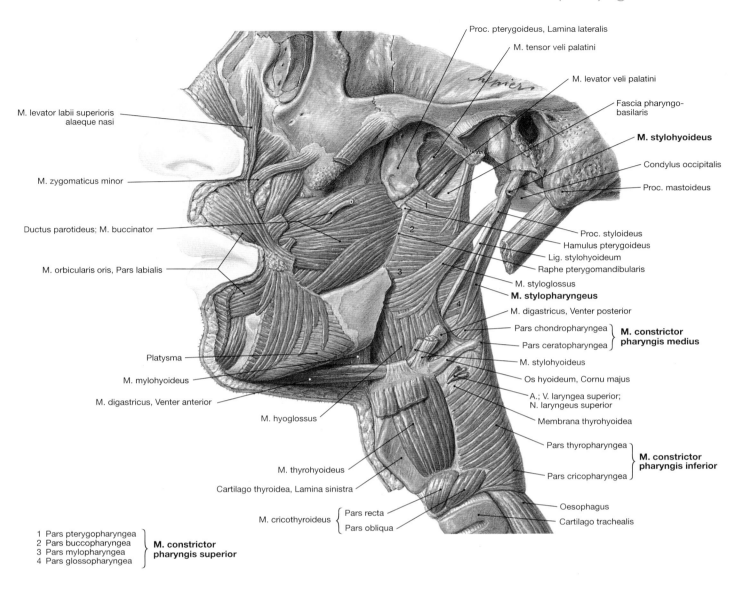

Proc. pterygoideus, Lamina lateralis
M. tensor veli palatini
M. levator veli palatini
Fascia pharyngo-basilaris
M. stylohyoideus
Condylus occipitalis
Proc. mastoideus
Proc. styloideus
Hamulus pterygoideus
Lig. stylohyoideum
Raphe pterygomandibularis
M. styloglossus
M. stylopharyngeus
M. digastricus, Venter posterior
Pars chondropharyngea
Pars ceratopharyngea } **M. constrictor pharyngis medius**
M. stylohyoideus
Os hyoideum, Cornu majus
A.; V. laryngea superior; N. laryngeus superior
Membrana thyrohyoidea
Pars thyropharyngea
Pars cricopharyngea } **M. constrictor pharyngis inferior**
Oesophagus
Cartilago trachealis

M. levator labii superioris alaeque nasi
M. zygomaticus minor
Ductus parotideus; M. buccinator
M. orbicularis oris, Pars labialis
Platysma
M. mylohyoideus
M. digastricus, Venter anterior
M. hyoglossus
M. thyrohyoideus
Cartilago thyroidea, Lamina sinistra
M. cricothyroideus { Pars recta / Pars obliqua }

1 Pars pterygopharyngea
2 Pars buccopharyngea
3 Pars mylopharyngea
4 Pars glossopharyngea
} **M. constrictor pharyngis superior**

Fig. 11.15 Pharyngeal muscles, Mm. pharyngis, and facial muscles, Mm. faciei, left side; lateral view. [S700]
The pharyngeal muscles divide into constrictor muscles (Mm. constrictores pharyngis superior, medius and inferior) and levator muscles (Mm. stylopharyngeus, salpingopharyngeus and palatopharyngeus). This lateral view displays the different parts of the Mm. constrictores pharyngis and the M. stylopharyngeus.

→ T 1.5, T 6, T 7

Fig. 11.16 Oropharyngeal muscle system; view from above. [S700-L127]
The muscles surrounding the oral cavity (M. orbicularis oris, Mm. buccinatores), together with the upper pharyngeal muscle (M. constrictor pharyngis superior), form an opposing muscle system which is crucially important for swallowing. The muscles form a closed ring. Points of attachment are the paired **Raphe pterygomandibularis,** stretching between the Proc. pterygoideus (Lamina lateralis), Hamulus pterygoideus and the Mandibula, as well as the occipitally located **Raphe pharyngis.**

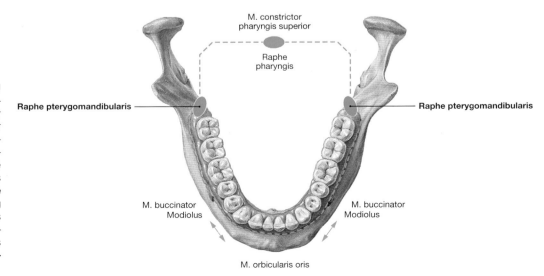

M. constrictor pharyngis superior
Raphe pharyngis
Raphe pterygomandibularis
Raphe pterygomandibularis
M. buccinator Modiolus
M. buccinator Modiolus
M. orbicularis oris

Topography

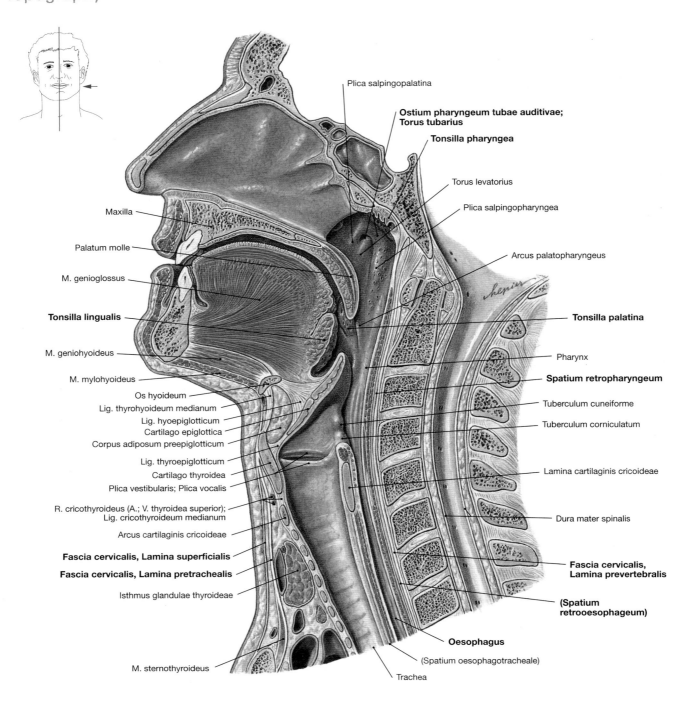

Plica salpingopalatina

**Ostium pharyngeum tubae auditivae;
Torus tubarius**

Tonsilla pharyngea

Torus levatorius

Plica salpingopharyngea

Maxilla

Palatum molle

M. genioglossus

Arcus palatopharyngeus

Tonsilla lingualis

Tonsilla palatina

M. geniohyoideus

Pharynx

M. mylohyoideus

Spatium retropharyngeum

Os hyoideum

Lig. thyrohyoideum medianum

Tuberculum cuneiforme

Lig. hyoepiglotticum

Tuberculum corniculatum

Cartilago epiglottica

Corpus adiposum preepiglotticum

Lig. thyroepiglotticum

Cartilago thyroidea

Lamina cartilaginis cricoideae

Plica vestibularis; Plica vocalis

R. cricothyroideus (A.; V. thyroidea superior);
Lig. cricothyroideum medianum

Dura mater spinalis

Arcus cartilaginis cricoideae

Fascia cervicalis, Lamina superficialis

**Fascia cervicalis,
Lamina prevertebralis**

Fascia cervicalis, Lamina pretrachealis

Isthmus glandulae thyroideae

**(Spatium
retrooesophageum)**

Oesophagus

(Spatium oesophagotracheale)

M. sternothyroideus

Trachea

Fig. 11.17 Oral cavity, Cavitas oris, pharynx, and larynx; midsagittal section. [S700]

Connections between the different sections of the pharynx with neighbouring structures:

- The **nasopharynx** (epipharynx, Pars nasalis pharyngis) connects with the nasal cavity via the choanae, and with the middle ear via the Tuba auditiva.
- The **oropharynx** (mesopharynx, Pars oralis pharyngis) represents the junction between the superior and inferior pharyngeal sections and connects with the oral cavity via the Isthmus faucium.

- The **laryngopharynx** (hypopharynx, Pars laryngea pharyngis) has an anterior connection with the larynx via the Aditus laryngis and transitions caudally into the oesophagus. Respiratory and digestive pathways cross each other within the pharynx.

At the transition from the nasal and oral cavities to the pharynx, the WALDEYER's tonsillar ring is made from lymphoepithelial tissue, which is part of the immune system. It is formed by the Tonsillae pharyngea, tubariae (not shown), palatinae and lingualis, as well as by lateral 'strands' of lymphatic tissue located on the Plicae salpingopharyngeae.

Clinical remarks

Foreign bodies that are swallowed often end up in the Valleculae epiglotticae at the base of the tongue and can displace the airways by pressure on the epiglottis or lead to **bolus death** (reflexive cardiovascular arrest by vagal stimulation of the sensitive nervous plexus of the pharynx and larynx by a foreign body). This can occur after a big bolus (bite of food) becomes jammed in the laryngopharynx so that even a forceful cough (expectoration) will not eject it. Smaller, pointed foreign bodies such as fish bones or pieces of chicken bone mostly get stuck in the Tonsilla palatina.

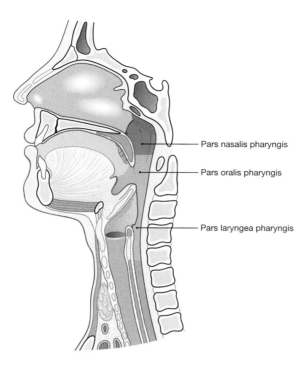

Pars nasalis pharyngis

Pars oralis pharyngis

Pars laryngea pharyngis

Fig. 11.18   Sections of the pharynx; midsagittal section. [S700-L126]
Corresponding with its openings, the pharynx can be divided into three sections:

• **upper section:** Pars nasalis pharyngis, epipharynx, nasopharynx (base of skull up to the upper margin of the Dens axis)

• **middle section:** Pars oralis pharyngis, mesopharynx, oropharynx (upper margin of the Dens axis up to the highest point of the epiglottis)

• **lower section:** Pars laryngea pharyngis, hypopharynx, laryngopharynx (highest point of the epiglottis up to the entrance of the oesophagus).

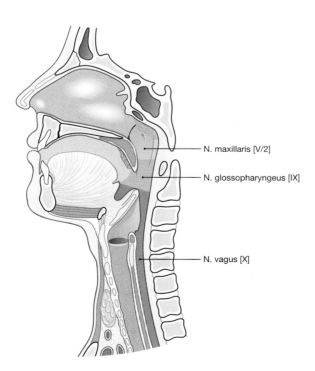

N. maxillaris [V/2]

N. glossopharyngeus [IX]

N. vagus [X]

Fig. 11.19   Sensory innervation of the pharynx; midsagittal section. [S700-L126]
Sensory fibres of the second trigeminal branch (R. pharyngeus, a branch of the Rr. ganglionares [Nn. pterygopalatini] of the N. maxillaris [V/2]) contribute to the innervation of the nasopharynx. Branches of the N. glossopharyngeus [IX] and the N. vagus [X] (N. laryngeus superior) innervate the rest of the pharynx. Together with autonomic nerve fibres of the Truncus sympathicus, these fibres form a neuronal network on the outer surface of the pharynx **(Plexus pharyngeus).** Afferent and efferent fibres of the Plexus pharyngeus are part of the vital swallowing and choking reflexes which remain active during sleep. The coordination of these complex reflexes takes place in the Medulla oblongata.

Act of swallowing

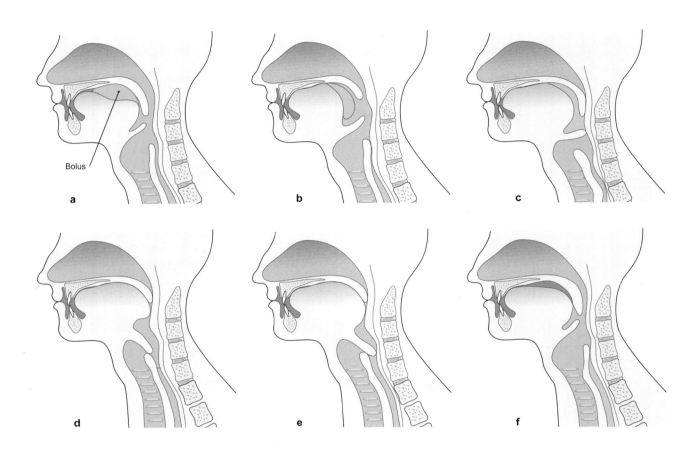

Bolus

a b c

d e f

Fig. 11.20a–f   Act of swallowing; median sagittal section. [R389-L106] The act of swallowing is divided into three phases:

- **Oral phase (1):** Hereby the food (green) is deliberately reduced in size in the oral cavity and insalivated **(a).** Subsequently, the tongue is pressed against the gums by contracting the floor of the mouth and the food bolus (green) is propelled in the direction of the Isthmus faucium **(b).**
- **Pharyngeal phase (2):** From this point the swallowing action continues reflexively and can no longer be interrupted. At the same time, the airways are protected during the coordinated transportation of food. Firstly, the M. tensor veli palatini and the M. constrictor pharyngis superior contract and form the PASSAVANT bar, which closes off the entrance to the nasopharynx **(c).** Because of the contraction

of the sphincter muscle system in the Isthmus faucium area and the tongue, the food bolus cannot return to the oral cavity and is pressed into the hypopharynx **(d).** Additionally, the laryngeal aperture and the glottis are closed off.

- **Oesophageal phase (3):** Peristaltic contractions of the pharyngeal musculature now follow, from cranial to caudal **(e).** At the same time, the pharyngeal muscles raise the larynx, and the pharynx is pulled across the food bolus, to some extent. In an upright position, fluids are propelled into the stomach by jerky movements of the floor of the mouth as well as by the M. constrictor pharyngis superior. Solid food components, as shown in the example, are transported with peristaltic contraction waves **(f).**

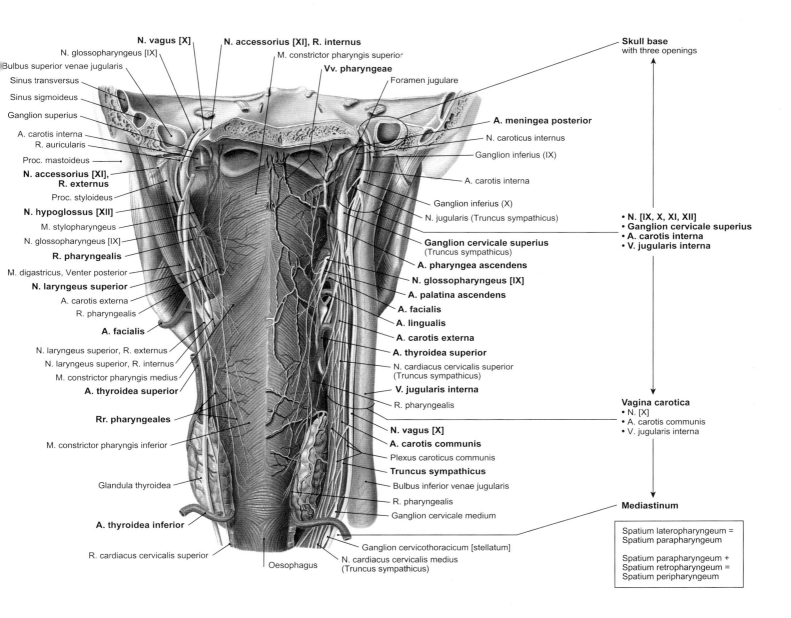

Fig. 11.21   Vessels and nerves of the pharynx and parapharyngeal space, Spatium lateropharyngeum; dorsal view. [S700]
The main source of the **blood supply** is the A. pharyngea ascendens. The artery ascends inside the parapharyngeal connective tissue, medial to the neurovascular bundle of the neck, upward to the cranial base. Its terminal branch, the A. meningea posterior, enters the posterior cranial fossa mostly via the Foramen jugulare. Additionally there are inflows in the area of the pharyngeal opening of the auditory tubes via the A. palatina ascendens and into the hypopharynx via the A. thyroidea inferior. The entire submucosa of the pharynx is permeated by a venous plexus (Plexus pharyngeus). The **venous draining** occurs via the Vv. pharyngeae into the V. jugularis interna, and in the area of the nasopharynx into the Vv. meningeae.

The **lymphatic drainage** of the Tonsilla pharyngea and the pharyngeal wall is directed to the Nodi lymphoidei retropharyngeales and Nodi lymphoidei cervicales profundi (not shown).
Innervation: In addition to the Plexus pharyngeus and the N. pharyngeus of the N. maxillaris [V/2] (see sensory innervation of the pharynx, → Fig. 11.19 and → Fig. 12.141), the N. glossopharyngeus [IX] provides motor innervation for the upper and also a part of the medial constrictor muscles, as well as for the levator muscles of the pharynx; the N. vagus [X] innervates the lower part of the medial pharyngeal constrictor muscle and the lower pharyngeal constrictor muscle.

Vessels and nerves of the parapharyngeal space

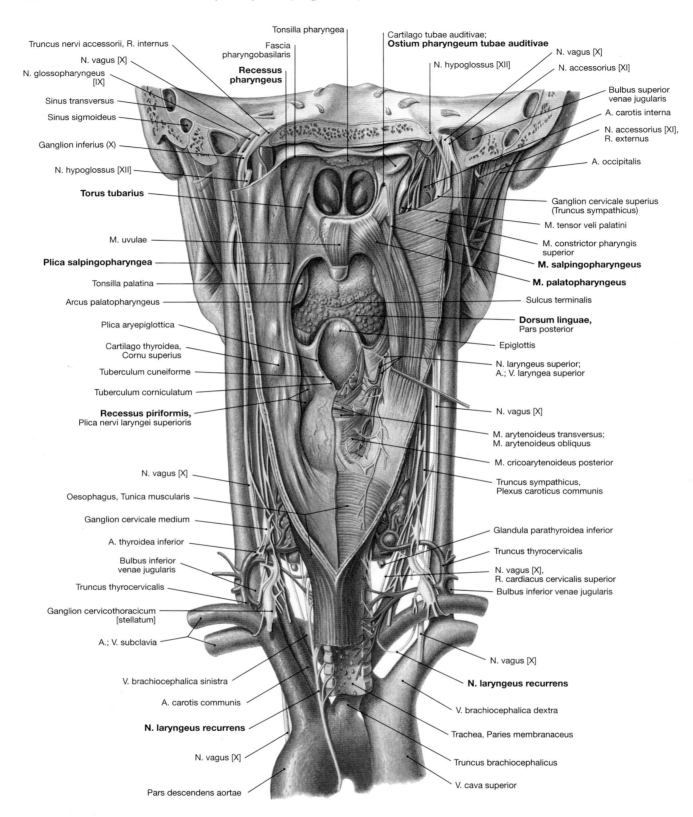

Truncus nervi accessorii, R. internus
N. vagus [X]
N. glossopharyngeus [IX]
Sinus transversus
Sinus sigmoideus
Ganglion inferius (X)
N. hypoglossus [XII]
Torus tubarius
M. uvulae
Plica salpingopharyngea
Tonsilla palatina
Arcus palatopharyngeus
Plica aryepiglottica
Cartilago thyroidea, Cornu superius
Tuberculum cuneiforme
Tuberculum corniculatum
Recessus piriformis, Plica nervi laryngei superioris
N. vagus [X]
Oesophagus, Tunica muscularis
Ganglion cervicale medium
A. thyroidea inferior
Bulbus inferior venae jugularis
Truncus thyrocervicalis
Ganglion cervicothoracicum [stellatum]
A.; V. subclavia
V. brachiocephalica sinistra
A. carotis communis
N. laryngeus recurrens
N. vagus [X]
Pars descendens aortae

Tonsilla pharyngea
Fascia pharyngobasilaris
Recessus pharyngeus

Cartilago tubae auditivae; **Ostium pharyngeum tubae auditivae**
N. hypoglossus [XII]
N. vagus [X]
N. accessorius [XI]
Bulbus superior venae jugularis
A. carotis interna
N. accessorius [XI], R. externus
A. occipitalis
Ganglion cervicale superius (Truncus sympathicus)
M. tensor veli palatini
M. constrictor pharyngis superior
M. salpingopharyngeus
M. palatopharyngeus
Sulcus terminalis
Dorsum linguae, Pars posterior
Epiglottis
N. laryngeus superior; A.; V. laryngea superior
N. vagus [X]
M. arytenoideus transversus; M. arytenoideus obliquus
M. cricoarytenoideus posterior
Truncus sympathicus, Plexus caroticus communis
Glandula parathyroidea inferior
Truncus thyrocervicalis
N. vagus [X], R. cardiacus cervicalis superior
Bulbus inferior venae jugularis
N. vagus [X]
N. laryngeus recurrens
V. brachiocephalica dextra
Trachea, Paries membranaceus
Truncus brachiocephalicus
V. cava superior

Fig. 11.22 Vessels and nerves of the pharynx and parapharyngeal space, Spatium lateropharyngeum; dorsal view; pharynx opened dorsally. [S700]

The opening of the auditory tube (Ostium pharyngeum tubae auditivae) is positioned approx. at the same level as the inferior nasal meatus. It is framed from the back and the top by the torus of the auditory tube **(Torus tubarius).** Caudally, the Torus tubarius extends into a longitudinal mucosal fold (Plica salpingopharyngea) which is created by the M. salpingopharyngeus. The inferior part of the Ostium pharyngeum tubae auditivae displays another elevation, the **Torus levatorius,** which forms on the M. levator veli palatini. This orifice is the entrance to the

Tuba auditiva (EUSTACHIAN tube) and connects the Pars nasalis pharyngis with the tympanic cavity. Directly behind the Torus tubarius is a depression (Recessus pharyngeus, fossa of ROSENMÜLLER) which extends cranially to the roof of the pharynx. The M. palatopharyngeus forms the lateral margin of the Isthmus faucium. Looking further down from the dorsal side at the dorsum of the tongue (Dorsum linguae), one can see the entrance into the oesophagus at the back of the larynx. On both sides of the posterior laryngeal wall is the Recessus piriformis. Note the different pathways of the N. laryngeus recurrens; on the left it winds around the Arcus aortae and on the right around the A. subclavia.

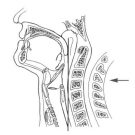

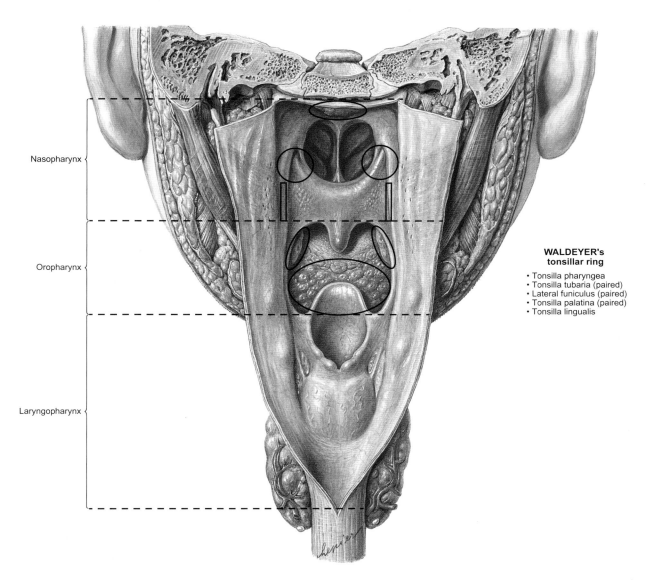

Nasopharynx

Oropharynx

WALDEYER's tonsillar ring

- Tonsilla pharyngea
- Tonsilla tubaria (paired)
- Lateral funiculus (paired)
- Tonsilla palatina (paired)
- Tonsilla lingualis

Laryngopharynx

Fig. 11.23 Lymphatic tissue in the region of the pharynx; dorsal view, pharynx opened dorsally. [S700]
In the region of the pharynx, lymphatic tissue is arranged in the shape of a lymphatic ring (lymphatic pharyngeal ring, WALDEYER's tonsillar ring). An aggregation of lymphoepithelial tissue is located at the transition from the oral to the nasal cavity in the pharynx. The lymphatic phar-

yngeal ring serves the immune defence and belongs to the mucosa-associated lymphatic tissue (MALT). The lymphatic pharyngeal ring surrounds the lingual tonsils (Tonsilla lingualis, unpaired), the palatine tonsils (Tonsilla palatina, paired), the lateral funiculi (paired), the tubal tonsils (Tonsilla tubaria, paired) and the pharyngeal tonsils (Tonsilla pharyngea, unpaired, compare table below, → Fig. 8.170).

Spatium peripharyngeum

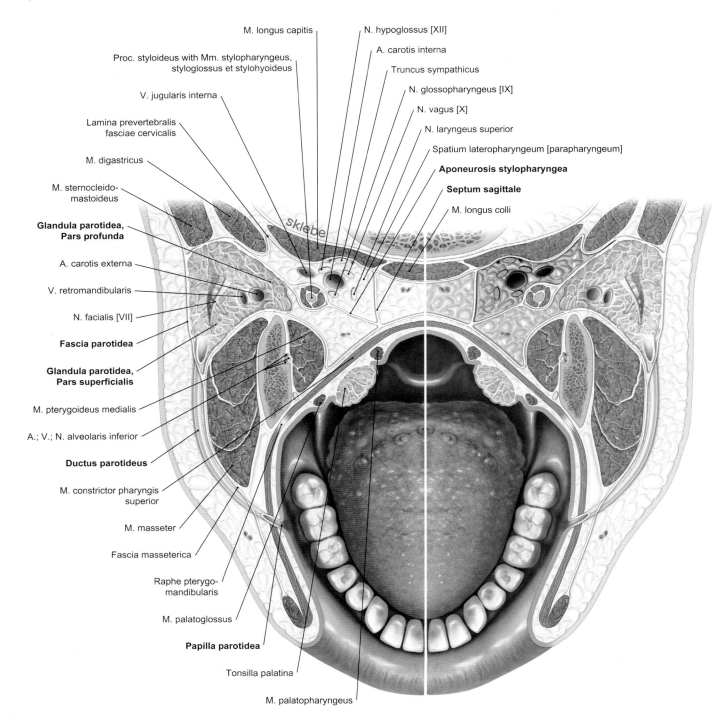

M. longus capitis

N. hypoglossus [XII]

Proc. styloideus with Mm. stylopharyngeus,
styloglossus et stylohyoideus

A. carotis interna

Truncus sympathicus

V. jugularis interna

N. glossopharyngeus [IX]

N. vagus [X]

Lamina prevertebralis
fasciae cervicalis

N. laryngeus superior

Spatium lateropharyngeum [parapharyngeum]

M. digastricus

Aponeurosis stylopharyngea

M. sternocleido-
mastoideus

Septum sagittale

M. longus colli

**Glandula parotidea,
Pars profunda**

A. carotis externa

V. retromandibularis

N. facialis [VII]

Fascia parotidea

**Glandula parotidea,
Pars superficialis**

M. pterygoideus medialis

A.; V.; N. alveolaris inferior

Ductus parotideus

M. constrictor pharyngis
superior

M. masseter

Fascia masseterica

Raphe pterygo-
mandibularis

M. palatoglossus

Papilla parotidea

Tonsilla palatina

M. palatopharyngeus

Fig. 11.24 Spatium lateropharyngeum and Spatium retropharyngeum; horizontal section at the level of the oral cavity. [S700-L238]/
[G1086]

Between the pharynx (M. constrictor pharyngis superior) and the prevertebral neck muscles (Mm. longus colli and longus capitis) is the **Spatium peripharyngeum** (green + purple). It includes the **Spatium lateropharyngeum** (purple) and the **Spatium retropharyngeum** (green), which are separated from each other sagittally by the septum, as well as by the Aponeurosis stylopharyngea. The Spatium retropharyngeum is divided into two sections. The deep part (Pars profunda) of the Glandula parotidea is laterally adjacent to the Spatium peripharyngeum, M. pterygoideus medialis and M. digastricus (Venter posterior). Passing

through the Spatium lateropharyngeum are the A. carotis interna, the V. jugularis interna, the N. glossopharyngeus [IX], the N. vagus [X] (as well as the N. laryngeus superior, after branching off), the N. accessorius [XI] (which leaves the space at an early point just below the cranial base), and the N. hypoglossus [XII]. The Truncus sympathicus runs inside the upper part of the neck, together with the aforementioned cranial nerves, in the Spatium lateropharyngeum, pierces the Lamina prevertebralis of the cervical fascia approx. in the middle of the neck and runs in the lower half on the prevertebral neck muscles. Between the Spatium lateropharyngeum and the Spatium retropharyngeum is the Proc. styloideus with the Mm. stylopharyngeus, styloglossus and stylohyoideus attached to it.

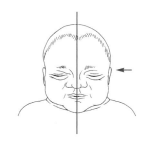

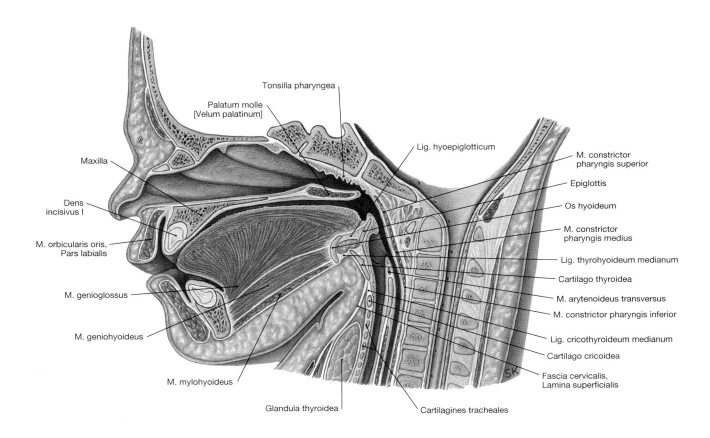

Fig. 11.25 Facial portion of the head, caput, and neck, collum, of a newborn; right paramedian sagittal section; medial view of the right side. [S700-L238]

In newborns and infants the larynx is much higher than in adults (→ Fig. 11.17). Unlike adults and children, babies can drink and breathe simultaneously (→ Fig. 11.26). Certainly within a few days or weeks after the birth, breathing and swallowing begin to synchronise and adjust in the sense of switching between breathing and swallowing.

In the clinic

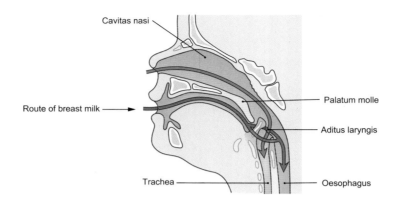

Fig. 11.26 Head of an infant; midsagittal section at the level of the nose and larynx. [S700-L126]/[E402-004]
Infants can drink and breathe at the same time. Since the larynx is located relatively high in the neck (Fig. 11.25), the epiglottis reaches as far as the nasopharynx. The liquids (breast milk) flow through the Recessus piriformis of the larynx into the oesophagus and do not pass into the lower respiratory tract. As part of the coordinated process between the different muscle groups of the oral cavity and the larynx, as well as the respiratory musculature, within a few days to weeks after the birth, synchronisation between breathing and the swallowing process takes place as part of a coordinated changeover, so that the descensus of the larynx (determined by the growing process) does not play a role in the swallowing process.

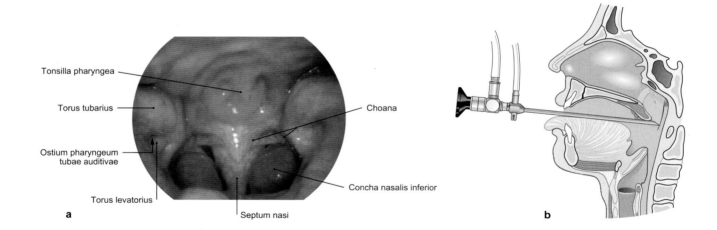

Fig. 11.27a and b Nasopharynx; endoscopy of the nasopharynx.
a Dorsal view on the choanae, the bilateral opening of the Tuba auditiva and the Tonsilla pharyngea. [S700-T720]
b Position and viewing angle of the endoscopy. [S700-L126]

The endoscopic view from posterior into the nasopharyngeal space shows the posterior ends of the inferior nasal concha and the entrance to the Tuba auditiva (Ostium pharyngeum tubae auditivae). Located at the roof of the pharynx is the inconspicuous Tonsilla pharyngea.

Clinical remarks

Compared to adults, the entrance to the Tuba auditiva in infants is approx. 1 cm deeper and thereby at the level of the palate. Bottle-feeding in particular, with the child lying horizontally, can lead to **Otitis media** if milk runs into the tympanic cavity.
Hyperplasia of the pharyngeal tonsils **(adenoids)** are common in childhood and often lead to recurrent middle ear infections due to an occlusion of the pharyngeal opening of the auditory tube. This can result in hearing impairment and subsequent developmental delays.

In such cases, a removal of the Tonsilla pharyngea **(adenoidectomy)** is indicated.
In front of the Tonsilla pharyngea, a **Hypophysis pharyngealis** (pharyngeal pituitary gland) may be present in the connective tissue on the lower surface of the sphenoid al bone, which is a remnant of the stalk of the embryonic RATHKE's pouch. In young people, the Hypophysis pharyngealis can be the starting point for a **craniopharyngeoma**.

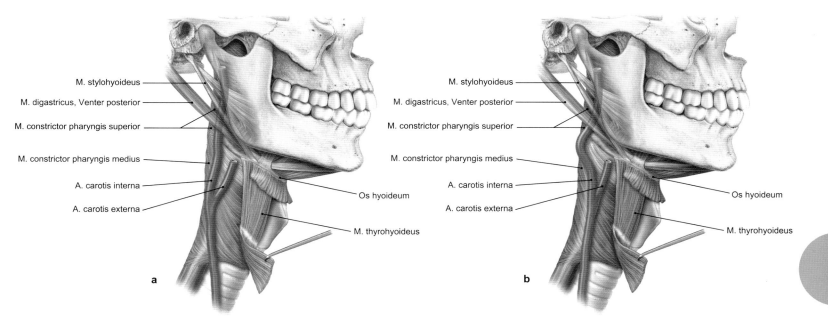

Straight variant of A. carotis interna

M. stylohyoideus
M. digastricus, Venter posterior
M. constrictor pharyngis superior
M. constrictor pharyngis medius
A. carotis interna
A. carotis externa

Os hyoideum
M. thyrohyoideus

a

Curved variant of A. carotis interna

M. stylohyoideus
M. digastricus, Venter posterior
M. constrictor pharyngis superior
M. constrictor pharyngis medius
A. carotis interna
A. carotis externa

Os hyoideum
M. thyrohyoideus

b

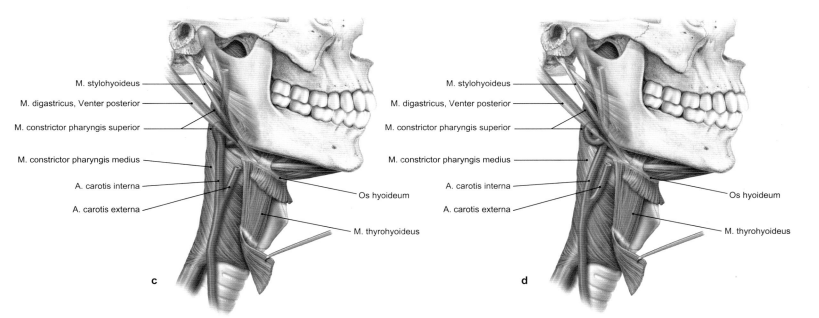

S-shaped pathway of A. carotis interna (kinking)

M. stylohyoideus
M. digastricus, Venter posterior
M. constrictor pharyngis superior
M. constrictor pharyngis medius
A. carotis interna
A. carotis externa

Os hyoideum
M. thyrohyoideus

c

Loop formation of A. carotis interna (coiling)

M. stylohyoideus
M. digastricus, Venter posterior
M. constrictor pharyngis superior
M. constrictor pharyngis medius
A. carotis interna
A. carotis externa

Os hyoideum
M. thyrohyoideus

d

Fig. 11.28a–d   Variants in the pathway of the Pars cervicalis of the A. carotis interna in relation to the pharyngeal wall. [S700-L238]
a Straight variant (frequency 66 %).
b Curved variant (frequency 26.2 %).

c S-shaped pathway (frequency 6 %, 2.8 % thereof in close association with the pharyngeal wall), regarded as **dangerous carotid loops.**
d Loop formation (frequency 1.8 %, 0.7 % thereof in close association with the pharyngeal wall), regarded as **dangerous carotid loops.**

Clinical remarks

Due to the close topographical relationship between the A. carotis interna and the tonsils (position of the Tonsilla palatina at the posterior margin of the Isthmus faucium) the presence of a so-called **dan-**gerous carotid loop** can result in the risk of injuries to the A. carotis interna with fatal bleeding during a tonsillectomy or the opening of a peritonsillar abscess.

Laryngeal skeleton

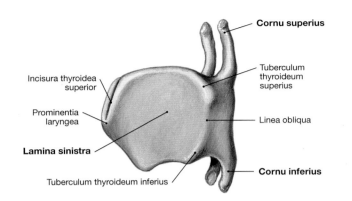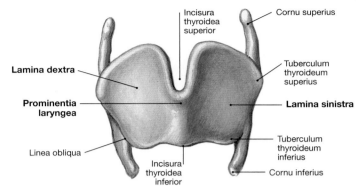

Fig. 11.29 **Thyroid cartilage, Cartilago thyroidea;** view from the left side. [S700]
The thyroid cartilage consists of two laminae (Lamina dextra and Lamina sinistra), each with a superior and inferior horn on the dorsal side.

Fig. 11.30 **Thyroid cartilage, Cartilago thyroidea;** ventral view. [S700]
Both of the lamina of the thyroid cartilage join at an angle of 90° in men and 120° in women.

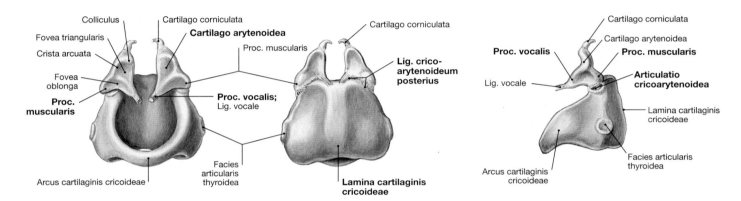

Fig. 11.31 **Cricoid cartilage, Cartilago cricoidea, and arytenoid cartilage, Cartilago arytenoidea;** ventral and dorsal views. [S700]
From the dorsal side, the Lig. cricoarytenoideum posterius can be seen between the cricoid and the arytenoid cartilages.

Fig. 11.32 **Cricoid cartilage, Cartilago cricoidea, and arytenoid cartilage, Cartilago arytenoidea;** view from the left side. [S700]
The cricoid and the arytenoid cartilages are connected via the Articulatio cricoarytenoidea, a diarthrosis.

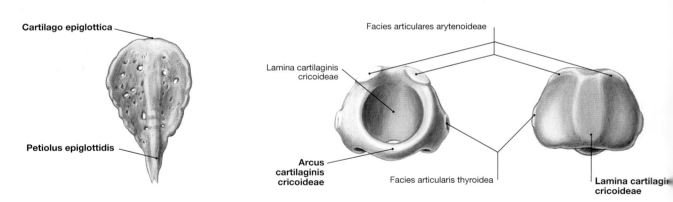

Fig. 11.33 **Epiglottic cartilage, Cartilago epiglottica;** dorsal view. [S700]
Unlike the other major hyaline laryngeal cartilages, the epiglottis is made of elastic cartilage.

Fig. 11.34 **Cricoid cartilage, Cartilago cricoidea;** ventral and dorsal views. [S700]
The cricoid cartilage is shaped like a signet ring.

Clinical remarks

From about 30 years of age, the ossification of the hyaline laryngeal cartilages (thyroid, cricoid and arytenoid cartilages) progresses in a gender-differentiated manner, and is very pronounced in men. **Fractures of the laryngeal skeleton** (e.g. car accidents) can result in severe obstruction of the airways, from difficulties in phonation through to danger of suffocation.

With surgical excision of the thyroid cartilage, for example because of a **hemilaryngectomy** due to a laryngeal carcinoma, the remaining laminae of the thyroid cartilage can be adjusted and connected with material used for osteosynthesis.
In rare cases, a congenital softening of the laryngeal cartilage (**laryngomalacia**) can cause difficulties in breathing (dyspnoea).

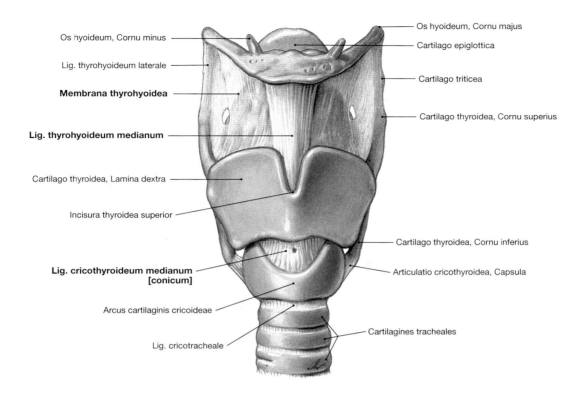

Os hyoideum, Cornu minus

Lig. thyrohyoideum laterale

Membrana thyrohyoidea

Lig. thyrohyoideum medianum

Cartilago thyroidea, Lamina dextra

Incisura thyroidea superior

**Lig. cricothyroideum medianum
[conicum]**

Arcus cartilaginis cricoideae

Lig. cricotracheale

Os hyoideum, Cornu majus

Cartilago epiglottica

Cartilago triticea

Cartilago thyroidea, Cornu superius

Cartilago thyroidea, Cornu inferius

Articulatio cricothyroidea, Capsula

Cartilagines tracheales

Fig. 11.35   Larynx and hyoid bone, Os hyoideum; ventral view. [S700]
Developmentally and functionally, the Os hyoideum has a close relationship with the laryngeal skeleton. The individual skeletal elements of the larynx are connected to each other by **syndesmosis** or by true joints **(diarthrosis).**

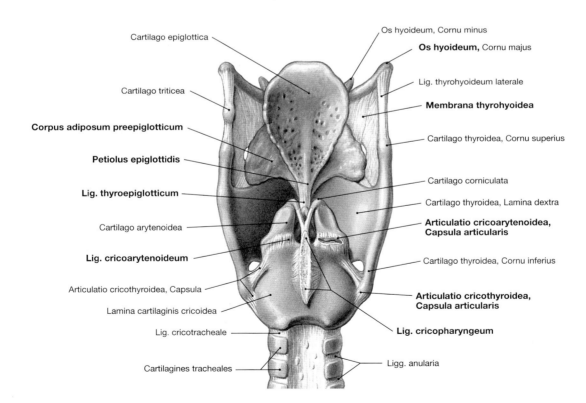

Cartilago epiglottica

Cartilago triticea

Corpus adiposum preepiglotticum

Petiolus epiglottidis

Lig. thyroepiglotticum

Cartilago arytenoidea

Lig. cricoarytenoideum

Articulatio cricothyroidea, Capsula

Lamina cartilaginis cricoidea

Lig. cricotracheale

Cartilagines tracheales

Os hyoideum, Cornu minus

Os hyoideum, Cornu majus

Lig. thyrohyoideum laterale

Membrana thyrohyoidea

Cartilago thyroidea, Cornu superius

Cartilago corniculata

Cartilago thyroidea, Lamina dextra

**Articulatio cricoarytenoidea,
Capsula articularis**

Cartilago thyroidea, Cornu inferius

**Articulatio cricothyroidea,
Capsula articularis**

Lig. cricopharyngeum

Ligg. anularia

**Fig. 11.36   Laryngeal cartilages, Cartilagines laryngis, and hyoid
bone, Os hyoideum;** dorsal view. [S700]
Behind the Membrana thyrohyoidea is a fat body (Corpus adiposum preepiglotticum), which reaches the Lig. hyoepiglotticum cranially and the front surface of the epiglottis dorsal-caudally. The epiglottis is attached by its stalk (Petiolus epiglottidis) via the Lig. thyroepiglotticum to the inside of the thyroid cartilage.

True joints of the larynx are the **Articulatio cricothyroidea,** the paired joint between the Cartilago cricoidea and the inferior horns of the thyroid cartilage (Cartilago thyroidea) as well as the **Articulatio cricoarytenoidea** between the cricoid and arytenoid cartilages. The Lig. cricoarytenoideum and the Lig. cricopharyngeum act as dorsal reins for the arytenoid cartilage.

Laryngeal skeleton

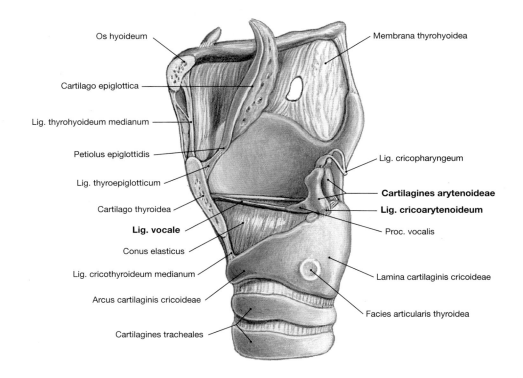

Fig. 11.37 Larynx and hyoid bone, Os hyoideum; view from the left side on Lig. vocale and arytenoid cartilage; the left lamina of the thyroid cartilage removed. [S700]
The cricoid (Cartilago cricoidea) and arytenoid cartilages (Cartilago arytenoidea) articulate within the Articulatio cricoarytenoidea. The articular surfaces of the Cartilago cricoidea are convex and oval in size (cylinder-shaped, → Fig. 11.34); the articular surface of the Cartilago arytenoidea is concave-shaped and rounder. Besides forming the articulating skeletal parts, a dorsal reinforcement of the capsule, the Lig. cricoarytenoideum (posterius) also ensures movements of the joint. Functionally, this ligament gives attachment to the arytenoid cartilage and counteracts the elastic force of the Lig. vocale.

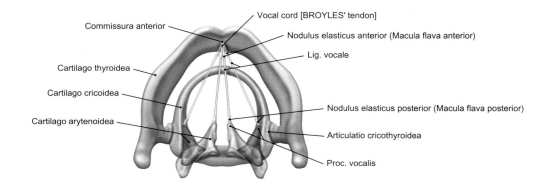

Fig. 11.38 Larynx; median section; superior view. [S700-L238]
The cricoarytenoid joint enables rotational and gliding motions parallel to the cylindrical axis; this joint primarily supports the opening and closing of the space between the Ligg. vocalia (glottis, Rima glottidis) and also tenses the vocal ligament (Lig. vocale). The rotation of the Cartilago arytenoidea, which is like a hinge moving outwards, leads to the raising and abduction of the Proc. vocalis and consecutively to the **opening of the glottis.** The inward rotation of the hinge as well as lowering and adducting the Proc. vocalis leads to the **closing of the glottis.** The hinge movements can be coupled with gliding movements. By doing so, the Cartilago arytenoidea moves with abduction and adduction ventrally or dorsally. The arytenoid and thyroid cartilages remain in contact with each other via the Lig. vocale and the Lig. vestibulare.

Clinical remarks

Endotracheal intubation and extubation, laryngoscopy or bronchoscopy can lead to dislocation of the arytenoid cartilage in the dorsolateral or medioventral direction. This is referred to as **arytenoid subluxation.** The patient has a hoarse voice as the Lig. vocale on the affected side is immobile. The displacement of the arytenoid cartilage leads to bleeding into the joint cavity or a reactive effusion after damage to the synovial membrane folds. The positional anomaly is maintained by muscle contractions. As a result, due to adherence of the joint surfaces, an ankylosis can occur. An arytenoid subluxation must be distinguished from a nerve lesion.

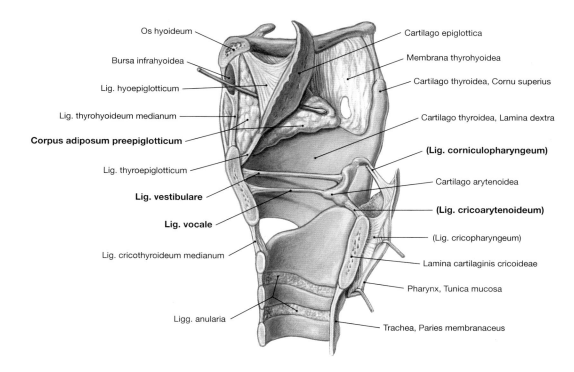

Fig. 11.39 Larynx and hyoid bone, Os hyoideum; median section, medial view. [S700]
The thyroid and cricoid cartilages are linked by the Articulationes cricothyroideae. The cricoid and arytenoid cartilages articulate via the Articulatio cricoarytenoidea. The thyroid and arytenoid cartilages remain in contact with each other via the Lig. vocale and the Lig. vestibulare. The Lig. cricoarytenoideum and the Lig. cricopharyngeum act as dorsal reins on the Cartilago arytenoidea. Laterally and in front of the epiglottis, the Corpus adiposum preepiglotticum can be seen.

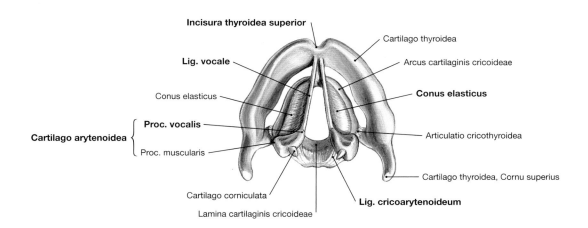

Fig. 11.40 Laryngeal cartilages, Cartilagines laryngis, and vocal ligament, Lig. vocale; superior view. [S700]
The paired Lig. vocale extends between the Proc. vocalis of the arytenoid cartilage and the inside of the thyroid cartilage just below the Incisura thyroidea superior. The Conus elasticus extends between the Lig. vocale and the upper rim of the cricoid cartilage. It is an elastic membrane which directs the air flow from the lungs in the direction of the Ligg. vocalia. The strong Lig. cricoarytenoideum can be seen dorsally behind the arytenoid cartilage.

Clinical remarks

Because the cricoarytenoid joint has an extracellular matrix comparable to limb joints, the same disorders such as those found in the major limb joints can occur. This can lead to degenerative cartilage changes **(degenerative arthritis)** in older people, affecting phona-tion and quality of voice due to improper occlusion of the glottis by the vocal ligaments. Also, joint infections **(infectious arthritis)** or rheumatism **(rheumatoid arthritis)** can occur.

Laryngeal muscles

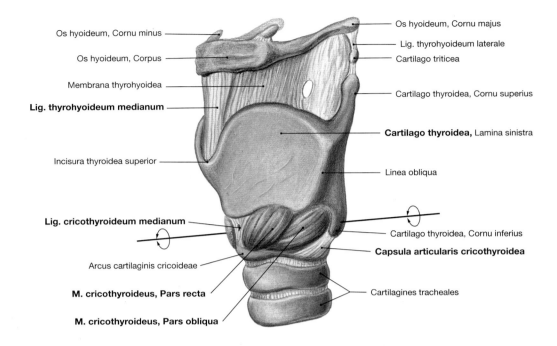

Fig. 11.41 **Cricothyroid muscle, M. cricothyroideus;** ventral view from the left side. [S700]
The cricoid cartilage (Cartilago cricoidea) and the thyroid cartilage (Cartilago thyroidea) articulate in the left and right Articulatio cricothyroidea. These are spheroidal (ball and socket) joints with a firm joint capsule.

This joint allows hinge movements around a transverse axis and small translational movements (shifting) in the sagittal plane. Contraction of the M. cricothyroideus increases the tension of the vocal folds → Fig. 11.42).

→ T 7

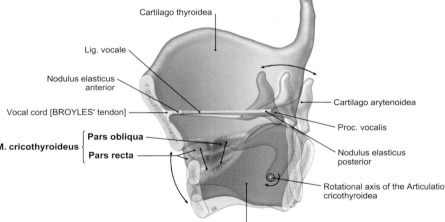

Fig. 11.42 **Cricothyroid muscle, M. cricothyroideus;** lateral view. [S702-L238]
During the contraction of the M. cricothyroideus, the anterior edge of the thyroid cartilage (Cartilago thyroidea) tilts in the direction of the cricoid cartilage arch (Arcus cartilaginis cricoideae). To an even greater extent, the anterior portion of the cricoid cartilage is pulled towards the lower front edges of the thyroid cartilage (excessive tension of the Plicae vocales with extension of the Lig. vocale). The arytenoid cartilages (Cartilagines arytenoideae) are stabilised in this movement by the M. cricoarytenoideus posterior and the Lig. cricoarytenoideum.

Biomechanics of the Plicae vocales: the structures at the attachment point of the vocal ligaments (**Noduli elastici anteriores** and **posteriores** as well as the BROYLES' ligament, → Fig. 11.63) perform biomechanical functions in the context of the oscillating vibrations of the Plicae vocales by adjusting the different elasticity modules of tendon, cartilage and bone. This prevents tearing (rupture) of the vocal ligaments from their point of attachment during oscillating vibrations.

→ T 7

Clinical remarks

Benign and malignant **changes in the area of the Plicae vocales** lead to incomplete closure of the glottis and are accompanied by hoarseness and, at an advanced stage, by shortness of breath. The Lig. cricothyroideum medianum [Lig. conicum] extends between the

thyroid and cricoid cartilages, and can be easily palpated there. In the event of an emergency, in order to maintain respiratory function, it can be split to insert a breathing tube (Clinical remarks for → Fig. 11.5).

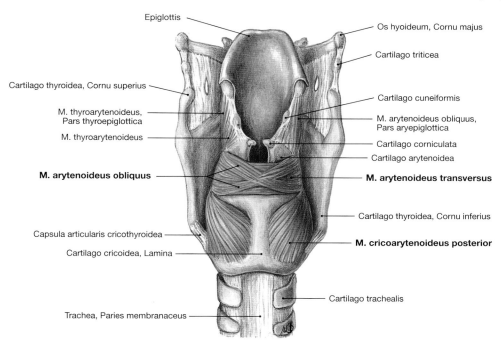

Fig. 11.43 Laryngeal muscles, Mm. laryngis; dorsal view. [S700]
Several laryngeal structures regulate the shape of the glottis (Rima glottides) and the tension of the vocal ligaments. The most important muscle is the **M. cricoarytenoideus posterior,** carrying out the abduction and elevation of the Proc. vocalis of the arytenoid cartilages, which results in the widening of the glottis when breathing in. The other muscles that attach at the arytenoid cartilages and facilitate the closing of the vocal ligaments are the **M. arytenoideus transversus** and the

M. arytenoideus obliquus as well as the **Mm. cricoarytenoidei laterales** (→ Fig. 11.44).
Whispering is also made possible by the isolated contraction of the M. cricoarytenoideus lateralis, which results in the so-called **'whispering triangle',** the formation of a small triangular opening in the posterior part of the Rima glottidis (→ Fig. 11.56).

→ T 7

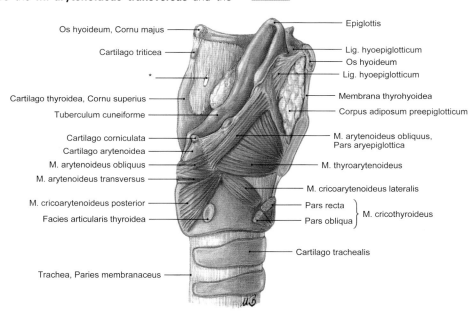

Fig. 11.44 Laryngeal muscles, Mm. laryngis; dorsal view obliquely from the right side, the posterior part of the right lamina of the thyroid cartilage with the horns is removed. [S700]
By removing the posterior part of the thyroid cartilage, the **M. thyroarytenoideus** becomes visible with its strong Pars externa (→ Fig. 11.46) and the Pars thyroepiglottica lying across it – the **Pars aryepiglottica** – which contributes to the lowering of the epiglottis, as well as the

muscular variant of a M. thyroarytenoideus superior. Coming below from the outside of the cricoid cartilage, the **M. cricoarytenoideus lateralis** extends to the Proc. muscularis of the arytenoid cartilage.
* point at which the Vasa laryngea superiora and the R. internus of the N. laryngeus superior pass through

→ T 7

Clinical remarks

After an isolated, unilateral **paralysis of the M. cricoarytenoideus posterior,** the Plica vocalis is in the paramedian position; a bilateral paralysis results in respiratory distress due to narrowing of the glottis and may even lead to death.

Dysphonia refers to all signs of a phonation ('speech sound') disorder. This also includes hoarseness in patients with a unilateral paralysis of the M. cricoarytenoideus posterior. **Aphonia** means the complete loss of voice.

Laryngeal muscles

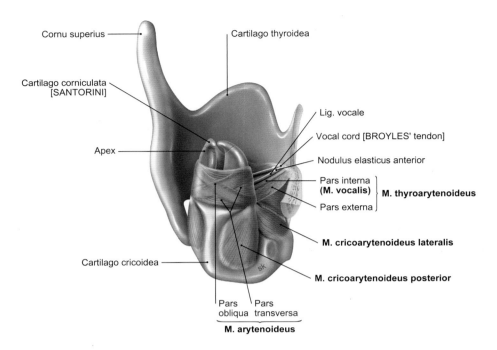

Fig. 11.45 Laryngeal muscles, Mm. laryngis; dorsal view. [S702-L238]
From this angle, the M. cricoarytenoideus lateralis and the Pars interna of the M. thyroarytenoideus (M. vocalis) can be seen. The M. cricoarytenoideus lateralis belongs to the arytenoid cartilages, narrowing the glottis. The **fine tension of the vocal folds** is due to the **M. vocalis** (Pars interna of the M. thyroarytenoideus), of which the muscle fibres run parallel to the Lig. vocale and Plica vocalis. The muscle creates a cushion which acts like the mouthpiece of a blowpipe. The tension of this mouthpiece is regulated by isometric muscle contractions and its length is shortened by isotonic muscle contractions. The M. vocalis thus has a decisive impact on the sound quality and the voice or vocalisation.

→ T 7

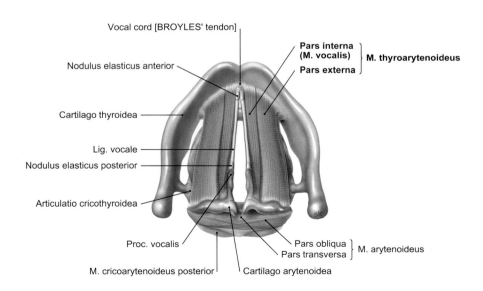

Fig. 11.46 Laryngeal muscles, Mm. laryngis; view from above. [S702-L238]
Lateral to the M. vocalis (Pars interna of the M. thyroarytenoideus) is the strong Pars externa of the M. thyroarytenoideus, which contracts to adduct and abduct the Proc. vocalis of the arytenoid cartilage, thus closing the Pars intermembranacea of the glottis (→ Fig. 11.50b).

→ T 7

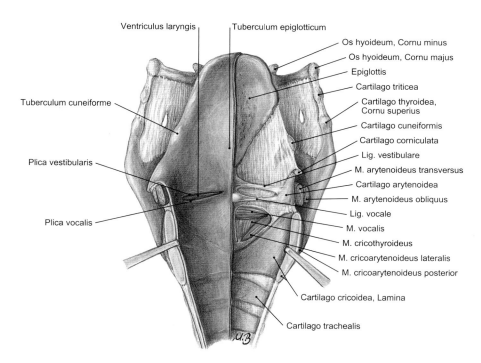

Ventriculus laryngis
Tuberculum epiglotticum
Os hyoideum, Cornu minus
Os hyoideum, Cornu majus
Epiglottis
Cartilago triticea
Cartilago thyroidea, Cornu superius
Cartilago cuneiformis
Cartilago corniculata
Lig. vestibulare
M. arytenoideus transversus
Cartilago arytenoidea
M. arytenoideus obliquus
Lig. vocale
M. vocalis
M. cricothyroideus
M. cricoarytenoideus lateralis
M. cricoarytenoideus posterior
Cartilago cricoidea, Lamina
Cartilago trachealis
Tuberculum cuneiforme
Plica vestibularis
Plica vocalis

Fig. 11.47 Larynx; dorsal view; the larynx was sectioned dorsally in the median plane and spread out with hooks. [S700]
On the left side, the mucosal lining is shown; on the right side, the laryngeal muscles (M. vocalis [= Pars interna of the M. thyroarytenoideus], M. cricothyroideus and M. cricoarytenoideus lateralis), the cartilages (epiglottis, arytenoid, cricoid and thyroid cartilages, as well as the small laryngeal cartilages), and the mucosal folds (Plicae vestibularis and vocalis) are depicted.

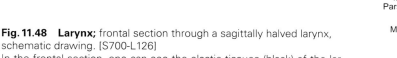

→ T 7

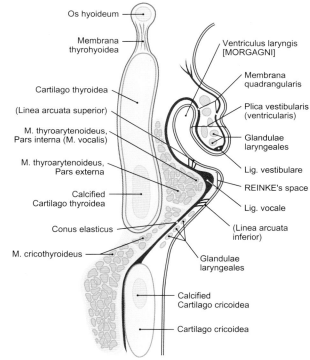

Os hyoideum
Membrana thyrohyoidea
Cartilago thyroidea
(Linea arcuata superior)
M. thyroarytenoideus, Pars interna (M. vocalis)
M. thyroarytenoideus, Pars externa
Calcified Cartilago thyroidea
Conus elasticus
M. cricothyroideus
Ventriculus laryngis [MORGAGNI]
Membrana quadrangularis
Plica vestibularis (ventricularis)
Glandulae laryngeales
Lig. vestibulare
REINKE's space
Lig. vocale
(Linea arcuata inferior)
Glandulae laryngeales
Calcified Cartilago cricoidea
Cartilago cricoidea

Fig. 11.48 Larynx; frontal section through a sagittally halved larynx, schematic drawing. [S700-L126]
In the frontal section, one can see the elastic tissues (black) of the larynx, which extend as a **Conus elasticus** from the top edge of the cricoid cartilage to the **Lig. vocale** of the Plica vocalis, and from here on as a **Membrana quadrangularis** below the mucosa of the Ventriculus laryngis to the top edge of the thyroid cartilage. In the vestibular fold or false vocal cord, the Membrana quadrangularis is thickened to the **Lig. vestibulare.** Below the mucosa of the Plica vocalis there is very loose connective tissue. It reaches cranially to the **Linea arcuata superior,** caudally to the **Linea arcuata inferior** and forms the **REINKE's space.** The loose connective tissue forms the base for the mucosal wave that takes place in phonation (→ Fig. 11.52). In the vestibular fold and below the mucosa of the subglottic area there are numerous bundles of glands that form a seromucous substance for moistening the Plicae vocales.

Clinical remarks

An accumulation of fluid in the REINKE's space creates a swelling of the Plicae vocales, which extends into the glottis and results in hoarseness and dyspnoea **(REINKE's oedema).** The REINKE's oedema must be distinguished from a **'glottic oedema'.** The latter means that fluid collects in the Lamina propria of the mucous membrane of the supraglottic space (e.g. in allergic reactions), and thus spreads out above the glottis. It leads to wheezing due to the narrowing of the lumen of the larynx, hoarseness and severe shortness of breath.

Inner surface of the larynx

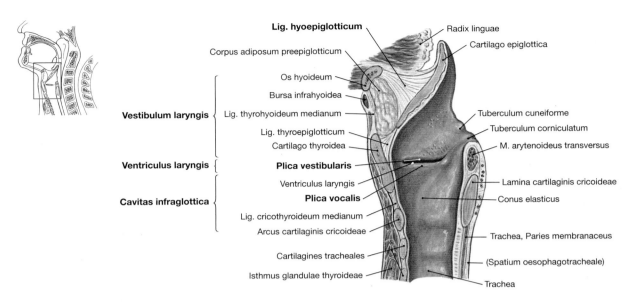

Fig. 11.49 **Larynx;** midsagittal section. [S700]

The paired vocal folds (Plicae vocales) are located below the paired vestibular folds (Plicae vestibulares) in the middle laryngeal section. The largest part of the Cavitas laryngis is lined by **respiratory epithelium.** In addition, there are some consistent areas of multilayered, non-keratinised **squamous epithelium,** which in other areas occurs only occasionally with interindividual variants. One can find it consistently on the Plicae vocales covering the Lig. vocale. It spreads further in the mucous membrane of the arytenoid cartilages and passes continuously into the squamous epithelium of the hypopharynx. The lingual surface of the epiglottis is covered with squamous epithelium. The distribution of both types of epithelium on the Plicae vestibulares and within the entire Cavitas laryngis can show significant individual variants. The expanse of the area of squamous epithelium changes in the course of a lifetime. With increasing age, laryngeal areas covered with squamous epithelium increase.

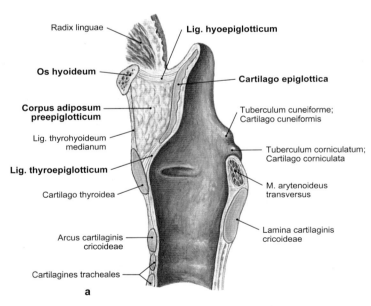

a

b

Fig. 11.50a and b **Larynx, position of the epiglottis;** midsagittal section. [S700]
a Epiglottis at rest.
b Epiglottis when swallowing.

During the swallowing process, the structures of the Aditus laryngis shift. The epiglottis is pushed downward by the food. This is supported by the M. aryepiglotticus (→ Fig. 11.44). The pre-epiglottic fat body moves dorsally, and the Aditus laryngis is narrowed.

Clinical remarks

The term 'vocal cords', used routinely in the clinical setting, is anatomically incorrect; the term should only be used to describe the Lig. vocale.

The squamous epithelium, which carries on growing within the larynx throughout one's life, can be the starting point of a **squamous cell carcinoma** of the larynx.

Fig. 11.51   Sections of the larynx. [S700-L238]

In clinical terms, the following areas of the larynx are differentiated:

Supraglottic space (supraglottis): It extends from the Aditus laryngis, up to the level of the Plicae vestibulares, and can be subdivided into the:

- epilarynx: laryngeal area of the epiglottis, Plicae aryepiglotticae and arytenoid cartilages
- Vestibulum laryngis: Petiolus epiglottidis, Plicae vestibulares = ventriculares, Ventriculus laryngis = ventricle of MORGAGNI.

Transglottic space (glottis): The glottis is an area containing the free margin of the Plicae vocales and is contrasted with the 'transglottic space', which surrounds the area containing the glottis, the vestibular folds and the Ventriculi laryngis. The anterior part of the glottis, including the anterior commissure (Commissura anterior) is known as the Pars intermembranacea; the dorsal part of the glottis between the arytenoid cartilages is the Pars intercartilaginea (→ Fig. 11.56) and constitutes two-thirds of the Rima glottidis. In their dorsal part, the Plicae vocales end at the transition of the Pars intercartilaginea into the Plica interarytenoidea (→ Fig. 11.56).

Subglottic space (subglottis): The subglottis is the space that extends below the Plicae vocales to the lower rim of the cricoid cartilage (Cartilago cricoidea). It is a conical space between the free margin of the Plica vocalis, the area below the Plica vocalis, and the lower margin of the cricoid cartilage. The cranial border of the subglottis is the macroscopically visible Linea arcuata inferior (→ Fig. 11.48) of the Plica vocalis. The caudal border is at the level of the lower rim of the subglottis. Craniolaterally, it is delimited by the Conus elasticus, and further caudally by the cricoid cartilage. The subglottic space which caudally has a cylindrical shape, narrows further cranially, corresponding to the shape of the Conus elasticus. The Lig. cricothyroideum [Lig. conicum] is defined as the ventral border, and the cricoid cartilage is defined as the dorsal border of the subglottic space.

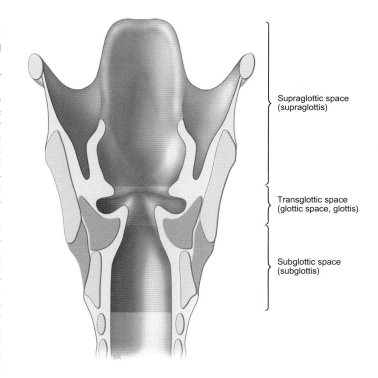

Supraglottic space
(supraglottis)

Transglottic space
(glottic space, glottis)

Subglottic space
(subglottis)

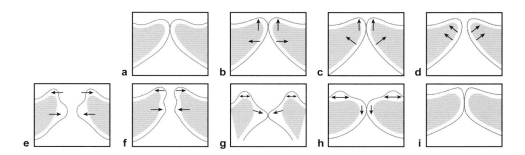

Fig. 11.52a–i   Mucosal waves of the vocal folds during the opening and closing phase; schematic drawing. [S702-L126]

For phonation, the mucosa of the Plicae vocales is set in motion by the forced airflow from the lungs, which is still bunched up by the shape of the Conus elasticus. This leads to harmonic motion (oscillating vibrations) of the Plicae vocales. The basis for this is the loose connective tissue of the REINKE's space. With sufficient tension of the vocal cords, **mucosal waves** are formed by the wave-shaped motion of the mucosa at the free margin of the Plicae vocales. When the 'mucosal wave' rolls towards the subglottic space and back again, the mucous membranes on both sides meet each other for a short period and completely stop the airflow. This increases the flow pressure and forces them to separate again. This results in a constant shift between the obstruction and release of the airflow (vibration): the Plicae vocales swing back and forth in the air stream.

a Starting position with closed Plicae vocales.

b–d The rising subglottic pressure reaches a threshold value, pushing the Plicae vocales apart. Initially there is a separation of the lower margins with an upward progression until both Plicae vocales are completely separated.

e–h The respiratory air is now directed (as if through a nozzle) into the supraglottis and the pharynx. The airflow leads sideways to a suction effect (BERNOULLI's principle), which results in the mucosal wave. The epithelium and the loose connective tissue of the REINKE's space (→ Fig. 11.48) is sucked in and contracted. The lower margins close first, and the upper margins follow once the airflow from the subglottic region is cut off (rolling of the epithelium on the Lig. vocale from bottom to top).

i The subglottic pressure forces the Plicae vocales to separate again, and a new cycle begins. Repeated cycles lead to rhythmic vibrations.

Clinical remarks

The subdivision of the larynx as described in → Fig. 11.51 is relevant for imaging techniques as part of the staging for **determining the spread of a tumour.** For the diagnostic imaging of the larynx, the recommended standard procedure is the spiral computed tomography (CT) in a thin-layered reconstruction. Although magnetic resonance imaging (MRI) is the most sensitive of all imaging techniques for tumour staging, this method is prone to significant motion artefacts due to patients' movements.

Laryngoscopy

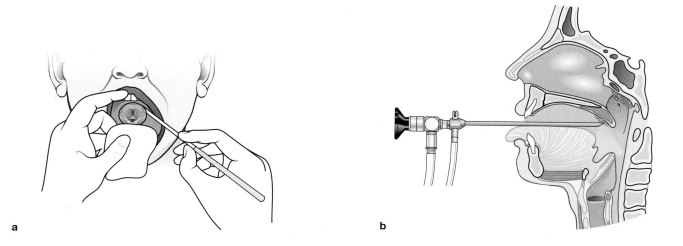

a

b

Fig. 11.53a and b   Laryngoscopy. [S700-L126]

a Indirect laryngoscopy.
b Direct endoscopic laryngoscopy.

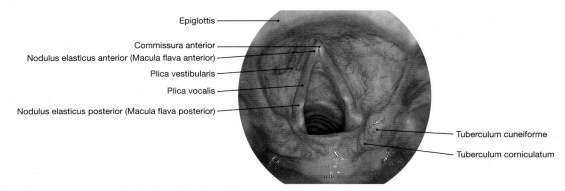

Epiglottis

Commissura anterior

Nodulus elasticus anterior (Macula flava anterior)

Plica vestibularis

Plica vocalis

Nodulus elasticus posterior (Macula flava posterior)

Tuberculum cuneiforme

Tuberculum corniculatum

Fig. 11.54   Direct laryngoscopy; respiration (breathing) position.
[S700-T719]

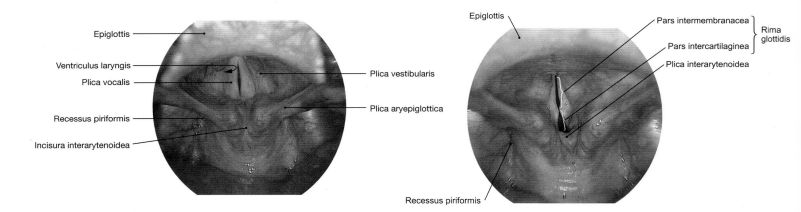

Epiglottis

Ventriculus laryngis

Plica vocalis

Recessus piriformis

Incisura interarytenoidea

Plica vestibularis

Plica aryepiglottica

Epiglottis

Pars intermembranacea

Pars intercartilaginea

} Rima glottidis

Plica interarytenoidea

Recessus piriformis

Fig. 11.55   Direct laryngoscopy; phonation (speaking) position.
[S700-T719]

Fig. 11.56   Direct laryngoscopy; whispering position. It is easy to recognise the 'whispering triangle' which is formed by the Partes inter-
cartilagineae and the Plica interarytenoidea. [S700-T719]

Clinical remarks

Overuse (in speaking professions) or misuse of the voice can lead to
the formation of **singer's nodules** on the free margin of the Plicae
vocales. Due to weakness of the M. arytenoideus, the Pars intercartilaginea of the Plica vocalis can no longer be closed (open whispering triangle). The voice sounds wheezy as a result.

The most frequently observed benign tumours of the Plicae vocales
are **polyps;** and **squamous cell carcinomas** are the most frequent
malignant tumours. In cases of longer-term intubation, **intubation
granuloma** may develop in the Pars intercartilaginea.

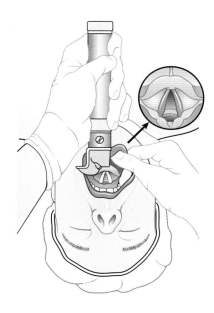

Fig. 11.57   Using a laryngoscope in preparation for an endotracheal intubation. [S701-L126]

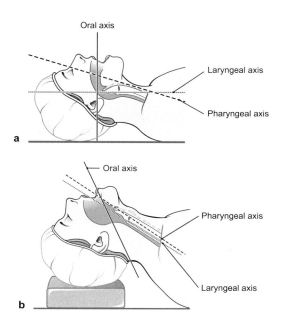

Fig. 11.58a and b   Position of the head during an endotracheal intubation. [S701-L126]
a Normal position of the head when lying down.
b For an endotracheal intubation, the head must be stretched back (by placing it on a cushion) so that the pharynx, larynx and oral cavity are positioned in an axis. In this way, one has a clear view of the endotracheal tube and can insert it into the trachea without causing injuries.

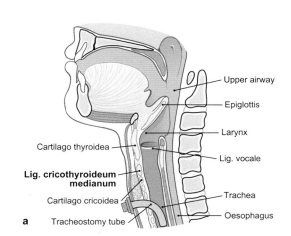

a

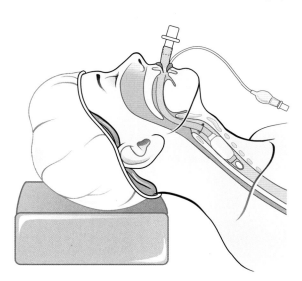

Fig. 11.59   Correct positioning of the endotracheal tube (with inflated balloon in the trachea). [S701-L126]

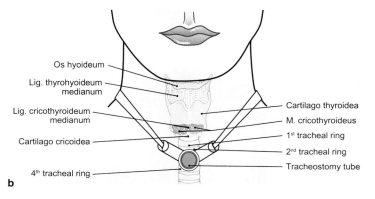

b

Fig. 11.60a and b   Performing a tracheostomy. [S701-L126]
a Lateral view.
b Anterior view.
The tracheal tube is placed below the larynx at the level of the third and fourth tracheal rings (lower tracheostomy). A tracheostomy can be necessary when the upper airways are obstructed (e.g. with a laryngeal carcinoma or with assisted ventilation). With a cricothyrotomy, however, the Lig. cricothyroideum medianum is severed (Clinical remarks below for → Fig. 11.5).

Arteries and nerves of the larynx

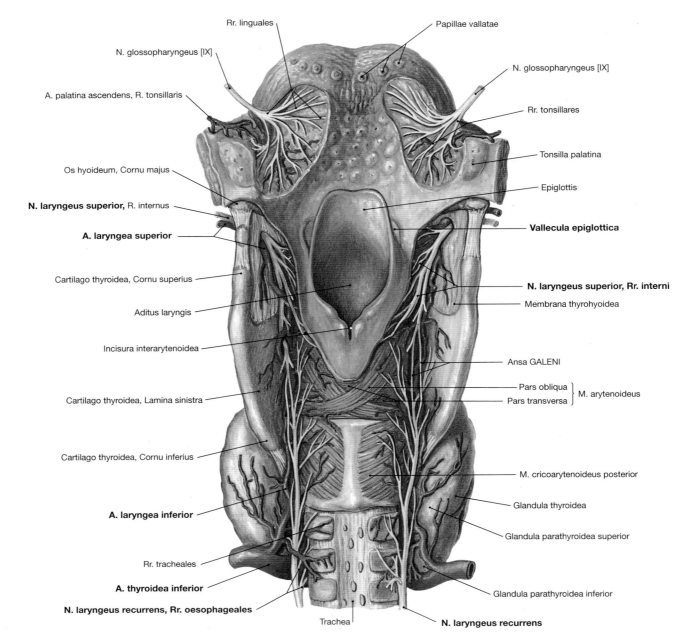

Rr. linguales

N. glossopharyngeus [IX]

Papillae vallatae

N. glossopharyngeus [IX]

A. palatina ascendens, R. tonsillaris

Rr. tonsillares

Tonsilla palatina

Os hyoideum, Cornu majus

Epiglottis

N. laryngeus superior, R. internus

Vallecula epiglottica

A. laryngea superior

Cartilago thyroidea, Cornu superius

N. laryngeus superior, Rr. interni

Membrana thyrohyoidea

Aditus laryngis

Incisura interarytenoidea

Ansa GALENI

Pars obliqua ⎫
⎬ M. arytenoideus
Pars transversa ⎭

Cartilago thyroidea, Lamina sinistra

Cartilago thyroidea, Cornu inferius

M. cricoarytenoideus posterior

Glandula thyroidea

Glandula parathyroidea superior

A. laryngea inferior

Rr. tracheales

Glandula parathyroidea inferior

A. thyroidea inferior

N. laryngeus recurrens, Rr. oesophageales

Trachea

N. laryngeus recurrens

Fig. 11.61 Arteries and nerves of the larynx and root of the tongue, Radix linguae; dorsal view. [S700]

The A. thyroidea superior originates from the A. laryngea superior. Below the Cornu majus of the Os hyoideum it penetrates the Membrana thyrohyoidea and bifurcates underneath the mucosa of the Recessus piriformis. There it forms numerous anastomoses and collaterals with the A. laryngea inferior.

The larynx receives bilateral innervation via **two branches of the N. vagus [X]:**

- The **N. laryngeus superior** is divided into a R. internus and a R. externus (→ Fig. 11.98). The R. internus runs laterally in the pharyngeal wall and passes together with the A. laryngea superior through the

Membrana thyrohyoidea into the larynx. Here it sensorily innervates the supraglottic mucosa, as well as the mucosa of the Valleculae epiglotticae and the epiglottis. The sensory innervation of the laryngeal mucosa is very dense (cough reflex). Apart from motor and sensory nerve fibres, the N. laryngeus superior also carries numerous parasympathetic fibres for the innervation of glands.

- The motor innervation of the inner laryngeal muscles is provided by the **N. laryngeus recurrens** [inferior]. Here the innervation of the two dorsal Mm. cricoarytenoideus posterior and arytenoideus can be seen. The connection between the N. laryngeus superior and N. laryngeus inferior is called GALEN's anastomosis. For the Nn. laryngei recurrentes pathway → Fig. 11.22 and → Fig. 11.72.

Clinical remarks

Damage to the N. laryngeus superior is accompanied by somatosensory disorders (frequent choking) and paralysis of the M. cricothyroideus. Insufficient tension of the Plicae vocales results in an incomplete glottic closure with speech or phonation disorders.

Acute oedema at the entrance to the larynx (e.g. due to allergic reactions) may fully extend into the loose connective tissue and lead to severe shortness of breath.

Acute bacterial infections of the epiglottis occur most frequently in children and can cause acute and life-threatening obstructions of the airways.

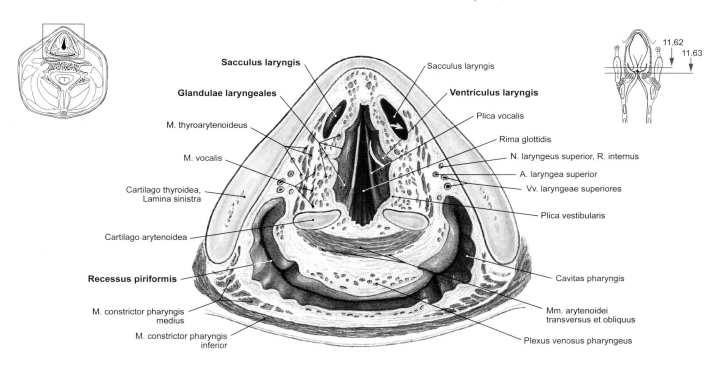

Sacculus laryngis

Glandulae laryngeales

M. thyroarytenoideus

M. vocalis

Cartilago thyroidea,
Lamina sinistra

Cartilago arytenoidea

Recessus piriformis

M. constrictor pharyngis
medius

M. constrictor pharyngis
inferior

Sacculus laryngis

Ventriculus laryngis

Plica vocalis

Rima glottidis

N. laryngeus superior, R. internus

A. laryngea superior

Vv. laryngeae superiores

Plica vestibularis

Cavitas pharyngis

Mm. arytenoidei
transversus et obliquus

Plexus venosus pharyngeus

Fig. 11.62 Larynx; transverse section at the level of the Plicae vestibulares. [S700]
The vestibular folds (Plicae vestibulares) contain multiple seromucous glands (Glandulae laryngeales) which serve to moisten the Plicae voca-

les. The white arrow indicates the connection between the Ventriculus laryngis and the Sacculus laryngis. Posterior to the larynx, the laryngopharynx can be seen along with the Recessus piriformis.

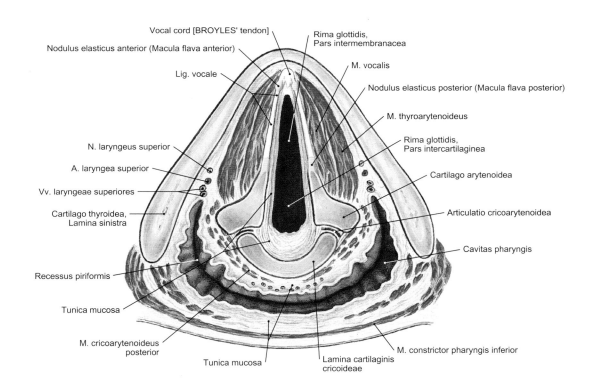

Vocal cord [BROYLES' tendon]

Nodulus elasticus anterior (Macula flava anterior)

Lig. vocale

N. laryngeus superior

A. laryngea superior

Vv. laryngeae superiores

Cartilago thyroidea,
Lamina sinistra

Recessus piriformis

Tunica mucosa

M. cricoarytenoideus
posterior

Tunica mucosa

Rima glottidis,
Pars intermembranacea

M. vocalis

Nodulus elasticus posterior (Macula flava posterior)

M. thyroarytenoideus

Rima glottidis,
Pars intercartilaginea

Cartilago arytenoidea

Articulatio cricoarytenoidea

Cavitas pharyngis

M. constrictor pharyngis inferior

Lamina cartilaginis
cricoideae

Fig. 11.63 Larynx; transverse section at the level of the vocal folds, Plicae vocales. [S700]
The section at the level of the true opening of the vocal ligaments (glottis, Rima glottidis) displays the mucosa (Tunica mucosa) of the vocal folds. Following from the inside to the outside: the vocal ligament (Lig. vocale), the M. vocalis (Pars interna of the M. thyroarytenoideus), and the Pars externa of the M. thyroarytenoideus. The cartilage-free part of the vocal fold is the Pars intermembranacea, the section between the

two arytenoid cartilages is the Pars intercartilaginea (→ Fig. 11.56). At the front, the vocal folds run towards the thyroid cartilage. The attachment point is referred to as the anterior commissure. Here, the vocal folds insert via Noduli elastici anteriores and the tendon of the Lig. vocale (BROYLES' tendon) in the thyroid cartilage. Dorsally, the Lig. vocale inserts via the Nodulus elasticus posterior on the Proc. vocalis of the arytenoid cartilage.

Position of the thyroid gland in relation to the larynx

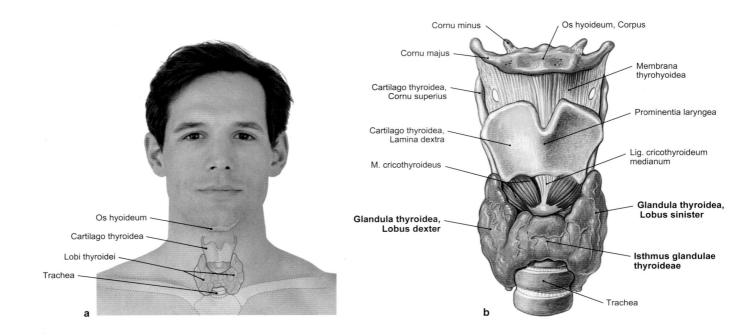

Fig. 11.64a and b   Position of the thyroid gland, Glandula thyroidea; ventral view.
a Position of the thyroid gland as projected onto the neck and the hyoid bone. [S700-J803/L126]

b Position of the thyroid gland below the larynx. The thyroid gland (weight in an adult 20–25 g) surrounds the upper part of the trachea on each side with a lobe (Lobus dexter and Lobus sinister) as well as at the front with an isthmus. [S700]

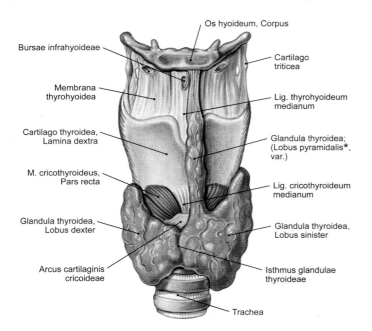

Fig. 11.65   Position of the thyroid gland, Glandula thyroidea, with Lobus pyramidalis; ventral view. [S700]
As an embryonic remnant of the descent of the thyroid gland, a Lobus pyramidalis often remains, spanning almost the centre and secured to the Os hyoideum by a strip of connective tissue. In a cricothyrotomy (Clinical remarks below for → Fig. 11.5) it can be a risk factor for unexpectedly severe bleeding.

* embryonic remnant of the Ductus thyroglossalis, present in approx. 30 % of the population

---

Clinical remarks

A **lobectomy** is the removal of the thyroid gland lobe, which can be necessary when removing the thyroid gland nodule; a complete removal of the thyroid gland (total thyroidectomy) is for instance carried out with patients with thyroid cancer.

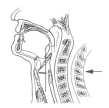

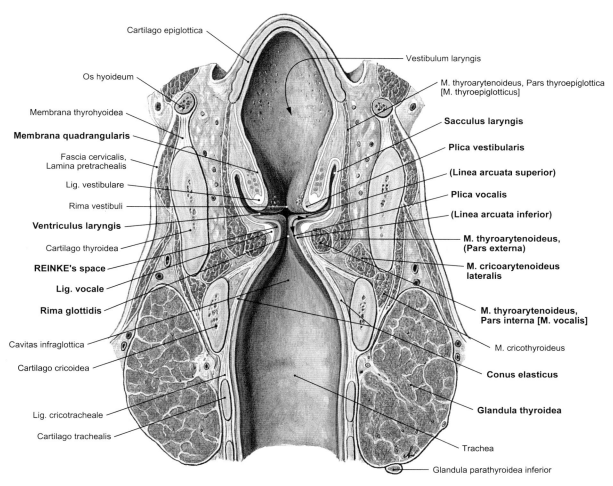

Cartilago epiglottica

Os hyoideum

Membrana thyrohyoidea

Membrana quadrangularis

Fascia cervicalis,
Lamina pretrachealis

Lig. vestibulare

Rima vestibuli

Ventriculus laryngis

Cartilago thyroidea

REINKE's space

Lig. vocale

Rima glottidis

Cavitas infraglottica

Cartilago cricoidea

Lig. cricotracheale

Cartilago trachealis

Vestibulum laryngis

M. thyroarytenoideus, Pars thyroepiglottica
[M. thyroepiglotticus]

Sacculus laryngis

Plica vestibularis

(Linea arcuata superior)

Plica vocalis

(Linea arcuata inferior)

**M. thyroarytenoideus,
(Pars externa)**

**M. cricoarytenoideus
lateralis**

**M. thyroarytenoideus,
Pars interna [M. vocalis]**

M. cricothyroideus

Conus elasticus

Glandula thyroidea

Trachea

Glandula parathyroidea inferior

Fig. 11.66   Thyroid gland, Glandula thyroidea, and larynx; frontal
section. [S700]
The two lobes of the thyroid gland are located at the transition between
the cricoid cartilage and the upper tracheal semicircular cartilages.
Normally, the Plicae vocales protrude further into the lumen of the larynx than the Plicae vestibulares, so that they can be assessed in a laryngoscopy (→ Fig. 11.53). The Plicae vocales are composed of an outer
mucosa, the Lig. vocale, the caudally adjacent Conus elasticus, and in
particular the M. vocalis (Pars interna of the M. thyroarytenoideus), and
the Pars externa of the M. thyroarytenoideus. The M. cricoarytenoideus

lateralis follows laterally. Together the Plicae vocales demarcate the
opening of the vocal ligaments (glottis, Rima glottidis) which represents
the part of the larynx responsible for phonation.
Subepithelial loose connective tissue above the Lig. vocale between
the Linea arcuata superior and the Linea arcuata inferior enables sliding
movements (REINKE's space, double arrow). The Ventriculus laryngis
extends between the Plicae vocales and the Plicae vestibulares. The
elastic connective tissue of the Membrana quadrangularis provides the
basis for the vestibular folds.

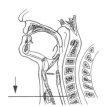

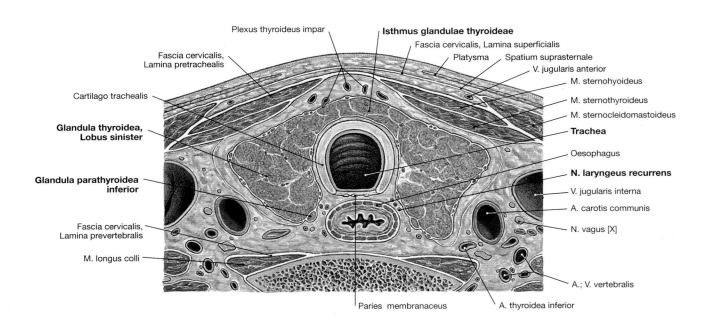

Fig. 11.67   Thyroid gland, Glandula thyroidea; horizontal section. [S700]
The thyroid gland covers the upper tracheal part laterally and ventrally. It is the largest endocrine gland in the body and secretes the hormones thyroxine (tetraiodothyronine, T4), tri-iodothyronine (T3), and calcitonin. The gland is ensheathed by its own capsule and, together with the larynx, trachea, oesophagus and pharynx, is surrounded by the general organ fascia.

Very variably, at the posterior side of each glandular lobe, there are two grain-sized epithelial bodies (parathyroid glands, **Glandulae parathyroideae**) weighing 12–50 mg each, which produce the parathyroid hormone (PTH). On both sides, the **N. laryngeus recurrens** runs between the trachea and the oesophagus. The nerve is located outside of the special organ fascia, but within the general organ fascia.

Clinical remarks

Thyroid gland surgery requires the ventral opening of the Fascia pretrachealis and the joined special and general organ fascia at the anterior side of the thyroid gland. Surgeons here refer to the outer (Fascia pretrachealis) and inner (organ fascia) thyroid capsule.

Hyperplasia, adenomas or carcinomas of the epithelial bodies may result in a glandular hyperactivity in the form of a primary **hyperparathyroidism.** The increased production of the parathyroid hormone leads to increased calcium levels in the serum and causes characteristic afflictions of the bones, kidneys and the gastrointestinal tract.

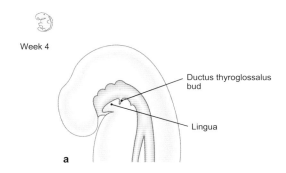

Week 4

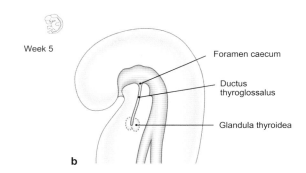

Week 5

Ductus thyroglossalus bud

Lingua

Foramen caecum

Ductus thyroglossalus

Glandula thyroidea

a

b

Fig. 11.68a and b Development of the thyroid gland. [E838]
a Development of the thyroid gland in the fourth week. From day 24, epithelium from the ectodermal stomodeum sprouts caudally in the median plane, bypassing the hyoid bone and the larynx, and forms the **Ductus thyroglossalis**).

b Development of the thyroid gland in the fifth week. When the Ductus thyroglossalis has reached its final position at the thyroid cartilage of the larynx in week 7, it forms the isthmus and the two lobes of the thyroid gland. The cranial part of the Ductus thyroglossalis regresses. The

proximal opening of the Ductus thyroglossalis persists as the **Foramen caecum** behind the Sulcus terminalis, and a **Lobus pyramidalis** (thyroid gland tissue) is frequently found along the passageway of the former Ductus thyroglossalis (→ Fig. 8.198).

The ultimobranchial body protrudes from the fifth pharyngeal pouch, from which the C-cells (producing calcitonin) develop, which then migrate into the thyroid gland. The epithelial bodies (producing the parathyroid hormone) develop from the third and fourth pharyngeal pouches.

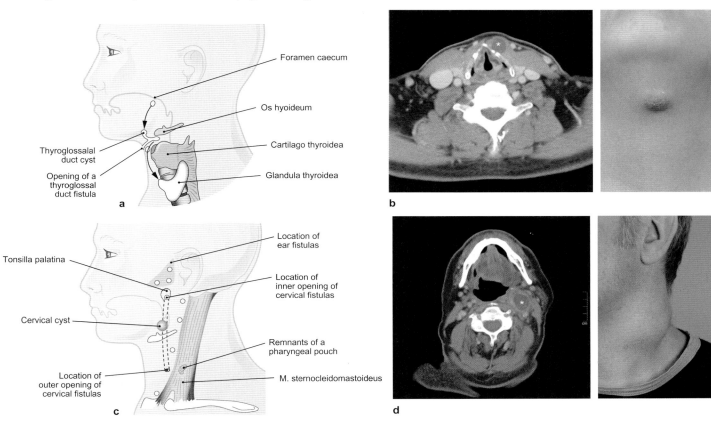

Foramen caecum

Os hyoideum

Cartilago thyroidea

Glandula thyroidea

Thyroglossalal duct cyst

Opening of a thyroglossal duct fistula

a

Tonsilla palatina

Cervical cyst

Location of outer opening of cervical fistulas

Location of ear fistulas

Location of inner opening of cervical fistulas

Remnants of a pharyngeal pouch

M. sternocleidomastoideus

c

b

d

Fig. 11.69a–d Cervical cysts and cervical fistulas. a, c [E347-09], b, d [S700-T882]
a Possible localisations of cysts of the Ductus thyroglossalis (arrows indicate the pathway of the Ductus thyroglossalis during the descent of the thyroid gland from the Foramen caecum to its final position in the Regio cervicalis anterior).

b Medial cervical cyst on the computed tomography (pictured on the left, * = cervical cyst) and clinically with a swelling in the neck (pictured on the right).
c Possible localisations of cervical cysts and cervical fistulas.
d Lateral cervical cysts on the computed tomography (pictured on the left, * = cervical cyst) and clinically with a swelling in the neck (pictured on the right).

Clinical remarks

It is possible that a portion of the Ductus thyroglossalis persists in the form of a **median cervical cyst** or, in the case of a connection to the outside, in the form of a **median cervical fistula** (→ Fig. 11.69a and b). Both have no clinical significance, as long as they are not inflamed. **Lateral cervical cysts** arise when the branchial clefts or the Sinus cervicalis are not completely obliterated.

Lateral cervical fistulas usually open at the anterior margin of the M. sternocleidomastoideus (→ Fig. 11.69c); the accumulation of fluid n **lateral cervical cysts** results in a visible swelling at the side of the neck (→ Fig. 11.69d).

Vessels and nerves of the thyroid gland

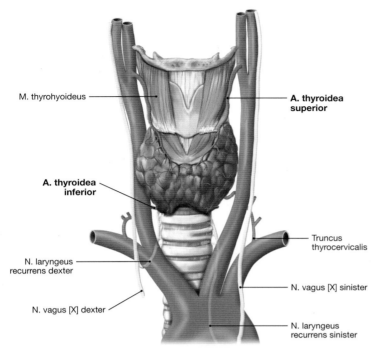

M. thyrohyoideus

A. thyroidea superior

A. thyroidea inferior

N. laryngeus recurrens dexter

N. vagus [X] dexter

Truncus thyrocervicalis

N. vagus [X] sinister

N. laryngeus recurrens sinister

Fig. 11.70 Arteries of the thyroid gland, Glandula thyroidea; ventral view. [S700-L266]
As an endocrine organ, the thyroid gland is very well perfused. It receives blood via the **A. thyroidea superior** (along with the Rr. glandulares anterior and posterior) from the A. carotis externa as well as via the **A. thyroidea inferior** from the Truncus thyrocervicalis. Sometimes, a small A. thyroidea ima from the Truncus brachiocephalicus or the Arcus aortae also contributes to the blood supply (not shown). The blood vessels also supply the epithelial bodies (→ Fig. 11.72).

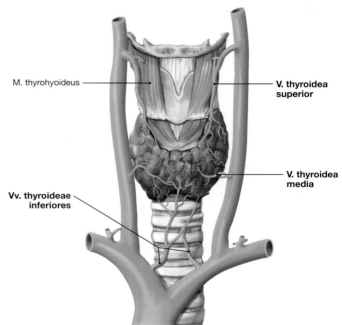

M. thyrohyoideus

V. thyroidea superior

V. thyroidea media

Vv. thyroideae inferiores

Fig. 11.71 Veins of the thyroid gland, Glandula thyroidea; ventral view. [S700-L266]
Three paired veins collect the blood of the thyroid gland. The **Vv. thyroideae superior and media** drain into the V. jugularis interna, and the **V. thyroidea inferior** passes its blood into the left V. brachiocephalica.

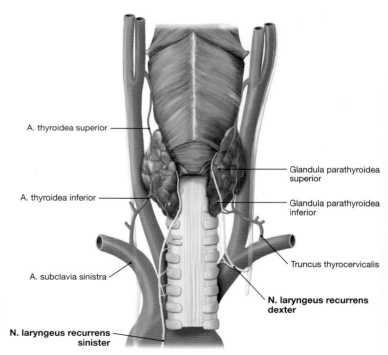

A. thyroidea superior

A. thyroidea inferior

Glandula parathyroidea superior

Glandula parathyroidea inferior

Truncus thyrocervicalis

A. subclavia sinistra

N. laryngeus recurrens dexter

N. laryngeus recurrens sinister

Fig. 11.72 Aa. thyroideae superior and inferior, as well as Nn. laryngei recurrentes sinister and dexter; dorsal view. [S700-L266]
The thyroid gland has close topographical relationships with the Nn. laryngei recurrentes (Nn. laryngei inferiores). These nerves run cranially to the larynx within the groove between the trachea and the oesophagus (→ Fig. 11.61).

Clinical remarks

The most common causes of **paralysis of the laryngeal muscles** are goitre operations (thyroidectomy, mostly subtotal strumectomies). The enlargement of the thyroid gland disrupts the normal topography of the N. laryngeus recurrens. Even in the case of a **goitre,** the nerve maintains a close relationship with the thyroid gland and the A. thyroidea inferior, but is more difficult to localise and is therefore at great risk of injuries. An enlarged thyroid gland can constrict the trachea or in an advanced stage may lead to breathing difficulties. An operation is therefore often unavoidable.

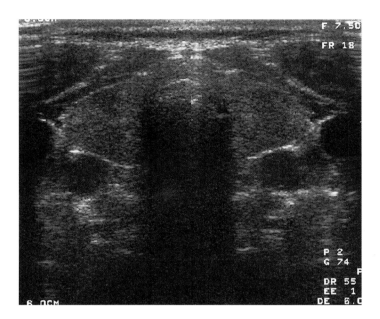

Fig. 11.73   Thyroid gland, Glandula thyroidea; ultrasound image, cross-section at the level of the thyroid gland. [R316-007] Normal finding.

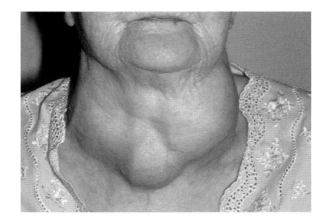

Fig. 11.74   Enlargement of the thyroid gland (Struma multinodosa). [S700] The thyroid gland is noticeably enlarged (on the left more than the right) with nodular changes (multinodular goitre).

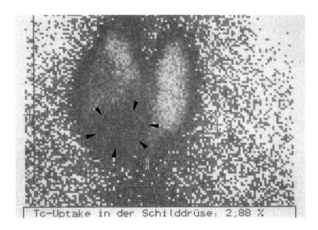

Fig. 11.75   Thyroid gland, Glandula thyroidea; scintigraphic scan, ventral view. [R132] Thyroid scintigraphy is a functional topographical examination procedure. This scan was taken 20 minutes after an intravenous injection of technetium-99 m-pertechnetate and shows a cold nodule (arrowheads) in the right thyroid lobe, extending into the isthmus. In the left thyroid lobe, a homogeneous distribution of nuclides is visible. There is no active thyroid tissue in the cold nodule.

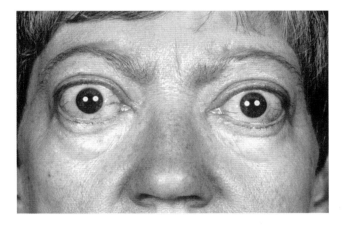

Fig. 11.76   Patient with endocrine ophthalmopathy. Exophthalmos (bulging eyes) and retraction of the upper eyelid due to hyperthyroidism. [T1127]

Clinical remarks

The pathology of the thyroid gland is complex. **Diffuse** (→ Fig. 11.74) and **focal** → Fig. 11.75) **changes in the thyroid gland** are the main distinctions. There are numerous causes for both. In addition, a deficiency **(hypothyroidism)** or overproduction **(hyperthyroidism)** of the hormones thyroxine and triiodothyronine can occur. An example of this is the hyperthyroidism in a diffuse goitre **(GRAVES' disease),** which is due to an immunological process. It is frequently associated with orbitopathy. This is likely the result of circulating antibodies against an antigen derived from the external ocular muscles. The antibodies will show a cross-reaction with the microsomal fraction of the follicular epithelial cells of the thyroid gland. An **exophthalmus** can result from a retro-orbital oedema, deposits of glycosaminoglycans, lymphocytic infiltrates and progressive fibrosis (→ Fig. 11.76).

Vessels and nerves of the neck

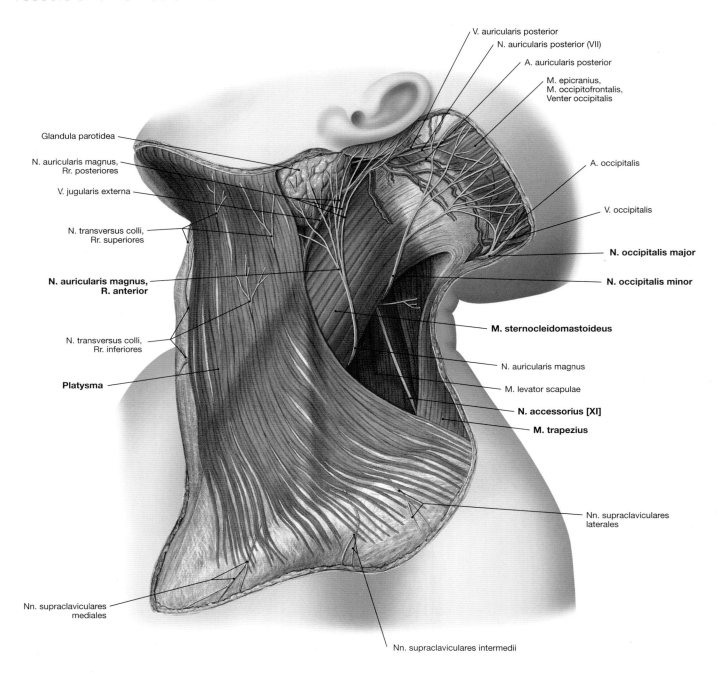

V. auricularis posterior

N. auricularis posterior (VII)

A. auricularis posterior

M. epicranius,
M. occipitofrontalis,
Venter occipitalis

Glandula parotidea

N. auricularis magnus,
Rr. posteriores

V. jugularis externa

N. transversus colli,
Rr. superiores

**N. auricularis magnus,
R. anterior**

N. transversus colli,
Rr. inferiores

Platysma

A. occipitalis

V. occipitalis

N. occipitalis major

N. occipitalis minor

M. sternocleidomastoideus

N. auricularis magnus

M. levator scapulae

N. accessorius [XI]

M. trapezius

Nn. supraclaviculares
laterales

Nn. supraclaviculares
mediales

Nn. supraclaviculares intermedii

Fig. 11.77   Vessels and nerves of the anterior and lateral cervical regions, Regiones cervicales anterior et lateralis; lateral view. [S700]
The superficial fascia of the neck is positioned dorsally to the platysma. The **N. auricularis magnus** and the **N. occipitalis minor** surround the M. sternocleidomastoideus from behind to the upper front. Both are sensory nerves derived from the Plexus cervicalis (C1–C4) and innervate the skin in front of and below the auricle to the occipital region. The

N. occipitalis major passes through the tendinous origin of the M. trapezius at the Linea nuchalis superior and continues the sensory innervation of the skin in the occipital region. It is the R. dorsalis of the spinal nerve C2. The **N. accessorius [XI]** runs through the lateral triangle of the neck on the M. levator scapulae, from the M. sternocleidomastoideus to the M. trapezius, and innervates the two muscles. The nerve has its origin in the brainstem and the upper cervical spinal cord (→ Fig. 12.169).

Clinical remarks

In the case of surgical interventions in the lateral cervical region (e.g. removal of a neck lymph node or during a neck dissection) the **N. accessorius [XI]** is at risk. Injury to the nerve in this region mostly

only leads to paralysis of the M. trapezius. The arm can then no longer be elevated above the horizontal plane.

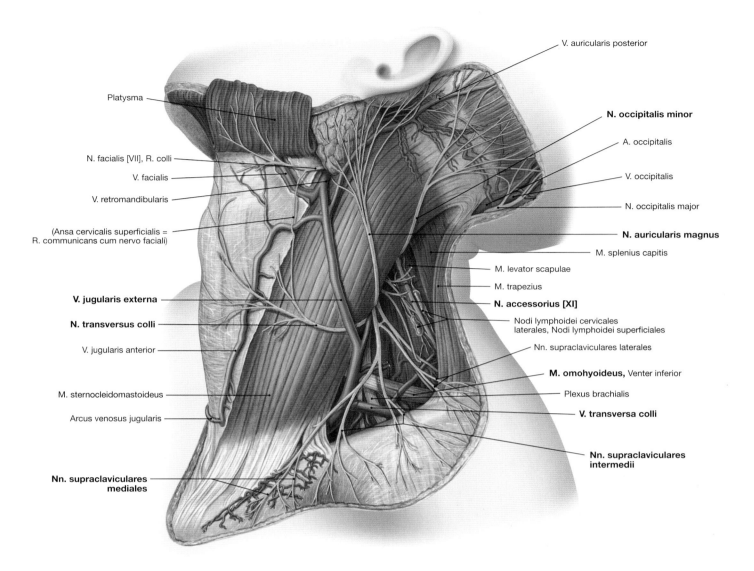

Platysma

N. facialis [VII], R. colli

V. facialis

V. retromandibularis

(Ansa cervicalis superficialis = R. communicans cum nervo faciali)

V. jugularis externa

N. transversus colli

V. jugularis anterior

M. sternocleidomastoideus

Arcus venosus jugularis

Nn. supraclaviculares mediales

V. auricularis posterior

N. occipitalis minor

A. occipitalis

V. occipitalis

N. occipitalis major

N. auricularis magnus

M. splenius capitis

M. levator scapulae

M. trapezius

N. accessorius [XI]

Nodi lymphoidei cervicales laterales, Nodi lymphoidei superficiales

Nn. supraclaviculares laterales

M. omohyoideus, Venter inferior

Plexus brachialis

V. transversa colli

Nn. supraclaviculares intermedii

Fig. 11.78 Vessels and nerves of the lateral cervical region, Regio cervicalis lateralis, left side; lateral view. Parts of the platysma folded upwards, Lamina superficialis of the Fascia cervicalis largely removed. [S700]
The sensory nerves of the Plexus cervicalis emerge at the posterior margin of the M. sternocleidomastoideus and penetrate the superficial fascia of the neck. The passageways of the Nn. supraclaviculares, the N. transversus colli and the N. auricularis magnus are located tightly

packed in the middle of the muscle. This location is called the **Punctum nervosum** (ERB's point). The Punctum nervosum also includes the N. occipitalis minor, although it exits significantly more cranially. In the posterior triangle of the neck the N. accessorius [XI], the M. omohyoideus and the V. transversa colli can also be seen, draining into the V. jugularis externa, which runs variably across the M. sternocleidomastoideus.

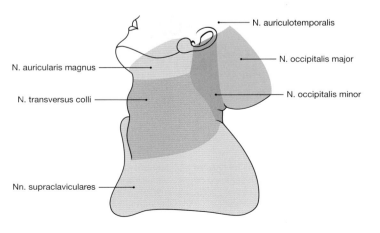

N. auriculotemporalis

N. auricularis magnus

N. occipitalis major

N. transversus colli

N. occipitalis minor

Nn. supraclaviculares

Fig. 11.79 Sensory innervation of the skin in the cervical region (cutaneous nerves). [S700-L126]
The sensory innervation of the skin of the neck is provided by the Nn. supraclaviculares, transversus colli, auricularis magnus, occipitalis minor, occipitalis major and occipitalis tertius (not visible).

Vessels and nerves of the neck

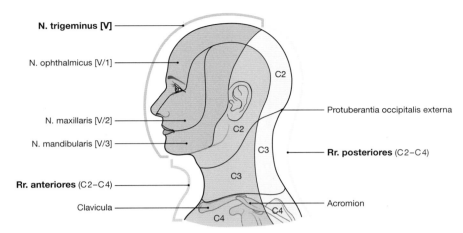

N. trigeminus [V]

N. ophthalmicus [V/1]

N. maxillaris [V/2]

N. mandibularis [V/3]

Rr. anteriores (C2–C4)

Clavicula

C2

C2

C3

C3

C4   C4

Protuberantia occipitalis externa

Rr. posteriores (C2–C4)

Acromion

Fig. 11.80 Sensory innervation of the skin of the neck and head, as well as segmental mapping of the cutaneous areas. [S700-L126]
The skin in the neck region is innervated from the cervical segments C2, C3 and C4. The Rr. anteriores of the spinal nerves innervate the ventral area of the neck, and the Rr. posteriores are responsible for the dorsal area.

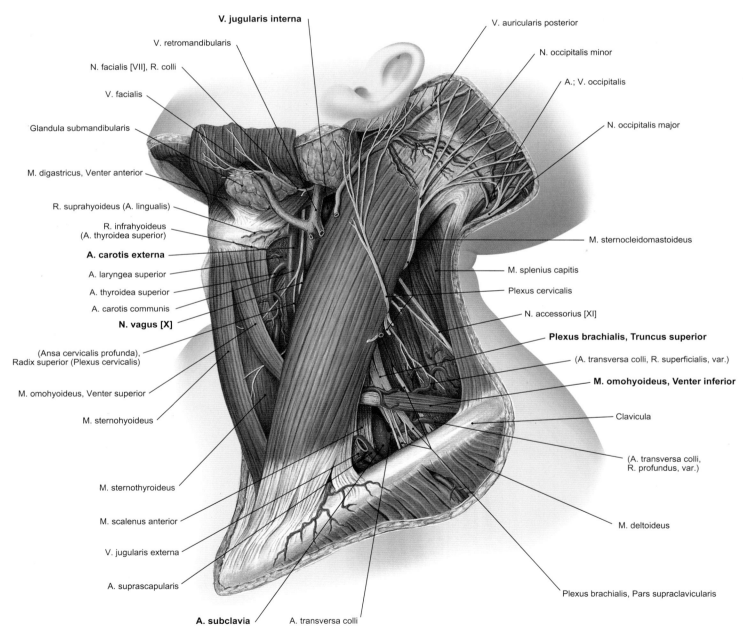

V. jugularis interna

V. retromandibularis

N. facialis [VII], R. colli

V. facialis

Glandula submandibularis

M. digastricus, Venter anterior

R. suprahyoideus (A. lingualis)

R. infrahyoideus
(A. thyroidea superior)

A. carotis externa

A. laryngea superior

A. thyroidea superior

A. carotis communis

N. vagus [X]

(Ansa cervicalis profunda),
Radix superior (Plexus cervicalis)

M. omohyoideus, Venter superior

M. sternohyoideus

M. sternothyroideus

M. scalenus anterior

V. jugularis externa

A. suprascapularis

A. subclavia   A. transversa colli

V. auricularis posterior

N. occipitalis minor

A.; V. occipitalis

N. occipitalis major

M. sternocleidomastoideus

M. splenius capitis

Plexus cervicalis

N. accessorius [XI]

Plexus brachialis, Truncus superior

(A. transversa colli, R. superficialis, var.)

M. omohyoideus, Venter inferior

Clavicula

(A. transversa colli,
R. profundus, var.)

M. deltoideus

Plexus brachialis, Pars supraclavicularis

Fig. 11.81 Vessels and nerves of the anterior and lateral cervical regions, Regiones cervicales anterior et lateralis, left side; lateral view; after removal of the superficial and the middle cervical fascia. [S700]

In the anterior triangle of the neck, structures are visible which are normally covered by the carotid sheath (A. carotis externa, N. vagus [X], V. jugularis interna); displayed in the posterior triangle of the neck are the Plexus brachialis and the A. subclavia in the scalene hiatus, which are crossed over by the Venter inferior of the M. omohyoideus.

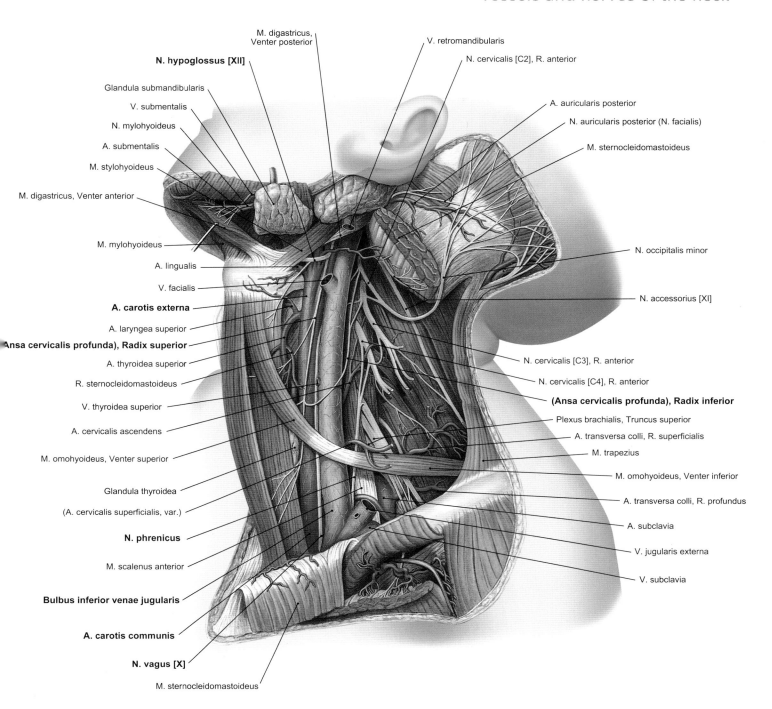

M. digastricus, Venter posterior

N. hypoglossus [XII]

Glandula submandibularis

V. submentalis

N. mylohyoideus

A. submentalis

M. stylohyoideus

M. digastricus, Venter anterior

M. mylohyoideus

A. lingualis

V. facialis

A. carotis externa

A. laryngea superior

Ansa cervicalis profunda), Radix superior

A. thyroidea superior

R. sternocleidomastoideus

V. thyroidea superior

A. cervicalis ascendens

M. omohyoideus, Venter superior

Glandula thyroidea

(A. cervicalis superficialis, var.)

N. phrenicus

M. scalenus anterior

Bulbus inferior venae jugularis

A. carotis communis

N. vagus [X]

M. sternocleidomastoideus

V. retromandibularis

N. cervicalis [C2], R. anterior

A. auricularis posterior

N. auricularis posterior (N. facialis)

M. sternocleidomastoideus

N. occipitalis minor

N. accessorius [XI]

N. cervicalis [C3], R. anterior

N. cervicalis [C4], R. anterior

(Ansa cervicalis profunda), Radix inferior

Plexus brachialis, Truncus superior

A. transversa colli, R. superficialis

M. trapezius

M. omohyoideus, Venter inferior

A. transversa colli, R. profundus

A. subclavia

V. jugularis externa

V. subclavia

Fig. 11.82 Vessels and nerves of the lateral cervical region, Regio cervicalis lateralis, left side; lateral view; after extensive removal of the M. sternocleidomastoideus. [S700]
The removal of the M. sternocleidomastoideus permits an unobstructed view of the **A. carotis communis** in the lower cervical region, the **A. carotis externa** in the upper cervical region as well as the **N. vagus [X]** and the **V. jugularis interna.** The **Ansa cervicalis (profunda)** is positioned in the upper cervical region with its Radices superior and inferior

lying around the V. jugularis interna. The Radices send branches to the infrahyoid muscles. Lateral to the V. jugularis interna, the **N. phrenicus** branches off the Plexus cervicalis and crosses the M. scalenus anterior in the lower cervical region to reach the upper thoracic aperture. In the upper cervical region, the **N. hypoglossus [XII]** passes forward across the A. carotis externa in the area of the outflow of the A. lingualis and disappears underneath the M. stylohyoideus.

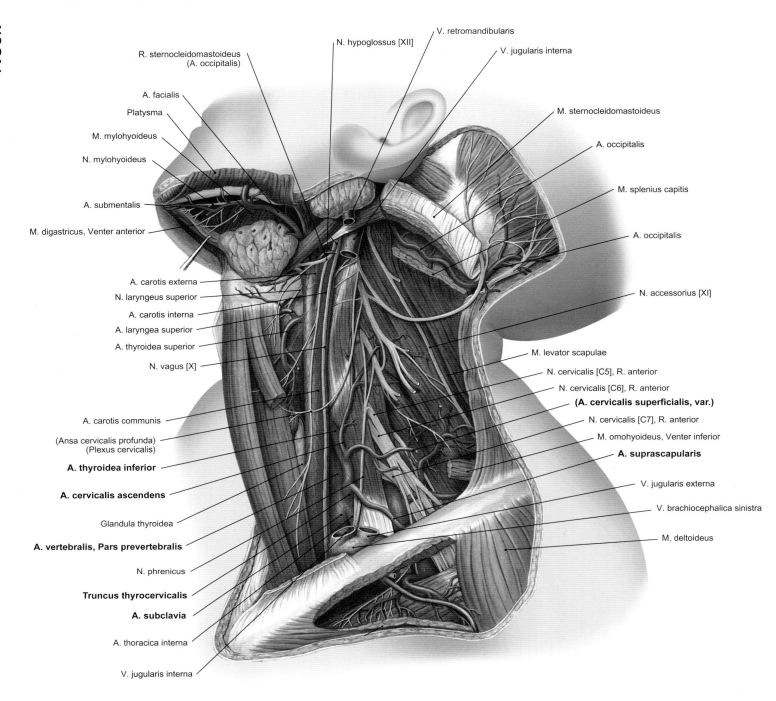

N. hypoglossus [XII]
V. retromandibularis
V. jugularis interna
R. sternocleidomastoideus (A. occipitalis)
A. facialis
Platysma
M. mylohyoideus
N. mylohyoideus
A. submentalis
M. digastricus, Venter anterior
A. carotis externa
N. laryngeus superior
A. carotis interna
A. laryngea superior
A. thyroidea superior
N. vagus [X]
A. carotis communis
(Ansa cervicalis profunda) (Plexus cervicalis)
A. thyroidea inferior
A. cervicalis ascendens
Glandula thyroidea
A. vertebralis, Pars prevertebralis
N. phrenicus
Truncus thyrocervicalis
A. subclavia
A. thoracica interna
V. jugularis interna

M. sternocleidomastoideus
A. occipitalis
M. splenius capitis
A. occipitalis
N. accessorius [XI]
M. levator scapulae
N. cervicalis [C5], R. anterior
N. cervicalis [C6], R. anterior
(A. cervicalis superficialis, var.)
N. cervicalis [C7], R. anterior
M. omohyoideus, Venter inferior
A. suprascapularis
V. jugularis externa
V. brachiocephalica sinistra
M. deltoideus

Fig. 11.83 Vessels and nerves of the lateral cervical region, Regio cervicalis lateralis, deep layer, left side; lateral view. [S700]
After removal of the V. jugularis interna it is possible to see the **A. subclavia,** the **A. vertebralis** and the **Truncus thyrocervicalis** originating from the A. subclavia. The A. subclavia runs dorsally of the M. scalenus anterior and, together with the Plexus brachialis, passes through the scalene hiatus.

Branches of the Truncus thyrocervicalis	
• A. thyroidea inferior – A. laryngea inferior – Rr. glandulares – Rr. pharyngeales – Rr. oesophageales – Rr. tracheales	• A. suprascapularis – R. acromialis
	• A. transversa colli – R. superficialis – R. profundus
• A. cervicalis ascendens – Rr. spinales	• (A. dorsalis scapulae)

Clinical remarks

A proximal high-grade stenosis (narrowing) of the A. subclavia sinistra, or less frequently of the A. subclavia dextra, can result in a retrograde (reversed) flow in the A. vertebralis of the affected side during intense physical activity of the arm **(subclavian steal syndrome; SSS).** The resulting reduction in the blood perfusion of the brain can cause dizziness and headaches.

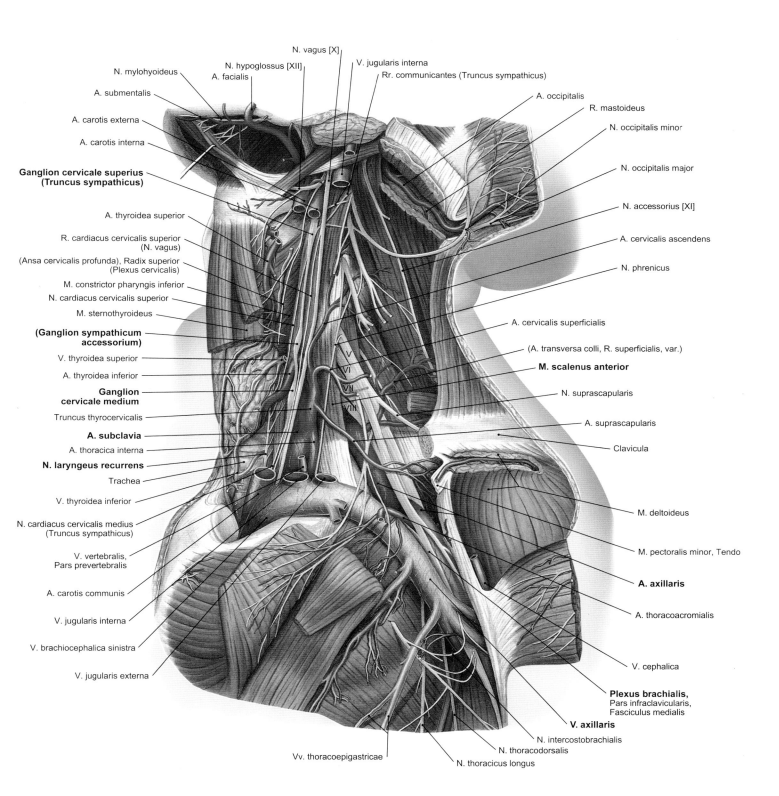

N. vagus [X]
N. hypoglossus [XII]
A. facialis
N. mylohyoideus
A. submentalis
A. carotis externa
A. carotis interna
Ganglion cervicale superius (Truncus sympathicus)
A. thyroidea superior
R. cardiacus cervicalis superior (N. vagus)
(Ansa cervicalis profunda), Radix superior (Plexus cervicalis)
M. constrictor pharyngis inferior
N. cardiacus cervicalis superior
M. sternothyroideus
(Ganglion sympathicum accessorium)
V. thyroidea superior
A. thyroidea inferior
Ganglion cervicale medium
Truncus thyrocervicalis
A. subclavia
A. thoracica interna
N. laryngeus recurrens
Trachea
V. thyroidea inferior
N. cardiacus cervicalis medius (Truncus sympathicus)
V. vertebralis, Pars prevertebralis
A. carotis communis
V. jugularis interna
V. brachiocephalica sinistra
V. jugularis externa

V. jugularis interna
Rr. communicantes (Truncus sympathicus)
A. occipitalis
R. mastoideus
N. occipitalis minor
N. occipitalis major
N. accessorius [XI]
A. cervicalis ascendens
N. phrenicus
A. cervicalis superficialis
(A. transversa colli, R. superficialis, var.)
M. scalenus anterior
N. suprascapularis
A. suprascapularis
Clavicula
M. deltoideus
M. pectoralis minor, Tendo
A. axillaris
A. thoracoacromialis
V. cephalica
Plexus brachialis, Pars infraclavicularis, Fasciculus medialis
V. axillaris
N. intercostobrachialis
N. thoracodorsalis
N. thoracicus longus
Vv. thoracoepigastricae

V
VI
VII
VIII

Fig. 11.84 Vessels and nerves of the lateral cervical region, Regio cervicalis lateralis, and the axillary region, Regio axillaris. [S700]
The numbers V to VIII mark the ventral branches of the corresponding cervical nerves.
After the removal of the anterior two-thirds of the clavicula, the **Plexus brachialis** and the **A. subclavia** become visible, passing through the scalene hiatus (between M. scalenus anterior and M. scalenus medius), as well as the V. subclavia (in front of the M. scalenus anterior) and its pathway across the first rib to the upper limb. In some cases, the upper part of the Plexus brachialis can penetrate the M. scalenus medius. In the cervical region, the Plexus brachialis delivers several

smaller branches and restructures itself – after multiple fibre exchanges – to fascicles, all of which lie just below the clavicula, laterally from the A. subclavia. Only in the middle of the axilla do they reach their topographically named position.
On the deep neck muscles lies the **Truncus sympathicus** with the Ganglia cervicalia superius and medium (in the upper cervical region, the Truncus sympathicus runs within the general organ fascia, and in the lower cervical region between the Fascia prevertebralis and the general organ fascia, not shown). Between the trachea and the oesophagus, the **N. laryngeus recurrens** is visible below the thyroid gland.

Plexus cervicalis

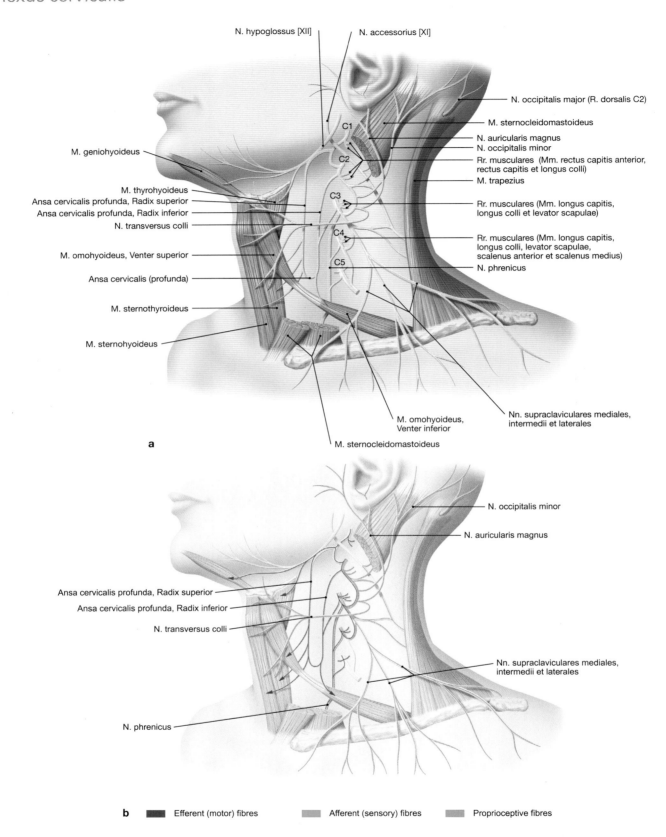

N. hypoglossus [XII]

N. accessorius [XI]

N. occipitalis major (R. dorsalis C2)

M. sternocleidomastoideus

M. geniohyoideus

N. auricularis magnus

N. occipitalis minor

Rr. musculares (Mm. rectus capitis anterior, rectus capitis et longus colli)

M. trapezius

M. thyrohyoideus

Ansa cervicalis profunda, Radix superior

Ansa cervicalis profunda, Radix inferior

N. transversus colli

Rr. musculares (Mm. longus capitis, longus colli et levator scapulae)

M. omohyoideus, Venter superior

Rr. musculares (Mm. longus capitis, longus colli, levator scapulae, scalenus anterior et scalenus medius)

Ansa cervicalis (profunda)

N. phrenicus

M. sternothyroideus

M. sternohyoideus

C1

C2

C3

C4

C5

M. omohyoideus, Venter inferior

Nn. supraclaviculares mediales, intermedii et laterales

a

M. sternocleidomastoideus

N. occipitalis minor

N. auricularis magnus

Ansa cervicalis profunda, Radix superior

Ansa cervicalis profunda, Radix inferior

N. transversus colli

Nn. supraclaviculares mediales, intermedii et laterales

N. phrenicus

b ▬ Efferent (motor) fibres ▬ Afferent (sensory) fibres ▬ Proprioceptive fibres

Fig. 11.85a and b Plexus cervicalis, sensory and motor branches.
Schematic drawing. [S700-L127]
a Depiction of the branches.
b Depiction of the functions.
For teaching purposes, nerves, muscles and bones in the figure are projected onto the body surface without regard to topographical layers. Thus, for example, the M. geniohyoideus appears to be on the outside of the Mandibula and the N. hypoglossus looks like a cutaneous nerve. The Ansa cervicalis profunda and the N. phrenicus constitute the motor branches of the Plexus cervicalis. The **Ansa cervicalis profunda,** consist-

ing of a Radix superior from segment C1 and a Radix inferior from segments C2 and C3, serves to innervate the infrahyoid muscles (Mm. thyrohyoideus, sternohyoideus, sternothyroideus, and omohyoideus). Additional motor branches innervate the suprahyoid M. geniohyoideus, the prevertebral muscles, the M. rectus capitis anterior, the Mm. scaleni anterior and medius, as well as parts of the M. levator scapulae. The **N. phrenicus** derives from the segments C3 to C5, runs caudally, and enters the thoracic cavity through the superior thoracic aperture.

→ T 8

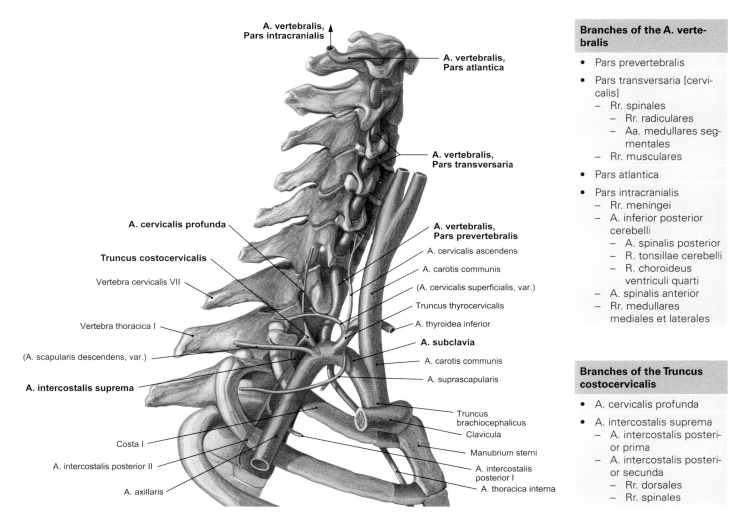

Branches of the A. vertebralis

- Pars prevertebralis
- Pars transversaria [cervicalis]
  - Rr. spinales
    - Rr. radiculares
    - Aa. medullares segmentales
  - Rr. musculares
- Pars atlantica
- Pars intracranialis
  - Rr. meningei
  - A. inferior posterior cerebelli
    - A. spinalis posterior
    - R. tonsillae cerebelli
    - R. choroideus ventriculi quarti
  - A. spinalis anterior
  - Rr. medullares mediales et laterales

Branches of the Truncus costocervicalis

- A. cervicalis profunda
- A. intercostalis suprema
  - A. intercostalis posterior prima
  - A. intercostalis posterior secunda
    - Rr. dorsales
    - Rr. spinales

Fig. 11.86 Branches of the Aa. subclavia and vertebralis, as well as the Truncus costocervicalis; lateral view. [S700]

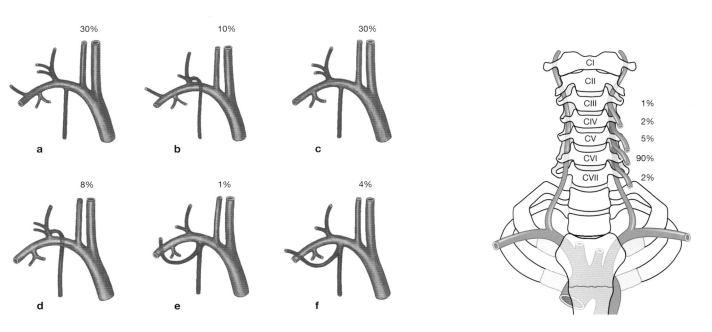

Fig. 11.87a–f Variants of branching types of the A. thyroidea inferior, A. suprascapularis, A. transversa colli and A. thoracica interna with separate outflow from the A. vertebralis and Truncus costocervicalis. [S700]

Fig. 11.88 Variants of the levels of entry of the A. vertebralis into the Foramina transversaria. [S700-L126]

Veins of the neck

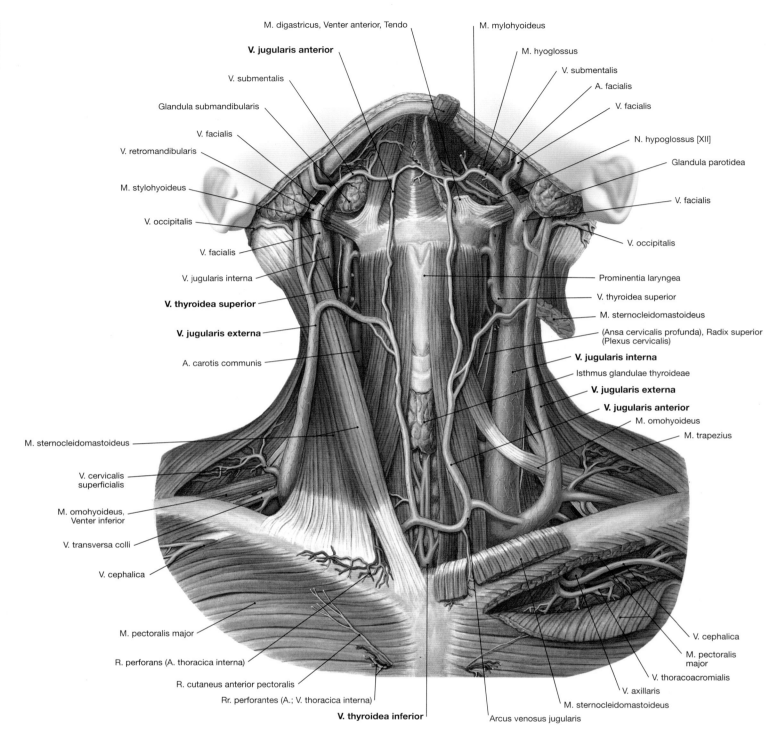

M. digastricus, Venter anterior, Tendo

M. mylohyoideus

V. jugularis anterior

V. submentalis

M. hyoglossus

Glandula submandibularis

V. submentalis

A. facialis

V. facialis

V. facialis

V. retromandibularis

N. hypoglossus [XII]

M. stylohyoideus

Glandula parotidea

V. occipitalis

V. facialis

V. facialis

V. occipitalis

V. jugularis interna

Prominentia laryngea

V. thyroidea superior

V. thyroidea superior

V. jugularis externa

M. sternocleidomastoideus

A. carotis communis

(Ansa cervicalis profunda), Radix superior (Plexus cervicalis)

V. jugularis interna

Isthmus glandulae thyroideae

V. jugularis externa

V. jugularis anterior

M. omohyoideus

M. trapezius

M. sternocleidomastoideus

V. cervicalis superficialis

M. omohyoideus, Venter inferior

V. transversa colli

V. cephalica

M. pectoralis major

V. cephalica

R. perforans (A. thoracica interna)

M. pectoralis major

R. cutaneus anterior pectoralis

V. thoracoacromialis

V. axillaris

Rr. perforantes (A.; V. thoracica interna)

M. sternocleidomastoideus

V. thyroidea inferior

Arcus venosus jugularis

Fig. 11.89 Veins of the neck, collum; ventral view. [S700]
The M. sternocleidomastoideus has mostly been removed on the left side. All cervical fasciae have been removed.
Superficial veins of the neck are the Vv. jugulares anteriores and the Vv. jugulares externae, which drain venous blood into the Vv. jugulares internae, subclaviae and brachiocephalicae. The **deep** cervical veins include the Vv. jugulares internae and thyroideae superiores, the V. thyroidea inferior and the Plexus thyroideus impar (not visible). The pathways of the superficial veins are very variable.

Clinical remarks

Gaining **intravenous access** is the most commonly used invasive technique in preclinical emergency care. The V. jugularis externa provides good accessibility for venipuncture, even where veins are in a poor condition. The guidelines for cardiovascular resuscitation recommend this as the first choice for an intravenous access route.

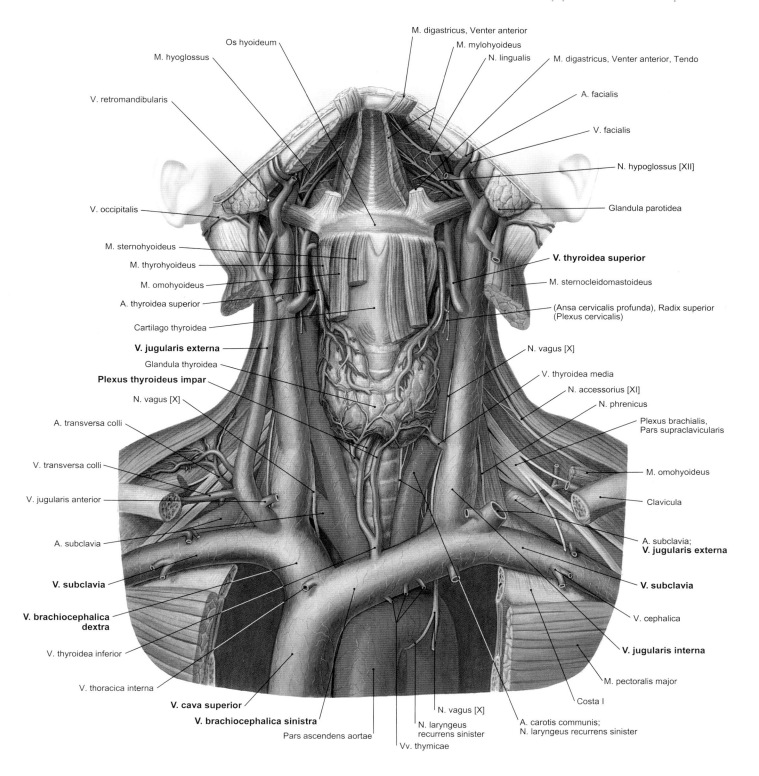

M. digastricus, Venter anterior

Os hyoideum

M. mylohyoideus

M. hyoglossus

N. lingualis

M. digastricus, Venter anterior, Tendo

A. facialis

V. retromandibularis

V. facialis

N. hypoglossus [XII]

V. occipitalis

Glandula parotidea

M. sternohyoideus

V. thyroidea superior

M. thyrohyoideus

M. sternocleidomastoideus

M. omohyoideus

(Ansa cervicalis profunda), Radix superior
(Plexus cervicalis)

A. thyroidea superior

Cartilago thyroidea

N. vagus [X]

V. jugularis externa

V. thyroidea media

Glandula thyroidea

N. accessorius [XI]

Plexus thyroideus impar

N. phrenicus

N. vagus [X]

Plexus brachialis,
Pars supraclavicularis

A. transversa colli

V. transversa colli

M. omohyoideus

V. jugularis anterior

Clavicula

A. subclavia

A. subclavia;
V. jugularis externa

V. subclavia

V. subclavia

V. brachiocephalica
dextra

V. cephalica

V. thyroidea inferior

V. jugularis interna

M. pectoralis major

V. thoracica interna

Costa I

V. cava superior

N. vagus [X]

V. brachiocephalica sinistra

A. carotis communis;
N. laryngeus recurrens sinister

N. laryngeus
recurrens sinister

Pars ascendens aortae

Vv. thymicae

Fig. 11.90 Vessels and nerves of the neck, collum, and upper thoracic aperture, Apertura thoracis superior; ventral view. [S700]
The sternum, parts of the claviculae, the M. sternocleidomastoideus, and parts of the infrahyoid muscles have been removed.
Presentation of the venous tributary of the **V. cava superior** (Vv. brachiocephalicae, jugulares internae, jugulares externae and subclaviae)

with particular emphasis on the venous drainage of the thyroid gland (→ Fig. 11.71). The passage of the Plexus brachialis, the A. and V. subclavia are also visible, running between the clavicula and the first rib, as well as the pathway of the N. phrenicus on the M. scalenus anterior, and the pathway of the left N. laryngeus recurrens around the Arcus aortae.

Lymph nodes and lymph vessels of the neck

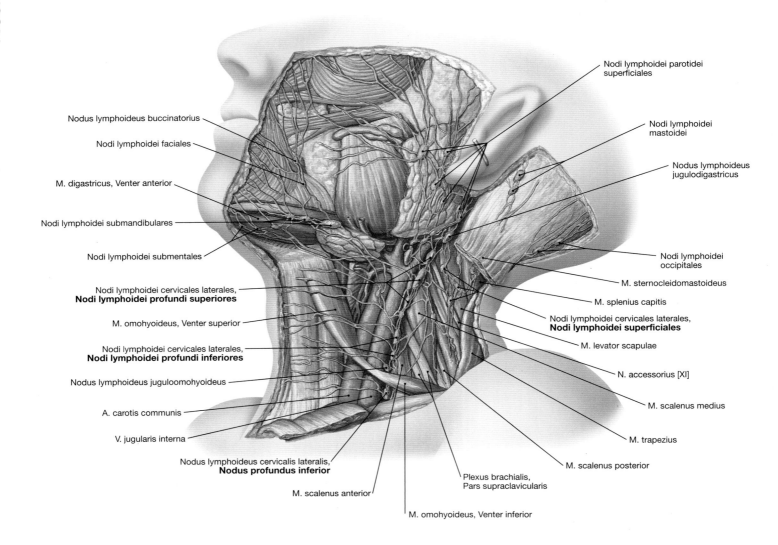

Nodi lymphoidei parotidei
superficiales

Nodi lymphoidei
mastoidei

Nodus lymphoideus buccinatorius

Nodi lymphoidei faciales

M. digastricus, Venter anterior

Nodi lymphoidei submandibulares

Nodi lymphoidei submentales

Nodi lymphoidei cervicales laterales,
Nodi lymphoidei profundi superiores

M. omohyoideus, Venter superior

Nodi lymphoidei cervicales laterales,
Nodi lymphoidei profundi inferiores

Nodus lymphoideus juguloomohyoideus

A. carotis communis

V. jugularis interna

Nodus lymphoideus cervicalis lateralis,
Nodus profundus inferior

M. scalenus anterior

Nodus lymphoideus
jugulodigastricus

Nodi lymphoidei
occipitales

M. sternocleidomastoideus

M. splenius capitis

Nodi lymphoidei cervicales laterales,
Nodi lymphoidei superficiales

M. levator scapulae

N. accessorius [XI]

M. scalenus medius

M. trapezius

M. scalenus posterior

Plexus brachialis,
Pars supraclavicularis

M. omohyoideus, Venter inferior

Fig. 11.91   Superficial lymph vessels, Vasa lymphatica superficialia, and lymph nodes, Nodi lymphoidei, of the head and neck of a child. [S700]
The cervical region contains 200 to 300 lymph nodes. The largest part of it is arranged along the neurovascular bundle (→ table, → Fig. 8.99).

Lymphatic fluid on the right side of the head and neck drains into the **Ductus lymphaticus dexter** (→ Fig. 8.100), whereas on the left side of the head and neck it drains into the **Ductus thoracicus.** To see where the Ductus thoracicus enters the left venous angle, → Fig. 11.98.

Lymph nodes of the neck (Nodi lyphoidei cervicales)	
Nodi lymphoidei cervicales anteriores	**Nodi lymphoidei cervicales laterales**
• Nodi lymphoidei superficiales	• Nodi lymphoidei superficiales
• Nodi lymphoidei profundi – Nodi lymphoidei infrahyoidei – Nodi lymphoidei prelaryngei – Nodi lymphoidei thyroidei – Nodi lymphoidei pretracheales – Nodi lymphoidei paratracheales – Nodi lymphoidei retropharyngeales	• Nodi lymphoidei profundi superiores – Nodus lymphoideus jugulodigastricus – Nodus lymphoideus lateralis – Nodus lymphoideus anterior
	• Nodi lymphoidei profundi inferiores – Nodi lymphoidei juguloomohyoidei – Nodus lymphoideus lateralis – Nodi lymphoidei anteriores
	• Nodi lymphoidei supraclaviculares
	• Nodi lymphoidei accessorii – Nodi lymphoidei retropharyngeales

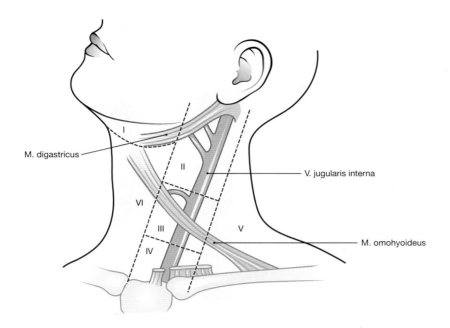

Fig. 11.92   Division of drainage areas of the head and neck into sections; according to the classification of the American Joint Committee of Cancer (AJCC). [S700-L126]

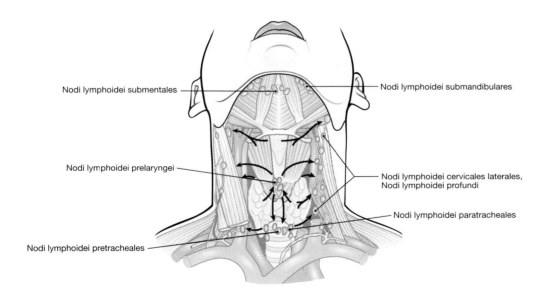

Fig. 11.93   Lymph vessels and lymph nodes of the larynx, thyroid gland, Glandula thyroidea, and trachea; ventral view. [S700-L126]
All three organs drain into the deep lymph nodes of the neck.

Clinical remarks

According to the classification of the American Joint Committee of Cancer (AJCC), the lymph nodes of the neck, in terms of the onset of regional **lymph node metastases,** are divided into six zones (**levels I–VI;** → Fig. 11.92). These serve as reference zones for the elective surgical removal of lymph nodes with metastases due to the lymphogenic spread of malignant tumours of the head and neck region (neck dissection).

Injuries to the Ductus thoracicus during surgery in the neck region can lead to the formation of a **chylous fistula.**

Vessels and nerves of the Trigonum submandibulare

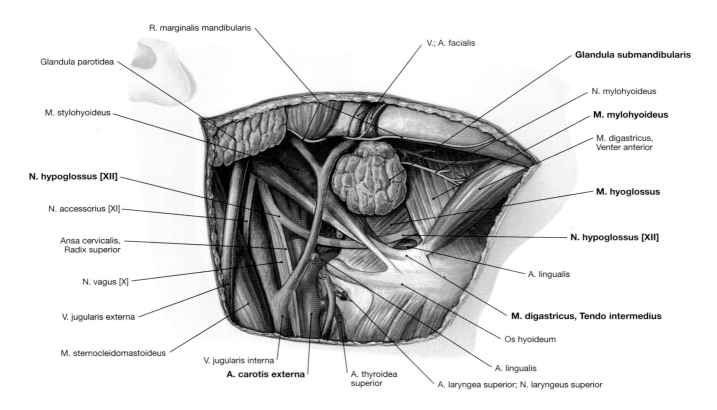

R. marginalis mandibularis

Glandula parotidea

M. stylohyoideus

N. hypoglossus [XII]

N. accessorius [XI]

Ansa cervicalis, Radix superior

N. vagus [X]

V. jugularis externa

M. sternocleidomastoideus

V. jugularis interna

A. carotis externa

V.; A. facialis

Glandula submandibularis

N. mylohyoideus

M. mylohyoideus

M. digastricus, Venter anterior

M. hyoglossus

N. hypoglossus [XII]

A. lingualis

M. digastricus, Tendo intermedius

Os hyoideum

A. lingualis

A. thyroidea superior

A. laryngea superior; N. laryngeus superior

Fig. 11.94 Vessels and nerves of the Trigonum submandibulare; inferolateral view. [S700]

After removal of all fascial layers to expose the Glandula submandibularis and the neurovascular pathways, the arc-shaped pathway of the **N. hypoglossus [XII]** can be seen; this nerve leaves the neurovascular bundle in the parapharyngeal space and passes forwards across the A. carotis externa, running between the M. hyoglossus and the intermediate tendon of the M. digastricus, until it disappears under the M. mylohyoideus.

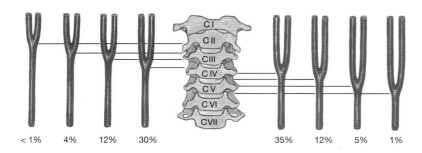

< 1%   4%   12%   30%   35%   12%   5%   1%

Fig. 11.95 Level of the bifurcation of the A. carotis communis, with regard to the cervical spine; frontal view. [S700]

Generally, the bifurcation of the A. carotis communis is located between CIII and CIV. In rare cases, it can also be positioned as high as CII, or as low as CV.

Clinical remarks

Inflammations in the area of the lower molars can lead to an **abscess formation in the fascial section of the Glandula submandibularis** and the sublingual section. Abscesses from the wisdom teeth can even extend into the fascial section of the Fossa retromandibularis and descend from here along the cervical fascia into the mediastinum to cause a life-threatening infection.

Damage to the N. hypoglossus [XII], e.g. due to tumour infiltration of a cervical lymph node metastasis, is easy to diagnose: when sticking out the tongue, it deviates to the diseased side since the muscles pushing it out on the healthy side no longer have any opposition on the diseased side.

The carotid bifurcation is often affected by **vascular changes** (extracranial arteriosclerosis: plaques, stenosis, obliteration). The Glomus caroticum located in the carotid bifurcation (not shown in → Fig. 11.94) is a paraganglion that contains chemoreceptors, which react to changes in the pH-value, and oxygen and carbon dioxide content of the blood.

A **carotid sinus syndrome** is defined as hypersensitivity of the pressoreceptors of the carotid sinus, which even triggers a reflex with rotating movements of the head, in turn strongly reducing the heart rate (vasovagal reflex). This can result in major circulatory complications and cardiac arrest.

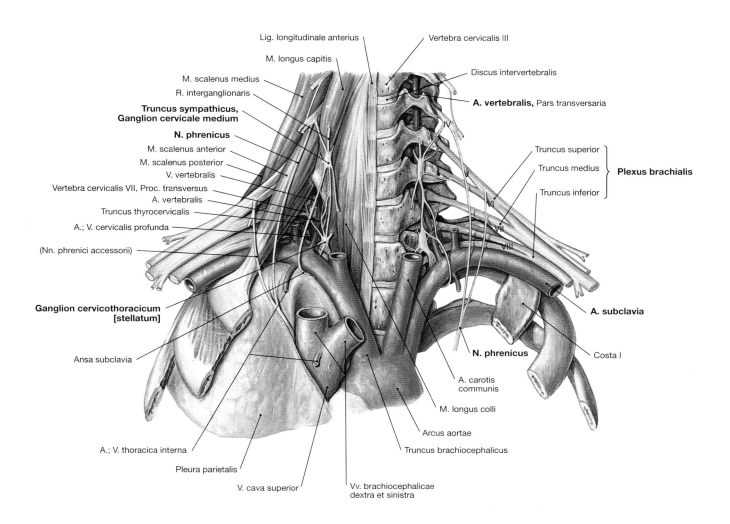

Lig. longitudinale anterius
M. longus capitis
M. scalenus medius
R. interganglionaris
Truncus sympathicus, Ganglion cervicale medium
N. phrenicus
M. scalenus anterior
M. scalenus posterior
V. vertebralis
Vertebra cervicalis VII, Proc. transversus
A. vertebralis
Truncus thyrocervicalis
A.; V. cervicalis profunda
(Nn. phrenici accessorii)
Ganglion cervicothoracicum [stellatum]
Ansa subclavia
A.; V. thoracica interna
Pleura parietalis
V. cava superior

Vertebra cervicalis III
Discus intervertebralis
A. vertebralis, Pars transversaria
Truncus superior
Truncus medius
Plexus brachialis
Truncus inferior
A. subclavia
Costa I
N. phrenicus
A. carotis communis
M. longus colli
Arcus aortae
Truncus brachiocephalicus
Vv. brachiocephalicae dextra et sinistra

Fig. 11.96 Vessels and nerves in the transition zone from the neck to the thorax and to the upper limb. [S700]
Visible are the pleural cupula with the scalene hiatus, the lower and middle sympathetic ganglia (Ganglion cervicale inferius/cervicothoracicum/stellatum on the head of rib I, and the Ganglion cervicale me-

dium on the M. longus colli), the pathway of the N. phrenicus and the A. vertebralis, as well as the trunci of the Plexus brachialis and the A. subclavia.
The numbers IV to VIII indicate the ventral branches of the corresponding spinal nerves.

Costae cervicales

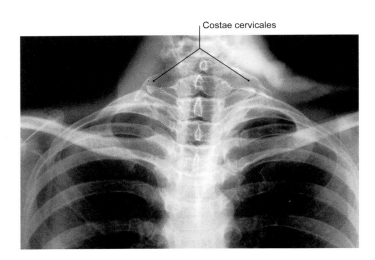

Fig. 11.97 Neck, collum; X-ray in anteroposterior (AP) projection. [E402]
A cervical rib (Costa cervicalis) can be seen on both sides.

Clinical remarks

Anatomic variants in the area of the scalene hiatus (cervical rib [cervical rib syndrome], narrow scalene hiatus, accessory M. scalenus minimus, or aberrant muscle fibres) are collectively called **scalenus anticus syndrome.** This is a form of thoracic outlet syndrome (TOS) that occurs when the space between rib I and the clavicula narrows

to cause the compression of the Plexus brachialis and the A. subclavia.

In the scalene hiatus, an **interscalene brachial plexus block** can be applied for the local anaesthesia of the Plexus brachialis.

Clinical remarks

A **PANCOAST tumour** (apical sulcus tumour) is a rapidly progressing peripheral bronchial carcinoma in the apex of the lung (Apex pulmonis; **a** schematic diagram, **b** MRI, **c** X-ray), which spreads relatively quickly into the ribs, soft tissues of the neck, Plexus brachialis, and vertebrae. Other affected structures can be the N. phrenicus, the

N. laryngeus recurrens, the A. and V. subclavia, as well as the Ganglion stellatum. In the case of the Ganglion stellatum being affected, it mostly leads to a HORNER's triad with an enophthalmus, miosis, narrow eyelid fissures (→ Fig. 12.213).
a [S701-L275], b [H084-001], c [E329]

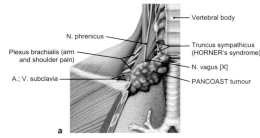

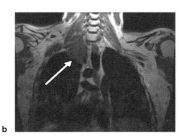

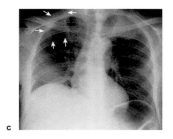

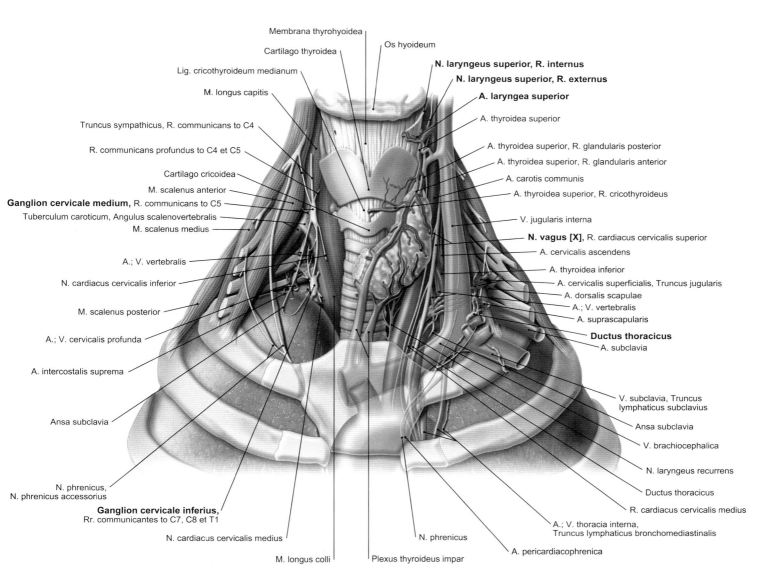

Membrana thyrohyoidea

Os hyoideum

Cartilago thyroidea

N. laryngeus superior, R. internus

Lig. cricothyroideum medianum

N. laryngeus superior, R. externus

M. longus capitis

A. laryngea superior

A. thyroidea superior

Truncus sympathicus, R. communicans to C4

A. thyroidea superior, R. glandularis posterior

R. communicans profundus to C4 et C5

A. thyroidea superior, R. glandularis anterior

Cartilago cricoidea

A. carotis communis

M. scalenus anterior

A. thyroidea superior, R. cricothyroideus

Ganglion cervicale medium, R. communicans to C5

V. jugularis interna

Tuberculum caroticum, Angulus scalenovertebralis

N. vagus [X], R. cardiacus cervicalis superior

M. scalenus medius

A. cervicalis ascendens

A.; V. vertebralis

A. thyroidea inferior

N. cardiacus cervicalis inferior

A. cervicalis superficialis, Truncus jugularis

A. dorsalis scapulae

M. scalenus posterior

A.; V. vertebralis

A. suprascapularis

A.; V. cervicalis profunda

Ductus thoracicus

A. subclavia

A. intercostalis suprema

V. subclavia, Truncus
lymphaticus subclavius

Ansa subclavia

Ansa subclavia

V. brachiocephalica

N. laryngeus recurrens

N. phrenicus,
N. phrenicus accessorius

Ductus thoracicus

Ganglion cervicale inferius,
Rr. communicantes to C7, C8 et T1

R. cardiacus cervicalis medius

A.; V. thoracica interna,
Truncus lymphaticus bronchomediastinalis

N. cardiacus cervicalis medius

N. phrenicus

M. longus colli

Plexus thyroideus impar

A. pericardiacophrenica

Fig. 11.98 Prevertebral and paravertebral structures of the neck and the upper thoracic aperture; ventral view. [S700-L238]/[Q300] On the right side of the body, the large blood vessels were removed to permit an unobstructed view of the pleural cupula and the Truncus sympathicus. One can see the **Ganglion cervicale inferius** (Ganglion cervicothoracicum [stellatum]) on the head of rib I as well as the **Ganglion cervicale medium** on the M. longus colli. The pleural cupula protrudes over the upper thoracic aperture. On the left side, the large blood vessels and the left thyroid lobe were left in place. It is possible to see the blood supply to the thyroid gland, the R. internus of the N. laryngeus superior and the Vasa laryngea superiora, the entry point of the Ductus thoracicus into the left venous angle as well as the pathway of the N. vagus [X] in between the A. carotis communis and the V. jugularis interna.

Sample exam questions

To check that you are completely familiar with the content of this chapter, sample questions from an oral anatomy exam are listed here.

Explain the structure of the neck:

- Which regions of the neck do you know and how are they delimited?
- How is the Regio cervicalis anterior subdivided and where are the boundaries?
- Which osseous parts of the skeleton are found in the neck?
- What is the function of the Os hyoideum?
- Are there any mimetic muscles located in the neck?
- Explain the pathway, function, blood supply and innervation of the M. sternocleidomastoideus.
- Where is the infrahyoid musculature situated? What is its function and how is it innervated?
- Which suprahyoid muscles do you know? Explain their position, function and innervation.
- What is the function of the prevertebral musculature, where is it located, what are the muscles called and how are they innervated?

Describe the structure of the Fascia cervicalis:

- How can the cervical fasciae be categorised?
- Name the muscles included in the superficial Fascia cervicalis?
- Which structures are located in the carotid sheath?
- Which cervical organs have their own fascia (organ fascia)?
- Name virtual spaces/sections within the connective tissue of the neck, which developed through the fasciae being adjoined.
- Which structures are located in the Spatium lateropharyngeum?
- How far does the Spatium retropharyngeum extend in the cranial and caudal direction?
- What is meant by the term Spatium peripharyngeum?

Describe the neurovascular pathways in the neck:

- Which branches usually emerge from the Truncus thyrocervicalis, and which from the Truncus costocervicalis?
- What pathway does the A. vertebralis follow through the neck?
- At what height does the carotid bifurcation usually lie? Which organ can be found in the bifurcation?
- Name branches of the A. carotis externa.
- Which large veins are located in the neck?

Explain the route of the nerves in the neck:

- What is the ERB's point? Where is it located and which branches does it provide? What is another name for it?
- What is meant by the Ansa cervicalis?
- Describe the pathway of the N. phrenicus through the neck.
- Which motor branches are in the Plexus cervicalis?
- Which muscle is innervated from the Plexus cervicalis via an anastomosis with the N. hypoglossus?
- What is the scalene hiatus? What passes through it?
- Describe the pathway of the N. accessorius. Which muscles does it innervate and what is their function?

- Where does the Truncus sympathicus run in the neck? Which ganglia do you know in the area of the neck?
- Describe the pathway of the N. hypoglossus. What does it innervate?
- Describe the pathway of the N. vagus from the point where it passes through the cranial base. Which branches run through the cervical region? What do they innervate here?

Explain the lymphatic drainage of the neck:

- How many lymph nodes are there in the area of the neck?
- Which lymph node groups are there in the area of the neck?
- Why is the neck divided into distinct regions (sections) of lymphatic drainage?
- Which structures drain their lymph into the cervical lymph nodes?

Describe the structure of the thyroid and the parathyroid glands:

- Explain the position, structure and function of the thyroid gland.
- How does the thyroid gland develop?
- What is a Lobus pyramidalis? What disruptive effect can it have?
- What can develop when a part of the Ductus thyroglossalis persists during its development? From what should it be differentiated?
- How is the thyroid gland supplied with blood?
- Where are the parathyroid glands usually located?
- Which structure is particularly vulnerable during thyroid gland surgery?

Explain the position and structure of the larynx:

- How is the larynx structured?
- Which muscles are involved in tensing the Plicae vocales?
- How is the larynx supplied with blood?
- Describe the innervation of the larynx.
- What is a cricothyrotomy? Where is it performed?
- Which muscle in particular is activated when breathing in and out deeply?
- What is the Conus elasticus, and the Membrana quadrangularis?
- Which structures form the vocal folds?
- What is the REINKE's space?
- What is the function of the vocal folds?
- What is the function of the Plica vestibularis?
- What is meant by the mucosal wave?
- Which sections of the larynx do you know?
- What is contained inside the transglottic space?
- What innervates the N. laryngeus superior?
- Describe the pathway of the N. laryngeus recurrens/inferior on the left and on the right side.
- How is the epiglottis structured and where is it attached? Are muscles involved in the movement of the epiglottis?
- Are you aware of changes in the laryngeal structures that contribute to voice alterations with age?
- Show the Recessus piriformis.

Brain and spinal cord

12

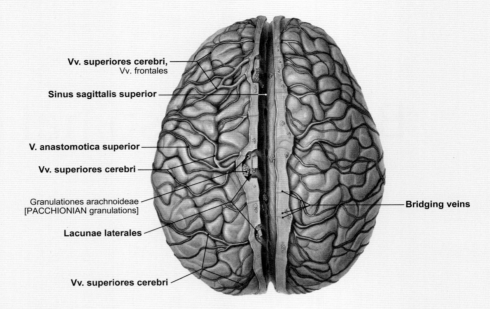

Vv. superiores cerebri,
Vv. frontales

Sinus sagittalis superior

V. anastomotica superior

Vv. superiores cerebri

Granulationes arachnoideae
[PACCHIONIAN granulations]

Lacunae laterales

Vv. superiores cerebri

Bridging veins

Overview

The human nervous system consists of 30–40 billion nerve cells, which come into contact with each other via synapses. Functionally, the somatic (voluntary) nervous system is separated from the autonomic (involuntary) nervous system. The **somatic nervous system** controls all the processes which are subject to the human will and consciousness; the **autonomic nervous system** regulates the sympathetic, parasympathetic and enteric nervous system, in particular the activities and functions of the internal organs during physical exertion, digestion, resting, but also in emergency situations. Topographically, a distinction is made between the central nervous system (CNS) and the peripheral nervous system. The CNS consists of the **spinal cord** (Medulla spinalis) and the **brain** (encephalon). The latter has five subdivisions in a cranial to caudal order: **cerebrum, diencephalon** ('intermediate' brain), **mesencephalon** (midbrain), **pons** and **Medulla oblongata** or myelencephalon. The **cerebellum,** which together with the Medulla oblongata and pons forms the **rhombencephalon,** is located on the dorsal side of the pons. The **brainstem** includes the Medulla oblongata, pons and mesencephalon. With the exception of two cranial nerves, all nerves outside the spinal cord and the brain belong to the peripheral nervous system (PNS).

Main topics

After working through this chapter, you should be able to:

- explain the principles of the development of the nervous system;
- name the internal structure of the cerebrum including the nuclei in sections/cuts of the brain;
- name the meninges, relate them to the brain and spinal cord, as well as to the surrounding bony structures, and explain their innervation and blood supply;
- explain the cerebrospinal fluid system in detail;
- identify the large blood vessels supplying the brain, describe their segments and their pathways, and find and name their main bifurcations and terminal branches;
- outline the Circulus arteriosus located at the cranial base and name its vessels;
- place the functional cortical areas relatively to the supply areas of the cerebral arteries;
- name the blood vessels of the Capsula interna;
- explain the venous system of the Sinus durae matris, bridging veins and cerebral veins as well as venous anastomoses;
- explain the fibre connections of the brain and their function;
- describe the parts of the neocortex;
- describe the areas of the hippocampus and explain how they connect to the ventricular system;
- explain the individual parts of the Cortex cinguli as well as the areas of the paleocortex, and the olfactory cortical areas and functions;
- explain the connections between the paleocortex and other areas of the brain, in particular the limbic system;

- explain the arrangement, location and function of the central subcortical nuclei;
- explain the components, organisational structure and functions of the diencephalon, thalamus, hypothalamus and epithalamus;
- explain the parts of the brainstem and describe its functional systems, including important brainstem reflexes;
- explain the surface, structure, blood supply, function and nuclei as well as the control and fibre systems of the cerebellum;
- correctly name the twelve pairs of cranial nerves, their nuclei, exit points, pathways, and fibre qualities, the special position of the cranial nerves I and II, the respective target organs as well as their topographical position;
- describe the segmentation of the spinal cord;
- define the pyramidal and extrapyramidal system;
- know the different neuronal functional systems;
- describe the olfactory and gustatory system;
- show a basic knowledge about different forms of pain;
- describe the circuits of the visceral motor system, the structure of sympathetic and parasympathetic systems, including paravertebral and prevertebral ganglia, and show these on the dissection;
- explain the enteric nervous system;
- describe the visceral sensory system and its importance for autonomic reflex arches and control loops;
- name parts of the autonomic nervous system, demonstrate the localisation of the centres, such as the respiratory centre and the cardiovascular centre, and describe the hypothalamus;
- explain the limbic system, including its connections.

Clinical relevance

In order not to lose touch with prospective everyday clinical life with so many anatomical details, the following describes a typical case that shows why the content of this chapter is so important.

Meningioma

Case study

A successful 48-year-old project manager from the financial sector has hardly ever been to see a doctor. Because she has been suffering from headaches for several weeks, sometimes without any relief, she has gone to her GP. After a thorough medical history and physical examination, he prescribed strong painkillers and advised her to reduce her workload and to take up sport if possible. The painkillers improved the symptoms, but the headaches remained. She was able to go on holiday two months later and followed the doctor's advice to practice sport (jogging). Nevertheless, the headaches persisted. On a cycling tour with her husband she suddenly fell from the bicycle and lay twitching on the ground. Her husband sought medical help immediately, as she was unresponsive. When the ambulance arrived, the woman had become responsive, but was still very groggy. The ambulance took her to the nearest hospital, with her husband accompanying her.

Result of examination

When examined in the ambulance, the woman reported no other complaints besides the headaches and two painful grazes on the chin and right forearm. However, she was still slightly dizzy. During the initial examination in the hospital, the doctor on duty observes that the woman appeared to have urinated spontaneously. He asks her husband about details of the fall and previous illnesses. The husband describes his wife's 'twitching' after the fall, but says that she is otherwise always healthy. In the past few months she had frequently complained about severe headaches, supposedly because of her work load and had already been to the doctor, who had prescribed painkillers. After conducting a thorough physical examination to exclude fractures and internal injuries, the doctor arranges for a computed tomography of the head.

Diagnostic procedure

The CT shows a round, smoothly margined mass with a strong and homogeneous uptake of contrast agent, making it look like a snowball (→ Fig. a). It is located at the cranial vault, in a parasagittal-right plane in the middle third of the Sinus sagittalis superior. Other pathologies or a trauma caused by the fall with the bicycle can now be ruled out. The CT finding and the seizure lead the radiologist to the suspected diagnosis of a meningioma.

Diagnosis

Meningioma.

Treatment

Due to the location, size and symptoms as well as the good general condition of the patient, she is advised to undergo immediate surgical removal of the tumour. She agrees and is transferred to the neurosurgery department, is given pre-operative information and is operated on the next day. After opening the cranium, the neurosurgeons can resect a confined, round, grey-white tumour of solid consistency, including the infiltrated dura mater, and thereby minimise the risk of relapse. For confirmation of the diagnosis, the resected tissue is brought to the pathology department.

The histopathologic examination with HE staining reveals grouped, uniform tumour cells, emerging from cells of the arachnoid mater and enveloped by collagenous septa.

 Many meningiomas contain small focal calcifications.

The result of the pathological-anatomical evaluation is a meningioma of the meningotheliomatous type, WHO grade I. This classification is especially important for the prognosis. Of all meningiomas, 90 % are of this type, i.e., they grow very slowly without infiltrating the brain and do not form metastases. The tumour is therefore classified as benign.

Dissection lab

The dissection lab is the best place to get an idea of the location of the meninges. The three meninges (dura mater, arachnoid mater and pia mater) are very closely interlinked. Observing the meninges shows how and where a meningioma can develop from the cells of the arachnoid. As the arachnoid also surrounds the spinal cord, meningiomas are found throughout the cranial-spinal axis.

 Nine percent of patients have multiple meningiomas.

Attention should be paid to the following intracranial predilection sites of meningiomas during dissection: the Falx cerebri, Sinus sagittalis superior, Alae ossis sphenoidalis, Tuberculum sellae, the olfactory groove and N. opticus.

 Blood supply is guaranteed via meningeal branches of the A. carotis externa.

Back in the clinic

The indication for surgery depends on factors such as location, size, symptoms and the health status of the patient. Because they are mostly benign tumours with slow growth rates, very small meningiomas without clinical symptoms must often only be controlled. In the case of faster growth rates or incipient clinical symptoms as in the above-mentioned patient, a surgical procedure is indicated.

 Further treatment options are fractionated or stereotactic radiation (radiotherapy), or the gamma knife.

The prognosis is particularly positive for grade I meningioma. Following complete removal of the tumour, the probability of relapse is approx. 9 % over the next five years. Long-term monitoring with MRI is often sufficient. The patient has already left the hospital and is now in a rehabilitation clinic. In eight weeks' time, she can expect to return to her professional life.

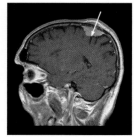

Fig. a Paramedian CT, right side; sagittal plane. The arrow points to a round mass with smooth margins, showing homogeneous enhancement with contrast agent. [R261-T534]

Development of the nervous system and brain

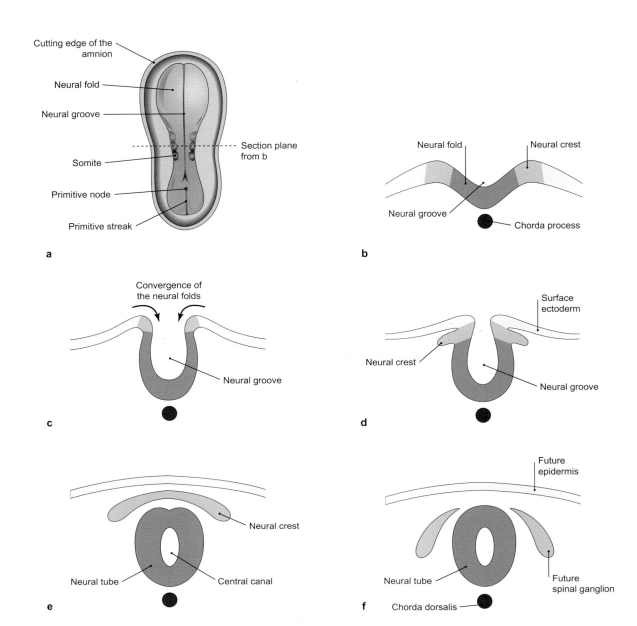

Fig. 12.1a–f   Formation of the neural groove, neural folds, neural tube and neural crests. [E347-09]
a Superior view after removal of the amniotic cavity.
b–f Cross-sections of embryos in sequential developmental stages.
The CNS and PNS originate from the ectoderm. The CNS develops via a neural plate, which forms a neural groove as well as two neural folds and neural crests on both its right and left side. While the neural groove deepens, the right and left neural folds move closer together and soon fuse to become the neural tube (starting from the fourth to sixth somites) that encloses the central canal. Initially, the neural tube is still open to the amniotic cavity via the Neuroporus anterior (rostralis) and the Neuroporus posterior (caudalis). On the 24th day, the Neuroporus anterior closes, and on the 26th day the Neuroporus posterior closes. The right and left neural crests also approach each other and fuse above the neural tube to become the neural crest, before separating again shortly afterwards. The PNS begins to differentiate from the neural crest cells.

Clinical remarks

If the rostral part of the neural tube does not close (open Neuroporus rostralis), the regular development of the three brain vesicles will not take place. Only a diffuse cluster of neural tissue is formed due to misdirected induction processes. The absence of brain development also results in an improper development of the skull. A facial skull is formed, but the brain and neurocranium are absent **(anencephaly)**. This developmental malformation is always fatal.

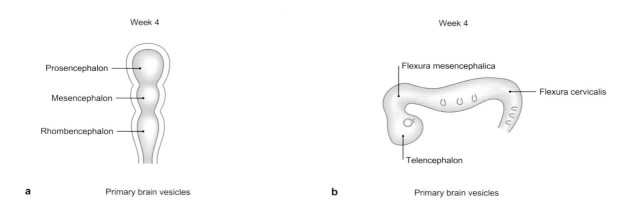

a Primary brain vesicles

b Primary brain vesicles

Fig. 12.2a and b   Development of the brain: primary brain vesicles. [E838]
a Schematic frontal section. In **week 4,** the neural tube is closed at both ends. The rostral end begins to enlarge and forms the three successive **primary brain vesicles:** forebrain (prosencephalon), midbrain (mesencephalon), and hindbrain (rhombencephalon).

b Schematic lateral view. **Also** during **week 4,** the **midbrain flexure** (Flexura mesencephalica) emerges between the forebrain (prosencephalon) and the midbrain (mesencephalon), and the **cervical flexure** (Flexura cervicalis) forms between the hindbrain (rhombencephalon) and the spinal cord.

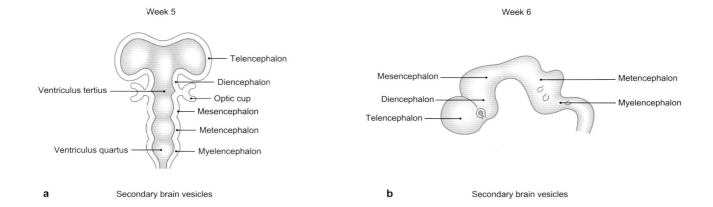

a Secondary brain vesicles

b Secondary brain vesicles

Fig. 12.3a and b   Development of the brain: secondary brain vesicles. [E838]
a Schematic frontal section. In **week 5,** a part of the prosencephalon expands on the right and left sides of the median line to become the **cerebrum,** from which the cerebral hemispheres emerge. Also, the diencephalon originates from the prosencephalon. The third ventricle is formed between the diencephalon and mesencephalon. Beneath the mesencephalon, the hindbrain **(metencephalon)** evolves, of which the main components will eventually be the pons and cerebellum. The posterior part of the hindbrain **(myelencephalon)** follows caudally; it includes the fourth ventricle and the Medulla oblongata and transitions into the spinal cord.

The three primary brain vesicles give rise to six **secondary brain vesicles** (paired vesicles of the cerebrum, as well as the diencephalon, mesencephalon, metencephalon and myelencephalon).
b Schematic lateral view. In **week 6,** the cerebrum, diencephalon, mesencephalon, metencephalon, and myelencephalon are clearly definable. The optic cups (or eye cups) become visible between the cerebrum and diencephalon. The development of the cerebellum starts with a lateral extension of the rhombencephalon. At the dorsal aspect of the metencephalon, the developing cerebellum can already be seen.

Development of the brain

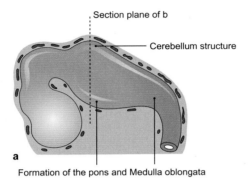

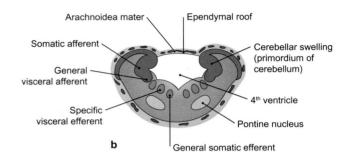

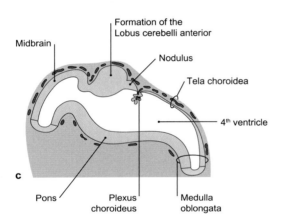

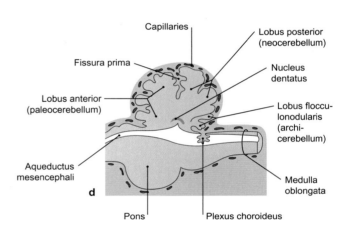

Fig. 12.4a–d   Development of the brain. [E347-09]
a Schematic lateral view. In **week 5,** the primordial pons, Medulla oblongata and cerebellum are formed (from the myelencephalon vesicle).
b Schematic cross-section. The central canal in the rhombencephalon expands and the dorsal alar plates fold outwards, so that the canal is only covered by a thin roofplate (formation of the rhomboid fossa). Hereby the alar and basal plates end up next to each other, separated by the Sulcus limitans. The future nuclei of the cranial nerves are located symmetrically next to each other. As a consequence, the primordial structures of the cerebellum expand further dorsally and, by uniting in the median line, they will later enclose the rhomboid fossa (not shown).
c, d Schematic sagittal sections. The sagittal sections through the rhombencephalon in **week 6 (c)** and in **week 17 (d)** clearly show the ongoing development of the pons and cerebellum.

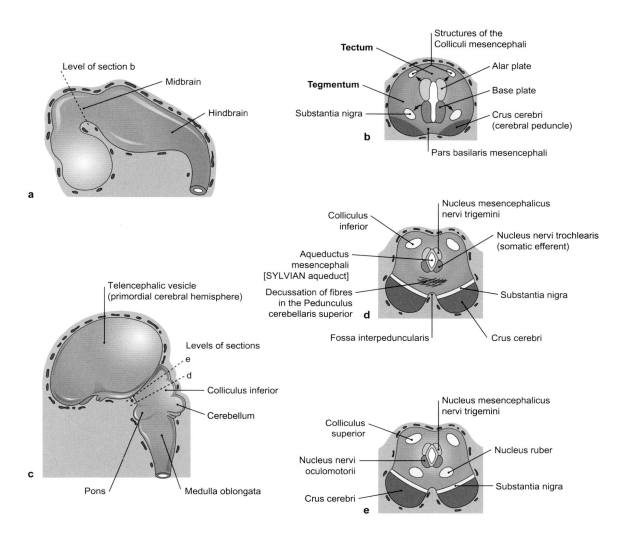

Fig. 12.5a–e   Development of the mesencephalon. [E347-09]
a Schematic lateral view. In **week 5,** the primordial mesencephalon emerges in the area of the Flexura mesencephalica. In comparison to other parts of the brain, the area of the mesencephalon vesicle undergoes only minimal changes.
b Schematic cross-section. The centrally located lumen narrows due to the strong growth of the lateral walls. This leads to the formation of the Aqueductus mesencephali [SYLVIAN aqueduct], a relatively thin structure as compared to other internal parts of the cerebrospinal fluid system, which connects the third ventricle to the fourth ventricle. The surrounding tissue forms a roofplate **(tectum)** and a larger ventral covering **(tegmentum),** which with its most anterior part as the **Pars basilaris mesencephali** includes the Crura cerebri. From the alar plates that

have arisen from the dorsal-lateral parts of the neural tube, neuroblasts migrate into the Tectum mesencephali and form the paired Colliculi superiores and inferiores here. It is debatable whether the Nucleus ruber and the Substantia nigra originate from differentiated neuroblasts of the alar plates or roofplates (presented here is the formation of the Substantia nigra from the basal plates).
c–e Schematic sagittal section **(c)** and schematic cross-sections **(d, e)** of the mesencephalon in **week 11.** Neuroblasts of the former basal plates migrate into the Tegmentum mesencephali and form groups of motor nuclei (e. g. Nucleus nervi oculomotorii) here. In week 11, the structure of the mesencephalon has already developed its definitive form.

Development of the brain

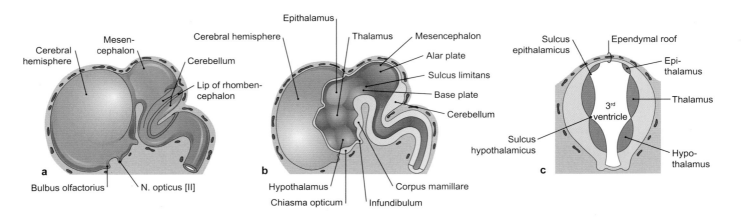

a Cerebral hemisphere — Mesen-cephalon — Cerebral hemisphere — Cerebellum — Lip of rhomben-cephalon — Bulbus olfactorius — N. opticus [II]

b Epithalamus — Thalamus — Mesencephalon — Alar plate — Sulcus limitans — Base plate — Cerebellum — Corpus mamillare — Infundibulum — Chiasma opticum — Hypothalamus

c Sulcus epithalamicus — Ependymal roof — Epi-thalamus — Thalamus — 3rd ventricle — Sulcus hypothalamicus — Hypo-thalamus

Fig. 12.6a–c   Development of the brain in week 7. [E347-09]
a Schematic view of the surface of the brain. Due to the increasing size/expansion of the cerebrum, the diencephalon is only visible at a few points from the outside.
b Schematic median section with prosencephalon and mesencephalon. The former vesicle of the diencephalon differentiates further into the parts of the diencephalon, including the hypothalamus with pituitary gland, thalamus, epithalamus and subthalamus. The primordial eyes also emerge from the diencephalon.
c Schematic cross-section through the diencephalon. The centrally located lumen enlarges to become the third ventricle. The epithalamus, thalamus and hypothalamus differentiate in the lateral wall of the neural tube. Grooves or depressions (Sulcus epithalamicus, Sulcus hypothalamicus) are formed between the areas of the nuclei.

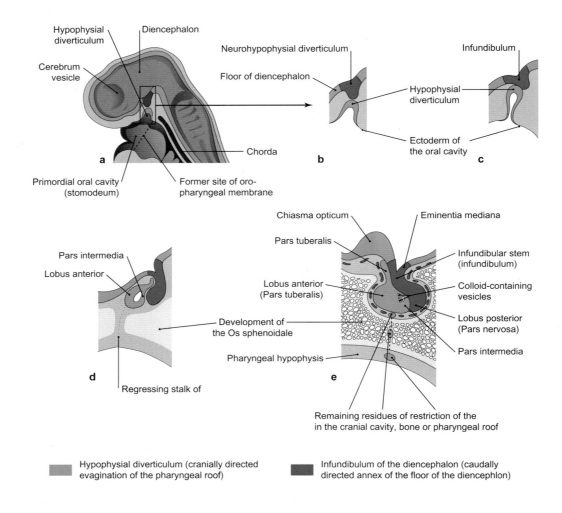

a Hypophysial diverticulum — Diencephalon — Cerebrum vesicle — Neurohypophysial diverticulum — Floor of diencephalon — Infundibulum — Hypophysial diverticulum — Chorda — Ectoderm of the oral cavity — Primordial oral cavity (stomodeum) — Former site of oro-pharyngeal membrane

b **c**

d Pars intermedia — Lobus anterior — Development of the Os sphenoidale — Regressing stalk of

e Chiasma opticum — Eminentia mediana — Pars tuberalis — Infundibular stem (infundibulum) — Lobus anterior (Pars tuberalis) — Colloid-containing vesicles — Lobus posterior (Pars nervosa) — Pars intermedia — Pharyngeal hypophysis — Remaining residues of restriction of the in the cranial cavity, bone or pharyngeal roof

Hypophysial diverticulum (cranially directed evagination of the pharyngeal roof)

Infundibulum of the diencephalon (caudally directed annex of the floor of the diencephlon)

Fig. 12.7a–e   Development of the pituitary gland. [E347-09]
a Schematic overview in the median section with the roof of the stomodeum and base of the diencephalon.
b–d Folding of the epithelium of the roof of the stomodeum (RATHKE's pouch, forms the future adenohypophysis) and fusion with the infundibulum (forms the later neurohypophysis). The pituitary gland emerges from two types of tissue: firstly, around the 36th day of development, the ectodermal epithelium of the roof of the stomodeum forms a fold or diverticulum (so-called RATHKE's pouch), which later becomes the adenohypophysis. Secondly, it grows towards the infundibulum, which is the primordial neurohypophysis, and within a short time both structures merge to form the pituitary gland.
e Position of the pituitary gland (hypophysis) in the Sella turcica.

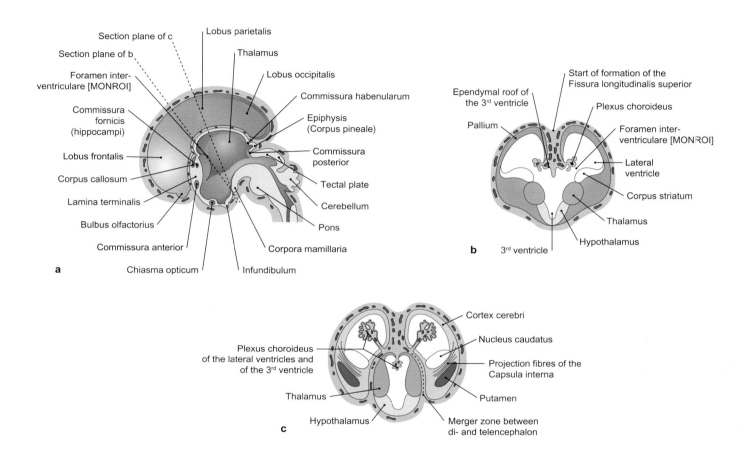

Fig. 12.8a–c   Development of the forebrain (mesencephalon).
[E347-09]
a Schematic lateral view of the medial surface of the mesencephalon in week 10. The cerebral vesicle develops into a median part and two lateral appendages. The latter differentiate to later become the adult cerebral hemispheres.
b Cross-section of the mesencephalon at the level of the Foramina interventricularia, showing the Corpus striatum and the Plexus choroideus of the lateral ventricles. Due to the considerably slower growth of the cover plate, the rapidly growing cerebral hemispheres arch over the cover plate. Thereby the Fissura longitudinalis superior is created between them; the former cover plate is located in the area of the later Corpus callosum. The basal and alar plates become the grey matter and form the pallium. Thickening of the basal plate gives rise to the basal ganglia at the bottom of the lateral ventricles. The inner (subarachnoid) spaces of the cerebrospinal fluid emerge from the lumen of the neural tube. The ventricles and their communicating ducts are created by the faster and slower growth rates in the different parts. In the cerebrum, the crescent- or C-shaped growth direction of the two cerebral hemispheres results in the typical structure of the first and second ventricles. The Plexus choroideus of the two lateral ventricles and of the third ventricle emerge from the cover plate.

c Comparable section in week 11. The ingrowing Capsula interna divides the Corpus striatum into the putamen and the Nucleus caudatus. All afferent and efferent nerve fibres to or from the cerebrum have to pass through the diencephalon. A majority of these fibres is therefore visible as Capsula interna. The nuclei of the subthalamus located here are pushed aside by the fibres. These lateral parts of the diencephalon are called Globus pallidus (pallidum). They lie in the cerebrum, but originate from the diencephalic basal plate.

Brain and spinal cord

Development of the brain

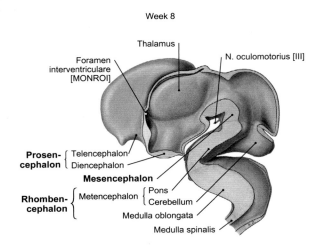

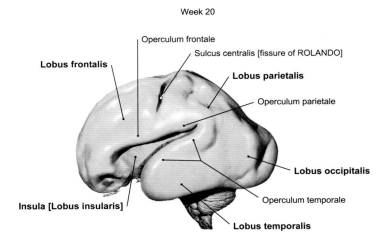

Fig. 12.9   Development of the brain; median section. [S700]
In **week 8,** the individual brain structures are already clearly definable. The cerebrum and diencephalon have emerged from the prosencephalon. The thalamus in the diencephalon can already be recognised. In the mesencephalon, the exiting N. oculomotorius [III] becomes visible. The rhombencephalon has differentiated into the metencephalon and the Medulla oblongata (myelencephalon). The pons and cerebellum emerge from the metencephalon. The Medulla oblongata is followed by the Medulla spinalis.

Fig. 12.10   Development of the brain; view from the left side. [S700]
The growth of the cerebrum is already far advanced in **week 20 of the fetal development** (crown-rump length 20 cm). In the area of the cerebral hemispheres, the Lobi frontalis, parietalis, occipitalis and temporalis have already been formed. However, the Lobus insularis is not yet completely covered by the Lobi frontalis, parietalis and temporalis. Only parts of the pons, cerebellum and Medulla oblongata are still visible structures of the brainstem.

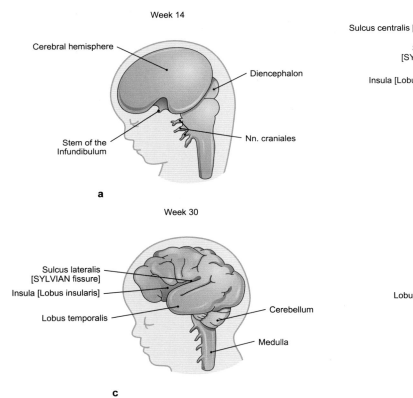

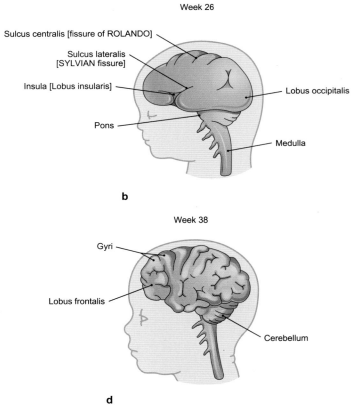

Fig. 12.11a–d   Development of the left cerebral hemisphere, diencephalon and brainstem; schematic representation; lateral view. [E347-09]
a Week 14 of fetal development. In week 14, the cerebrum still has a completely smooth surface.

b–d Weeks 26, 30 and 38 of fetal development. Subsequently, convolutions (gyri) and grooves (sulci) develop incrementally (**gyrification,** surface enlargement), the insula is formed and is progressively overlaid by the Lobi frontalis, parietalis and temporalis.

Clinical remarks

The term **encephalocele** (hernia cerebri, cerebral hernia, outer brain prolapse, cranium bifidum) summarises defective developmental malformations with a median gap of the skull (at the root of the nose, or the forehead, cranial base, or occiput) (→ Fig. a). Protruding from this gap can be parts of the meninges (**meningocele,** → Fig. b), or the brain (**meningoencephalocele,** → Fig. c) without involvement of the cerebrospinal fluid spaces (**encephalocele,** or d) including parts of the brain ventricles (**encephalocystocele,** → Fig. d, **meningohydroencephalocele**).

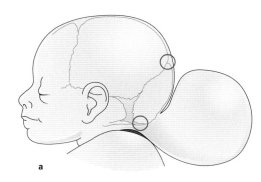

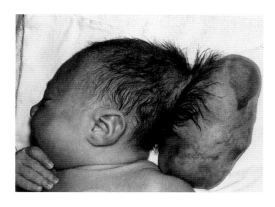

Head of a newborn with an extensive herniation in the occipital region. The upper red circle marks the defect in the area of the small fontanelle, the lower red circle indicates the defect in the area of the Foramen magnum. [E347-09]

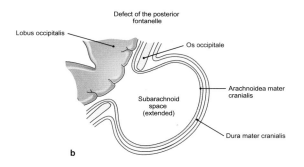

The hernial sac of a **meningocele** is formed by the skin and meninges and is filled with cerebrospinal fluid. [E347-09]

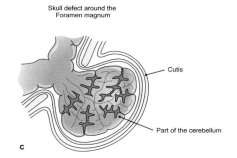

The hernial sac of a **meningoencephalocele** contains parts of the cerebellum and is covered by the meninges and skin. [E347-09]

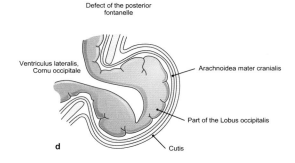

The hernial sac of this **encephalocystocele** is formed by parts of the Lobus occipitalis and part of the posterior horn of the lateral ventricle. [E347-09]

Development of the spinal cord

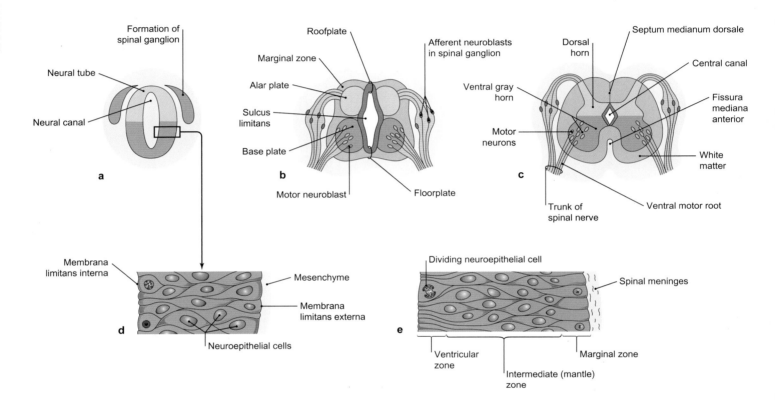

Fig. 12.12a–e   Development of the spinal cord from the caudal portion of the neural tube, schematic representation. [E347-09]
a Day 23. In the caudal portion of the neural tube, the lateral parts of the alar and basal plates begin to thicken.
b Week 6. The efferent fibres emerge from the basal plate (the future motor anterior horn) and form the Radix anterior. Afferent fibres assemble in the direction of the alar plate (the future sensory posterior horn) and form the Radix posterior.

c Week 9. Due to the growth processes of other structures and the simultaneous growth retardation of the basal and roofplates, the latter are shifted into a deeper position. This results in the formation of the Fissura mediana anterior and of the Sulcus medianus posterior. The lumen of the neural tube hardly enlarges and remains as the central canal (Canalis centralis).
d, e The wall of the neural tube thickens (**d**), and differentiates into three zones (**e**): (1) ventricular zone, (2) intermediate zone, (3) marginal zone.

Clinical remarks

Spina bifida is a congenital cleft formation of the spine and the spinal cord caused by teratogenic substances (e. g. alcohol, medication) or the failed induction of the Chorda dorsalis.

In the case of a **Spina bifida occulta** (→ Fig. a) only the vertebral arches are affected. A vertebral cleft usually results from the failed fusion of one or two vertebrae. Hairy and strongly pigmented skin often covers the area of the defect. There are usually no clinical symptoms.

In the case of a **Spina bifida cystica** (→ Fig. b), the incomplete development of several adjacent vertebrae leaves a gap through which the meninges covering the spinal cord protrude cyst-like into the defect (meningocele). If the cyst also contains spinal cord and nerve tissue it is considered a meningomyelocele (usually associated with deficits).

A **Spina bifida aperta** (rhachischisis, myeloschisis, myelocele; → Fig. c) is the most severe form of a cleft disorder of the vertebral arches and is combined with the inability of the neural folds to fuse. The undifferentiated neural plate is not covered by skin and lies fully exposed on the back. Newborns affected by such defects usually die shortly after birth. If the defect extends to the rostral end of the neural groove, the primordial brain does not develop (anencephaly).

a, b [E347-09], c [G617]

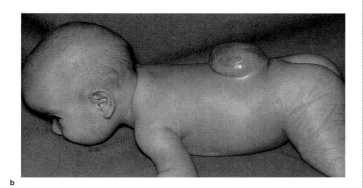

b

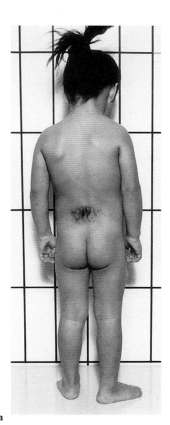

a

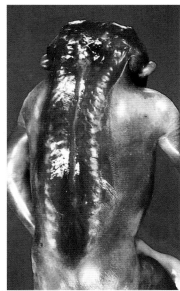

c

General principles

Nervous system, organisation

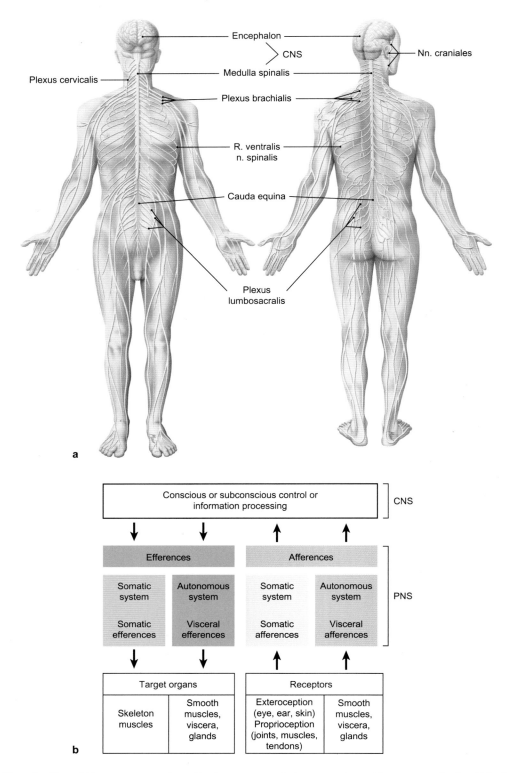

Fig. 12.13a and b   Organisation of the nervous system, Systema nervosum.
a Morphological organisation, ventral and dorsal views. The nervous system is divided into the central (CNS) and the peripheral nervous system (PNS). The **CNS** consists of the brain and spinal cord, and accomplishes complex functions such as storage of experience (memory), development of ideas (thinking) as well as emotions, and enables the rapid adjustment of the whole organism to extrinsic and intrinsic changes in the external environment and within the body. The CNS is well protected in the skull and the Canalis vertebralis. The **PNS** is mainly composed of spinal nerves (with connections to the spinal cord) and cranial nerves (with connections to the brain). It enables communication between the organs and the CNS, controls the activity of muscles and viscera, and provides communication links between the environment and the internal human body. The structures of the PNS leave the protective vertebral canal through the Foramina intervertebralia of the spine. [S702-L127]
b Functional organisation. Functionally, the nervous system is divided into an **autonomic** (visceral, for the control of visceral activity, mostly involuntary) and a **somatic** (for the innervation of skeletal muscles, voluntary perception of sensory input, communication with the environment) nervous system. Both systems are closely interlinked and interact with each other. The functional structure is not identical to the morphological structure in all the parts.
In addition to the nervous system, the endocrine system also participates in the regulation of the entire organism. [S702-L126]

12 cranial nerves (Nn. craniales)
• paired
• non-segmental structure
• heterogeneous structure
• each has its own name

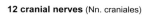

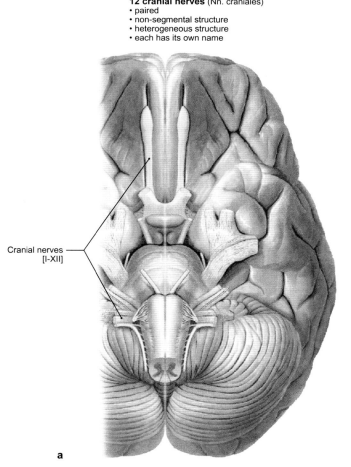

Cranial nerves
[I-XII]

31 spinal nerves (Nn. spinales)
• paired
• segmental structure
• uniform structure
• don't have a separate name

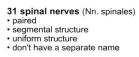

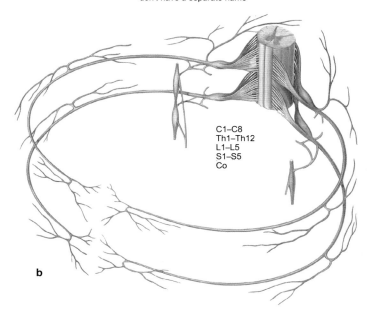

C1–C8
Th1–Th12
L1–L5
S1–S5
Co

b

a

Fig. 12.14a and b   Comparison of cranial nerves, Nn. craniales, and spinal nerves, Nn. spinales. [S700]
a Ventral view onto the caudal base of the brain.
b Oblique view from above left onto two spinal nerves with their corresponding spinal cord segments.

There are 12 paired **cranial nerves, Nn. craniales.** They are non-segmental, heterogeneous in structure, and all individually named. The 31 **spinal nerves, Nn. spinales,** are also paired nerves but, contrary to cranial nerves, follow a segmental order, are more homogeneous in structure, and are not individually named.

Brain and spinal cord

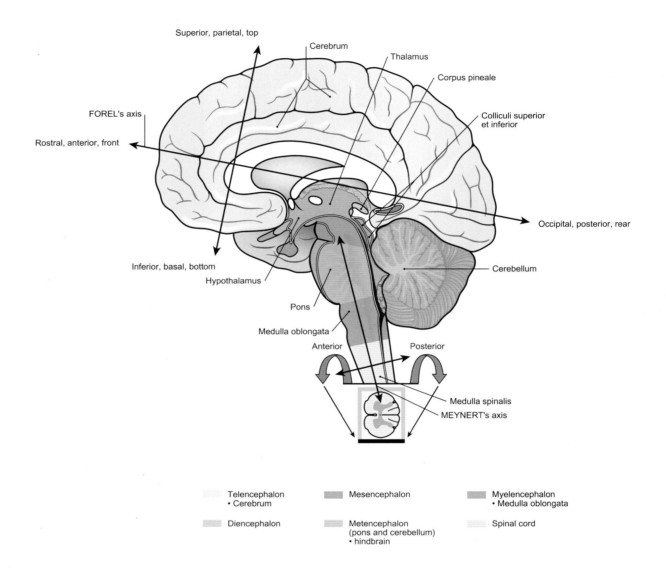

Superior, parietal, top

Cerebrum

Thalamus

Corpus pineale

FOREL's axis

Colliculi superior
et inferior

Rostral, anterior, front

Occipital, posterior, rear

Inferior, basal, bottom

Cerebellum

Hypothalamus

Pons

Medulla oblongata

Anterior   Posterior

Medulla spinalis

MEYNERT's axis

Telencephalon • Cerebrum	Mesencephalon	Myelencephalon • Medulla oblongata
Diencephalon	Metencephalon (pons and cerebellum) • hindbrain	Spinal cord

Fig. 12.15   Positional and directional terms for the CNS and spinal cord; median section. [S700-L126]

In the course of the development of the brain, a bending of the neural tube occurs. Thereby the longitudinal axis of the forebrain (prosencephalon = diencephalon and cerebrum) tilts forward. Consequently, a unique nomenclature was created for the brain, as is shown in the figure. For example, although former occipital parts, e.g. the metencephalon, shifted in a parietal direction, they are still referred to as occipital.

The topographical axis between the cerebrum and diencephalon is referred to as **FOREL's axis,** and the axis through the centre of the brainstem (Truncus encephali) is called **MEYNERT's axis.**

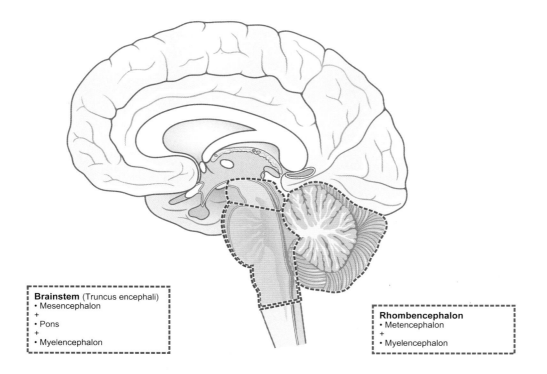

Brainstem (Truncus encephali)
· Mesencephalon
+
· Pons
+
· Myelencephalon

Rhombencephalon
· Metencephalon
+
· Myelencephalon

Fig. 12.16   Organisation of the brainstem, Truncus cerebri, Truncus encephali, versus the rhombencephalon; median section [S700-L126] The brainstem, Truncus cerebri or Truncus encephali, comprises the midbrain, mesencephalon, the pons, and the afterbrain, myelencephalon (red dotted lines). The rhombencephalon is composed of the hindbrain, metencephalon and the afterbrain, myelencephalon (blue dotted line).

Clinical remarks

The **clinical neurological examination** includes a physical examination and the taking of a medical history to obtain information in particular on previous neurological diseases, cranial-cerebral trauma, congenital or familial neurological disorders, risk factors and autonomic functions. This is complemented by taking a symptom-focused history and specific diagnostic techniques to evaluate the cranial nerves and their corresponding functional systems. In addition, the physician should try a preliminary assessment of the patient's consciousness, orientation in space and time, memory function, concentration and basic mood. **Disorders of the consciousness** are clinically divided into **somnolence** (abnormal sleepiness but easy to wake up, delayed reaction to verbal communication, immediate response to pain stimuli), **sopor** (abnormally deep sleepiness and difficult to wake up, delayed but targeted defensive reaction to pain stimuli), and **coma** (cannot be woken up by external stimuli). A quantitative assessment of impaired states of consciousness, e.g. within the context of a follow-up, can be attained with the **Glasgow coma scale.** The severity of a consciousness disorder is quantitatively evaluated by testing the patient's spontaneous activity, and his or her response to verbal requests and pain stimuli, and scoring these reactions with points. Disorientation, confusion and perception disorders (e.g. in the context of an alcoholic or drug delirium) can lead to substantial disturbance of consciousness.

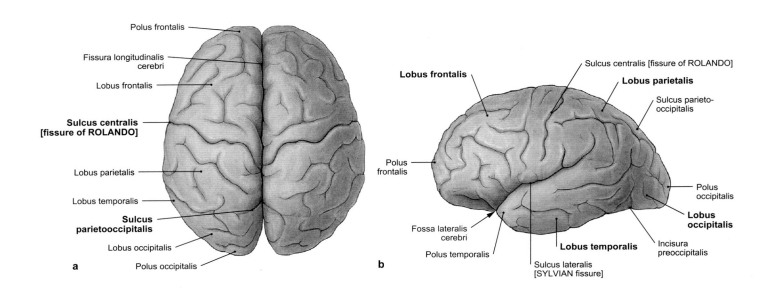

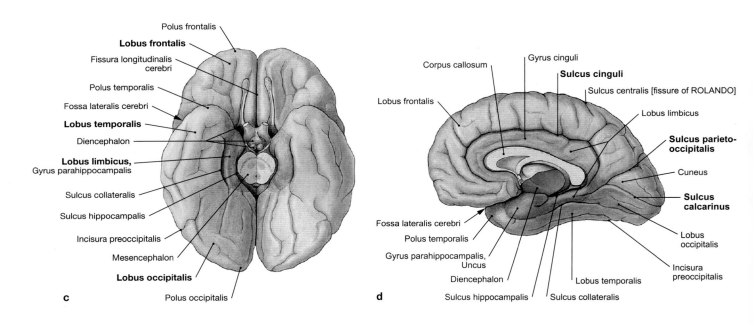

Fig. 12.17a–d   Lobes of the cerebrum, Lobi cerebri. [S700]
a Superior view.
b Lateral view from the outer left side.
c Inferior view.
d Medial view from the left side of the sagittal section of the right hemisphere.

Towards the end of the eighth embryonic month, the primary grooves of the cerebrum are developed. These are consistently present in all humans. Each cerebral hemisphere is divided into **four lobes:**

* frontal lobe (Lobus frontalis)
* parietal lobe (Lobus parietalis)
* temporal lobe (Lobus temporalis)
* occipital lobe (Lobus occipitalis).

In addition to the four cerebral lobes, the **Lobus limbicus** (composed mainly of the Gyrus cinguli, together with the Gyrus parahippocampalis and the uncus) and the **Lobus insularis** (insula, not visible, as it is covered by the opercula of the frontal, parietal, and temporal lobes) can be distinguished (→ Fig. 12.18). Secondary and tertiary grooves of the cerebrum develop in an individually variable pattern. So the boundaries between the individual lobes are arbitrary in many parts (e.g. Incisura preoccipitalis).

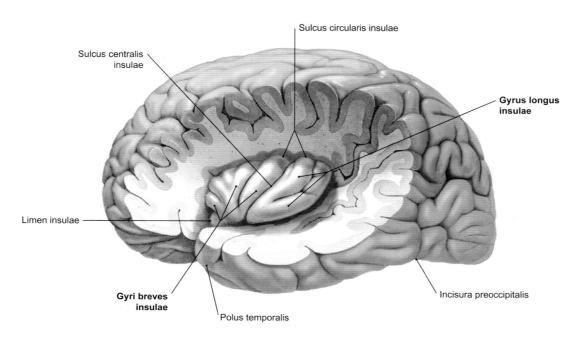

Sulcus circularis insulae

Sulcus centralis insulae

Gyrus longus insulae

Limen insulae

Gyri breves insulae

Polus temporalis

Incisura preoccipitalis

Fig. 12.18 Convolutions, gyri, and grooves, sulci, of the cerebral hemispheres; view from the left side; after removal of the parts of the frontal, parietal and temporal lobes covering the insula. [S700-L238]

The cortical regions of the Lobi frontalis, parietalis and temporalis that surround the Sulcus lateralis are called the opercula and have been removed to expose the insula (→ Fig. 12.17). The processing of olfactory, gustatory and visceral information takes place in the insula. It is usually considered an independent lobe.

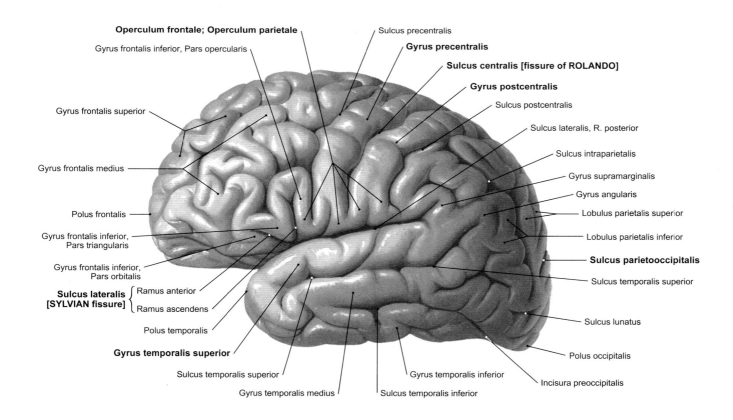

Operculum frontale; Operculum parietale

Gyrus frontalis inferior, Pars opercularis

Gyrus frontalis superior

Gyrus frontalis medius

Polus frontalis

Gyrus frontalis inferior, Pars triangularis

Gyrus frontalis inferior, Pars orbitalis

Sulcus lateralis [SYLVIAN fissure] { Ramus anterior / Ramus ascendens }

Polus temporalis

Gyrus temporalis superior

Sulcus temporalis superior

Gyrus temporalis medius

Sulcus precentralis

Gyrus precentralis

Sulcus centralis [fissure of ROLANDO]

Gyrus postcentralis

Sulcus postcentralis

Sulcus lateralis, R. posterior

Sulcus intraparietalis

Gyrus supramarginalis

Gyrus angularis

Lobulus parietalis superior

Lobulus parietalis inferior

Sulcus parietooccipitalis

Sulcus temporalis superior

Sulcus lunatus

Polus occipitalis

Incisura preoccipitalis

Gyrus temporalis inferior

Sulcus temporalis inferior

Fig. 12.19 Convolutions, gyri, and grooves, sulci, of the cerebral hemispheres; view from the left side. [S700]
Although the labelled gyri and sulci can be identified in each human brain (e.g. Sulcus centralis, Sulcus lateralis or Gyrus temporalis supe-

rior), an identical pattern of gyri and sulci are not even displayed by both of the hemispheres of the same brain. The individual singularity of the brain surface is comparable to a fingerprint.

Brain

Cerebrum, cerebral cortex

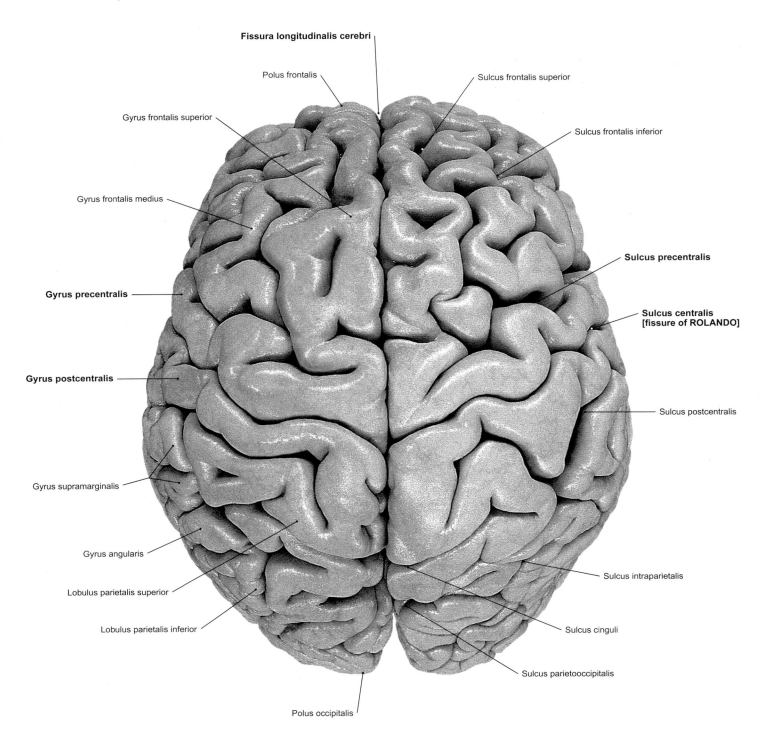

Fissura longitudinalis cerebri

Polus frontalis

Sulcus frontalis superior

Gyrus frontalis superior

Sulcus frontalis inferior

Gyrus frontalis medius

Sulcus precentralis

Gyrus precentralis

Sulcus centralis
[fissure of ROLANDO]

Gyrus postcentralis

Sulcus postcentralis

Gyrus supramarginalis

Gyrus angularis

Sulcus intraparietalis

Lobulus parietalis superior

Sulcus cinguli

Lobulus parietalis inferior

Sulcus parietooccipitalis

Polus occipitalis

Fig. 12.20 Cerebrum; superior view; after removal of the Leptomeninx. [S700]

The cerebrum constitutes the main part of the brain. It is composed of **two hemispheres** which are separated by the **Fissura longitudinalis cerebri.** During early development, the surface of the brain is still smooth. Its strong growth results in the quite variable formation of grooves **(sulci)** and convolutions **(gyri). Due** to this folding, the surface area of the brain is significantly increased. Of the cerebral surface, an area of two-thirds is thus not visible from the outside at all.

Clinical remarks

Atrophy of the brain develops with advanced age. This is associated with a widening of the sulci and a narrowing of the gyri. However, the decreasing memory function which accompanies advanced age is not directly linked to this atrophy of the brain, but is caused above all by a shorter duration of the deep sleep phases. With ageing, the proportion of deep sleep will diminish significantly. Up to the 26th year of life, 19 % of total sleep duration is spent in deep sleep phases. Between 36 and 50 years of life this percentage drops to 3 %. Studies have shown that this correlates to significant decreases in memory function.

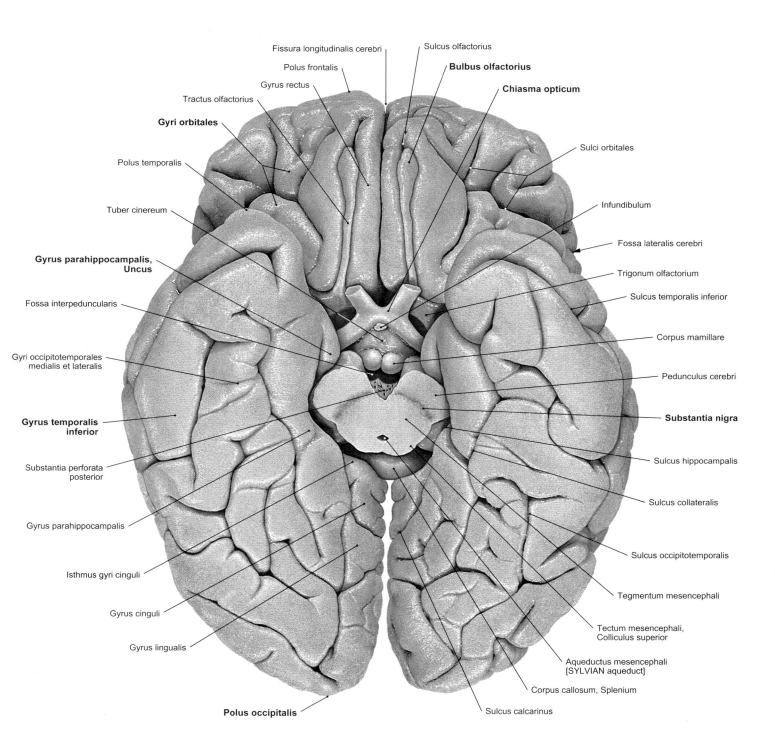

Fissura longitudinalis cerebri

Sulcus olfactorius

Polus frontalis

Bulbus olfactorius

Gyrus rectus

Tractus olfactorius

Chiasma opticum

Gyri orbitales

Sulci orbitales

Polus temporalis

Infundibulum

Tuber cinereum

Fossa lateralis cerebri

Gyrus parahippocampalis, Uncus

Trigonum olfactorium

Sulcus temporalis inferior

Fossa interpeduncularis

Corpus mamillare

Gyri occipitotemporales medialis et lateralis

Pedunculus cerebri

Gyrus temporalis inferior

Substantia nigra

Substantia perforata posterior

Sulcus hippocampalis

Gyrus parahippocampalis

Sulcus collateralis

Isthmus gyri cinguli

Sulcus occipitotemporalis

Gyrus cinguli

Tegmentum mesencephali

Gyrus lingualis

Tectum mesencephali, Colliculus superior

Aqueductus mesencephali [SYLVIAN aqueduct]

Corpus callosum, Splenium

Polus occipitalis

Sulcus calcarinus

Fig. 12.21 Convolutions, gyri, and grooves, sulci, of the cerebral hemispheres; inferior view; after cutting through the midbrain (mesencephalon). [S700]

The cerebrum accounts for the largest part of the cranial base. Here the Gyri orbitales are located with the overlying Bulbi and Tractus olfactorii.

In addition to the Chiasma opticum, the Gyrus parahippocampalis in the Lobus temporalis with its characteristic anterior bend (uncus), the Gyri temporales and the Polus occipitalis are visible. In the mesencephalon, the dark Substantia nigra can be clearly differentiated.

Cerebrum, cerebral cortex

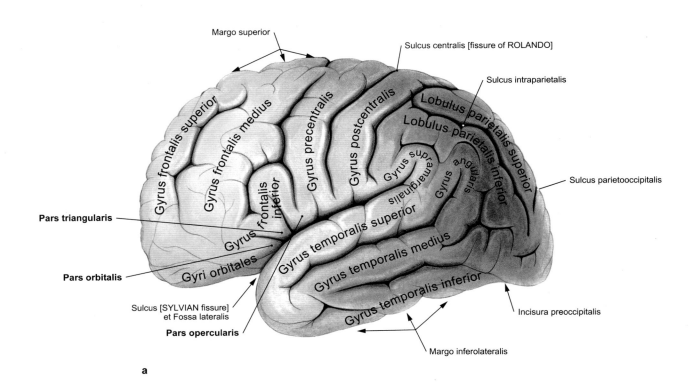

a

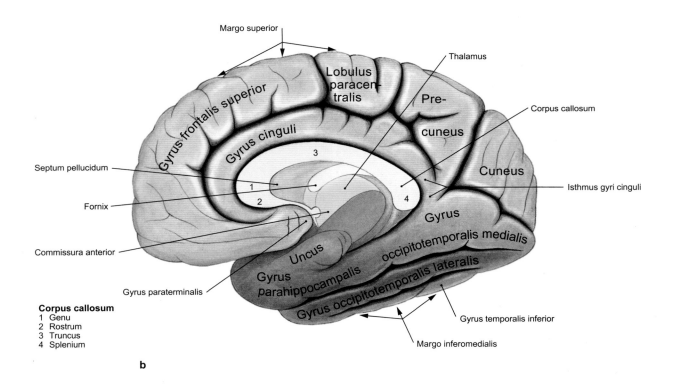

Corpus callosum
1 Genu
2 Rostrum
3 Truncus
4 Splenium

b

Fig. 12.22a and b Convolutions, gyri, of the cerebral hemispheres. [S700]
a View from the left side. The Gyrus frontalis inferior is divided into a Pars orbitalis, a Pars triangularis and a Pars opercularis.

b Medial view. The Corpus callosum is composed of the rostrum, genu, truncus and splenium. In addition, the fornix, the Commissura anterior, the thalamus and the Septum pellucidum are visible.

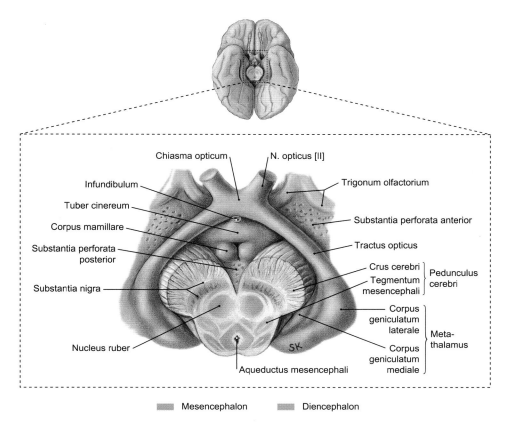

Chiasma opticum
N. opticus [II]
Infundibulum
Trigonum olfactorium
Tuber cinereum
Corpus mamillare
Substantia perforata anterior
Substantia perforata posterior
Tractus opticus
Substantia nigra
Crus cerebri
Tegmentum mesencephali
Pedunculus cerebri
Corpus geniculatum laterale
Nucleus ruber
Meta-thalamus
Aqueductus mesencephali
Corpus geniculatum mediale
SK

Mesencephalon   Diencephalon

Fig. 12.23 Diencephalon; inferior view; the brainstem was removed at the level of the mesencephalon (see dotted line of incision in → Fig. 12.24). [S702-L238]
The diencephalon does not only control the link between the brainstem and cerebrum, but also coordinates the neuronal and endocrine systems. It is barely visible from the outside, as it is almost completely covered by the cerebrum due to the embryological development. Only in the inferior view are some of its parts visible, such as the N. opticus [II], Chiasma opticum, Tractus opticus, Corpus geniculatum laterale, Corpus geniculatum mediale, Substantia perforata anterior, infundibulum of the pituitary gland (infundibular stalk), Tuber cinereum and Corpora mamillaria.

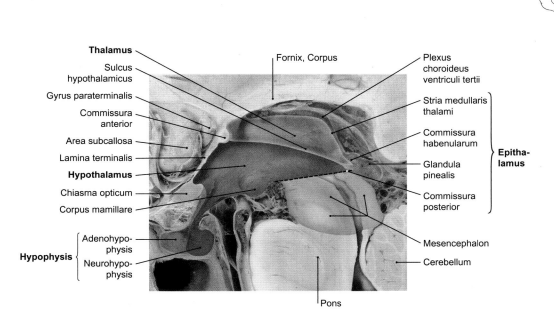

Thalamus
Sulcus hypothalamicus
Gyrus paraterminalis
Commissura anterior
Area subcallosa
Lamina terminalis
Hypothalamus
Chiasma opticum
Corpus mamillare
Fornix, Corpus
Plexus choroideus ventriculi tertii
Stria medullaris thalami
Commissura habenularum
Epitha-lamus
Glandula pinealis
Commissura posterior
Mesencephalon
Hypophysis { Adenohypo-physis / Neurohypo-physis }
Cerebellum
Pons

Fig. 12.24 Third ventricle, Ventriculus tertius, and parts of the di-encephalon; median section. [S700]
The diencephalon can be divided into different parts:
• epithalamus
• thalamus
• hypothalamus
• subthalamus.

The subthalamus is not visible in this section, since it comprises several accumulations of nerve cell bodies, which were shifted laterally during the development of the third ventricle (→ Fig. 12.8).

Mesencephalon and brainstem

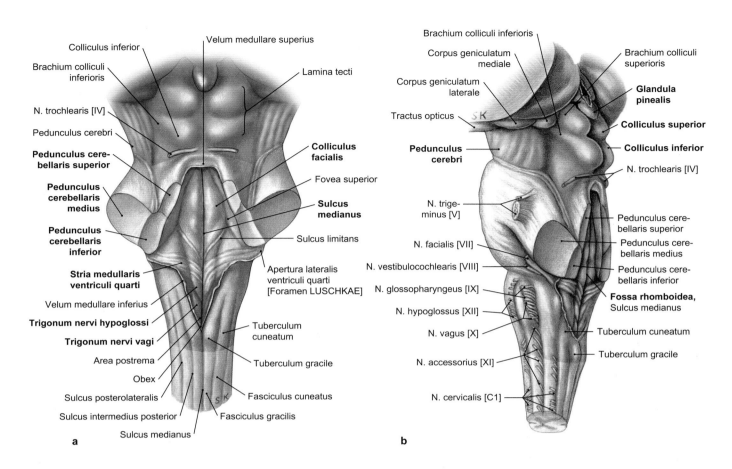

Colliculus inferior
Brachium colliculi inferioris
N. trochlearis [IV]
Pedunculus cerebri
Pedunculus cerebellaris superior
Pedunculus cerebellaris medius
Pedunculus cerebellaris inferior
Stria medullaris ventriculi quarti
Velum medullare inferius
Trigonum nervi hypoglossi
Trigonum nervi vagi
Area postrema
Obex
Sulcus posterolateralis
Sulcus intermedius posterior
Sulcus medianus

Velum medullare superius
Lamina tecti
Colliculus facialis
Fovea superior
Sulcus medianus
Sulcus limitans
Apertura lateralis ventriculi quarti [Foramen LUSCHKAE]
Tuberculum cuneatum
Tuberculum gracile
Fasciculus cuneatus
Fasciculus gracilis

a

Brachium colliculi inferioris
Corpus geniculatum mediale
Corpus geniculatum laterale
Tractus opticus
Pedunculus cerebri
N. trigeminus [V]
N. facialis [VII]
N. vestibulocochlearis [VIII]
N. glossopharyngeus [IX]
N. hypoglossus [XII]
N. vagus [X]
N. accessorius [XI]
N. cervicalis [C1]

Brachium colliculi superioris
Glandula pinealis
Colliculus superior
Colliculus inferior
N. trochlearis [IV]
Pedunculus cerebellaris superior
Pedunculus cerebellaris medius
Pedunculus cerebellaris inferior
Fossa rhomboidea, Sulcus medianus
Tuberculum cuneatum
Tuberculum gracile

b

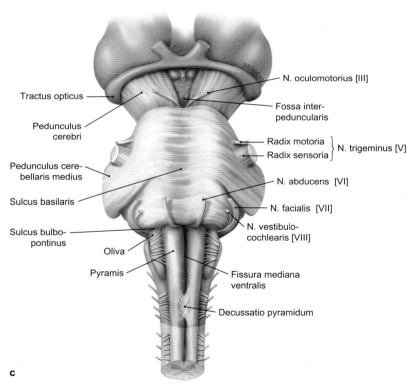

Tractus opticus
Pedunculus cerebri
Pedunculus cerebellaris medius
Sulcus basilaris
Sulcus bulbopontinus
Oliva
Pyramis

N. oculomotorius [III]
Fossa interpeduncularis
Radix motoria
Radix sensoria } N. trigeminus [V]
N. abducens [VI]
N. facialis [VII]
N. vestibulocochlearis [VIII]
Fissura mediana ventralis
Decussatio pyramidum

c

Fig. 12.25a–c Brainstem, Truncus encephali. [S702-L238]
a Dorsal view.
b Lateral view.
c Ventral view.

The brainstem consists of the **mesencephalon** (midbrain, green), the **pons** (blue) and the **Medulla oblongata** (red). The **mesencephalon** extends from the diencephalon to the upper margin of the pons. The **cerebellum** was detached at the cerebellar peduncles (Pedunculi cerebellares). The exit points of the cranial nerves III to XII, with their nuclei located in the brainstem, are also visible.

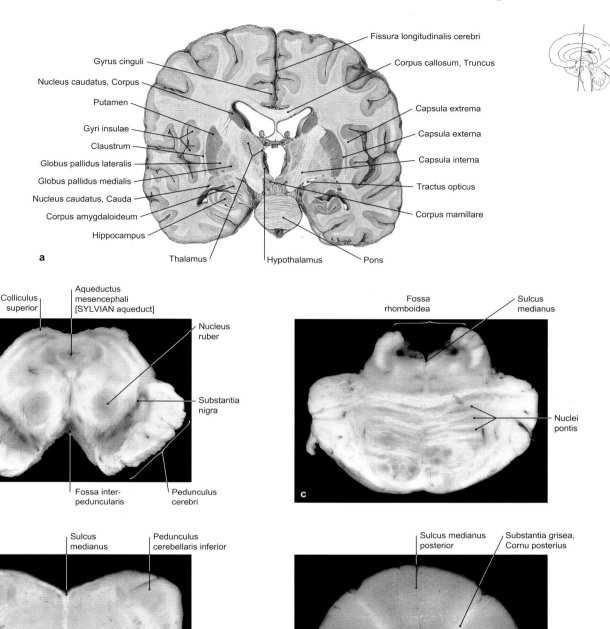

Fig. 12.26a–e   Distribution of the Substantiae grisea and alba in the central nervous system. a [S700], b–e [R247-L318]
a Cerebrum (frontal section at the level of the Corpora mamillaria).
b Mesencephalon.
c Pons.
d Medulla oblongata.
e Medulla spinalis.
Along the gyri and sulci of the cerebrum, there is an approx. 0.5 cm broad layer of grey matter (Substantia grisea), which is known as the Cortex cerebri. Here the neuronal perikarya and glial cells are arranged in six layers, known as the isocortex. Its counterpart is the allocortex with only three to four layers. Developmentally, the latter is characteristic for the older parts of the brain, such as the paleocortex (e. g. olfactory cortex) and the archicortex (e. g. hippocampus). Adjacent to the inner

side of this 0.5 cm broad layer is the white matter (Substantia alba). Deep inside the white matter of the cerebrum are embedded areas of the nuclei (Nucleus caudatus, claustrum, putamen, Globus pallidus and amygdala) or the thalamus in the diencephalon. In the brainstem, the external white matter is interspersed with accumulations of grey matter, e. g. the Substantia nigra and the Nucleus ruber in the mesencephalon, the Nuclei pontis in the pons, the Nucleus olivaris inferior in the Medulla oblongata. In the brainstem, the white and grey matter are more or less clearly distinct and arranged in zones: ventral fibres (white matter, e. g. Crura cerebri), in the middle nuclei of the cranial nerves, and dorsal superior centres of the reflexes (tectum, cerebellum). Therefore, in the mesencephalon these are called the base, tegmentum and Tectum mesencephali.

Association and commissural fibres

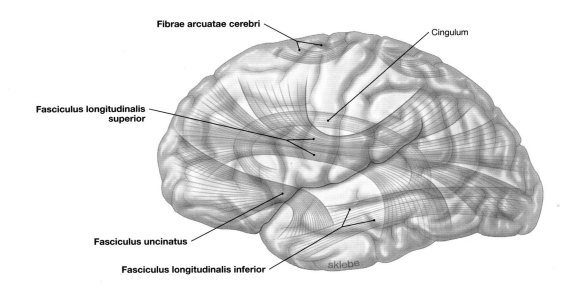

Fibrae arcuatae cerebri

Cingulum

Fasciculus longitudinalis
superior

Fasciculus uncinatus

Fasciculus longitudinalis inferior

sklebe

Fig. 12.27 Association fibres, Neurofibrae associationes, and arcuate fibres, Fibrae arcuatae; overview; view from the left side. [S700-L238]
Association fibres (→ table for → Fig. 12.29) account for the largest part of the fibre pathways of the white matter. They connect different areas of a cerebral hemisphere and thus enable associative and integrative functions through interlinking the functionally different areas.

Short association fibres are also referred to as arcuate fibres (Fibrae arcuatae cerebri). They are located near the cortex and connect adjacent gyri in a U-shaped manner. **Long association fibres** are located deeper in the medulla and connect the cerebral lobes with each other.
Functionally important **bundles of association fibres** are the Fasciculi longitudinalis superior, longitudinalis inferior and uncinatus as well as the Fibrae arcuatae cerebri and the cingulum.

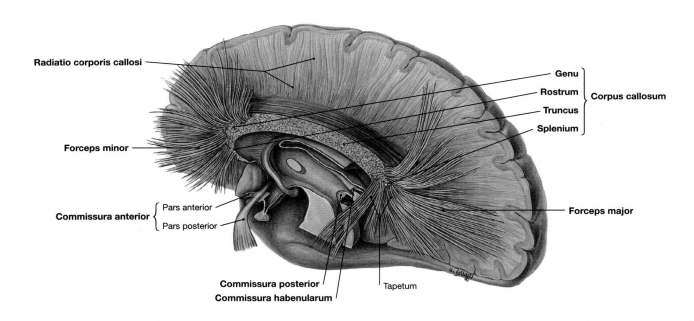

Radiatio corporis callosi

Genu

Rostrum

Corpus callosum

Truncus

Splenium

Forceps minor

Commissura anterior { Pars anterior / Pars posterior

Forceps major

Commissura posterior

Tapetum

Commissura habenularum

Fig. 12.28 Commissural fibres, Neurofibrae commissurales; topographical overview; view from the left side; the Corpus callosum was largely severed next to the median plane, and individual fibres are presented here. [S700]
Commissural fibres (→ table for → Fig. 12.29) serve to exchange information between the two cerebral hemispheres, for example to process the visual (optical) information arriving in both hemispheres into an overall visual impression. While **homotopic** commissural fibres connect corresponding regions of the brain, **heterotopic** fibres serve to exchange information between non-corresponding areas of the brain.

Each phylogenetic part of the cerebrum has its own commissure: the paleocortex possesses the Commissura anterior, the archicortex the Commissura fornicis and the neocortex the Corpus callosum. The latter consists of the rostrum, genu, truncus and Splenium corporis callosi. Because the Corpus callosum is shorter than the hemispheres, its rostral and occipital fibres radiate in a fan-like manner into the respective lobes (**Radiatio corporis callosi,** with Forceps minor and Forceps major).
There are however also homotopic areas of the brain which are not connected by commissural fibres. These include the primary visual cortex, the primary auditory cortex, and the somatosensory cortical fields of the hand and foot.

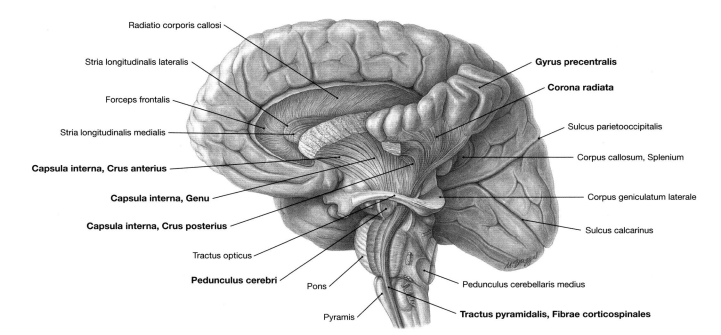

Fig. 12.29 Projection fibres, Neurofibrae projectiones; view from the left side; after exposing the internal capsule and the pyramidal tract. [S700]

Projection tracts consist of projection fibres connecting the cortex with deeper structures of the CNS (e.g. thalamus, brainstem). In the area of the striatum and pallidum, the fibres must pass through narrow passages inside which they have to converge. These constrictions are formed by the Capsula interna and Capsula externa between the Nucleus lentiformis and the claustrum as well as by the Capsula extrema between the insular cortex and the claustrum. The **Capsula interna** is the main route for projection fibres, in contrast to the **Capsula externa** and **Capsula extrema,** along which mainly long association fibres pass. The radially arranged projection fibres between the cerebral cortex and the Capsula interna are called **Corona radiata.**

Fibre systems in the Substantia alba	
Fibre system	**Connection**
Association fibres	
Fasciculus longitudinalis superior	Lobus frontalis with Lobus parietalis and Lobus occipitalis
Fasciculus longitudinalis inferior	Lobus occipitalis with Lobus temporalis
Fasciculus arcuatus	Lobus frontalis with Lobus temporalis (BROCA's area with WERNICKE's area)
Fasciculus uncinatus	Lobus frontalis with basal Lobus temporalis
Cingulum	lower parts of the Lobus frontalis with lower parts of the Lobus parietalis and Lobus parahippocampalis
Commissural fibres	
Corpus callosum	Frontal, parietal and occipital lobes of both hemispheres
Commissura anterior	Tractus olfactorius; anterior parts of the Lobus temporalis (amygdala; Gyrus parahippocampalis) of both hemispheres
Commissura posterior	Nuclei commissurae posteriores of both hemispheres
Commissura fornicis	Hippocampus of both hemispheres
Projection fibres	
Tractus corticospinalis	Cortex (especially Gyrus precentralis) with spinal cord
Tractus corticopontinus	Cortex with nuclei of the pons (Nuclei pontis)
Tractus corticonuclearis	Cortex with nuclei of the cranial nerves in the mesencephalon, pons and Medulla oblongata
Fornix	Hippocampus with parts of the limbic system and the diencephalon
Fasciculi thalamocorticales	Thalamus with cortex

Clinical remarks

The developmental **failure of the primordial structure (agenesis) of the Corpus callosum** is, with three to seven cases per 1,000 births, a relatively common malformation in humans. It can have a wide range of causes and may be associated with absent or underdeveloped connections between the left and right hemispheres, without inevitably leading to changes in behaviour. The clinical signs and symptoms depend largely on the cause. It often presents with neuropsychiatric deficits and difficulties in problem-solving behaviour, in the understanding of language and grammar, or in the verbal description of emotions (alexithymia).

Although the neurosurgical resection of the Corpus callosum **(callosotomy)** is a treatment option in patients with therapy-resistant epilepsy, it is only practised in exceptional cases. In patients who have undergone this treatment **(split-brain patients)**, the information processed in the right half of the brain can no longer be transmitted to the left dominant hemisphere and thereby to the cortical language centres. They can recognise and also describe such information, but are not able to name it precisely.

Menges and blood supply

Meninges

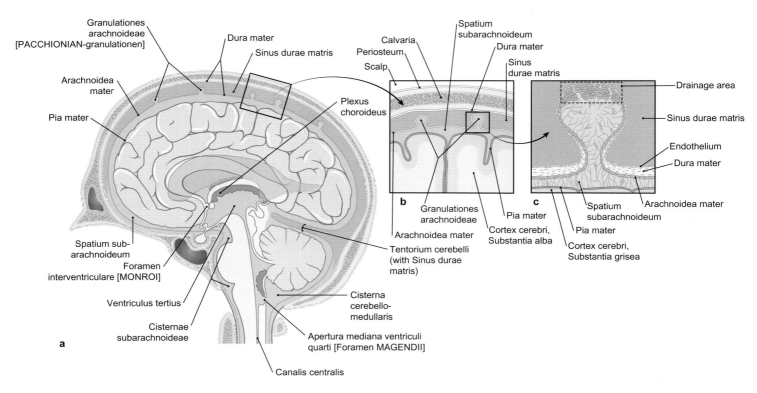

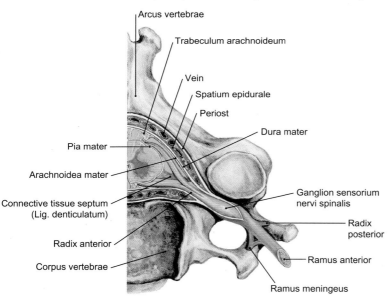

Fig. 12.30a–c Positional relationships of the meninges in the bony skull; sagittal section, medial view. a, b [S700-L126], c [S700-L126]~[F1082-001]

The brain and the spinal cord are surrounded by a fibrous system of membranes (meninges). The meninges consist of a solid part **(Pachymeninx)** and a soft part **(Leptomeninx);** the Leptomeninx is divided further into two components. The most exterior hard membrane **(dura mater,** Pachymeninx) is made of tight interlaced fibres of connective tissue and is fused with the periosteum inside the skull. The Leptomeninx joins it underneath. It consists of a complex system of meningeal cells and thin collagen fibres.

In the course of its development, a space forms within the Leptomeninx and a distinction is made between two laminae, the outer **Arachnoidea mater** which is directly adjacent to the dura mater, and the inner **pia mater** which is directly adjacent to the brain tissue, drawing everything into the gyri and sulci. The space between the arachnoid mater and the pia mater, the **subarachnoid space (Spatium subarachnoideum),** is filled with cerebrospinal fluid and traversed by arachnoid trabeculae. So the brain and spinal cord are completely surrounded by cerebrospinal fluid.

From the Spatium subarachnoideum, in particular along the Sinus sagittalis superior, fungal or villiform **arachnoidal granulations** (Granulationes arachnoideae) evert into the lumen of the sinus and partially up to the cranial bone. It was previously assumed that the granulations present the most important drainage pathway for the fluid in the venous system, but there are now many substantiated indications that the main drainage pathway for the fluid takes place perineurally via the extracranial parts of the cranial nerves and the spinal nerves (close to the dorsal root ganglia) into the lymphsystem in the dura mater. Some authors therefore ascribe intracranial pressure valves to the Granulationes arachnoideae, which are able to open up under increased intracranial pressure as a type of safety valve **(c).** However, further evidence in support of this is needed.

Fig. 12.31 Topographical relationships of the meninges in the vertebral canal; cross-section at the level of the fourth cervical vertebra. [S702-L126]

In contrast to the dura mater inside the skull, which is fused with the cranial periosteum (→ Fig. 12.30), the dura mater of the spinal cord (Dura mater spinalis) forms a tubular sac, which surrounds the spinal cord but is not fused with the bony vertebral canal, except for its anchorage around the Foramen magnum and at the Os sacrum. The dural sac is located in the epidural space (Spatium epidurale; syn. epidural space), which is filled with adipose tissue and a dense venous plexus (Plexus venosus vertebralis internus).

Clinical remarks

If a cerebrocranial trauma is accompanied by rupture of the dura mater and the arachnoid mater, e.g. in the area of the nose or ear, this can lead to a **fistula of cerebrospinal fluid (CSF fistula)**. This means that cerebrospinal fluid runs out of the nose **(rhinoliquorrhoea)** or out of the ear **(otoliquorrhoea).** To test for the presence of a CSF fistula, a small amount of the fluid is collected to determine its content of glycoprotein β_2-transferrin, as this isoform only occurs in the CSF.

Epidural anaesthesia (epidural) is a standard anaesthetic method. After the insertion of a cannula into the epidural space (without penetrating the dura), local anaesthetics can be injected. These anaesthetics act on the spinal roots and spinal ganglia. The epidural is used for the regional elimination of pain, for example in obstetrics, when surgical procedures cannot or do not need to be conducted under general anaesthesia.

Fig. 12.32 Dura mater cranialis and dural septa; lateral view. [S700]

In the skull, the dura mater consists of two laminae: (1) the **Lamina externa** is firmly attached to the periosteum, and (2) the **Lamina interna** is adjacent to the Arachnoidea mater. In several areas, the two laminae are split to form elongated cavities with an endothelial lining **(Sinus durae matris)**, into which the venous blood of the brain is drained. The sinuses form a vascular system around the brain, in which the great majority of the venous blood flows to the V. jugularis interna. The Lamina interna also forms strong plate-like dural septa, which separate individual parts of the brain from each other and stabilise the entire brain in the skull. The dural septa/dural duplications include the crescent-shaped **Falx cerebri,** the tent-shaped **Tentorium cerebelli,** the crescent-shaped **Falx cerebelli** and the **Diaphragma sellae.** A slit-like gap **(Incisura tentorii)** between the legs (crura) of the Tentorium cerebelli enables the passage of the brainstem.

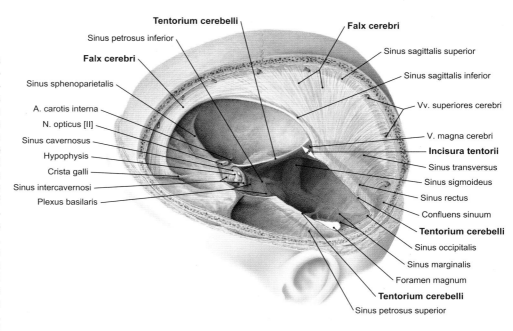
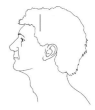

Fig. 12.33 Roof of the skull, calvaria, meninges, and venous sinuses, Sinus durae matris; frontal section. [S700]

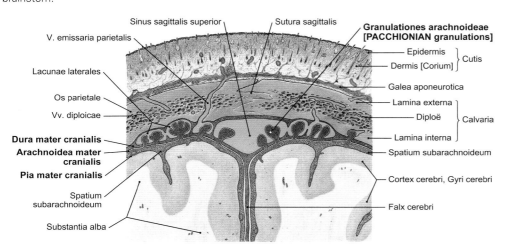

In adults, the **arachnoid or PACCHIONIAN granulations** (Granulationes arachnoideae, arachnoid protrusions in the Sinus sagittalis superior or the Lacunae laterales) along the Sinus sagittalis superior reabsorb most of the cerebrospinal fluid (CSF) (→ Fig. 12.30). Additionally, CSF is drained via the lymphatic sheaths of small vessels in the pia mater and the perineural sheaths of cranial and spinal nerves (not shown).

Fig. 12.34 Meninges; oblique superior view [S701-L285]

The brain is enveloped by membranes which are devided into a hard part **(Pachymeninx)** and a soft part **(Leptomeninx).** The outermost Pachymeninx, the **dura mater,** is a tough, tearproof, shiny membrane which is attached to the periosteum on the inside of the skull. There are slight differences with the arrangement of the membranes in the spinal cord (→ Fig. 12.31, see also → Fig. 2.144). The Leptomeninx is covered by the dura mater and is composed of the cobweb-like **arachnoid mater** and the soft meninges, the **pia mater,** which adheres directly to the brain. The **subarachnoid space, Spatium subarachnoideum,** spans the space between the arachnoid and pia mater, and is filled with CSF, Liquor cerebrospinalis.

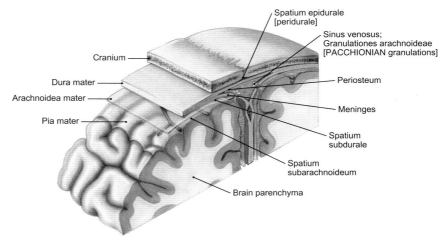

Brain and spinal cord

Leptomeninx

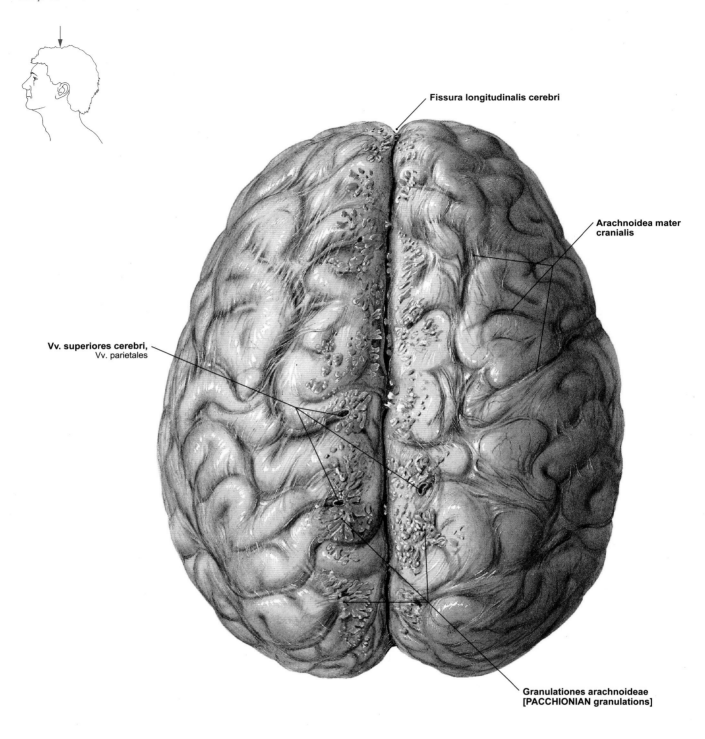

Fissura longitudinalis cerebri

Arachnoidea mater
cranialis

Vv. superiores cerebri,
Vv. parietales

Granulationes arachnoideae
[PACCHIONIAN granulations]

Fig. 12.35   Brain, encephalon, with arachnoid mater, Arachnoidea mater cranialis; superior view. [S700]
The brain is covered by the cobweb-like Arachnoidea mater. The **Fissura longitudinalis cerebri** normally contains the Falx cerebri (a duplication of the Dura mater cranialis; → Fig. 12.32), which divides the two cerebral hemispheres into a right and a left half and extends deep down to the Corpus callosum (not shown here). On both sides of the Fissura longitudinalis cerebri, numerous arachnoid or PACCHIONIAN granulations (Granulationes arachnoideae) are visible, reaching beyond the level of the arachnoid mater. In addition, several cerebral veins (Vv. superiores cerebri, Vv. parietales) are visible, which were torn off from the bridging veins (small veins piercing the Dura mater cranialis and flowing to the Sinus sagittalis superior) during the removal of the brain from the skull.

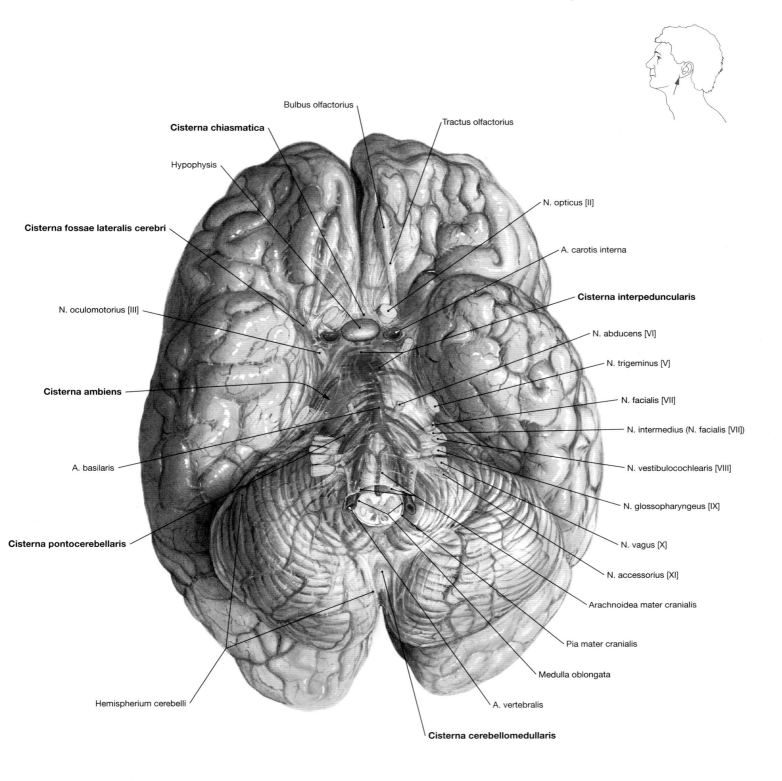

Bulbus olfactorius

Cisterna chiasmatica

Tractus olfactorius

Hypophysis

N. opticus [II]

Cisterna fossae lateralis cerebri

A. carotis interna

N. oculomotorius [III]

Cisterna interpeduncularis

N. abducens [VI]

N. trigeminus [V]

Cisterna ambiens

N. facialis [VII]

N. intermedius (N. facialis [VII])

A. basilaris

N. vestibulocochlearis [VIII]

N. glossopharyngeus [IX]

Cisterna pontocerebellaris

N. vagus [X]

N. accessorius [XI]

Arachnoidea mater cranialis

Pia mater cranialis

Hemispherium cerebelli

Medulla oblongata

A. vertebralis

Cisterna cerebellomedullaris

Fig. 12.36   Brain, encephalon, with arachnoid mater, Arachnoidea mater cranialis; inferior view. [S700]
The brain is surrounded by the cobweb-like Arachnoidea mater. Nerves and blood vessels run in the Spatium subarachnoideum. The inferior view shows the frontal, temporal and occipital lobes, as well as the cerebellum. The Circulus arteriosus cerebri [WILLIS] (→ Fig. 12.56) is preserved but only partially visible. The arachnoid mater does not cover all of the brain evenly so that superficial irregularities of the brain or the cranial base can lead to enlargements of the subarachnoid space. Partic-

ularly wide expansions of the subarachnoid space are called cisterns (CSF cisterns). The most important cisterns are:
* Cisterna cerebellomedullaris (Cisterna magna)
* Cisterna chiasmatica
* Cisterna interpeduncularis
* Cisterna ambiens
* Cisterna fossae lateralis cerebri
* Cisterna pontocerebellaris.

Meninges and blood supply

Ventricles of the brain

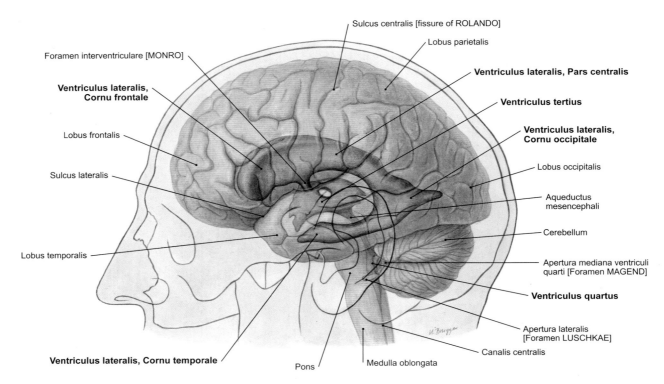

Sulcus centralis [fissure of ROLANDO]

Lobus parietalis

Foramen interventriculare [MONRO]

Ventriculus lateralis, Pars centralis

Ventriculus lateralis, Cornu frontale

Ventriculus tertius

Lobus frontalis

Ventriculus lateralis, Cornu occipitale

Sulcus lateralis

Lobus occipitalis

Aqueductus mesencephali

Cerebellum

Lobus temporalis

Apertura mediana ventriculi quarti [Foramen MAGEND]

Ventriculus quartus

Apertura lateralis [Foramen LUSCHKAE]

Ventriculus lateralis, Cornu temporale

Canalis centralis

Pons

Medulla oblongata

a

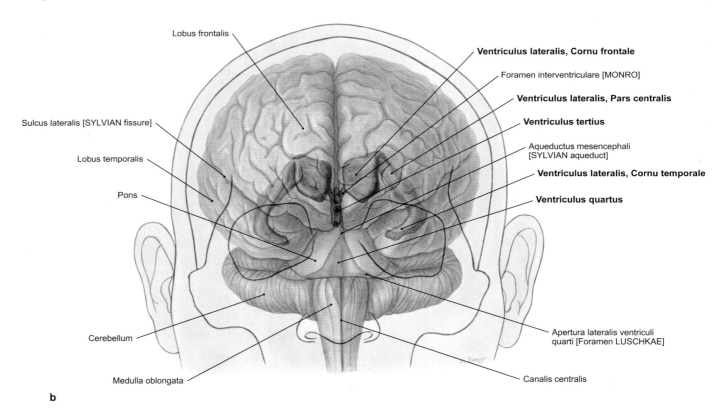

Lobus frontalis

Ventriculus lateralis, Cornu frontale

Foramen interventriculare [MONRO]

Ventriculus lateralis, Pars centralis

Ventriculus tertius

Sulcus lateralis [SYLVIAN fissure]

Aqueductus mesencephali [SYLVIAN aqueduct]

Lobus temporalis

Ventriculus lateralis, Cornu temporale

Pons

Ventriculus quartus

Apertura lateralis ventriculi quarti [Foramen LUSCHKAE]

Cerebellum

Medulla oblongata

Canalis centralis

b

Fig. 12.37a and b   Ventricles of the brain, Ventriculi encephali. [S700]

a View from the left side. The inner subarachnoid (CSF) space consists of the ventricular system and the central canal (Canalis centralis) of the spinal cord. The ventricular system comprises the **paired lateral ventricles** (Ventriculi laterales) with Cornu frontale, Pars centralis, Cornu occipitale and Cornu temporale, the **third ventricle** (Ventriculus tertius), the Aqueductus mesencephali [SYLVIAN aqueduct] and the **fourth ventricle** (Ventriculus quartus).

b Anterior view. The anterior view shows the paired lateral ventricles, as well as the third and fourth ventricles located in the median line, in the projection onto the brain.

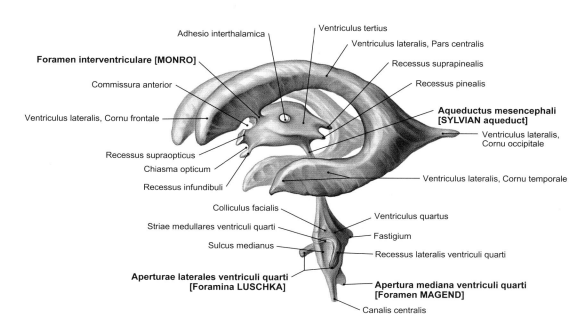

Foramen interventriculare [MONRO]
Commissura anterior
Ventriculus lateralis, Cornu frontale
Recessus supraopticus
Chiasma opticum
Recessus infundibuli
Adhesio interthalamica
Ventriculus tertius
Ventriculus lateralis, Pars centralis
Recessus suprapinealis
Recessus pinealis
Aqueductus mesencephali [SYLVIAN aqueduct]
Ventriculus lateralis, Cornu occipitale
Ventriculus lateralis, Cornu temporale
Colliculus facialis
Striae medullares ventriculi quarti
Sulcus medianus
Aperturae laterales ventriculi quarti [Foramina LUSCHKA]
Ventriculus quartus
Fastigium
Recessus lateralis ventriculi quarti
Apertura mediana ventriculi quarti [Foramen MAGEND]
Canalis centralis

Fig. 12.38   Inner subarachnoid spaces, Ventriculi encephali; corrosion cast specimen; oblique view from the left side. [S700]
Each lateral ventricle is connected to the third ventricle via a **Foramen interventriculare [MONRO].** The **Aqueductus mesencephali** [SYLVIAN aqueduct] connects the third ventricle to the fourth ventricle. The fourth ventricle has three openings (aperturae) to the outer subarachnoid (CSF) space: the Apertura mediana (Foramen MAGENDIE) and the paired Aperturae laterales (Foramina LUSCHKA).

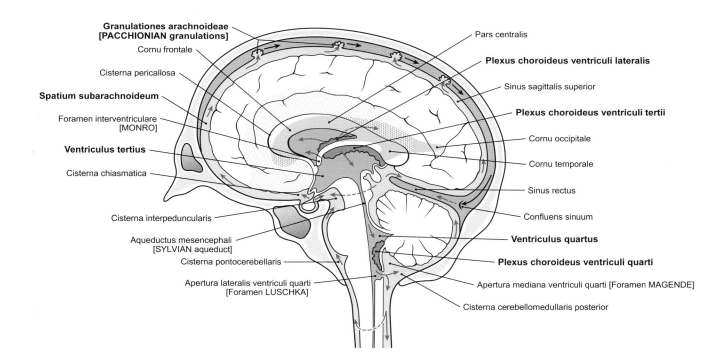

Granulationes arachnoideae [PACCHIONIAN granulations]
Cornu frontale
Cisterna pericallosa
Spatium subarachnoideum
Foramen interventriculare [MONRO]
Ventriculus tertius
Cisterna chiasmatica
Cisterna interpeduncularis
Aqueductus mesencephali [SYLVIAN aqueduct]
Cisterna pontocerebellaris
Apertura lateralis ventriculi quarti [Foramen LUSCHKA]
Pars centralis
Plexus choroideus ventriculi lateralis
Sinus sagittalis superior
Plexus choroideus ventriculi tertii
Cornu occipitale
Cornu temporale
Sinus rectus
Confluens sinuum
Ventriculus quartus
Plexus choroideus ventriculi quarti
Apertura mediana ventriculi quarti [Foramen MAGENDE]
Cisterna cerebellomedullaris posterior

Fig. 12.39   Ventricles of the brain, Ventriculi encephali, and subarachnoid space, Spatium subarachnoideum; schematic representation of the CSF circulation (arrows) from the inner to the outer subarachnoid spaces. [S700-L126]/[G1060-003]
The outer subarachnoid space is located between the arachnoid mater and pia mater. This space surrounds the brain as well as the spinal cord. The major part of the cerebrospinal fluid (Liquor cerebrospinalis) is secreted by the Plexus choroidei in the ventricles.

The circulating fluid volume (150 ml) is permanently being exchanged (daily production of approx. 500 ml).
Functionally, the cerebrospinal fluid (CSF) serves as a protective cushion of the CNS against mechanical forces, as a means of weight reduction of the CNS (by creating a buoyancy it lowers the weight by 97 % from 1,400 g to 45 g), and it also supports the metabolism of the CNS, the removal of toxic substances, and the transport of hormones (e.g. leptin).

Blood supply of the dura mater

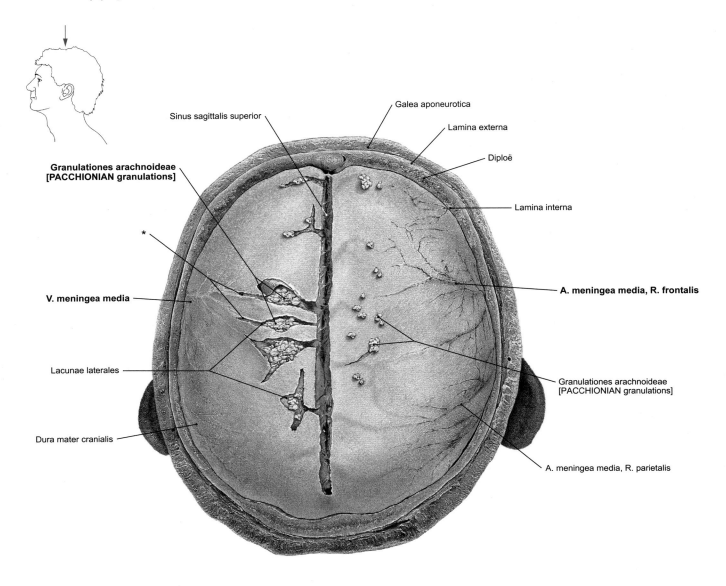

Sinus sagittalis superior

Granulationes arachnoideae
[PACCHIONIAN granulations]

*

V. meningea media

Lacunae laterales

Dura mater cranialis

Galea aponeurotica

Lamina externa

Diploë

Lamina interna

A. meningea media, R. frontalis

Granulationes arachnoideae
[PACCHIONIAN granulations]

A. meningea media, R. parietalis

**Fig. 12.40   Dura mater cranialis, and Sinus sagittalis superior
with several Lacunae laterales;** superior view. [S700]
The calvaria is removed and on the left side of the head the Dura mater
cranialis (hard meningeal membrane) has been opened along the **Lacunae laterales,** and the openings of the **Vv. meningeae mediae** into the
lacunae are visible. The arachnoid or PACCHIONIAN granulations (Granulationes arachnoideae) lie in the lacunae. On the right side, some

elevated Granulationes arachnoideae are visible, rising above the level
of the dura. These arachnoid granulations extend into the bones of the
skull where they leave impressions and are in contact with the Vv. diploicae.

* openings of the Vv. meningeae mediae into the Lacunae laterales

---

Clinical remarks

Meningiomas are slow-growing, usually benign intracranial tumours. They develop predominantly in the area of the PACCHIONIAN
granulations (Granulationes arachnoideae), along the Falx cerebri, in
the area of the sphenoidal wings, and in the olfactory groove. They
mostly originate from mesothelial cells in the arachnoid mater. Initially, they often remain unnoticed because the surrounding tissue
can adapt to the tumour growth rate. So they can achieve a significant size before causing symptoms, e.g. a sudden seizure or increasing headaches. If a surgical resection is possible, the prognosis is
very good.
In contrast to the brain and spinal cord, the **meninges** are extremely
well innervated and therefore very pain-sensitive. This is particularly

apparent in patients with meningitis, who suffer from severe headaches, accompanied by stiffness of the neck and overextension of
the spine **(meningismus).** A suspected meningismus can be diagnosed with two tests:
(1) If the head of a supine patient is passively bent forward, and this
leads to a reflexive flexion of the legs for pain relief (decompression
of the meninges), the **BRUDZINSKI's sign is positive.**
(2) For a positive **KERNIG's sign,** the passive lifting of the straight-
ened leg triggers an active flexion of the knee joint due to irritation of
the meninges.

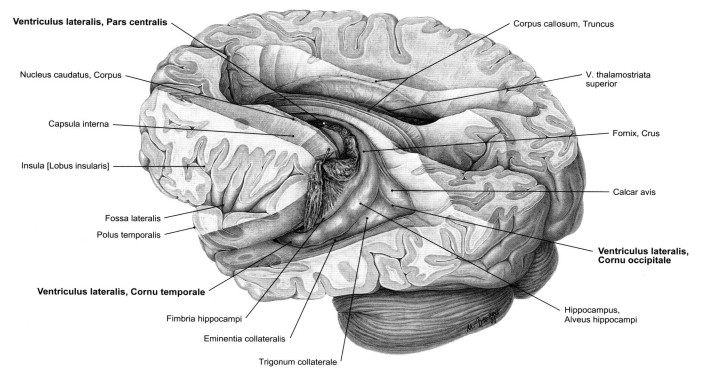

Ventriculus lateralis, Pars centralis

Nucleus caudatus, Corpus

Capsula interna

Insula [Lobus insularis]

Fossa lateralis

Polus temporalis

Ventriculus lateralis, Cornu temporale

Fimbria hippocampi

Eminentia collateralis

Trigonum collaterale

Corpus callosum, Truncus

V. thalamostriata superior

Fornix, Crus

Calcar avis

Ventriculus lateralis, Cornu occipitale

Hippocampus, Alveus hippocampi

Fig. 12.41   Lateral ventricles, Ventriculi laterales; posterior-superior view from the left side; after removal of the upper parts of the cerebral hemispheres. [S700]
This is a view into both the lateral ventricles. In the left lateral ventricle, the **Plexus choroideus** is visible, lifted up by a probe at the transition

from the Pars centralis to the Cornu temporale of the lateral ventricle.
Fluid production takes place in the Plexus choroideus.
The walls of the ventricles are presented in the table below.

Topography of the lateral ventricles			
Ventricle, section	**Wall**	**Adjacent structures**	**Plexus choroideus**
Ventriculi laterales, Cornu frontale	Roof	Corpus callosum (truncus)	No
	Anterior wall	Corpus callosum (genu)	
	Medial wall	Septum pellucidum	
	Lateral wall	Caput nuclei caudati	
Ventriculi laterales, Pars centralis	Roof	Corpus callosum	Yes
	Floor	Thalamus	
	Medial wall	Septum pellucidum, Fornix	
	Lateral wall	Corpus nuclei caudati	
Ventriculi laterales, Cornu occipitale	Roof	Medullary body of the Lobus occipitalis	No
	Floor	Medullary body of the Lobus occipitalis	
	Medial wall	Calcar avis	
	Lateral wall	Radiatio optica	
Ventriculi laterales, Cornu temporale	Roof	Cauda nuclei caudati	Yes
	Floor	Hippocampus	
	Medial wall	Fimbria hippocampi	
	Lateral wall	Cauda nuclei caudati	
	Anterior wall	Amygdala	
Ventriculus tertius	Roof	Tela choroidea ventriculi tertii	Yes
	Floor	Hypothalamus	
	Anterior wall	Lamina terminalis ventriculi tertii	
	Lateral wall	Thalamus, epithalamus	
Ventriculus quartus	Roof	Velum medullare superius cerebelli and Velum medullare inferius cerebelli	Yes
	Floor	Fossa rhomboidea	
	Lateral wall	Pedunculi cerebelli	

Depiction of the ventricles

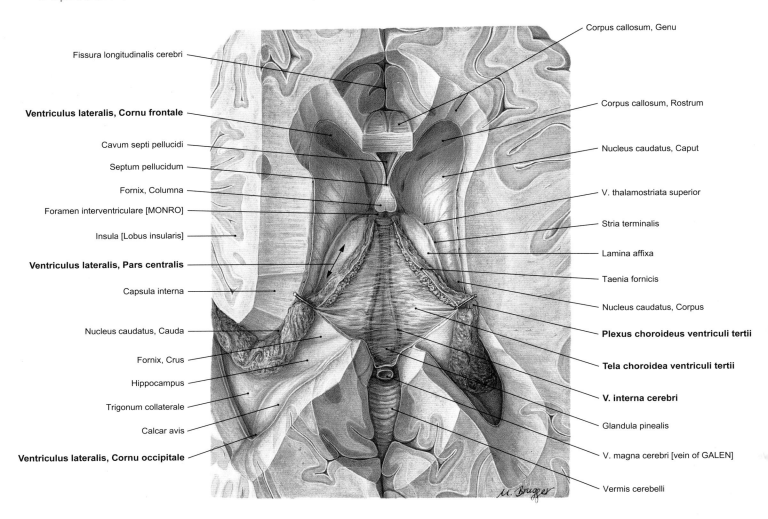

Fissura longitudinalis cerebri

Ventriculus lateralis, Cornu frontale

Cavum septi pellucidi

Septum pellucidum

Fornix, Columna

Foramen interventriculare [MONRO]

Insula [Lobus insularis]

Ventriculus lateralis, Pars centralis

Capsula interna

Nucleus caudatus, Cauda

Fornix, Crus

Hippocampus

Trigonum collaterale

Calcar avis

Ventriculus lateralis, Cornu occipitale

Corpus callosum, Genu

Corpus callosum, Rostrum

Nucleus caudatus, Caput

V. thalamostriata superior

Stria terminalis

Lamina affixa

Taenia fornicis

Nucleus caudatus, Corpus

Plexus choroideus ventriculi tertii

Tela choroidea ventriculi tertii

V. interna cerebri

Glandula pinealis

V. magna cerebri [vein of GALEN]

Vermis cerebelli

Fig. 12.42 Lateral ventricles, Ventriculi laterales; superior view; after removal of the central part of the Corpus callosum and the column (crura) of the fornix. [S700]
The **Tela choroidea** spans the third ventricle, as shown here. The Vv. internae cerebri, which shimmer through, drain to the V. magna cerebri. The Cornu frontale, the Pars centralis and the Cornu occipitale of the lateral ventricles can be seen. On the side, the **Plexus choroideus** continues on the hippocampus into the Cornu temporale.

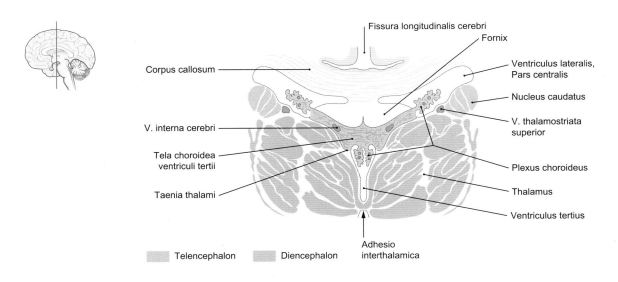

Fissura longitudinalis cerebri

Fornix

Corpus callosum

Ventriculus lateralis, Pars centralis

Nucleus caudatus

V. interna cerebri

V. thalamostriata superior

Tela choroidea ventriculi tertii

Plexus choroideus

Taenia thalami

Thalamus

Ventriculus tertius

Adhesio interthalamica

Telencephalon   Diencephalon

Fig. 12.43 Plexus choroideus in the lateral ventricles, Ventriculi laterales, and in the third ventricle, Ventriculus tertius; schematic frontal section. [S702-L126]/[B500-M282/L132]
A **Plexus choroideus,** which produces the cerebrospinal fluid (CSF), is present in the paired lateral ventricles (the first on the left side and the second on the right side) as well as in the third and the fourth ventricles (not shown). In the Plexus choroidei, the capillary blood and subarachnoid space are separated by a **blood-CSF barrier.**

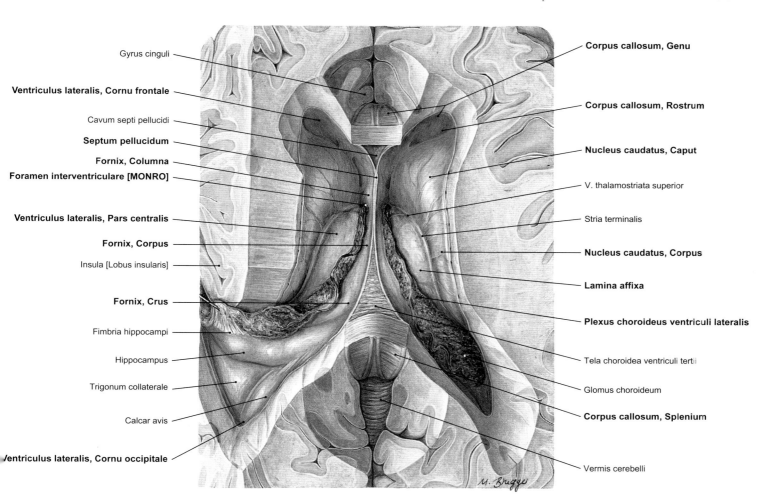

Gyrus cinguli

Ventriculus lateralis, Cornu frontale

Cavum septi pellucidi

Septum pellucidum

Fornix, Columna

Foramen interventriculare [MONRO]

Ventriculus lateralis, Pars centralis

Fornix, Corpus

Insula [Lobus insularis]

Fornix, Crus

Fimbria hippocampi

Hippocampus

Trigonum collaterale

Calcar avis

Ventriculus lateralis, Cornu occipitale

Corpus callosum, Genu

Corpus callosum, Rostrum

Nucleus caudatus, Caput

V. thalamostriata superior

Stria terminalis

Nucleus caudatus, Corpus

Lamina affixa

Plexus choroideus ventriculi lateralis

Tela choroidea ventriculi tertii

Glomus choroideum

Corpus callosum, Splenium

Vermis cerebelli

M. Brugge

Fig. 12.44 Lateral ventricles, Ventriculi laterales; superior view; after removal of the upper parts of the cerebral hemispheres and the central part of the Corpus callosum. [S700]
This view shows the Cornu frontale, the Pars centralis and the Cornu occipitale as well as the transition to the Cornu temporale of both lateral ventricles. The **Cornu frontale** is bordered by the genu of the Corpus callosum (anterior wall), the truncus of the Corpus callosum (the roof is not visible because the Corpus callosum has been separated at the genu and splenium), the Septum pellucidum (medial wall), the caput of

the Nucleus caudatus (lateral wall), as well as by the rostrum of the Corpus callosum (floor). In addition, the **Foramina interventricularia [foramina MONRO]** are visible in the Cornu frontale. Like the roof of the Pars frontalis, the roof of the **Pars centralis** is also formed by the truncus of the Corpus callosum (removed). The commissure of the fornix and the Septum pellucidum form the medial wall, the corpus of the Nucleus caudatus forms the lateral wall, whereas the floor consists of the Lamina affixa of the Plexus choroideus as well as of the commissure of the fornix.

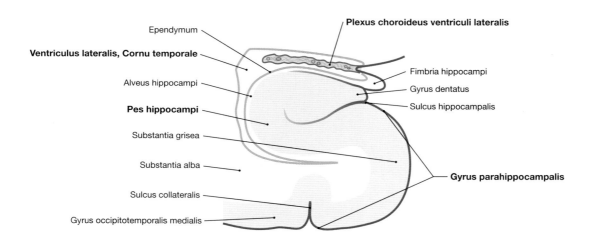

Ependymum

Ventriculus lateralis, Cornu temporale

Alveus hippocampi

Pes hippocampi

Substantia grisea

Substantia alba

Sulcus collateralis

Gyrus occipitotemporalis medialis

Plexus choroideus ventriculi lateralis

Fimbria hippocampi

Gyrus dentatus

Sulcus hippocampalis

Gyrus parahippocampalis

Fig. 12.45 Temporal horn, Cornu temporale, of the lateral ventricle, Ventriculus lateralis; schematic frontal section. [S700-L126]
The schematic representation shows how the lateral ventricle is arranged around the hippocampal formation. The Plexus choroideus pro-

trudes into the lateral ventricle. The walls of the ventricle are marked with light green lines, and the fluid or inner ventricular space is white.

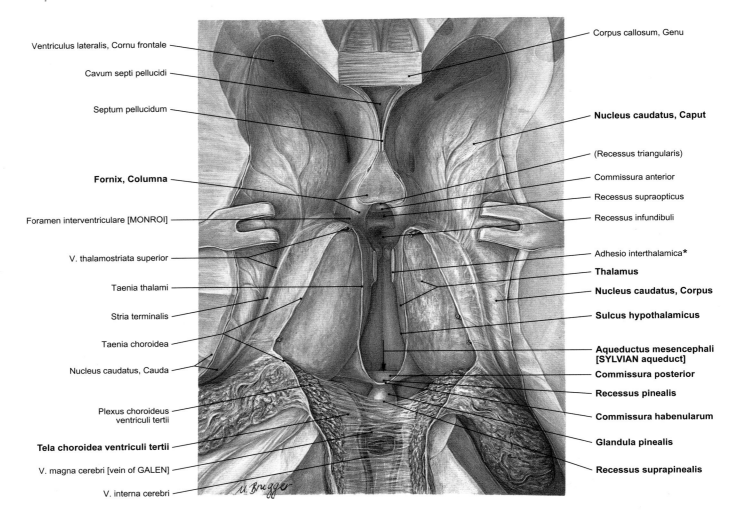

Ventriculus lateralis, Cornu frontale

Cavum septi pellucidi

Septum pellucidum

Fornix, Columna

Foramen interventriculare [MONROI]

V. thalamostriata superior

Taenia thalami

Stria terminalis

Taenia choroidea

Nucleus caudatus, Cauda

Plexus choroideus ventriculi tertii

Tela choroidea ventriculi tertii

V. magna cerebri [vein of GALEN]

V. interna cerebri

Corpus callosum, Genu

Nucleus caudatus, Caput

(Recessus triangularis)

Commissura anterior

Recessus supraopticus

Recessus infundibuli

Adhesio interthalamica*

Thalamus

Nucleus caudatus, Corpus

Sulcus hypothalamicus

Aqueductus mesencephali [SYLVIAN aqueduct]

Commissura posterior

Recessus pinealis

Commissura habenularum

Glandula pinealis

Recessus suprapinealis

Fig. 12.46 Lateral ventricles, Ventriculi laterales, and third ventricle, Ventriculus tertius; superior view; after removal of parts of the cerebral hemispheres and the central part of the Corpus callosum, the fornix and the Plexus choroideus; the Tela choroidea of the third ventricle is folded back. [S700]

The boundaries of the third ventricle are listed in the table for → Fig. 12.41.

* Adhesio interthalamica severed in the median plane

Arterial blood supply of the Plexus choroideus (→ Fig. 12.61)	
Ventricle	**Artery**
Ventriculi laterales	• A. choroidea anterior (from the A. carotis interna) • A. choroidea posterior lateralis (from the A. cerebri posterior)
Ventriculus tertius	A. choroidea posterior medialis (from the A. cerebri posterior)
Ventriculus quartus	• A. inferior posterior cerebelli (from the A. vertebralis) • A. inferior anterior cerebelli (from the A. basilaris)

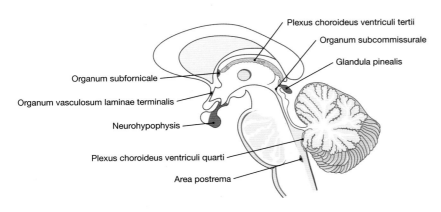

Plexus choroideus ventriculi tertii

Organum subcommissurale

Glandula pinealis

Organum subfornicale

Organum vasculosum laminae terminalis

Neurohypophysis

Plexus choroideus ventriculi quarti

Area postrema

Fig. 12.47 Circumventricular organs; median sagittal section. [S700-L126]/[B500~T1189/L316]
Characteristic features of the circumventricular organs (CVOs) are their rich vascularisation, modified ependyma (tanycytes with tight junctions), and a blood-CSF barrier instead of a blood-brain barrier.
The CVOs are divided into sensory and secretory organs: secretory CVOs include the neurohypophysis, the Eminentia mediana of the (pituitary) infundibulum, and the pineal gland (Glandula pinealis). Sensory CVOs in the narrow sense are the Organum vasculosum laminae terminalis and the Organum subfornicale (both: regulation of blood volume and arterial pressure, release of hormones such as angiotensin, somatostatin, inducing fever), the Organum subcommissurale (only present in the fetal and newborn phase; release of a glycoprotein-rich secretion) and the Area postrema (trigger zone of nausea/vomiting).

Clinical remarks

Due to their blood-CSF barrier instead of a blood-brain barrier, the circumventricular organs serve as pharmacological access routes. In the case of fever, for example, **acetylsalicylic acid (ASA)** has an antipyretic action as inhibitor of cyclooxygenase by reducing the production of prostaglandin. In the case of fever, the temperature-sensitive neurons of the Organum vasculosum laminae terminalis have a reduced sensitivity for intrinsic prostaglandins. These neurons normally initiate cooling mechanisms, which in the case of fever only function to a minor extent or not at all. By reducing the prostaglandin formation, ASA can therefore increase the sensitivity of neurons. As a result, the downregulation of the set-point caused by the fever is readjusted to the standard value – and the high temperature/fever is lowered. Central vomiting (emesis), e.g. due to opioids, can be treated with **neuroleptic drugs,** which bind to dopamine receptors in the Area postrema and thus have an antiemetic effect.

Clinical remarks

Obstructions of CSF drainage (→ Fig. a CT scan image) can be caused by tumours, malformations, bleeding or other factors, and due to increased intracranial pressure they can lead to headaches, nausea and a papilloedema (→ Fig. c image of ocular fundus). In the case of a blockage in the inner CSF space, a **hydrocephalus internus** will occur and impaired drainage in the outer CSF or subarachnoid space will lead to a **hydrocephalus externus. Hydrocephalus e vacuo** is the term for a condition when ventricular size considerably increases because of a loss of brain substance, e.g. as in ALZHEIMER's disease.

The circumventricular organs (→ Fig. 12.47) **lack the blood-brain barrier** and are thus capable of monitoring the plasma-blood milieu: as such they are of more interest than at a purely pharmacological level. The Area postrema for example contains numerous dopamine and serotonin receptors. Highly promising anti-emetic effects can be achieved by using dopamine or serotonin antagonists. In addition, the excitability of biochemical receptors in the Area postrema is a protective mechanism for the whole body, for example by centrally triggered vomiting after the ingestion of spoiled food, so that the major part of the potentially harmful substance is eliminated from the body.

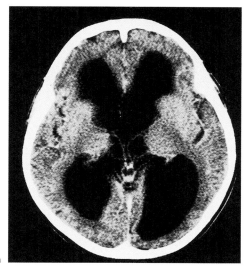

a

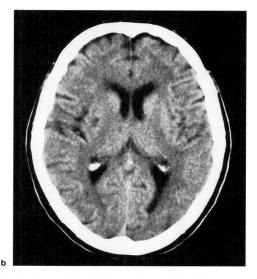

b

Computed tomographic (CT) cross-section of the head of a female patient with impaired CSF drainage (→ Fig. a) due to a narrowing of the Aqueductus mesencephali [SYLVIAN aqueduct]. The ventricles are significantly enlarged at the expense of the parenchyma of the brain (hydrocephalus). The patient suffered from massive intellectual deficits and significant gait disorders. For comparison, a CT scan of a healthy person is shown (→ Fig. b). [R317]

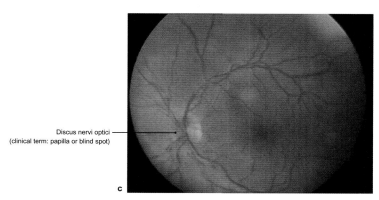

Discus nervi optici
(clinical term: papilla or blind spot)

c

Ocular fundus, Fundus oculi; left side; anterior view; ophthalmoscopic image of the central area showing a congested Papilla nervi optici due to increased cranial pressure. A congested Papilla nervi optici (optic disc) is visible on the ocular fundus as a clinical sign of an intraventricular neurocytoma WHO grade II. As the N. opticus [II] is surrounded by meninges and fluid, the optic disc bulges in the eyeball. [S700]

Meninges and blood supply

Arteries of the head

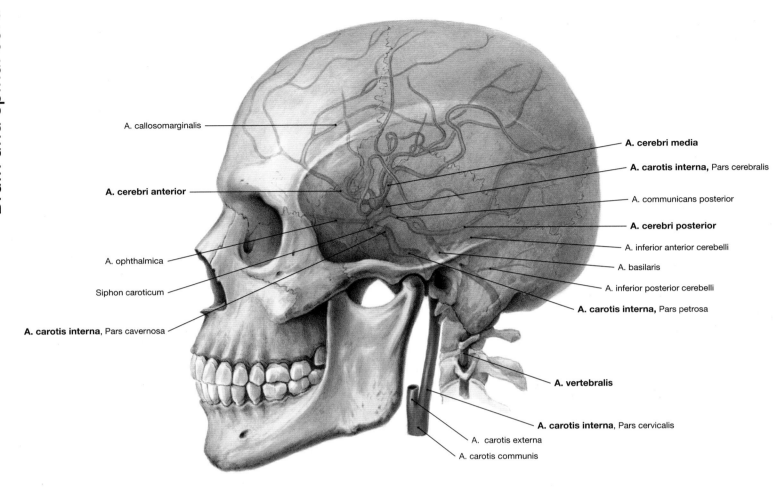

A. callosomarginalis

A. cerebri media

A. carotis interna, Pars cerebralis

A. cerebri anterior

A. communicans posterior

A. cerebri posterior

A. inferior anterior cerebelli

A. ophthalmica

A. basilaris

Siphon caroticum

A. inferior posterior cerebelli

A. carotis interna, Pars petrosa

A. carotis interna, Pars cavernosa

A. vertebralis

A. carotis interna, Pars cervicalis

A. carotis externa

A. carotis communis

Fig. 12.48   Internal arteries of the head. [S700]
The blood supply to the brain is provided by four major arteries: the two Aa. carotides internae and the two Aa. vertebrales. The four vessels supply the **Circulus arteriosus cerebri [WILLIS]** (→ Fig. 12.56), located at the base of the brain and forming the anastomosis between the Aa. carotides internae and the Aa. vertebrales, from which the paired cerebral arteries (Aa. cerebri anterior, cerebri media and cerebri posterior) exit.
The anastomotic vessels of the Circulus arteriosus cerebri [WILLIS] are often so thin that no important blood exchange takes place via them. In most cases, under normal conditions of intracranial pressure, each hemisphere is supplied with blood by the ipsilateral **A. carotis interna** and the ipsilateral **A. cerebri posterior.** In 10 % of the cases, both Aa. cerebri anteriores originate from the A. carotis interna on one side. Also in 10 % of the cases, the A. cerebri posterior originates from the A. carotis interna via the A. communicans posterior. The A. carotis interna originates together with the A. carotis externa from the A. carotis communis. The Glomus caroticum sits in this bifurcation.

Clinical remarks

The cerebral blood flow has great clinical relevance. Lack of oxygen will irreversibly damage brain tissue **(ischaemia tolerance)** within a maximum time of 7–10 min. This must be taken into account in the cardiovascular resuscitation of patients in cardiac arrest. The importance of brain circulation is immediately clear when standing up too quickly leads to a blackout, because the brain is momentarily not sufficiently supplied with blood. The same occurs with fainting (syncope). The brain is not supplied with enough blood, and as a result, the patient drops to the floor. When lying down, the cerebral blood flow improves and the brain functions return.

Vascular changes (extracranial arteriosclerosis: plaques, stenosis, obliteration) are often located in the carotid bifurcation. The Glomus caroticum (not shown in → Fig. 12.48, → Fig. 12.158) is a paraganglion located in the carotid bifurcation; it contains chemoreceptors, which react to changes of the pH, oxygen and carbon dioxide levels of the blood.
The **carotid sinus syndrome** is defined as a hypersensitivity of pressure receptors in the carotid sinus and may often be triggered in response to a rotation of the head. This initiates a reflex that strongly lowers the heart rate (vasovagal reflex) which can result in cardiovascular collapse and cardiac arrest.

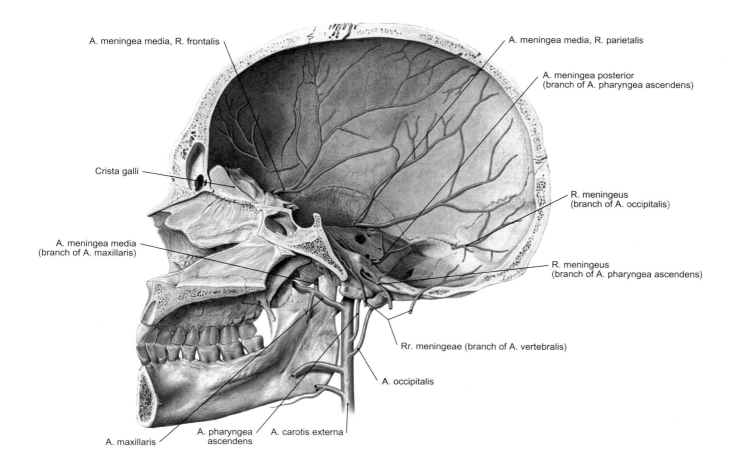

A. meningea media, R. frontalis

A. meningea media, R. parietalis

A. meningea posterior
(branch of A. pharyngea ascendens)

Crista galli

R. meningeus
(branch of A. occipitalis)

A. meningea media
(branch of A. maxillaris)

R. meningeus
(branch of A. pharyngea ascendens)

Rr. meningeae (branch of A. vertebralis)

A. occipitalis

A. pharyngea
ascendens

A. carotis externa

A. maxillaris

Fig. 12.49 Intracranial arteries of the head; sagittal section of the skull, medial view. [S700-L127]

Blood supply to the meninges derives mainly from branches of the A. carotis externa.

Meninges and blood supply

Intracranial arteries of the head

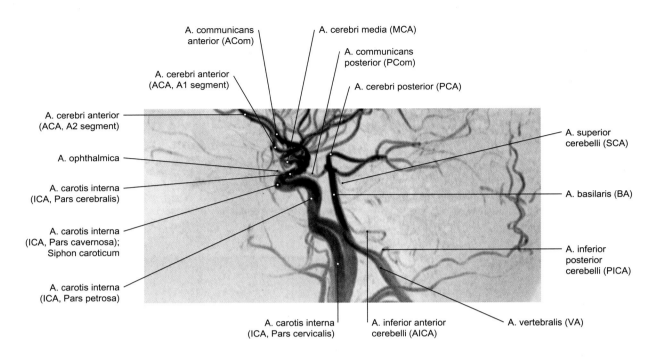

A. communicans anterior (ACom)

A. cerebri media (MCA)

A. communicans posterior (PCom)

A. cerebri anterior (ACA, A1 segment)

A. cerebri posterior (PCA)

A. cerebri anterior (ACA, A2 segment)

A. ophthalmica

A. carotis interna (ICA, Pars cerebralis)

A. carotis interna (ICA, Pars cavernosa); Siphon caroticum

A. carotis interna (ICA, Pars petrosa)

A. superior cerebelli (SCA)

A. basilaris (BA)

A. inferior posterior cerebelli (PICA)

A. carotis interna (ICA, Pars cervicalis)

A. inferior anterior cerebelli (AICA)

A. vertebralis (VA)

Fig. 12.50 MR angiography of the arteries supplying the brain; lateral view. [S702-T786]

The figure shows the carotid siphon (Siphon caroticum; → Fig. 12.52).

Clinical (radiological) terms for segmental branches of large arteries supplying the brain		
Artery	**Segment**	**Topography/anatomical structures**
A. carotis interna, ICA = internal carotid artery	C1 – cervical	Pars cervicalis
	C2 – petrous	Pars petrosa up to the end of the Canalis caroticus
	C3 – lacerum	up to a ligament between Lingula sphenoidalis and the apex of the Os petrosum ('Lig. petrolingualis')
	C4 – cavernous	in the Sinus cavernosus until exiting the dura below the Proc. clinoideus
	C5 – clinoid	between Proc. clinoideus anterior and the base of the Os sphenoidale
	C6 – ophthalmic	up to the outlet of the A. communicans posterior; outlet of the A. ophthalmica
	C7 – communicating	up to the bifurcation of the ICA into the Aa. cerebri anterior et media
A. cerebri anterior, ACA = anterior cerebral artery	A1	Pars precommunicalis; from its origin to the outlet of the A. communicans anterior
	A2	Pars postcommunicalis; from the outlet of the A. communicans anterior to the outlet of the A. callosomarginalis; also: Pars infracallosa
	A3	Pars postcommunicalis; distally of the outlet of the A. callosomarginalis (A. pericallosa); some authors differentiate even more segments (A4 and A5)
A. cerebri media, MCA = middle cerebral artery	M1	Pars sphenoidalis; from its outlet to the bifurcation in two or three main branches
	M2	Pars insularis; in the Fossa lateralis, above the insula
	M3	Pars opercularis; in the Fossa lateralis, lateral branches in the direction of the cortical surface
	M4	Pars terminalis; after the exit of all vessels from the Sulcus lateralis
A. cerebri posterior, PCA = posterior cerebral artery	P1	Pars precommunicalis; from its outlet to the A. communicans posterior; passes through the Cisterna interpeduncularis
	P2	Pars ambiens; from the A. communicans posterior to the outlet of the Rr. temporales anteriores (at the level of the Cisterna ambiens)
	P3	Pars quadrigeminalis; from the Rr. temporales anteriores to the bifurcation into the Aa. occipitales medialis and lateralis (at the level of the Cisterna quadrigeminalis)
	P4	Pars calcarina; terminal branches: A. occipitalis medialis and A. occipitalis lateralis
A. vertebralis, VA = vertebral artery	V1	Pars prevertebralis
	V2	Pars transversaria
	V3	Pars atlantica
	V4	Pars intracranialis

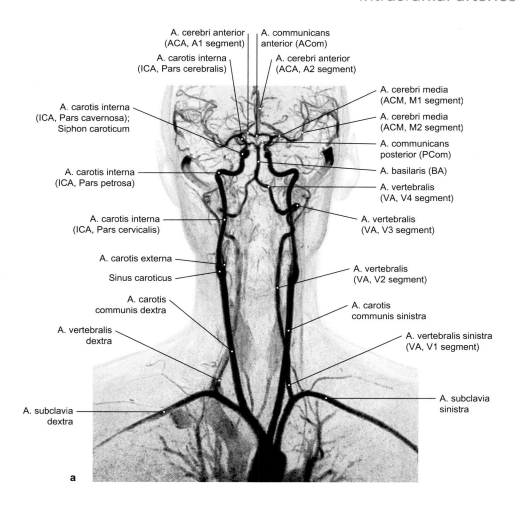

A. cerebri anterior
(ACA, A1 segment)

A. communicans
anterior (ACom)

A. carotis interna
(ICA, Pars cerebralis)

A. cerebri anterior
(ACA, A2 segment)

A. cerebri media
(ACM, M1 segment)

A. cerebri media
(ACM, M2 segment)

A. carotis interna
(ICA, Pars cavernosa);
Siphon caroticum

A. communicans
posterior (PCom)

A. carotis interna
(ICA, Pars petrosa)

A. basilaris (BA)

A. vertebralis
(VA, V4 segment)

A. carotis interna
(ICA, Pars cervicalis)

A. vertebralis
(VA, V3 segment)

A. carotis externa

Sinus caroticus

A. vertebralis
(VA, V2 segment)

A. carotis
communis dextra

A. carotis
communis sinistra

A. vertebralis
dextra

A. vertebralis sinistra
(VA, V1 segment)

A. subclavia
sinistra

A. subclavia
dextra

a

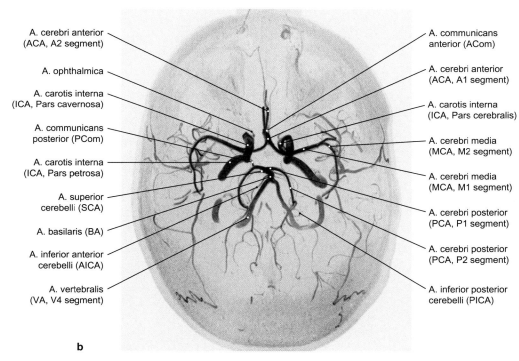

A. cerebri anterior
(ACA, A2 segment)

A. communicans
anterior (ACom)

A. ophthalmica

A. cerebri anterior
(ACA, A1 segment)

A. carotis interna
(ICA, Pars cavernosa)

A. carotis interna
(ICA, Pars cerebralis)

A. communicans
posterior (PCom)

A. cerebri media
(MCA, M2 segment)

A. carotis interna
(ICA, Pars petrosa)

A. cerebri media
(MCA, M1 segment)

A. superior
cerebelli (SCA)

A. cerebri posterior
(PCA, P1 segment)

A. basilaris (BA)

A. inferior anterior
cerebelli (AICA)

A. cerebri posterior
(PCA, P2 segment)

A. vertebralis
(VA, V4 segment)

A. inferior posterior
cerebelli (PICA)

b

Fig. 12.51a and b   MR angiography of the arteries supplying the brain. [S702-T786]

a Frontal view.
b Caudal view.

Sinus cavernosus

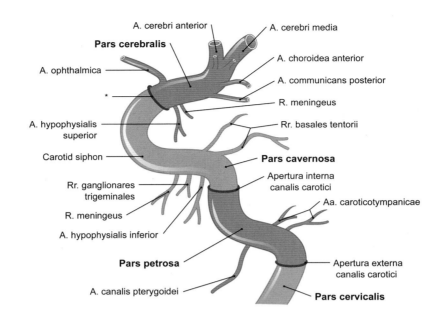

Fig. 12.52 Segments of the A. carotis interna. [S700-L126]/[E633-003]

The A. carotis interna forms an S-shaped loop system (Siphon caroticum) and can be divided into four segments: Pars cervicalis, Pars petrosa, Pars cavernosa and Pars cerebralis. Along its pathway in the region of the cranial base, the A. carotis interna passes through the Apertura externa canalis carotici, the Apertura interna canalis carotici and the dura mater. In the Pars cervicalis no vessels branch off. The first larger branch is the A. ophthalmica. The A. carotis interna ends by bifurcating

into the A. cerebri anterior and the A. cerebri media. It supplies the pituitary gland, the trigeminal ganglion, the eye, and the anterior parts of the cerebrum and of the diencephalon. A frequent variation of the vascular pattern is the outlet of the A. canalis pterygoidei from the Pars petrosa of the A. carotis interna. In most cases, the A. canalis pterygoidei originates from the Pars sphenopalatina of the A. maxillaris.

* passage through the Dura mater cranialis in the area of the Diaphragma sellae

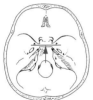

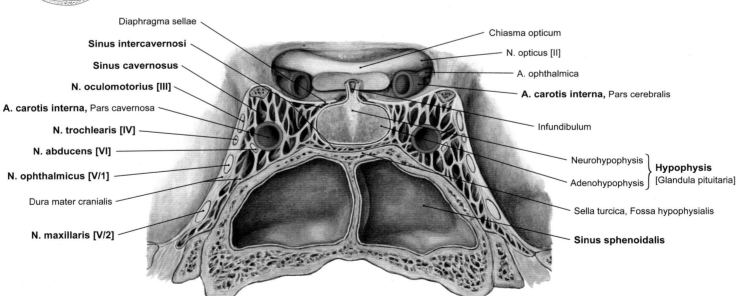

Fig. 12.53 A. carotis interna, Pars cavernosa; frontal section; posterior view. [S700]

The pituitary gland (hypophysis) is surrounded by the right and left Sinus cavernosus, which communicate via the Sinus intercavernosi. The Pars cavernosa of the A. carotis interna and the laterally adjacent N. abdu-

cens [VI] run through the centre of the Sinus cavernosus; the N. oculomotorius [III], N. trochlearis [IV], N. ophthalmicus [V/1], and N. maxillaris [V/2] are located in its wall. The Sinus sphenoidalis is located beneath the Sella turcica which contains the pituitary gland.

12

In the clinic, Circulus arteriosus

Clinical remarks

Arteriosclerotic changes in vascular walls are relatively common findings at the outlet of the A. carotis interna from the A. carotis communis, as well as in the Pars cavernosa.

More than 90 % of all **cerebral aneurysms** occur in the basal cerebral vessels of the Circulus arteriosus cerebri [WILLIS] (→ figure). Most often, the A. communicans anterior (ACA, up to 40 %) and the A. carotis interna are affected. During the surgical removal of an aneurysm in the A. communicans anterior, care must be taken not to sever the A. centralis longa (syn.: A. striata medialis distalis, A. striata longa, A. recurrens, HEUBNER's artery). This artery is a branch which mostly originates laterally descending from the proximal A2 segment or the distal A1 segment of the A. cerebri anterior (→ Fig. 12.63) and runs anti-parallel back to the initial segment of the A. cerebri anterior. In addition, care should be taken to avoid the other branches of the A. communicans anterior, as otherwise postoperative disorders of

the memory function could occur (syndrome of the A. communicans anterior). [G749]

Normally, (→ Fig. a) blood flows cranially from the aortic arch (caudal) through both arterial systems supplying the brain (black arrows) to reach the circle of WILLIS, Circulus arteriosus cerebri [WILLIS]. A patient with **subclavian steal syndrome (b)** frequently has a proximal high grade stenosis of the left A. subclavia. Intense physical activity with the left arm results in retrograde (reverse) blood flow in the left A. vertebralis (affected side, red arrows, → Fig. b). This causes the brain to receive less blood (thin arrows, → Fig. b) which may mean dizziness and headaches. The A. subclavia sinistra is usually affected in patients with subclavian steal syndrome. [S701-L126]

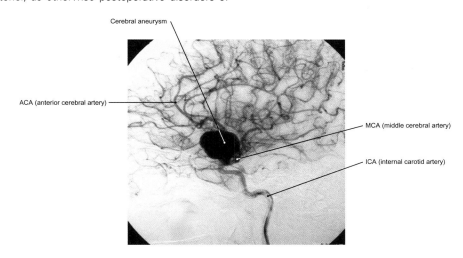

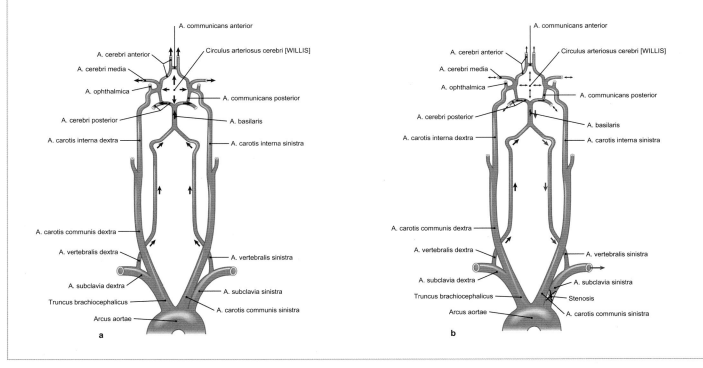

325

Meninges and blood supply

Arteries of the cranial base

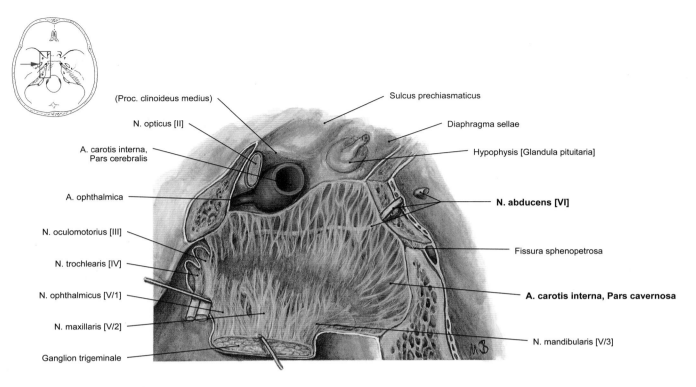

(Proc. clinoideus medius)

N. opticus [II]

A. carotis interna, Pars cerebralis

A. ophthalmica

N. oculomotorius [III]

N. trochlearis [IV]

N. ophthalmicus [V/1]

N. maxillaris [V/2]

Ganglion trigeminale

Sulcus prechiasmaticus

Diaphragma sellae

Hypophysis [Glandula pituitaria]

N. abducens [VI]

Fissura sphenopetrosa

A. carotis interna, Pars cavernosa

N. mandibularis [V/3]

Fig. 12.54   A. carotis interna, Pars cavernosa, and Sinus caverno-sus, on the left side; lateral view; after removal of the lateral wall-forming part of the dura; the Ganglion trigeminale folded back laterally. [S700]

The pathway of the Pars cavernosa of the A. carotis interna and of the N. abducens [VI] in the Sinus cavernosus are visible here.

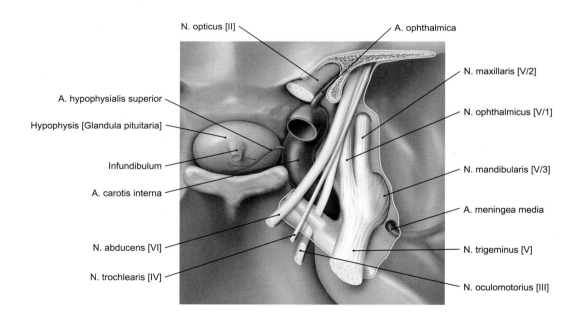

N. opticus [II]

A. ophthalmica

A. hypophysialis superior

Hypophysis [Glandula pituitaria]

Infundibulum

A. carotis interna

N. abducens [VI]

N. trochlearis [IV]

N. maxillaris [V/2]

N. ophthalmicus [V/1]

N. mandibularis [V/3]

A. meningea media

N. trigeminus [V]

N. oculomotorius [III]

Fig. 12.55   A. carotis interna, Pars cavernosa, right side; cranial view; Sinus cavernosus removed to allow a view of the structures running within and at the margins of the sinus. [S700-L275]

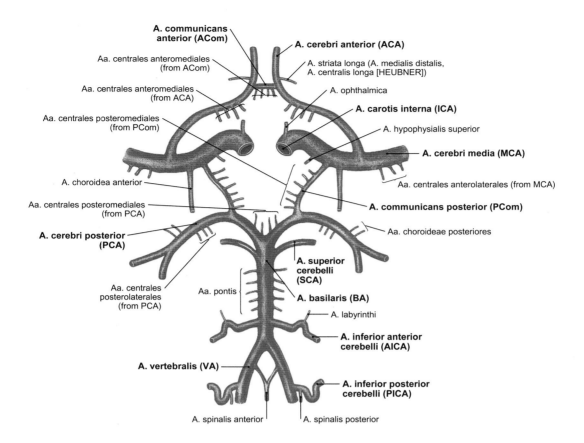

A. communicans anterior (ACom)

A. cerebri anterior (ACA)

Aa. centrales anteromediales (from ACom)

A. striata longa (A. medialis distalis, A. centralis longa [HEUBNER])

Aa. centrales anteromediales (from ACA)

A. ophthalmica

Aa. centrales posteromediales (from PCom)

A. carotis interna (ICA)

A. hypophysialis superior

A. cerebri media (MCA)

A. choroidea anterior

Aa. centrales anterolaterales (from MCA)

Aa. centrales posteromediales (from PCA)

A. communicans posterior (PCom)

A. cerebri posterior (PCA)

Aa. choroideae posteriores

A. superior cerebelli (SCA)

Aa. centrales posterolaterales (from PCA)

Aa. pontis

A. basilaris (BA)

A. labyrinthi

A. inferior anterior cerebelli (AICA)

A. vertebralis (VA)

A. inferior posterior cerebelli (PICA)

A. spinalis anterior

A. spinalis posterior

Fig. 12.56 Arterial circle of the brain, circle of WILLIS, Circulus arteriosus cerebri [WILLIS]; superior view. [S702-L127]
The Aa. communicantes posteriores connect the Aa. cerebri posteriores with the Partes cerebrales of the Aa. carotides internae on both sides. In the anterior part, the A. communicans anterior connects both Aa. cerebri anteriores to generate a closed arterial ring (the circle of WILLIS), which connects the Aa. carotides internae with each other and with the vertebral arterial system.

Clinical remarks

Most cerebral aneurysms are congenital defects of the Tunica media in the vascular wall at the points where it branches out. Often, aneurysms are associated with other diseases, such as polycystic kidneys or fibromuscular dysplasia. Cerebral aneurysms are usually asymptomatic. However, the pressure of the aneurysmal sac can lead to a cranial nerve compression.

Cerebral aneurysms have a tendency to **rupture** and are the most frequent cause of subarachnoid bleeding (haemorrhage). In the case of a rupture, sudden severe headaches occur, combined with vomiting and impaired consciousness.

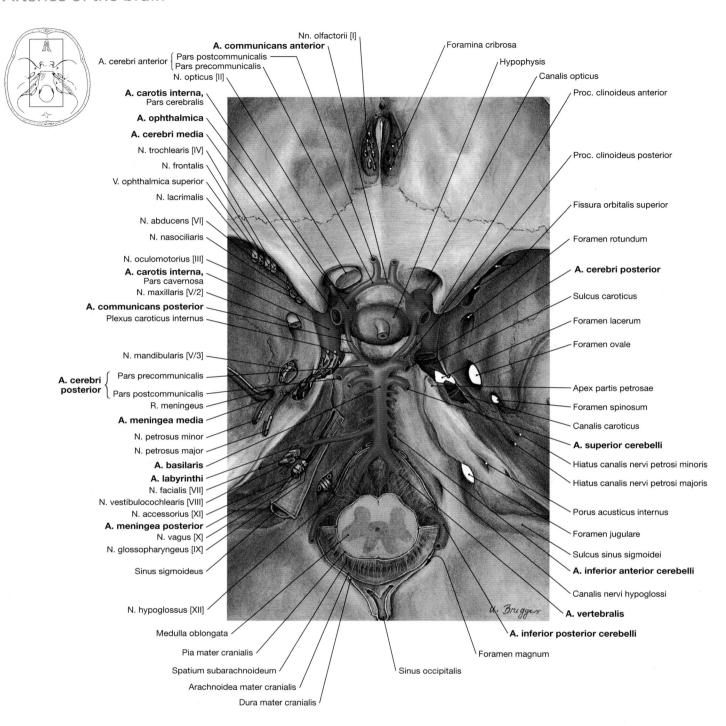

Nn. olfactorii [I]

A. communicans anterior

A. cerebri anterior { Pars postcommunicalis / Pars precommunicalis }

N. opticus [II]

A. carotis interna, Pars cerebralis

A. ophthalmica

A. cerebri media

N. trochlearis [IV]

N. frontalis

V. ophthalmica superior

N. lacrimalis

N. abducens [VI]

N. nasociliaris

N. oculomotorius [III]

A. carotis interna, Pars cavernosa

N. maxillaris [V/2]

A. communicans posterior

Plexus caroticus internus

N. mandibularis [V/3]

A. cerebri posterior { Pars precommunicalis / Pars postcommunicalis }

R. meningeus

A. meningea media

N. petrosus minor

N. petrosus major

A. basilaris

A. labyrinthi

N. facialis [VII]

N. vestibulocochlearis [VIII]

N. accessorius [XI]

A. meningea posterior

N. vagus [X]

N. glossopharyngeus [IX]

Sinus sigmoideus

N. hypoglossus [XII]

Medulla oblongata

Pia mater cranialis

Spatium subarachnoideum

Arachnoidea mater cranialis

Dura mater cranialis

Foramina cribrosa

Hypophysis

Canalis opticus

Proc. clinoideus anterior

Proc. clinoideus posterior

Fissura orbitalis superior

Foramen rotundum

A. cerebri posterior

Sulcus caroticus

Foramen lacerum

Foramen ovale

Apex partis petrosae

Foramen spinosum

Canalis caroticus

A. superior cerebelli

Hiatus canalis nervi petrosi minoris

Hiatus canalis nervi petrosi majoris

Porus acusticus internus

Foramen jugulare

Sulcus sinus sigmoidei

A. inferior anterior cerebelli

Canalis nervi hypoglossi

A. vertebralis

A. inferior posterior cerebelli

Foramen magnum

Sinus occipitalis

Fig. 12.57 Passageways of vessels and nerves through the internal surface of the cranial base, Basis cranii interna, and arterial circle of the brain, Circulus arteriosus cerebri [WILLIS]; superior view. [S700]

The Circulus arteriosus cerebri projects from above around the Fossa hypophysialis. The A. ophthalmica originates from the **A. carotis interna** at the Canalis nervi optici and, together with the N. opticus [II], pass-

es through this bony canal into the orbita. The **A. basilaris** runs along the top of the clivus. The **A. inferior anterior cerebelli** branches off the A. basilaris and runs past the Porus acusticus internus or enters it in a loop-like manner, and then provides the **A. labyrinthi**.

For an overview of the passageways through the cranial base → Fig. 8.22 and → Fig. 8.23.

Clinical remarks

The blood vessels supplying the brain show relatively great variations in their pattern, which correspond to the variability of the supplied areas. Disorders of the blood flow in these **'atypical' vessels**

can therefore lead to stroke symptoms that cannot be explained in terms of the normal 'textbook' anatomy. Not without reason do we say: 'The exception proves the rule.'

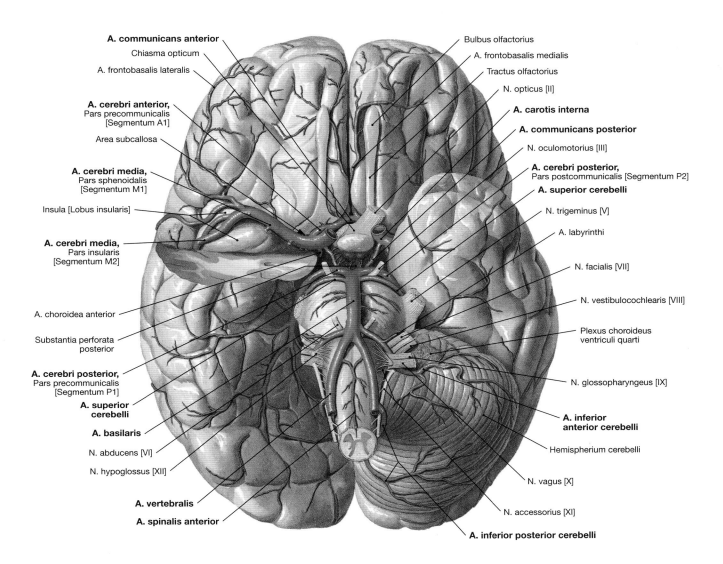

A. communicans anterior
Chiasma opticum
A. frontobasalis lateralis
A. cerebri anterior,
Pars precommunicalis
[Segmentum A1]
Area subcallosa
A. cerebri media,
Pars sphenoidalis
[Segmentum M1]
Insula [Lobus insularis]
A. cerebri media,
Pars insularis
[Segmentum M2]
A. choroidea anterior
Substantia perforata
posterior
A. cerebri posterior,
Pars precommunicalis
[Segmentum P1]
A. superior
cerebelli
A. basilaris
N. abducens [VI]
N. hypoglossus [XII]
A. vertebralis
A. spinalis anterior

Bulbus olfactorius
A. frontobasalis medialis
Tractus olfactorius
N. opticus [II]
A. carotis interna
A. communicans posterior
N. oculomotorius [III]
A. cerebri posterior,
Pars postcommunicalis [Segmentum P2]
A. superior cerebelli
N. trigeminus [V]
A. labyrinthi
N. facialis [VII]
N. vestibulocochlearis [VIII]
Plexus choroideus
ventriculi quarti
N. glossopharyngeus [IX]
A. inferior
anterior cerebelli
Hemispherium cerebelli
N. vagus [X]
N. accessorius [XI]
A. inferior posterior cerebelli

Fig. 12.58 Arteries of the brain; inferior view. [S700]
The figure shows the location of the arteries at the cranial base. The Aa. vertebrales converge to form the A. basilaris, which gives rise to the Aa. cerebri posteriores, as well as to the blood vessels supplying the brainstem, the cerebellum and the inner ear **(vertebral arterial system).** Via small connecting arteries (Aa. communicantes posteriores), the Aa. cerebri posteriores are linked with the two Aa. carotides inter-nae. Each of the latter contributes an A. cerebri media and an A. cerebri anterior, which together supply the largest part of the hemispheres with blood **(carotid arterial system).** Both Aa. cerebri anteriores are connected to each other via the A. communicans anterior. Clinically, the Aa. cerebri anterior, media and posterior are divided into segments (→ table for → Fig. 12.50). Some segments are visible in this figure.

─ **Clinical remarks** ───────────────────────────

One of the most frequent types of cerebral circulatory disorders (ischaemia) in the vertebral arterial system is the so-called **WALLEN-BERG's syndrome** (dorsal-lateral Medulla oblongata syndrome). In this case, an occlusion or impaired blood flow in the A. inferior posterior cerebelli (PICA = posterior inferior cerebellar artery) causes a broad range of symptoms, including nystagmus, vestibular disorder, dizziness (Nuclei vestibulares, inferior olive), ipsilateral hemiataxia (Pedunculus cerebellaris inferior, cerebellum), contralateral dissociat-ed sensations (Nuclei gracilis et cuneatus, Tractus spinothalamicus), swallowing difficulties, an attack of hiccups (singultus) and dyspho-nia (Nucleus ambiguus), HORNER's syndrome and a rapid pulse (central sympathetic system and cardiovascular centre in the rostral-ventrolateral Medulla oblongata), as well as respiratory disorders (respiratory centre in the ventrolateral Medulla oblongata with pre-BÖTZINGER complex).

Arteries of the brain

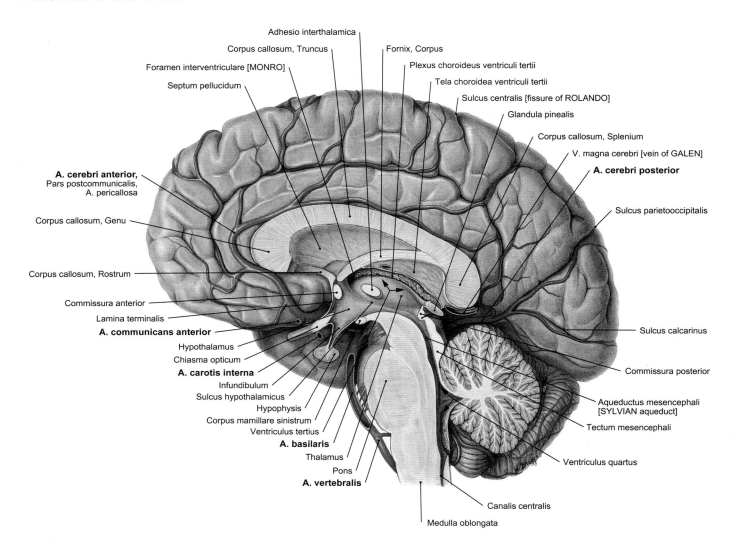

Adhesio interthalamica
Corpus callosum, Truncus
Foramen interventriculare [MONRO]
Septum pellucidum
Fornix, Corpus
Plexus choroideus ventriculi tertii
Tela choroidea ventriculi tertii
Sulcus centralis [fissure of ROLANDO]
Glandula pinealis
Corpus callosum, Splenium
V. magna cerebri [vein of GALEN]
A. cerebri posterior
A. cerebri anterior,
Pars postcommunicalis,
A. pericallosa
Corpus callosum, Genu
Sulcus parietooccipitalis
Corpus callosum, Rostrum
Commissura anterior
Lamina terminalis
A. communicans anterior
Hypothalamus
Chiasma opticum
A. carotis interna
Infundibulum
Sulcus hypothalamicus
Hypophysis
Corpus mamillare sinistrum
Ventriculus tertius
A. basilaris
Thalamus
Pons
A. vertebralis
Sulcus calcarinus
Commissura posterior
Aqueductus mesencephali [SYLVIAN aqueduct]
Tectum mesencephali
Ventriculus quartus
Canalis centralis
Medulla oblongata

Fig. 12.59   Medial surface of the brain, Facies medialis hemisphe-rii cerebri, diencephalon, and brainstem, Truncus encephali; staggered median section; view from the left side. [S700]
After providing the A. communicans anterior, the **A. cerebri anterior** passes with its Pars postcommunicalis (A. pericallosa) around the rostrum and the genu of the Corpus callosum, and continues along the surface of the Corpus callosum. Its branches extend to the Sulcus pa-rietooccipitalis. The A. cerebri anterior supplies the medial surface of the frontal and parietal lobes, as well as the rim of the hemisphere and a smaller area alongside thereof at the cerebral convexity (→ Fig. 12.66). The **A. cerebri posterior** flows to the occipital lobe, the basal part of the temporal lobe, the lower part of the striatum (not visible), and to the thalamus.

Clinical remarks

In most cases a **stroke** is caused by an acute circulation disorder in a smaller or larger brain area supplied by the affected cerebral artery (ischaemia, brainstem infarction (BSI), 80–90 % of cases). Acute bleeding in the brain (intracerebral haemorrhage) accounts for nearly 10 % of all strokes, followed by subarachnoid haemorrhages (approx. 3 %). The first diagnostic measure to confirm or exclude a haemor-rhage, ischaemia or a totally different cause of the neurological symptoms, is a **CT of the brain.** The speed of the CT-imaging makes it the preferred choice over MRI-imaging. With modern equipment, CT scans of the brain can now be obtained in less than half a minute. If the ischaemia is caused by a thrombus, a pharmacological therapy **(thrombolysis)** can be attempted. The outcome is largely deter-

mined by how much time has lapsed since the stroke ('time is brain'). Many clinical centres therefore have specialised stroke departments (stroke units). For patients with an intracerebral haemorrhage, how-ever, a thrombolysis is contraindicated. The rapid diagnostic evalua-tion therefore plays a crucial role in stroke treatment.
In the fetal period, all three cerebral arteries are fed by the ipsilateral A. carotis interna. Once the connection of the **A. cerebri posterior** to the A. vertebrobasilaris arterial system is established, the original (primary) vessel atrophies and becomes the predominantly thin A. communicans posterior. However, in 20 % of the cases this does not happen, so that in adults (just like in the fetus) an A. cerebri pos-terior persists which is fed by the A. cerebri posterior.

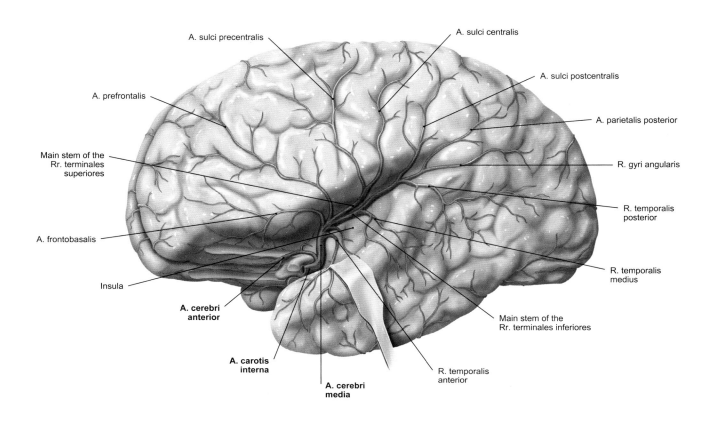

A. sulci precentralis

A. sulci centralis

A. prefrontalis

A. sulci postcentralis

A. parietalis posterior

Main stem of the
Rr. terminales
superiores

R. gyri angularis

R. temporalis
posterior

A. frontobasalis

R. temporalis
medius

Insula

A. cerebri
anterior

Main stem of the
Rr. terminales inferiores

A. carotis
interna

R. temporalis
anterior

A. cerebri
media

Fig. 12.60   A. cerebri media on the Facies lateralis cerebri; view from the left side. [S700-L127]/[B500]

The **A. cerebri media** supplies the major part of the lateral surface of the hemisphere, the insula and, with central branches, also the Capsula interna (parts of the Crus anterius, genu) as well as the basal ganglia.

Clinical remarks

Occlusions in the bifurcation area of the A. cerebri media due to arteriosclerosis or an embolism result in **cerebral infarction** (stroke, apoplexy) with severe deficits. These include a contralateral, predominantly brachiofacial hemiplegia with hypaesthesia (circumscribed or general decrease of touch and pressure sensations of the skin). If the dominant hemisphere is affected, this results in aphasia (speech disorder), agraphia (inability to write words and text despite having the necessary mobility of the hand, as well as the intellectual ability) and alexia (inability to read). In patients with high blood pressure (hypertension), changes in the walls of cerebral vessels can cause a

vascular rupture and bleeding into the cerebral parenchyma (possibly leading to massive bleeding). The basal ganglia in particular are commonly affected by this.

Arteriosclerosis-induced changes in the wall of vessels are often found in the A. carotis interna. Small thrombi emerging from these plaques can cause an occlusion of the A. centralis retinae via the A. ophthalmica, and thus lead to a sudden painless unilateral blindness. If the thrombus dissolves within a short time it is called **amaurosis fugax** (short-term blindness). As a frequent sign of cerebral circulatory disorders, it can be a red flag for an impending stroke.

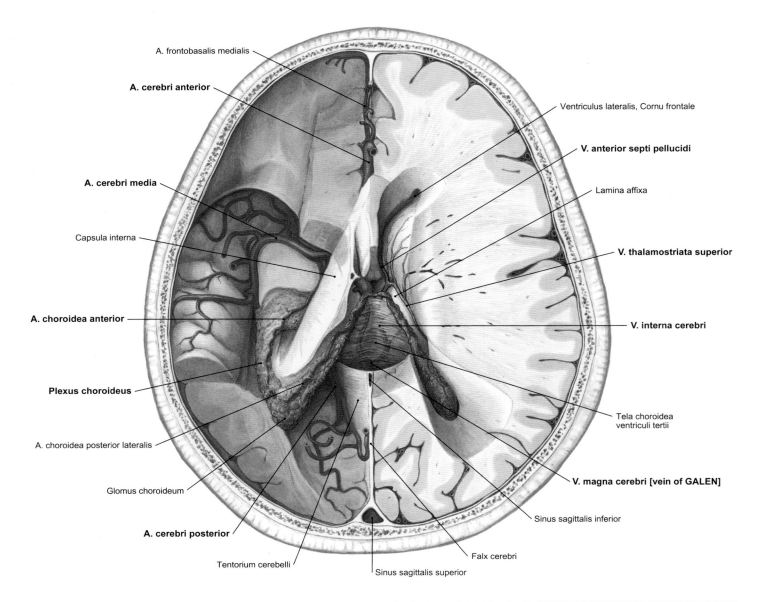

A. frontobasalis medialis

A. cerebri anterior

A. cerebri media

Capsula interna

A. choroidea anterior

Plexus choroideus

A. choroidea posterior lateralis

Glomus choroideum

A. cerebri posterior

Tentorium cerebelli

Ventriculus lateralis, Cornu frontale

V. anterior septi pellucidi

Lamina affixa

V. thalamostriata superior

V. interna cerebri

Tela choroidea ventriculi tertii

V. magna cerebri [vein of GALEN]

Sinus sagittalis inferior

Falx cerebri

Sinus sagittalis superior

Fig. 12.61 Branching of the A. cerebri media in the insular region and the outer cerebral surface, choroid arteries and internal cerebral veins; after removal of large areas of the brain with exposure of the Fossa lateralis (left) and the lateral ventricles. [S700]

The **A. cerebri media** passes laterally into the Fossa lateralis and divides into four segments (→ Fig. 12.58):

- **Pars sphenoidalis** (M1), where the A. choroidea anterior branches off (→ table)
- **Pars insularis** with short branches to the insular cortex (M2)
- **Pars opercularis** for the cortex of the temporal lobe (Aa. frontobasalis laterales and temporales; M3)
- **Pars terminalis** (M4) with the Rr. terminales inferiores and superiores for cortical areas of the Sulcus centralis and parietal lobe.

In the lateral ventricles, the **A. choroidea anterior** (from anterior below; originating from the A. cerebri interna) and the **Aa. choroideae posteriores laterales** (from dorsal above; originating from the A. cerebri posterior) form a plexus of vessels. On the right side, the inner venous system can also be seen in the vicinity of the Tela choroidea of the third ventricle.

Choroid arteries		
Vessel	**Origin**	**Flow region**
A. choroidea anterior	A. carotis interna	• Tractus opticus • Capsula interna (Crus posterius) • anterior hippocampus • Crura cerebri, Tegmentum mesencephali • Plexus choroideus
Aa. choroideae posteriores	A. cerebri posterior	• Corpus geniculatum laterale • hippocampus and fornix • thalamus (posterior parts) • dorsal mesencephalon • Glandula pinealis

---

Clinical remarks

The **anterior choroid artery syndrome** is caused by circulatory disorders in the area of the A. choroidea anterior and is associated with a triad of symptoms, including motor, sensory and visual dysfunctions: hemiplegia (failure of motor fibres in the Crura cerebri), hemi-sensory disorders (failure of the Crus posterius of the Capsula interna) and hemianopsia (failure of the Tractus opticus and parts of the Radiatio optica). **Circulatory disorders of the A. cerebri posterior** lead to visual failures, but can also be associated with temporary deficits of memory function (amnesia), as parts of the hippocampal formation are also supplied with blood from here (→ Fig. 12.81).

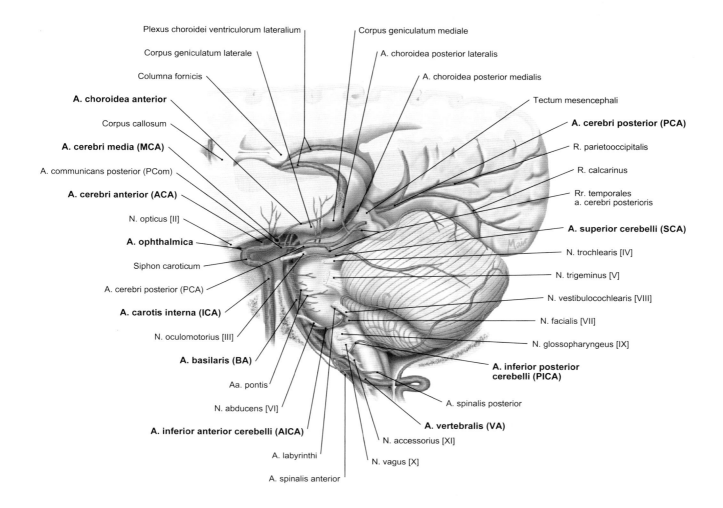

Plexus choroidei ventriculorum lateralium
Corpus geniculatum mediale
Corpus geniculatum laterale
A. choroidea posterior lateralis
Columna fornicis
A. choroidea posterior medialis
A. choroidea anterior
Tectum mesencephali
Corpus callosum
A. cerebri posterior (PCA)
A. cerebri media (MCA)
R. parietooccipitalis
A. communicans posterior (PCom)
R. calcarinus
A. cerebri anterior (ACA)
Rr. temporales
a. cerebri posterioris
N. opticus [II]
A. superior cerebelli (SCA)
A. ophthalmica
N. trochlearis [IV]
Siphon caroticum
N. trigeminus [V]
A. cerebri posterior (PCA)
N. vestibulocochlearis [VIII]
A. carotis interna (ICA)
N. facialis [VII]
N. oculomotorius [III]
N. glossopharyngeus [IX]
A. basilaris (BA)
A. inferior posterior cerebelli (PICA)
Aa. pontis
A. spinalis posterior
N. abducens [VI]
A. vertebralis (VA)
A. inferior anterior cerebelli (AICA)
N. accessorius [XI]
A. labyrinthi
N. vagus [X]
A. spinalis anterior

Fig. 12.62 Arteries of the posterior cranial fossa: A. vertebralis, A.basilaris and its branches; view from the left side. [S702-L127]/ [G343]

The posterior parts of the cortex, cerebellum and of the Truncus encephali are mainly supplied via blood vessels of the vertebrobasilar arterial system. The **A. vertebralis** branches off the A. subclavia at the level of the first thoracic vertebra and can be divided into four segments (→ table for → Fig. 12.63):

- **Pars prevertebralis** (V1), from the outlet of the A. subclavia (at the level of the first thoracic vertebra) up to the Foramen transversarium of the fourth cervical vertebra
- **Pars transversaria** (V2), within the Foramina transversaria of the sixth to second cervical vertebrae
- **Pars atlantica** (V3), from the transition to the atlas and arch of the atlas to the passage through the Foramen magnum
- **Pars intracranialis** (V4), the intracranial part up to the confluence with the A. basilaris.

Along its pathway, the A. vertebralis sends a number of branches to the neck muscles, the meninges, the cerebellum and spinal cord. The two most important branches are the **A. inferior posterior cerebelli** (which often gives rise to an A. spinalis posterior) and the A. spinalis anterior. Both Aa. vertebrales unite at the level of the pontomedullary transition to the unpaired, centrally located **A. basilaris** (→ Fig. 12.58). It runs in the middle of the pons and supplies large parts of the brainstem and the cerebellum with its branches. The branches of the A. basilaris are the **A. inferior anterior cerebelli** (giving rise to the A. labyrinthi which supplies the inner ear), the Aa. pontis and the A. superior cerebelli. At the approximate level of the mesencephalon (Cisterna interpeduncularis), the A. basilaris bifurcates into the Aa. cerebri posteriores. The latter supply large parts of the mesencephalon and occipitotemporal parts of the hemispheres. Branches of the **A. cerebri posterior** are the **Aa. centrales posteromediales,** the **Aa. centrales posterolateralis** (→ table for → Fig. 12.63) and the **Aa. choroideae posteriores** (→ table for → Fig. 12.61).

Clinical remarks

The A. vertebralis can be assessed in the so-called vertebral artery triangle (→ Fig. 2.92) between the M. obliquus capitis superior, the M. obliquus capitis inferior and the M. rectus capitis posterior major; with the head bent forward, the blood flow is determined with a **DOPPLER ultrasound examination.**

In the case of a stroke, very unusual symptoms can develop due to the blood supply to certain regions. So it is possible that, for example, **circulatory disorders of the Aa. pontis** lead to failures of motor

fibre tracts in ventral parts of the pons, which may be associated with an acute paraplegia. As the dorsal parts of the pons are supplied by branches of the A. superior cerebelli, important areas of awareness such as the Formatio reticularis and also the eye movements remain intact. Patients with **locked-in syndrome** are despite their paraplegia fully conscious without cognitive impairment, but they can only communicate with eye movements and blinking.

Arteries of the brain

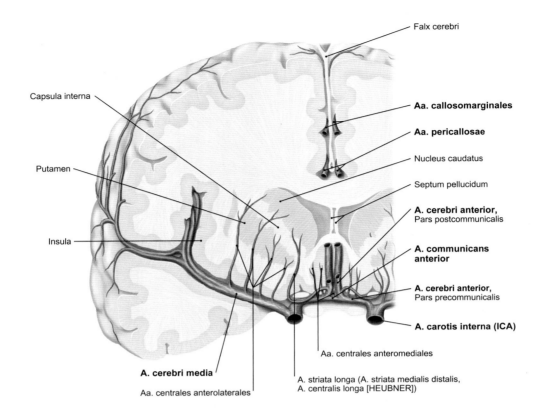

Falx cerebri

Capsula interna

Aa. callosomarginales

Aa. pericallosae

Nucleus caudatus

Putamen

Septum pellucidum

A. cerebri anterior,
Pars postcommunicalis

Insula

A. communicans anterior

A. cerebri anterior,
Pars precommunicalis

A. carotis interna (ICA)

Aa. centrales anteromediales

A. cerebri media

Aa. centrales anterolaterales

A. striata longa (A. striata medialis distalis,
A. centralis longa [HEUBNER])

Fig. 12.63 Central arteries; frontal section at the level of the bifurcation of the A. carotis interna. [S702-L127]/[G343]
The so-called central arteries provide the anterior inner part of the brain with the subcortical nuclei, the Corpus medullare which includes the Capsula interna, and the diencephalon. These penetrating vessels form vascular groups which enter the brain at the Basis cerebri, thereby perforating the tissue (Substantia perforata; → table). They are the:
- Aa. centrales anteromediales, the anterior-medial structures such as the Nucleus caudatus
- Aa. centrales anterolaterales (= Aa. lenticulostriatae), the anterior-lateral structures such as the Globus pallidus and the putamen

- Aa. centrales posteromediales and Aa. centrales posterolaterales, the posterior structures such as the thalamus and the hypothalamus.

In addition, interior parts of the brain are supplied by the choroid blood vessels (→ table for → Fig. 12.61). The choroid blood vessels of the lateral ventricles are connected via the Plexus choroideus and form a vascular corona or plexus (→ Fig. 12.61), which connects the tributaries of the A. carotis interna with those of the A. vertebralis/basilaris.

Arterial blood supply to the Capsula interna		
Capsula interna	**Arteries**	**Origin**
Crus anterius	Aa. centrales anteromediales	A. cerebri anterior
	A. striata longa (A. centralis longa [HEUBNER], A. striata medialis distalis, A. recurrens)	A. cerebri anterior
	Aa. centrales anterolaterales	A. cerebri media
Genu	Aa. centrales anterolaterales	A. cerebri media
Crus posterius	Aa. centrales anterolaterales	A. cerebri media
	A. choroidea anterior	A. carotis interna

Clinical remarks

As the **Aa. centrales anterolaterales** branch off the A. cerebri media almost at a right angle, this part is particularly prone to turbulent blood flow and to secondary arteriosclerotic changes. In patients with high blood pressure (hypertension), **occlusions** can therefore frequently be found at these bifurcations. Occlusions as well as **haem-** orrhages from these blood vessels can lead to tissue necrosis in the nuclear region of the cerebrum (basal ganglia) and the Capsula interna with resulting (contralateral) hemiplegia. Depending on their location, **lesions of the nuclei in the cerebrum** can cause severe hyperkinetic or hypokinetic disorders (dystonia).

Topography of arteries supplying the brain

Artery	Topography and characteristics
A. carotis interna (ICA, internal carotid artery)	• four topographic-anatomical defined segments: Pars cervicalis, Pars petrosa, Pars cavernosa, Pars cerebralis • exits the Sinus cavernosus lateral of the Chiasma opticum
A. ophthalmica	• first major vessel of the A. carotis interna • originates below the N. opticus [II] and passes through the Canalis nervi optici into the orbit of the eye • anastomosis (A. dorsalis nasi) with the A. facialis (A. angularis)
A. choroidea anterior	• vascular branch of the A. carotis interna • passes along the Tractus opticus to the inferior horn of the lateral ventricle
A. cerebri anterior (ACA, anterior cerebral artery)	• runs laterally to the Chiasma opticum to rostral • enters the Fissura longitudinalis cerebri • runs above the Corpus callosum occipitally
A. communicans anterior (ACOM, anterior communicating artery)	• between the Aa. cerebri anteriores • located in front of the Chiasma opticum
A. cerebri media (MCA, middle cerebral artery)	• passes around the Polus temporalis to the Fossa lateralis cerebri • bifurcation via the insula, leaving the Sulcus lateralis, with branches running on the lateral surface of the cerebrum
A. vertebralis (VA, vertebral artery)	• four topographic-anatomical defined segments: Pars prevertebralis, Pars transversaria, Pars atlantis, Pars intracranialis • passes ventrally and forms the A. basilaris (at the lower rim of the pons)
A. inferior posterior cerebelli (PICA, posterior inferior cerebellar artery)	• flows out of the A. vertebralis at the level of the olive (may be absent) • forms a loop at the level of the cerebellar tonsils (radiological feature) • enters the Vallecula cerebelli above the vermis
A. basilaris (BA, basilar artery)	• runs in the Sulcus basilaris of the pons • bifurcation into the Aa. cerebri posteriores (at the level of the mesencephalon)
A. inferior anterior cerebelli (AICA, anterior inferior cerebellar artery)	• flows out of the lower segment of the A. basilaris, ventrally of the cranial nerves VI, VII, VIII • runs to the Meatus acusticus internus, provides the A. labyrinthi (usually) and from there passes to the underside of the cerebellum
A. superior cerebelli (SCA, superior cerebellar artery)	• flows caudally out of the N. oculomotorius [III] from the A. basilaris • runs below the Tentorium cerebelli • passes posteriorly to the surface of the cerebellum
A. cerebri posterior (PCA, posterior cerebral artery)	• arises cranially of the N. oculomotorius [III] • runs above the Tentorium cerebelli • passes posteriorly to the occipital-basal surface of the cerebrum
A. communicans posterior (PCOM, posterior communicating artery)	• connects the A. carotis interna and the A. cerebri posterior • runs laterally of the pituitary gland and the Corpora mamillaria

Central arteries

Vessel/vascular group	Passage	Origin	Supply area (e.g.)
Aa. centrales anteromediales	Substantia perforata anterior	• A. cerebri anterior • A. communicans anterior	• Caput nuclei caudati • Globus pallidus • Commissura anterior • Capsula interna
Aa. centrales anterolaterales (Aa. lenticulostriatae)	Substantia perforata anterior	A. cerebri media	• Nucleus caudatus • Putamen • Globus pallidus • Capsula interna (medial vessels)
Aa. centrales posteromediales	Substantia perforata posterior	• A. cerebri posterior • A. communicans posterior	• Thalamus • Hypothalamus • Globus pallidus
Aa. centrales posterolaterales	Substantia perforata posterior	A. cerebri posterior (Pars postcommunicalis)	• Thalamus • Corpus geniculatum mediale • Colliculi • Glandula pinealis

Arteries of the brain

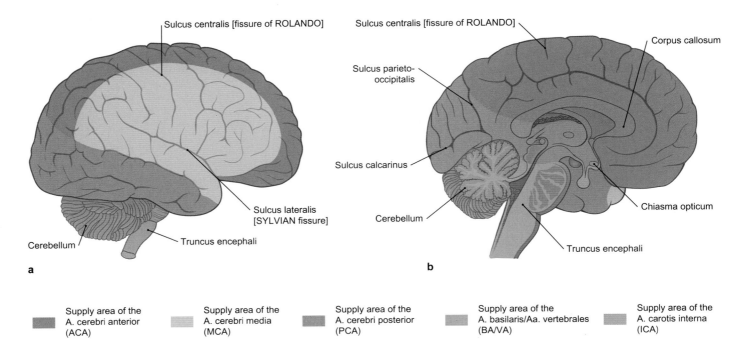

Fig. 12.64a and b   Areas supplied by the cerebral arteries (cerebrum). [S702-L126]/[R247-L318]

a Lateral view of the brain. The **A. cerebri anterior** supplies the frontal and parietal areas of the cerebral cortex approx. 1 cm beyond the hemispherical rim (→ table for → Fig. 12.63). The **A. cerebri posterior** provides blood to the occipital pole and the lower margin of the temporal lobe. The outer surface of the remaining cortical area is supplied by the **A. cerebri media.** The blood supply in the area of the Gyri precentralis

and postcentralis is fed in part by the A. cerebri anterior and in part by the A. cerebri media.

b Medial view onto a sagittal section of the brain. In the medial view, the A. cerebri anterior supplies the medial surface of the frontal and parietal lobes beyond the hemispherical rim up to the Sulcus parieto-occipitalis. The occipital lobe and the base of the temporal lobe are supplied by the **A. cerebri posterior.** The blood supply of the cerebellum and brainstem is provided by the vertebrobasilar arterial system.

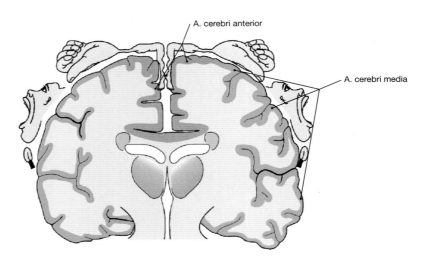

Fig. 12.65   Arteries in the region of the Gyrus precentralis and their projection onto the homunculus of the primary motor cortex. [S700-L238]

The **A. cerebri anterior** supplies the cortex of the Gyrus precentralis approx. 1 cm beyond the hemispherical rim with blood, taking on the

cortical representation areas of the lower limb, the pelvis and the rib cage. The cortical representation areas of the upper limb and the entire head are supplied via the **A. cerebri media.**

Clinical remarks

Due to the blood supply in the region of the Gyrus precentralis, circulatory disorders of the A. cerebri anterior are associated predominantly with **leg paralysis** and circulatory disorders of the A. cerebri media with **brachiofacial paralysis.** The patient's clinical picture (leg or brachiofacial paralysis) therefore allows conclusions about the affected vessel.

Strokes or haemorrhages in the area of the Capsula interna frequently involve the A. striata longa (A. striata medialis distalis, A. centralis longa, HEUBNER's artery, A. recurrens) as a branch of the A. cerebri anterior (belonging to the Aa. centrales anteromediales), or to the A. lenticulostriata as a branch of the A. cerebri media (belonging to the Aa. centrales anterolaterales) (→ Fig. 12.63).

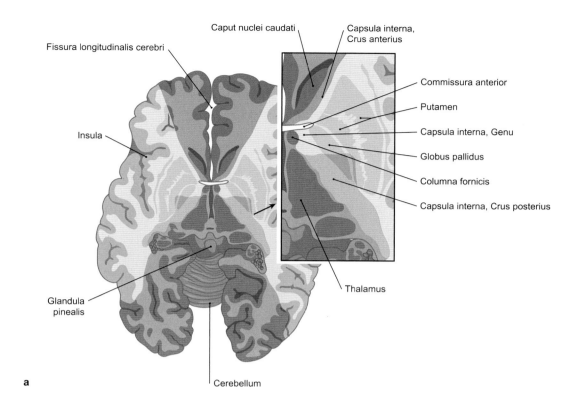

Caput nuclei caudati

Capsula interna, Crus anterius

Fissura longitudinalis cerebri

Commissura anterior

Putamen

Insula

Capsula interna, Genu

Globus pallidus

Columna fornicis

Capsula interna, Crus posterius

Thalamus

Glandula pinealis

Cerebellum

a

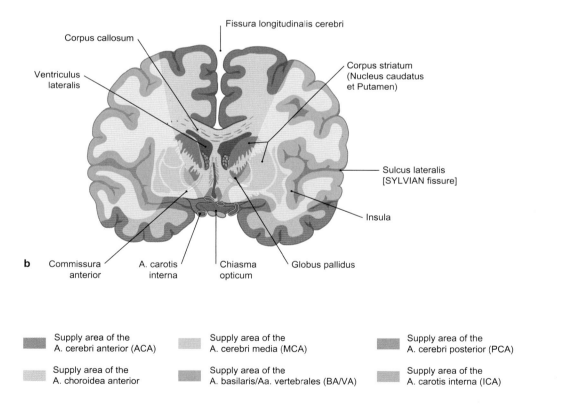

Fissura longitudinalis cerebri

Corpus callosum

Ventriculus lateralis

Corpus striatum (Nucleus caudatus et Putamen)

Sulcus lateralis [SYLVIAN fissure]

Insula

b

Commissura anterior

A. carotis interna

Chiasma opticum

Globus pallidus

Supply area of the A. cerebri anterior (ACA)

Supply area of the A. cerebri media (MCA)

Supply area of the A. cerebri posterior (PCA)

Supply area of the A. choroidea anterior

Supply area of the A. basilaris/Aa. vertebrales (BA/VA)

Supply area of the A. carotis interna (ICA)

Fig. 12.66a and b   Areas supplied by the cerebral arteries (cerebrum). [S702-L126]/[R247-L318]

a Horizontal section.
b Frontal section.

Meninges and blood supply

Arteries of the brain

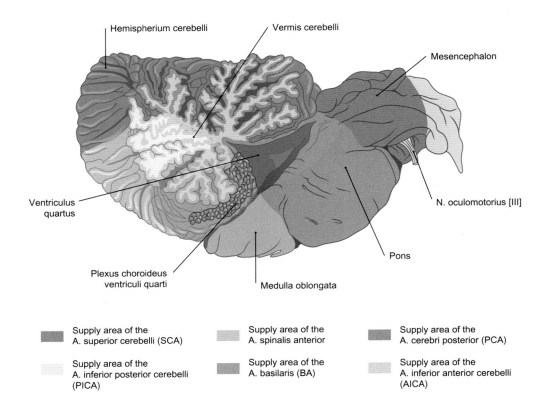

Fig. 12.67 **Areas supplied by the cerebral arteries (brainstem and cerebellum);** sagittal section. [S702-L126]/[R247-L318]

Arterial supply of the brainstem		
Parts of the brainstem	**Medial supply area**	**Lateral supply area**
Mesencephalon	A. cerebri posterior	• A. superior cerebelli • A. cerebri posterior
Pons	A. basilaris (Aa. pontis)	• A. superior cerebelli • A. inferior anterior cerebelli (very variable)
Medulla oblongata	• Aa. vertebrales • A. spinalis anterior • Aa. spinales posteriores	A. inferior posterior cerebelli

Arterial supply of the cerebellum					
Artery	**Clinical term**	**Cortical area**	**Central area**	**Other supply areas**	**Origin**
A. superior cerebelli	SCA (constant)	Major part of the cerebellum, upper part of the vermis	Nucleus dentatus	Upper parts of the pons	A. basilaris
A. inferior anterior cerebelli	AICA (variable)	Part of the anterior cerebellar hemispheres		Lateral pons, branching of the A. labyrinthi to the inner ear in 85 %	A. basilaris
A. inferior posterior cerebelli	PICA (variable)	Major part of the lower cerebellar hemispheres, flocculus	Nuclei emboliformis, globosus and fastigii	Posterior and lateral Medulla oblongata	A. vertebralis

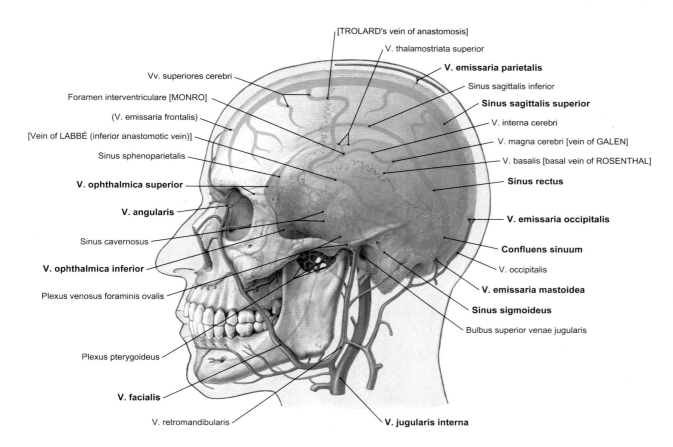

Fig. 12.68   Internal and external veins of the head. [S700]
The internal and external veins of the head are connected to each other via numerous anastomoses. These include the Vv. emissariae and ophthalmicae, as well as the Plexus venosi.

Passageways of Vv. emissariae through the skull

V. emissaria	Passageway
V. emissaria parietalis	Foramen parietale
V. emissaria mastoidea	Foramen mastoideum
V. emissaria occipitalis	Opening near the Protuberantia occipitalis externa
V. emissaria condylaris	Canalis condylaris
Plexus venosus canalis nervi hypoglossi	Canalis nervi hypoglossi
Plexus venosus foraminis ovalis	Foramen ovale
Plexus venosus caroticus internus	Canalis caroticus

Pathway of the Sinus durae matris

Sinus durae matris	Pathway and characteristics
Sinus sagittalis superior	• in the anterior-posterior direction in the Sulcus sinus sagittalis of the cranial bones • bridging veins, draining into the sinus or its lateral lacunae • flows toward the Confluens sinuum
Sinus sagittalis inferior	along the inferior margin of the falx to the Sinus rectus
Sinus rectus	originates from the Sinus sagittalis inferior and the V. magna cerebri at the intersection of the falx and tentorium
Confluens sinuum	confluence of the Sinus rectus, sagittalis superior and occipitalis and drainage from here into the Sinus transversi
Sinus occipitalis	flows toward the Confluens sinuum
Sinus marginalis	• surrounds the Foramen magnum • connected to the Sinus occipitalis and Plexus venosus vertebralis internus
Sinus transversus	passes laterally from the Confluens sinuum to the Sinus sigmoideus
Sinus sigmoideus	S-shaped pathway via the Pars mastoidea of the Os temporale to the Foramen jugulare and V. jugularis
Sinus cavernosus	• chambered venous space on both sides of the Sella turcica • connected to the Sinus cavernosus on the opposite side via the Plexus basilaris
Sinus petrosi superior et inferior	• passes along the upper or lower edge of the Pars petrosa ossis temporalis • connection between the Sinus cavernosus and the Sinus sigmoideus

Clinical remarks

Due to a lack of venous valves in this area, scalp injuries can lead to a reversed blood flow, and thus to a **spreading of bacteria via the Vv. emissariae** and via veins located in the diploë (Vv. diploicae, → Fig. 12.69) into the Sinus durae matris and subsequently the interior of the skull.

Meninges and blood supply

Veins of the head

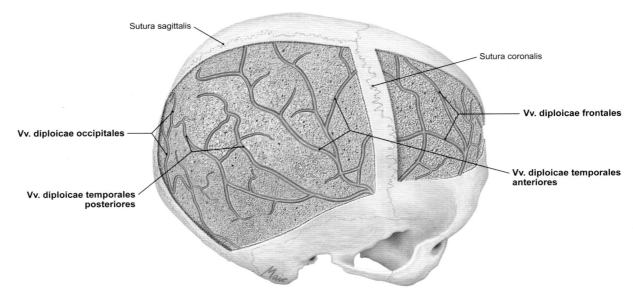

Fig. 12.69 Diploic canals, Canales diploici, and diploic veins, Vv. diploicae, of the calvaria, right side; oblique superior view; after removal of the outer layer of the calvaria. [S700-L127]

The diploë is traversed by diploic canals, in which the Vv. diploicae run. They are connected to the Vv. emissariae and the Sinus durae matris.

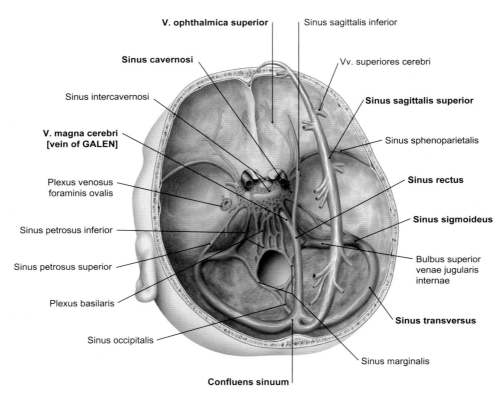

Fig. 12.70 Sinus durae matris projected onto the cranial base; oblique superior view; after removal of the calvaria. [S700-L127]/[B500]

The Sinus durae matris are large venous blood vessels around the brain, derived from dural folds or duplications (→ Fig. 12.33 and → table for → Fig. 12.68).

Clinical remarks

Altitude sickness refers to suddenly occurring headaches, dizziness and nausea when ascending heights of 2,500 metres above sea-level within a short period of time and without prior acclimatisation (e.g. to travel from Germany to La Paz/Bolivia with an altitude of 3,600 meters). Up to 25 % of all people are affected. It is assumed that due to the lower partial oxygen pressure at high altitude, the arterial blood flow to the brain is increased, in order to supply it with more oxygen. The larger amount of blood can only be drained if the cerebral veins are able to strongly dilate, but they are only capable of

doing this to a limited extent; the resulting congestion of blood explains the symptoms.

Sinus thrombosis (a thrombosis in a Sinus durae matris) is always a serious condition. Possible causes are, e.g. protracted infections of the face (cavernous sinus thrombosis) or a middle ear infection (sigmoid sinus thrombosis, septic sinus thromboses), but also coagulopathies with increased clotting. The patients suffer from headaches, seizures, paralysis and clouding of consciousness.

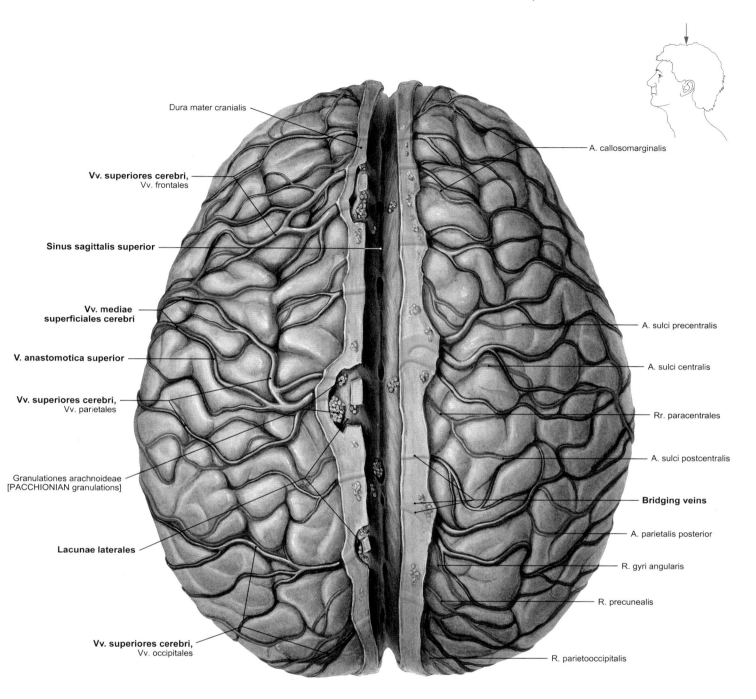

Dura mater cranialis

Vv. superiores cerebri,
Vv. frontales

Sinus sagittalis superior

Vv. mediae
superficiales cerebri

V. anastomotica superior

Vv. superiores cerebri,
Vv. parietales

Granulationes arachnoideae
[PACCHIONIAN granulations]

Lacunae laterales

Vv. superiores cerebri,
Vv. occipitales

A. callosomarginalis

A. sulci precentralis

A. sulci centralis

Rr. paracentrales

A. sulci postcentralis

Bridging veins

A. parietalis posterior

R. gyri angularis

R. precunealis

R. parietooccipitalis

Fig. 12.71 Superficial arteries and veins of the brain; superior view; after removal of the dura mater, and opening of the Sinus sagittalis superior, arachnoid mater also removed. [S700]
The superficial arteries and veins supply the cerebral cortex and the subjacent basal ganglia. The superficial veins include the Vv. superiores cerebri, the V. media superficialis cerebri and the Vv. inferiores cerebri (not visible here). The large veins are generally connected via anastomoses (V. anastomotica superior [TROLARD's vein] and V. anastomotica inferior [Vein of LABBÉ]; → Fig. 12.68). The Vv. superiores cerebri drain into the Sinus sagittalis superior via small bridging veins, which pass through the Dura mater cranialis, or are connected by bridging veins to the Lacunae laterales, which then drain into the Sinus sagittalis superior.

Clinical remarks

Injuries of the bridging veins can lead to bleeding between the dura mater and arachnoid mater, and thus cause a subdural haematoma (Clinical remarks for → Fig. 12.74). In particular, elderly patients with age-related atrophy of the brain and fragile bridging veins tend to develop a **chronic subdural haematoma,** which can easily be overlooked due to the insidious venous bleeding after a minor trauma that the patient often cannot remember.

Veins of the brain

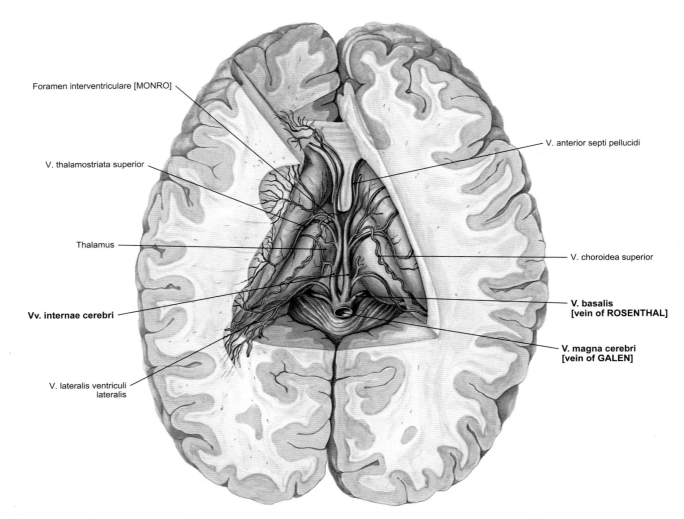

Foramen interventriculare [MONRO]

V. thalamostriata superior

Thalamus

Vv. internae cerebri

V. lateralis ventriculi lateralis

V. anterior septi pellucidi

V. choroidea superior

V. basalis [vein of ROSENTHAL]

V. magna cerebri [vein of GALEN]

Fig. 12.72   Deep cerebral veins, Vv. profundae cerebri; superior view. [S700]
The Vv. internae cerebri run within the Tela choroidea ventriculi tertii. The veins of the ventricular system, of the basal ganglia, and of the in-

ternal capsule also belong to the deep cerebral veins. The blood from these structures flows via the Vv. thalamostriatae superiores to the Vv. internae cerebri, and from here it is drained into the V. magna cerebri (vein of GALEN).

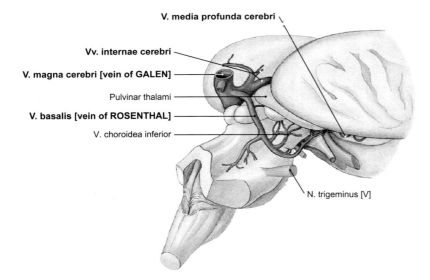

V. media profunda cerebri

Vv. internae cerebri

V. magna cerebri [vein of GALEN]

Pulvinar thalami

V. basalis [vein of ROSENTHAL]

V. choroidea inferior

N. trigeminus [V]

Venous branches merging with the V. magna cerebri		
Vein	**Most important tributaries**	**Areas of the brain**
V. interna cerebri	V. choroidea superior	Plexus choroideus, hippocampus
	V. septi pellucidi	Septum pellucidum
	V. thalamostriata	Nucleus caudatus
V. basalis [vein of ROSENTHAL]	V. anterior cerebri	Corpus callosum and adjacent gyri
	V. profunda cerebri	Putamen, Globus pallidus

Fig. 12.73   Deep cerebral veins, Vv. profundae cerebri; posterior view from the right side. [S700]
After removal of the cerebellum, the basal cerebral veins which drain the venous blood from the rhombencephalon, mesencephalon and in-

sula, are visible. Venous vessels of this region are the paired V. media profunda cerebri and the V. basalis (vein of Rosenthal), which just like the Vv. internae cerebri drain the blood into the V. magna cerebri (vein of GALEN).

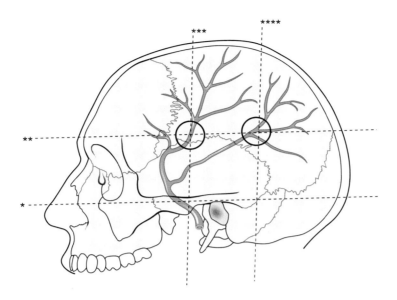

Fig. 12.74 Projection of the Rr. frontalis and parietalis of the A. meningea media onto the lateral cranial wall. Circles mark the projections of the main branches of the A. meningea media. [S700-L127]
The main branches of the A. meningea media run at the intersections of the upper horizontal line with the vertical line passing through the middle of the zygomatic arch, and through the posterior part of the Proc. mastoideus.

*   clin.: Linea horizontalis auriculo-orbitalis (Frankfort horizontal plane)
**   clin.: Linea horizontalis supraorbitalis
***   vertical plane through the middle of the Arcus zygomaticus
**** vertical plane through the posterior part of the Proc. mastoideus

Clinical remarks

Blunt cranial trauma with forces acting on the skull from the side often leads in the area of the marked interfaces above (→ Fig. 12.74) to **fractures of the calvaria.** This can easily cause ruptures of the R. frontalis or R. parietalis of the A. meningea media, which supplies the dura mater with blood. Often, the patient has no apparent injuries or does not develop symptoms during the first 30 minutes. The arterial bleeding induces a detachment of the dura mater from the calvaria and the formation of an **epidural haematoma** (→ figure) which

can lead to shifting of parts of the brain and increased pressure on the brain, brainstem and cranial nerves. Serious deficits with pathological reflexes can be the result. The cranial CT scan shows an area of hyperdensity (i.e. denser than the surrounding tissue), which is biconvex and does not extend beyond the sutures. The latter is due to the attachment of the dura mater to the sutures. Surgery with ligation of the bleeding vessel as soon as possible and relief of the intracranial pressure (by decompression) are crucial prognostic factors.

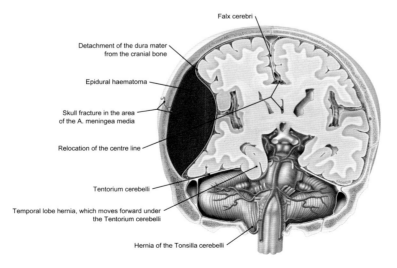

Falx cerebri

Detachment of the dura mater from the cranial bone

Epidural haematoma

Skull fracture in the area of the A. meningea media

Relocation of the centre line

Tentorium cerebelli

Temporal lobe hernia, which moves forward under the Tentorium cerebelli

Hernia of the Tonsilla cerebelli

Epidural haematoma; frontal section; anterior view. An injury to the A. meningea media on the right side of the body has resulted in arterial bleeding between the calvaria and dura mater. The haematoma induced a shift of the midline; in addition a part of the temporal

lobe was pushed through the Incisura tentorii underneath the Tentorium cerebelli. [S700-L238]

Meninges and blood supply

Intracranial bleeding

Clinical remarks

Compared to the veins of younger people, the veins of elderly people are less resilient. In the elderly, minor injuries can more readily cause rupture or tearing of the bridging veins (connecting veins between cerebral veins and Sinus durae matris) with subsequent development of a **subdural haematoma** (→ figures). In this acute or insidious process (sometimes taking weeks), venous blood collects between the dura mater and arachnoid mater, which is associated with nonspecific symptoms such as dizziness, headache, fatigue, lack of energy or confusion. Subdural haematoma can also occur with intracerebral bleeding and cause acute neurological deficits (e.g. headaches, nausea, vomiting, impaired consciousness, hemiplegia). In CT scans, subdural haematomas appear as hyperdense, crescent-shaped areas, extending beyond the sutures. The therapy consists of a surgical procedure with insertion of an outflow drainage pathway. **Subarachnoid haematomas** can usually be traced back to ruptures of aneurysms (pathological bulging of arteries). Aneurysms are particularly common in the area of the Circulus arteriosus [circle of WILLIS] and their rupture causes bleeding into the subarachnoid space. Subarachnoid haemorrhages also appear as hyperdense areas in the CT scan, but are strictly limited to the affected parts of the subarachnoid space, which can be especially clearly seen in the respective cisterns. An early intervention with surgical ligation of the blood source is prognostically important.

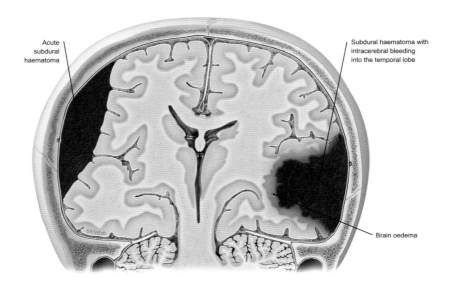

Acute subdural haematoma

Subdural haematoma with intracerebral bleeding into the temporal lobe

Brain oedema

Subdural haematoma and intracerebral haemorrhage; frontal section; anterior view. Ruptures of bridging veins have caused an acute subdural haematoma on the right side of the head and a subdural haematoma with intracerebral bleeding into the temporal lobe on the left side. [S700-L238]

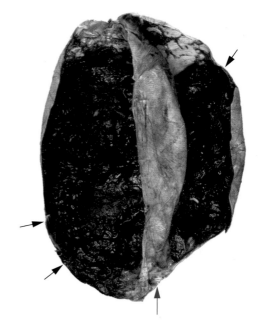

Subdural haematomas; superior view onto the brain. Extended bilateral acute traumatic subdural haematoma (arrows) on the inner side of the dura mater (red arrow = Falx cerebri). The dura above the haematoma was folded upwards. [R235]

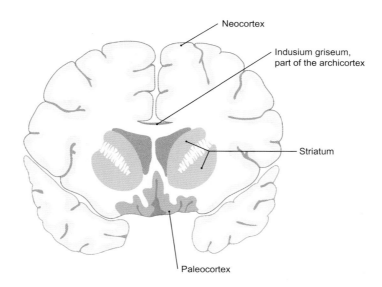

Fig. 12.75 **Parts of the cerebrum;** frontal section, schematic representation. [S702-L126]~[R317]
The cortical areas of the cerebrum can be divided into three parts:
* neocortex – mainly consists of six layers and accounts for the largest part

* archicortex – comprises the mostly three-layered parts (allocortex) of the limbic system
* paleocortex – also mostly three-layered (allocortex), and essentially encompassing the olfactory lobe (rhinencephalon).
The subcortical nuclei also belong to the cerebrum, e.g. the striatum.

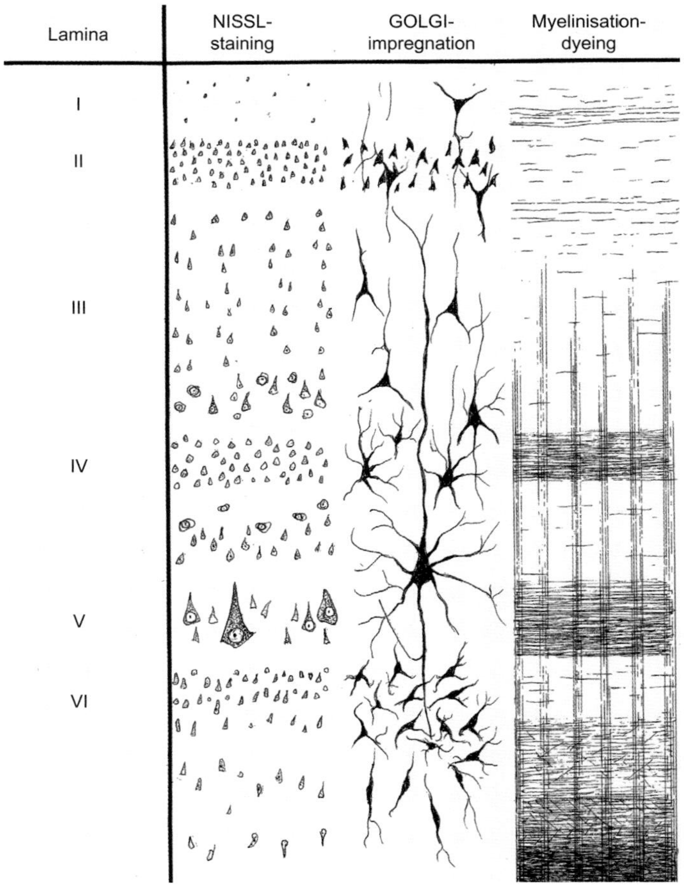

Lamina	NISSL-staining	GOLGI-impregnation	Myelinisation-dyeing
I			
II			
III			
IV			
V			
VI			

Fig. 12.76 **Lamination of the isocortex (neocortex);** schematic representation. [R170-5-L240]/[H234-001]
The laminar structure of the cerebral cortex, which consists of six layers and is usually ca. 4 mm thick (but only 2 mm in the primary visual cortex, for instance), is clearly visible in histological preparations obtained by perpendicular incisions to the surface of the brain. The layers are numbered from outside to inside:
* Lamina I – molecular layer (Lamina molecularis) – a few neurons, no pyramidal cells, but CAJAL-RETZIUS cells
* Lamina II – external granular layer (Lamina granularis externa) – tightly packed, small 'non-pyramidal cells' (granular cells), a few glutamatergic pyramidal cells
* Lamina III – external pyramidal layer (Lamina pyramidalis externa) – consists of three sublaminae and small pyramidal cells
* Lamina IV – internal granular layer (Lamina granularis interna) – tightly packed, small 'non-pyramidal cells' (granular cells)
* Lamina V – internal pyramidal layer (Lamina pyramidalis interna) – pyramidal cells of varying sizes, including giant BETZ' cells
* Lamina VI – multiform layer (Lamina multiformis) – often composed of Lamina VIa (dense in cells) and Lamina VIb (poor in neurons, with small pyramidal cells).

Cerebral areas

Cerebrum, neocortex

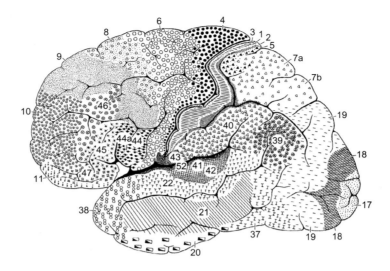

Fig. 12.77   BRODMANN areas; view from the left side, schematic representation. [G1085]
The brain is divided into so-called BRODMANN areas according to histological criteria.

The six-layered structure of the isocortex varies extremely by region. In the past, the layered structure has been extensively analysed and mapped to the cortical areas (BRODMANN areas). The numbering begins with the Gyrus postcentralis. The individual cortical areas are not only similar in their histology, but also assume functionally similar tasks.

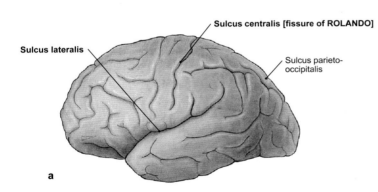

Fig. 12.78a and b   Primary grooves of the cortex. [S700]
a View from the left side.
b Medial view.

Primary grooves (→ table) as well as sulci which are developed and identifiable in each brain, divide the neocortex into five lobes (lobi) visible from the outside.

Sulci of the cortex	
Sulcus	**Position/pathway**
Sulcus centralis [fissure of ROLANDO]	extends between the frontal and parietal lobes; separates the (motor) Gyrus precentralis from the (sensory) Gyrus postcentralis
Sulcus lateralis [SYLVIAN fissure]	separates the frontal, parietal and temporal lobes from each other; Fossa lateralis and insula are located in the depths
Sulcus parieto-occipitalis	passes from the parasagittal cortex at the medial hemispherical surface to the Sulcus calcarinus; separates the parietal and occipital lobes
Sulcus calcarinus	runs like the Sulcus parietooccipitalis along the medial surface, and both together limit the cuneus
Sulcus cinguli	separates the Gyrus cinguli (Lobus limbicus) from the frontal and parietal lobes

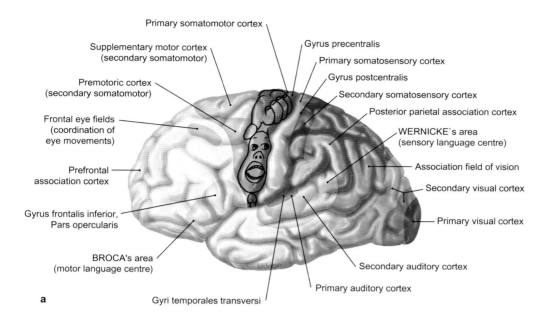

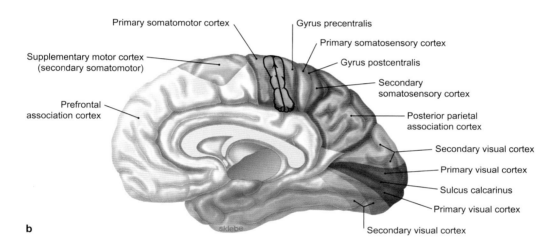

Fig. 12.79a and b Functional cortical areas of the cerebral hemispheres. [S702-L238]
a View from the left side. The homunculus (inserted manikin) roughly reflects the somatotopic map of the primary somatomotor cortex.
b Medial view. Primary and secondary auditory cortex as well as the WERNICKE's area extend beyond the superior margin of the temporal lobe to its inner surface.
Higher cortical functions such as speech are only possible through the interaction of various cortical areas. At the neocortex, primary fields or areas (e.g. Gyrus precentralis, primary somatomotor cortex) are distinguished from secondary and association fields (e.g. premotor cortex, supplementary motor cortex). Primary and secondary cortical areas serve a certain sensory function (e.g. perception and interpretation of visual stimuli by the visual cortex in the occipital lobe), whereas association areas (e.g. the prefrontal association cortex) occupy the largest part of the neocortex and help to integrate diverse complex information.

Clinical remarks

BROCA's aphasia is caused by failure of the BROCA's area (e.g. due to a stroke). Although the speech (language) production is severely restricted, the ability to name objects and speech comprehension are often preserved. The syntax is usually no longer correct and mixed with defective articulation.
Unilateral **lesions of the primary auditory cortex** lead to impairment of the directional hearing, as well as to problems in differentiating between frequencies and intensities. If the adjacent WERNICKE's area is affected, this will have a strong impact on speech comprehension **(WERNICKE's aphasia)**. Although speech production and melody are preserved, the verbal language is often senseless and lacks sentence structure (syntax).
Damage to the primary visual cortex on one side leads to **cortical blindness** with a homonymous hemianopsia. The visual field on the opposite side fails completely. If the secondary cortical areas are affected, the patient can still receive visual stimuli, but not interpret and coordinate them **(visual agnosia)**. Lesions in the frontal visual field that are associated with a loss in function of the BRODMANN area 8 (BA8) result in a deviation of the gaze of both eyes to the affected side **(déviation conjuguée)**.

Cerebrum, archicortex

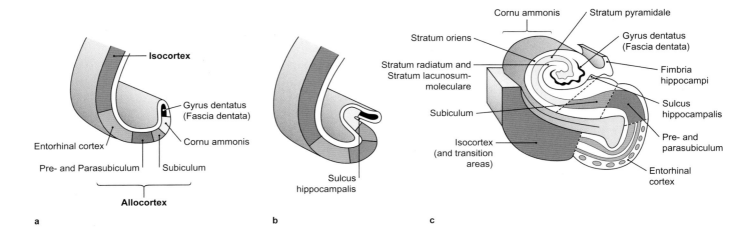

Fig. 12.80a–c Development of the hippocampal formation; schematic frontal sections. [S702-L126]

The hippocampus falls under the umbrella term of **hippocampal formation,** which summarises several cortical regions: Area entorhinalis (entorhinal cortex), Fascia dentata (Gyrus dentatus), Cornu ammonis (CA1, Hippocampus proprius), subiculum, presubiculum and parasubiculum. These regions of the brain are largely unidirectionally connected and form a functional unit. The development of the hippocampus begins as early as in week 9 of gestation **(a).** As the S-shaped folding of

the mediobasal cortex resembles the mythical creature hippocampus (a type of sea horse; **b and c**), it was named accordingly. Throughout one's life, new neural cells can be produced in the Fascia dentata (niche of neurogenic tissue with up to 700 new neural cells/day). The archicortex is part of the limbic system and functionally important for learning and memory processes. Via the limbic system it is connected intensely with cerebral regions, which are important for the control of autonomic and emotional processes.

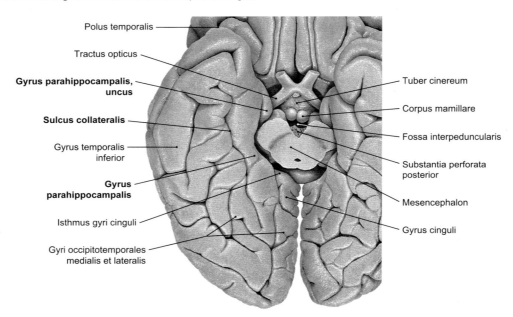

Fig. 12.81 Functional cortical areas of the hippocampus; inferior view; after dissection of the mesencephalon. [S700]

Due to its folding formation (→ Fig. 12.80), the position of the hippocampal formation can only partially be understood in a dorsomedial view of the surface of the brain (→ Fig. 12.82). The hippocampus is only macro-

scopically visible after opening the inferior horn of the lateral ventricle (→ Fig. 12.83). This view from below onto the gyri and sulci of the cerebral hemispheres shows the Gyrus parahippocampalis with the uncus and the neighbouring Sulcus collateralis.

Clinical remarks

The **hippocampus** has great clinical relevance. It plays an important role in neurodegenerative diseases with memory loss (e.g. ALZHEIMER's disease), in neuropsychiatric diseases (e.g. schizophrenia, depression, autism) and in temporal lobe epilepsy (the most common form of epilepsy).

Temporal lobe epilepsy (TLE) usually begins with an aura (an abnormal sensation that announces a seizure, e.g. seeing flashes of

light), followed by motor symptoms (e.g. smacking and chewing buccal motions up to convulsive movements of the whole body in the case of focal seizures) and loss of consciousness. Therapy is administered with drugs, and in therapy-resistant cases, the unilateral removal of the hippocampus can also be considered.

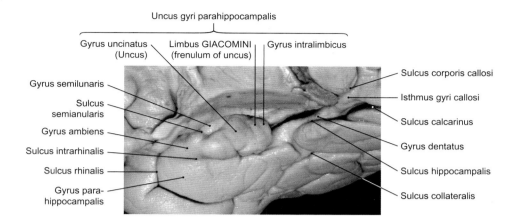

Uncus gyri parahippocampalis

Gyrus uncinatus (Uncus) — Limbus GIACOMINI (frenulum of uncus) — Gyrus intralimbicus

Gyrus semilunaris

Sulcus semianularis

Gyrus ambiens

Sulcus intrarhinalis

Sulcus rhinalis

Gyrus para-hippocampalis

Sulcus corporis callosi

Isthmus gyri callosi

Sulcus calcarinus

Gyrus dentatus

Sulcus hippocampalis

Sulcus collateralis

Fig. 12.82   Functional cortical areas of the hippocampus; temporal lobe in the dorsomedial view. [R247-L318]
Due to its folding formation (→ Fig. 12.80), the position of the hippocampal formation can only partially be understood in a caudal view of the brain surface (→ Fig. 12.81). The hippocampus is only macroscopically

visible after opening the inferior horn of the lateral ventricle (→ Fig. 12.83). The dorsomedial view shows parts of the Uncus, the Gyrus dentatus, Gyrus semilunaris, Gyrus ambiens, Gyrus parahippocampalis and the adjacent sulci.

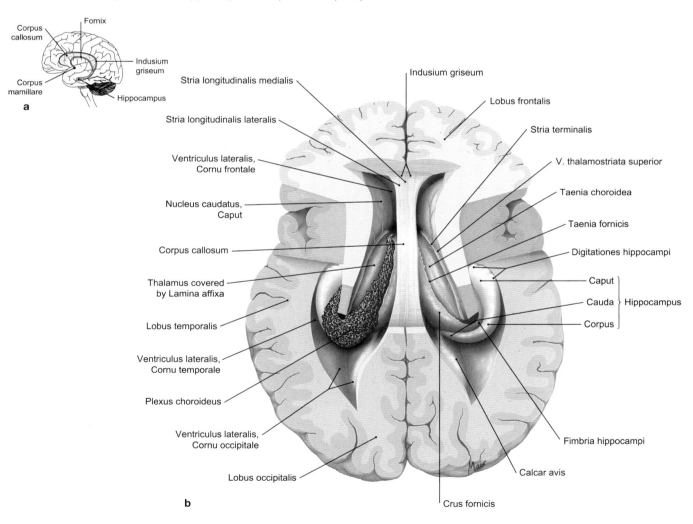

Corpus callosum — Fornix — Indusium griseum — Corpus mamillare — Hippocampus

a

Stria longitudinalis medialis

Stria longitudinalis lateralis

Ventriculus lateralis, Cornu frontale

Nucleus caudatus, Caput

Corpus callosum

Thalamus covered by Lamina affixa

Lobus temporalis

Ventriculus lateralis, Cornu temporale

Plexus choroideus

Ventriculus lateralis, Cornu occipitale

Lobus occipitalis

Indusium griseum

Lobus frontalis

Stria terminalis

V. thalamostriata superior

Taenia choroidea

Taenia fornicis

Digitationes hippocampi

Caput
Cauda } Hippocampus
Corpus

Fimbria hippocampi

Calcar avis

b

Crus fornicis

Fig. 12.83a and b   Opened lateral ventricle with hippocampus. [S702-L127]

a View from the left side. The brain is depicted transparently to visualise the three-dimensional structure of the hippocampus.
b View from above after opening of the lateral ventricles from dorsal and lateral.
The hippocampal formation lies in the medial temporal lobe and arches above the Corpus callosum. Depending on the topographical relationships to the Corpus callosum, a distinction is made between three macroscopic parts:

• Hippocampus retrocommissuralis (cortex of the temporal lobe) = 'hippocampus' in the proper sense and as a clinical term
• Hippocampus supracommissuralis (above the Corpus callosum)
• Hippocampus precommissuralis (beneath the Genu corporis callosi)
The caput, corpus and cauda of the hippocampus are located at the bottom of the inferior horn of the lateral ventricle, and covered by the Plexus choroideus on the left side. The plexus on the right side has been removed.

Cerebrum, archicortex

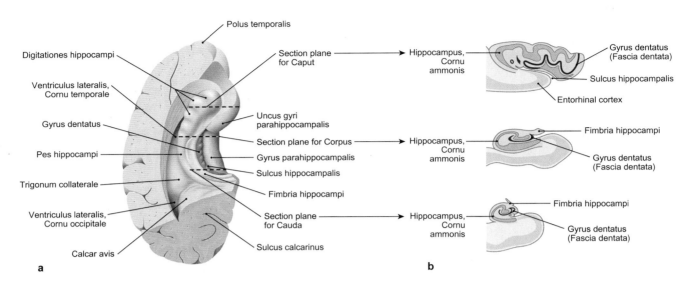

Fig. 12.84a and b   Hippocampus. [S700-L127]
a Superior posterior view onto the inferior horn of the opened lateral ventricle.
b Cross-sections through the hippocampus in the areas of the caput, corpus and cauda.

Significant differences in the arrangement of the principal cells are observed in the Gyrus dentatus (purple). Anterior frontal sections reveal several regions of the hippocampus; in the areas of its body and tail the 'classical' arrangement of hippocampus regions is displayed.

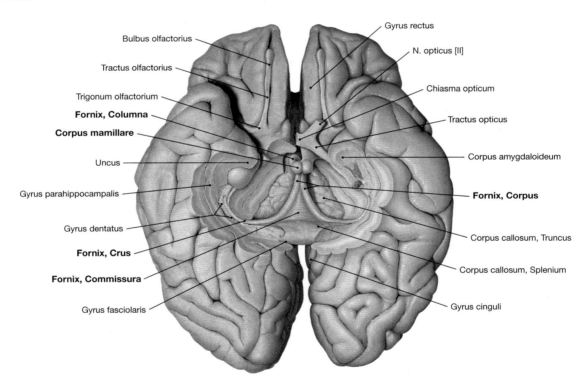

Fig. 12.85   Fornix; inferior view; after removal of the basal parts of the brain. [S700]
The fornix is a paired structure composed of the crus, commissura, corpus and Columna fornicis. From its origin at the hippocampus and the subiculum in the temporal lobe it forms an arch above the third ventricle towards the Corpus mamillare. Before reaching the Corpora mamillaria, the two fornices unite (Commissura fornicis). At this point, an **exchange of fibres** between both sides takes place (→ Fig. 12.86).

Clinical remarks

Neurodegenerative diseases are associated with an insidious destruction of nerve cells. If the hippocampal formation is affected, this is combined with disorders of the spatial memory and orientation functions. New knowledge and new experiences can no longer be stored. **ALZHEIMER's disease** is the most well-known of the neurodegenerative diseases. It is associated with the formation of extracellular protein deposits ('amyloid plaques') and intracellular protein aggregations in the brain. The hippocampal formation is affected at an early stage. In addition to spatial disorientation, there is a loss of memory function. If the neocortex is involved later on, the remaining memories will also be deleted. Thus, in advanced stages, patients cannot remember themselves as a person/personality nor the life events they have experienced.

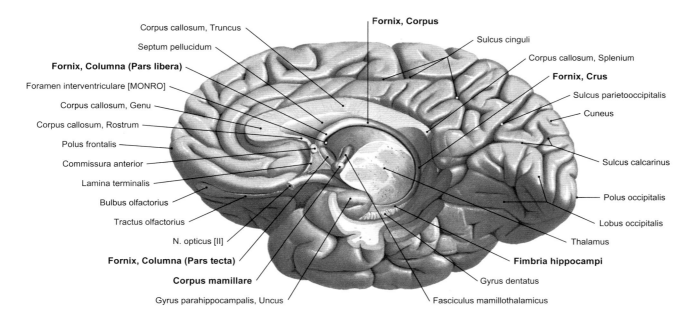

Corpus callosum, Truncus
Septum pellucidum
Fornix, Columna (Pars libera)
Foramen interventriculare [MONRO]
Corpus callosum, Genu
Corpus callosum, Rostrum
Polus frontalis
Commissura anterior
Lamina terminalis
Bulbus olfactorius
Tractus olfactorius
N. opticus [II]
Fornix, Columna (Pars tecta)
Corpus mamillare
Gyrus parahippocampalis, Uncus

Fornix, Corpus
Sulcus cinguli
Corpus callosum, Splenium
Fornix, Crus
Sulcus parietooccipitalis
Cuneus
Sulcus calcarinus
Polus occipitalis
Lobus occipitalis
Thalamus
Fimbria hippocampi
Gyrus dentatus
Fasciculus mamillothalamicus

Fig. 12.86   Fornix; medial view from below. [S700]
The fornix is an important tract of the limbic system. There are **fibre connections** to the anterior hypothalamic nuclei, the thalamus, and the habenulae. The figure shows the topographical relationships of the fornix.

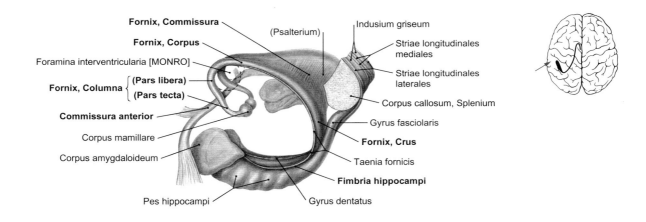

Fornix, Commissura
(Psalterium)
Fornix, Corpus
Foramina interventricularia [MONRO]
Fornix, Columna {
(Pars libera)
(Pars tecta) }
Commissura anterior
Corpus mamillare
Corpus amygdaloideum
Pes hippocampi

Indusium griseum
Striae longitudinales mediales
Striae longitudinales laterales
Corpus callosum, Splenium
Gyrus fasciolaris
Fornix, Crus
Taenia fornicis
Fimbria hippocampi
Gyrus dentatus

Fig. 12.87   Anterior commissure, Commissura anterior, fornix and hippocampal formation, Indusium griseum; view from the left side. [S700]
All structures shown here are part of the **limbic system,** a functional concept with input from numerous structures in the cerebrum, diencephalon and mesencephalon. The most relevant structures are both hippocampi, the Corpora amygdaloidea, the Gyri cinguli and the Nuclei septales. The limbic system controls functions such as impulse, learning, memory, emotions, but also the autonomic regulation of food intake, digestion and reproduction.
The **Commissura anterior** (→ Fig. 12.28 and → table for → Fig. 12.29) is a system of commissural fibres, composed of a Pars anterior and a Pars posterior. The Pars anterior connects the olfactory tracts and the olfactory cortices of both sides. The Pars posterior connects the anterior parts of the temporal lobes (particularly the cortex and Corpora amygdaloidea). The Corpus amygdaloideum is in contact with the hippocampus.
Visible structures of the **hippocampus** are the Digitationes hippocampi of the Pes hippocampi and the Fimbria hippocampi, which transition into the crus of the fornix. In the region of the columna, an exchange of fibres occurs between both sides. In the rostral direction, the fornix continues via the corpora in the columnae, which respectively consist of a Pars libera and a Pars tecta. The Pars tecta is connected to the Corpus mamillare.

Clinical remarks

Like the fornix and the hippocampus, the Corpora mamillaria are part of the limbic system. They probably play a role in memory function. However, precise details are not yet known. A lack of thiamine (vitamin B_1), e. g. due to chronic alcohol abuse, may lead to the destruction of the Corpora mamillaria, which is associated with the most severe form of memory loss **(amnesia),** disorders of movement coordination **(ataxia),** as well as disorientation and false story-telling **(confabulations; WERNICKE-KORSAKOFF syndrome).** The patient creates fake 'stories' to conceal memory gaps.

Cerebrum, archicortex

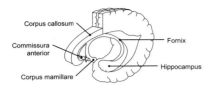

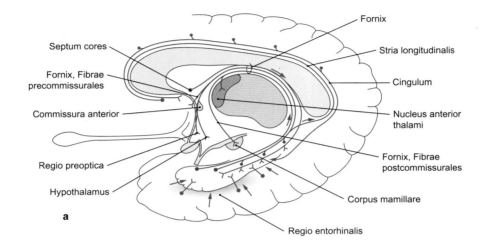

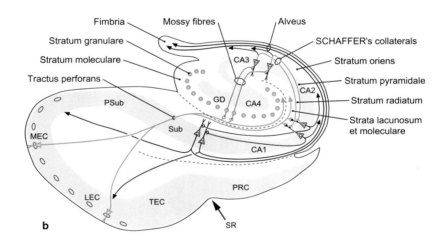

Fig. 12.88a and b   Connections of the hippocampal formation.
a PAPEZ circuit. [S702-L127]

b Regions of the hippocampal formation and their intrinsic interconnections. Frontal section through the corpus of the hippocampus. [S700-L141]/[B500-T1190/T1189]

CA = Cornu ammonis, GD = Gyrus dentatus, Sub = subiculum, PSub = presubiculum, MEC/LEC = medial/lateral entorhinal cortex, TEC = transentorhinal cortex, PRC = perirhinal cortex, SR = Sulcus rhinalis.
Connections of the hippocampal formation are:

* neocortical (via entorhinal cortex, the 'gateway to the hippocampus'; subiculum complex)
* intrinsic (entorhinal cortex – Fascia dentata – CA3 – CA1 – subiculum complex – entorhinal cortex)

* commissural (especially entorhinal cortex and subiculum)
* subcortical (septal nuclei, Corpora mamillaria, amygdala, brainstem, etc.)

Broadly speaking, the neuronal circle **(PAPEZ circuit)** connects the hippocampus via the fornix to the Corpora mamillaria, and continues via the mamillothalamic bundle to the Nucleus anterior of the thalamus, and then to the Gyrus cinguli. The Gyrus cinguli projects via the cingulum to the Regio entorhinalis of the Gyrus parahippocampalis, and this in turn via the Tractus perforans to the hippocampus, so that the circuit is closed. Today, it is assumed that the PAPEZ circuit supports the storage of memory, by transferring the content of the primary memory in the form of the secondary memory and tertiary memory.

Clinical remarks

Sometimes the affected parts of the hippocampal formation are surgically removed on one side, as a treatment in the case of severe and **drug therapy-resistant temporal lobe epilepsy.** While this strategy apparently does not lead to memory impairment, the resection of both hippocampi results in a severe, mainly anterograde amnesia (inability to store and recall new memory contents).
Lesions of cingulate cortical areas lead to cognitive changes, which also occur in complex neuropsychiatric diseases (depression, schizophrenia, anxiety disorder, lethargy).

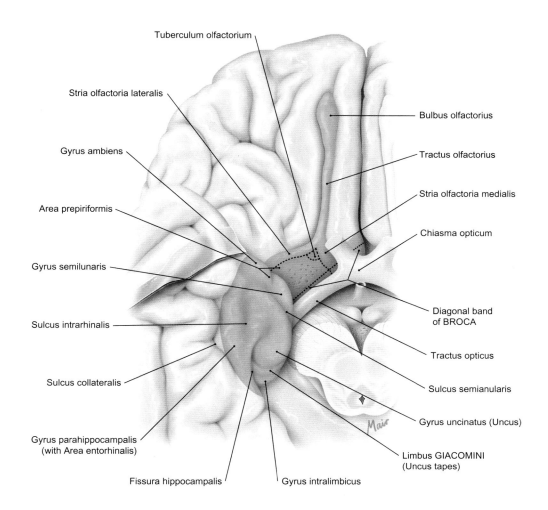

Tuberculum olfactorium

Stria olfactoria lateralis

Gyrus ambiens

Area prepiriformis

Gyrus semilunaris

Sulcus intrarhinalis

Sulcus collateralis

Gyrus parahippocampalis
(with Area entorhinalis)

Fissura hippocampalis

Gyrus intralimbicus

Bulbus olfactorius

Tractus olfactorius

Stria olfactoria medialis

Chiasma opticum

Diagonal band
of BROCA

Tractus opticus

Sulcus semianularis

Gyrus uncinatus (Uncus)

Limbus GIACOMINI
(Uncus tapes)

Fig. 12.89 Structures of the paleocortex (green) and the adjacent archicortex (purple); inferior view. [S702-L127]/[E633-002]
The paleocortex is the oldest cortical part in terms of phylogeny. It includes the Bulbus olfactorius, Tractus olfactorius, Nucleus olfactorius anterior, Tuberculum olfactorium, the septal nuclei, the Regio periamygdalaris and Regio prepiriformis. The Bulbus and Tractus olfactorius show clear histological differences to the six-layered isocortex. Therefore they belong to the allocortex (allo = different, as opposed to the six-layered isocortex). The paleocortex is responsible for the sense of smell. The olfactory sensations of the receptor cells in the nasal mucosa (→ Fig. 12.127) are passed directly via the Bulbus olfactorius to the primary olfactory cortex without being switched in the thalamus. This distinguishes the sense of smell from all other senses or sensations. However, there are close connections to different parts of the limbic system. Olfactory cortical areas exert their effects on other areas of the brain via connections to the thalamus and the insula.

Clinical remarks

As **neurodegenerative diseases** such as ALZHEIMER's and PARKINSON's are often associated with smell disorders at an early stage, an evaluation of the sense of smell by using standardised (olfactory) tests is discussed as an early diagnostic marker for these diseases.

Cerebrum, subcortical nuclei

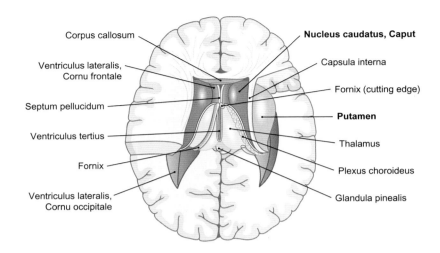

Corpus callosum

Ventriculus lateralis, Cornu frontale

Septum pellucidum

Ventriculus tertius

Fornix

Ventriculus lateralis, Cornu occipitale

Nucleus caudatus, Caput

Capsula interna

Fornix (cutting edge)

Putamen

Thalamus

Plexus choroideus

Glandula pinealis

Fig. 12.90 Basal ganglia, thalamus and lateral ventricles; overview; superior view after dorsal and lateral opening of the lateral ventricles. [S702-L126]/[G1084]

The basal ganglia belong to the group of subcortical nuclei. Further subcortical nuclei are the amygdala and the Nucleus basalis MEYNERT (neither is shown). The basal ganglia (nuclei) are involved in the configuration of movement sequences, as well as in the regulation of higher brain functions such as learning, memory, motivation and emotion. They primarily belong to the extrapyramidal motor system (EPMS). The basal ganglia include the:

* striatum (Corpus striatum) consisting of the Nucleus caudatus and putamen
* pallidum (Globus pallidus; not visible).

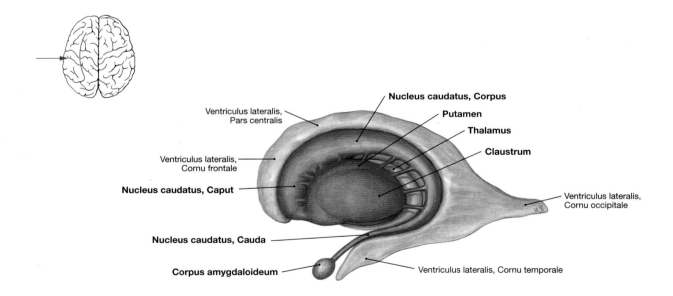

Ventriculus lateralis, Pars centralis

Ventriculus lateralis, Cornu frontale

Nucleus caudatus, Caput

Nucleus caudatus, Cauda

Corpus amygdaloideum

Nucleus caudatus, Corpus

Putamen

Thalamus

Claustrum

Ventriculus lateralis, Cornu occipitale

Ventriculus lateralis, Cornu temporale

Fig. 12.91 Basal ganglia and thalamus; view from the left side. [S700]

The illustration shows the topographical relationship between the Ventriculus lateralis, Nucleus caudatus, amygdala, putamen, Globus pallidus and thalamus. Many nuclei of the cerebrum are summarised under the generic term **basal ganglia.** The basal ganglia include the striatum (Nucleus caudatus and putamen, shown here) and the pallidum, as well as the Nucleus subthalamicus and Substantia nigra (none of these three structures is shown) in the mesencephalon.

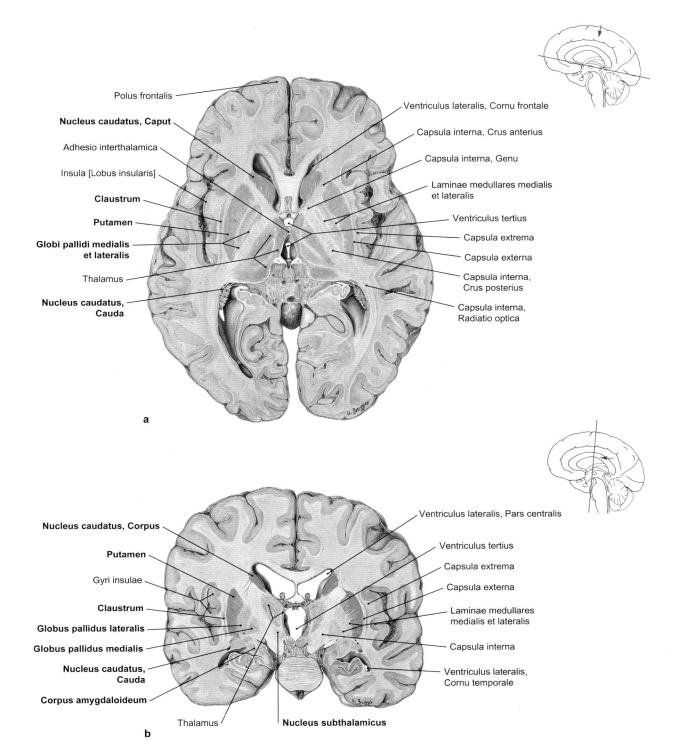

Polus frontalis

Nucleus caudatus, Caput

Adhesio interthalamica

Insula [Lobus insularis]

Claustrum

Putamen

Globi pallidi medialis et lateralis

Thalamus

Nucleus caudatus, Cauda

Ventriculus lateralis, Cornu frontale

Capsula interna, Crus anterius

Capsula interna, Genu

Laminae medullares medialis et lateralis

Ventriculus tertius

Capsula extrema

Capsula externa

Capsula interna, Crus posterius

Capsula interna, Radiatio optica

a

Nucleus caudatus, Corpus

Putamen

Gyri insulae

Claustrum

Globus pallidus lateralis

Globus pallidus medialis

Nucleus caudatus, Cauda

Corpus amygdaloideum

Thalamus

Nucleus subthalamicus

Ventriculus lateralis, Pars centralis

Ventriculus tertius

Capsula extrema

Capsula externa

Laminae medullares medialis et lateralis

Capsula interna

Ventriculus lateralis, Cornu temporale

b

Fig. 12.92a and b Subcortical nuclei. [S700]
a Horizontal section through the centre of the third ventricle.
b Frontal section at the level of the Corpora mamillaria.

Clinical remarks

PARKINSON's disease is caused by a degeneration of dopaminergic neurons and can thus be traced back to a loss of nigrostriatal fibres (fibres between the Substantia nigra and the striatum). The result is a general inhibition of motor activity with restrictions of movement (ranging from hypokinesia through to akinesia = absence of movement). This is characterised by small stumbling steps accompanied by a lack of arm swinging. Furthermore, there is usually a unilateral tremor (trembling of the hand) when at rest, as well as a general muscle stiffness (rigour, e.g. lack of facial expression). In addition, these patients suffer from an increased secretion of saliva, tears, sweat, and sebum, and mentally they are also slower and emotionally more unstable. The disease affects 1 % of the age group over 60 years. Similar conditions to PARKINSON's disease can occur after suffering from encephalitis, poisoning, long-term use of psychotropic drugs, etc.

Cerebrum, subcortical nuclei

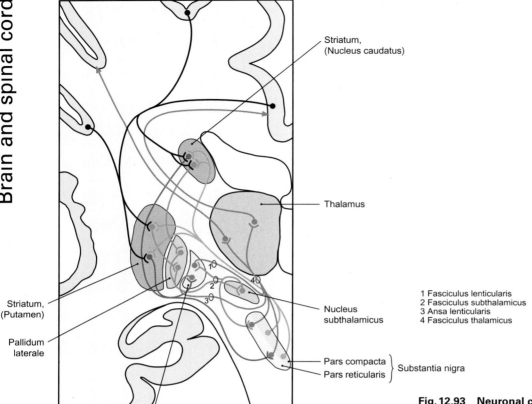

Striatum,
(Nucleus caudatus)

Thalamus

Striatum,
(Putamen)

Pallidum
laterale

Nucleus
subthalamicus

1 Fasciculus lenticularis
2 Fasciculus subthalamicus
3 Ansa lenticularis
4 Fasciculus thalamicus

Pars compacta } Substantia nigra
Pars reticularis }

Pallidum mediale

Fig. 12.93   Neuronal circuits of the subcortical nuclei; schematic representation, frontal section. [B500-T1189/L316]
Internal structure and fibre connections of the basal ganglia. The striatum is the main entry point into the basal ganglia (→ Fig. 12.94).

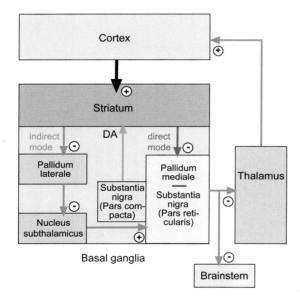

Fig. 12.94   Neuronal circuits of the subcortical nuclei; schematic representation. [B500-T1189/L316]
The basal ganglia are involved in the **planning of movement programmes** via their integration into various cortical feedback loops (cortex – basal ganglia – thalamus – cortex) Their main task is the modulation of movements (force, direction, deviation). The impulses entering the basal ganglia are processed either in a direct mode, promoting movement, or in an indirect mode, inhibiting movement.
DA = dopamine

Clinical remarks

Changes in the huntingtin (HTT) gene lead to autosomal-dominant inherited **HUNTINGTON's disease.** This neurodegenerative disorder is associated with a degeneration of striatal GABAergic projection neurons, in particular with the indirect processing mode, and leads to exaggerated involuntary movements with reduced muscle tone (choreatic hyperkinesia).

Damage to the Nucleus subthalamicus causes disorders of the indirect processing mode. The patients perform proximally accentuated, wild flinging movements **(hemiballism)** with the unaffected limb on the contralateral side of the body.

Brain and spinal cord

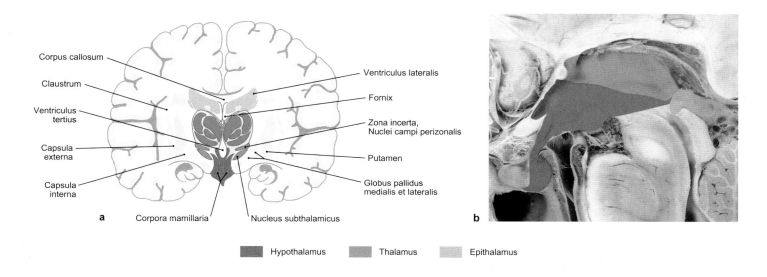

Corpus callosum

Claustrum

Ventriculus tertius

Capsula externa

Capsula interna

Ventriculus lateralis

Fornix

Zona incerta, Nuclei campi perizonalis

Putamen

Globus pallidus medialis et lateralis

a Corpora mamillaria   Nucleus subthalamicus   **b**

Hypothalamus   Thalamus   Epithalamus

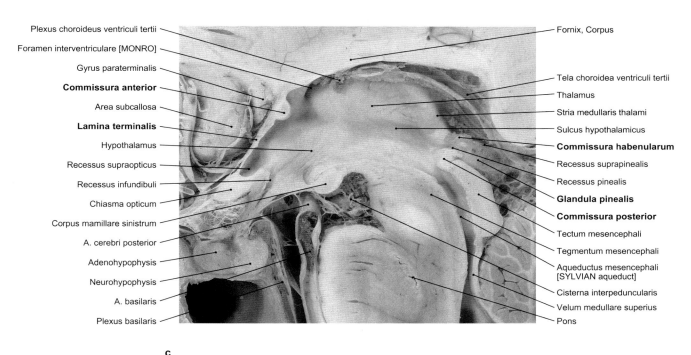

Plexus choroideus ventriculi tertii

Foramen interventriculare [MONRO]

Gyrus paraterminalis

Commissura anterior

Area subcallosa

Lamina terminalis

Hypothalamus

Recessus supraopticus

Recessus infundibuli

Chiasma opticum

Corpus mamillare sinistrum

A. cerebri posterior

Adenohypophysis

Neurohypophysis

A. basilaris

Plexus basilaris

Fornix, Corpus

Tela choroidea ventriculi tertii

Thalamus

Stria medullaris thalami

Sulcus hypothalamicus

Commissura habenularum

Recessus suprapinealis

Recessus pinealis

Glandula pinealis

Commissura posterior

Tectum mesencephali

Tegmentum mesencephali

Aqueductus mesencephali [SYLVIAN aqueduct]

Cisterna interpeduncularis

Velum medullare superius

Pons

c

Fig. 12.95a–c   Parts of the diencephalon.
a Frontal section, schematic representation. [S702-L126]/[B500-T1189/ L316]/[G1081]
b Mid-sagittal section. [S702]
c Original image of b. [S700]
The diencephalon is divided structurally and functionally into four parts:
* epithalamus (upper part on top of the thalamus, includes Corpus pineale, habenulae and Commissura posterior)
* Thalamus dorsalis (large, tightly packed nuclear complex, extends bean-shaped on both sides of the third ventricle; this includes the Corpora geniculata = metathalamus)
* subthalamus (Thalamus ventralis, transition zone between diencephalon and mesencephalon, motor zone of the diencephalon, nu-

clei for the control of motoric functions such as the Globus pallidus and Nucleus subthalamicus)
* hypothalamus (lowest part, nuclei and fibre tracts at the bottom of the third ventricle and in the lower parts of the lateral ventricles).
In terms of phylogeny, the diencephalon belongs to the prosencephalon and is located between the cerebrum and the mesencephalon. It surrounds the third ventricle. Rostrally, the diencephalon is bordered by the Commissura anterior (reaching up to the Chiasma opticum) and the Lamina terminalis. The posterior border is formed by the Commissura posterior, the Commissura habenularum and the pineal gland (Glandula pinealis).

Diencephalon, epithalamus and thalamus

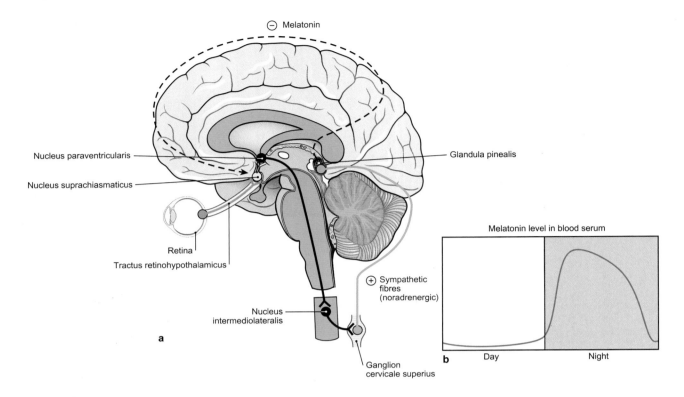

Fig. 12.96a and b Circuit for controlling the pineal gland, Glandu-la pinealis; schematic median section. [S700-L126]/[B500-T1188]
The epithalamus comprises the Striae medullares thalami, the habenu-lae, the Nuclei habenulares, the Commissura habenularum, the Commissura posterior (epithalamica), the Area pretectalis and the Glandula pinealis. The synthesis of **melatonin** in organotypical pinealocytes within the Glandula pinealis is light-dependent. Melatonin regulates the circadian rhythm in other endocrine organs. In addition, the effect of the

melatonin feeds back onto the Nucleus suprachiasmaticus, which synchronises endogenous with exogenous environmental rhythms.
The **circuit** starts at the photoreceptors of the retina **(a)** which send signals to the Nucleus suprachiasmaticus in the hypothalamus (Tractus retinohypothalamicus). From there, the information is transmitted via the Nucleus paraventricularis of the hypothalamus to the sympathetic Ganglion cervicale superius, and then to the pinealocytes of the Glandu-la pinealis. Melatonin is produced in larger quantities at night **(b)**.

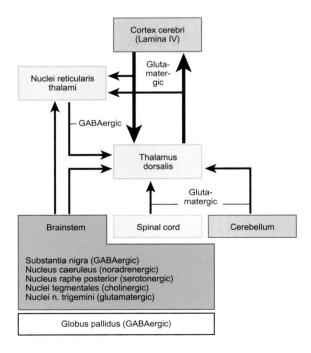

Fig. 12.97 Afferent and efferent connections of the Thalamus dorsalis; schematic representation. [S702-L126]/[B500-M492/L316]
The Thalamus dorsalis performs key tasks in the communication of cortical areas with the periphery and from the periphery to central cerebral regions **('gateway to consciousness')**. All sensations, with the excep-

tion of smell, are relayed through the thalamus, like a switchboard. Furthermore, specialised nuclei/nuclear areas are involved in the motor (movement) control and are integrated into different subcortical feedback circuits, such as the limbic system. Finally, the thalamus also participates in autonomic and motor activities.

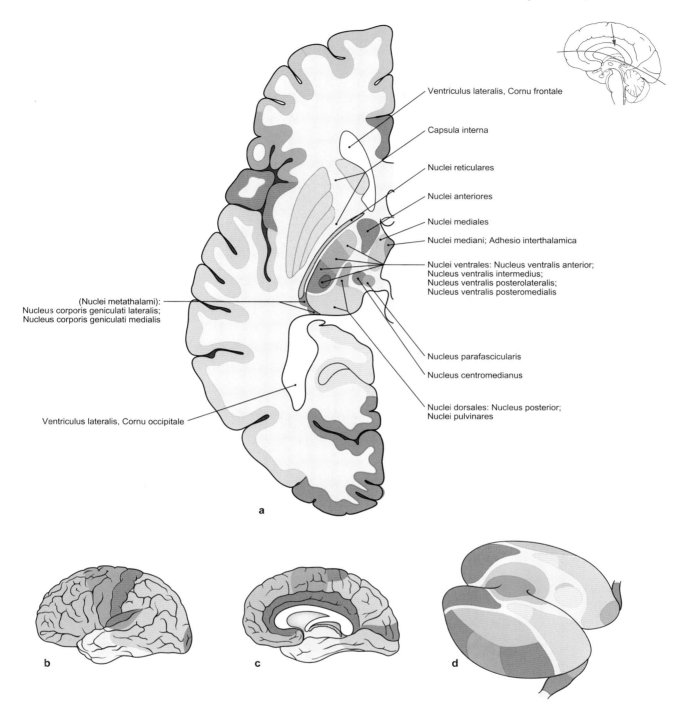

Ventriculus lateralis, Cornu frontale

Capsula interna

Nuclei reticulares

Nuclei anteriores

Nuclei mediales

Nuclei mediani; Adhesio interthalamica

Nuclei ventrales: Nucleus ventralis anterior;
Nucleus ventralis intermedius;
Nucleus ventralis posterolateralis;
Nucleus ventralis posteromedialis

(Nuclei metathalami):
Nucleus corporis geniculati lateralis;
Nucleus corporis geniculati medialis

Nucleus parafascicularis

Nucleus centromedianus

Nuclei dorsales: Nucleus posterior;
Nuclei pulvinares

Ventriculus lateralis, Cornu occipitale

a

b   c   d

Fig. 12.98a–d   Nuclei and cortical projection of the thalamus.
Corresponding nuclei and cortical regions are marked with the same
colours, respectively. [S700-L126]
a Horizontal section through the left cerebral hemisphere.
b Left lateral view of the left cerebral hemisphere.
c Medial view of the right cerebral hemisphere.
d Oblique superior view of both thalami.
All sensory impulses from the body enter the thalamus, where they are
relayed (exception: smell), integrated and sent on to the cortex. In addition, the thalamus participates in autonomic and motor activities. Its
various groups of nuclei are structurally divided by lamellae **(Lamina
medullaris medialis interna)** into three nuclear areas:

- ventrolateral group **(Nuclei ventrolaterales)**
- medial group **(Nuclei mediani)**
- anterior group **(Nuclei anteriores).**

Furthermore, a distinction is made between the Nuclei mediani embedded in the Lamina medullaris medialis interna, the occipital pulvinar, and
the Nuclei reticulares. The respective groups of nuclei can be subdivided
into smaller functional units (more than 100 nuclear areas). Thereby specific nuclei (palliothalamus) control defined cortical areas (primary cortical
projection and association fields/areas); non-specific nuclei (truncothala-
mus) project to the brainstem and to some more diffuse cortical areas.

Clinical remarks

Damage in the area of the non-specific thalamic nuclei, e.g. in
the case of circulatory disorders, often leads to a reduced state of
consciousness with impaired awareness. Depending on the location,
damage to **specific thalamic nuclei** may cause sensory impairment

(Nucleus ventralis posterolateralis), hemianopsia, pain (thalamic
pain), or motor disorders such as paralysis, ataxia (Nucleus anterior
ventrolateralis) as well as personality changes.

Diencephalon, thalamus and hypothalamus

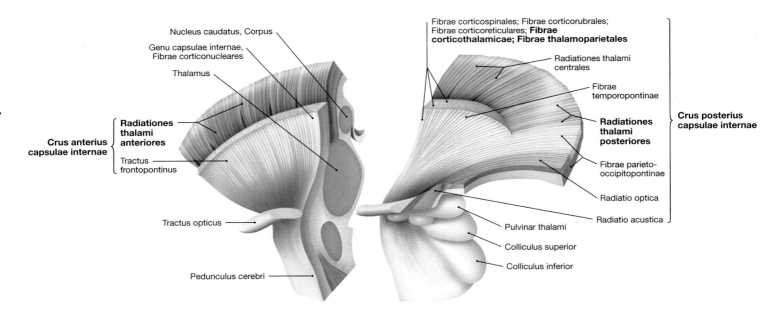

Nucleus caudatus, Corpus

Genu capsulae internae, Fibrae corticonucleares

Thalamus

Radiationes thalami anteriores

Crus anterius capsulae internae

Tractus frontopontinus

Tractus opticus

Pedunculus cerebri

Fibrae corticospinales; Fibrae corticorubrales; Fibrae corticoreticulares; **Fibrae corticothalamicae; Fibrae thalamoparietales**

Radiationes thalami centrales

Fibrae temporopontinae

Radiationes thalami posteriores

Crus posterius capsulae internae

Fibrae parieto-occipitopontinae

Radiatio optica

Radiatio acustica

Pulvinar thalami

Colliculus superior

Colliculus inferior

Fig. 12.99 Radiation from the thalamus, Radiationes thalami, and internal capsule, Capsula interna; view from the left side; cut into two parts by a frontal section. [S700-L275]

The thalamic nuclei project mainly to the cortex. Their tracts form parts of the Crus anterius and the Crus posterius of the Capsula interna. The tracts include the Radiationes thalami anteriores and posteriores. Other tracts are the Fibrae corticothalamicae and the Fibrae thalamoparietales.

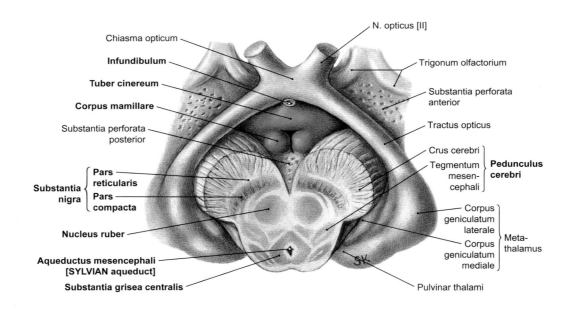

Chiasma opticum

Infundibulum

Tuber cinereum

Corpus mamillare

Substantia perforata posterior

Substantia nigra
— **Pars reticularis**
— **Pars compacta**

Nucleus ruber

Aqueductus mesencephali [SYLVIAN aqueduct]

Substantia grisea centralis

N. opticus [II]

Trigonum olfactorium

Substantia perforata anterior

Tractus opticus

Crus cerebri

Tegmentum mesencephali } **Pedunculus cerebri**

Corpus geniculatum laterale

Corpus geniculatum mediale } Meta-thalamus

Pulvinar thalami

Fig. 12.100 Parts of the hypothalamus; inferior (basal) view. [S700-L238]

Parts of the hypothalamus, extending between the Chiasma opticum, the Tractus optici and the Corpora mamillaria, can be seen from the base of the brain.

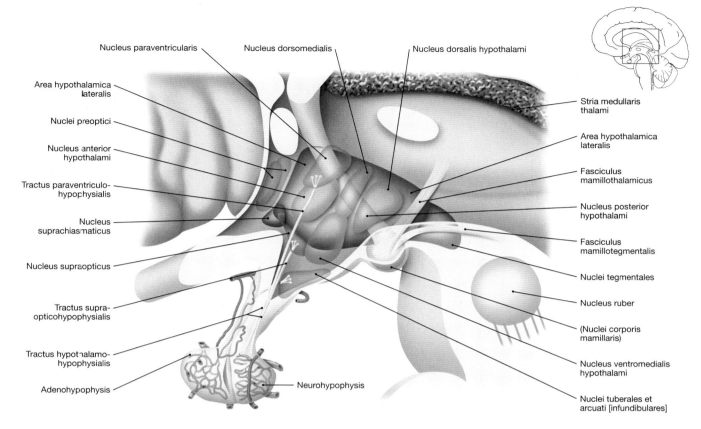

Fig. 12.101 Hypothalamus; medial view; overview, nuclear areas (nuclei) illustrated transparently. [S700-L127]

Forming the floor of the diencephalon, the hypothalamus is the supervisory regulatory centre of the autonomic nervous system.

The hypothalamus has a number of nuclear areas divided according to their location into the anterior, middle and posterior nuclei regions:

- The nuclei of the **anterior or preoptic region** include the Nucleus suprachiasmaticus (central pacemaker for circadian rhythms, sleep-wake cycle, body temperature, blood pressure), the Nuclei paraventricularis and supraopticus (production of antidiuretic hormone [ADH] and oxytocin, axonal transport [Tractus hypothalamohypophysialis] in the neurohypophysis), and the Nuclei preoptici (participate in the regulation of blood pressure, body temperature, sexual behaviour, menstrual cycle, gonadotropin).
- The nuclei of the **intermediate or tuberal region** include the Nuclei tuberales, dorsomedialis, ventromedialis and arcuatus [infundibularis = semilunaris] (production and secretion of releasing and release-inhibiting hormones, participation in the regulation of water and food intake).

- The nuclei of the **posterior or manillary region** include the Nuclei corporis mamillaris in the Corpora mamillaria, which are integrated in the limbic system by afferent fibres from the fornix and efferent fibres to the thalamus (Fasciculus mamillothalamicus). They modulate sexual functions and play an important role in activities related to memory and emotions. They are connected to the Tegmentum mesencephali via the Fasciculus mamillotegmentalis.

The hypothalamus continues downwards (caudally) via the infundibulum into the pituitary gland, which consists of the neurohypophysis and the adenohypophysis. The portal vein system of the pituitary gland receives blood from the A. hypophysialis superior, a branch of the Pars cerebralis of the A. carotis interna. The blood flow then passes through two venous tributaries. The first is located on the Eminentia mediana of the hypothalamus (zone with neurosecretory axon endings of parvocellular neurons). Here, these neurons release statins and liberins (= releasing and inhibiting hormones) into the venous blood. The second venous system, lying in the adenohypophysis, takes up the hormones produced here (→ table), and transports them throughout the body.

Structure of the hypothalamus based on regions, zones, important areas and nuclei		
Periventricular zone	**Medial (intermediate) zone**	**Lateral zone**
Preoptic (chiasmatic) region		
• Nucleus preopticus medianus • Nuclei periventriculares, preopticus et anterior hypothalami • Nucleus suprachiasmaticus	• Area preoptica medialis (Nucleus preopticus medialis) • Area hypothalamica anterior (Nucleus anterior hypothalami) • Nucleus paraventricularis • Nucleus supraopticus • Nuclei interstitiales hypothalami anteriores	• Area preoptica lateralis • Area hypothalamica lateralis • Nuclei interstitiales hypothalami anteriores
Intermediate (tuberal) region		
Nucleus arcuatus	• Nucleus ventromedialis • Nucleus dorsomedialis	• Area hypothalamica lateralis • Nuclei tuberales laterales • Nucleus tuberomamillaris
Posterior (mamillary) region		
• Nucleus periventricularis posterior • Area hypothalamica posterior (Nucleus posterior hypothalami)	Nuclei mamillares medialis et lateralis	• Area hypothalamica lateralis • Nucleus tuberomamillaris

Cerebral areas

Diencephalon, hypothalamus and pituitary gland

Afferent and efferent fibres of the hypothalamus	
Important afferent fibres of the hypothalamus	**Important efferent fibres of the hypothalamus**
• Limbic system • Hippocampus • Corpus amygdaloideum • Septal region • Olfactory cortex • Formatio reticularis, posterior horn of the spinal cord, sensory nuclei of the cranial nerves • Retina • Within the hypothalamus • Insular cortex	• Cerebral cortex, thalamic nuclei • Nuclei of the cranial nerves, Formatio reticularis • Spinal cord • Within the hypothalamus • As part of the magnocellular system of the neurohypophysis

Hormones of the adenohypophysis (anterior pituitary)			
Hormone	**Staining characteristics**	**Function**	**Hypothalamic regulation via**
Pars distalis			
Prolactin (PRL)	Acidophil	Milk synthesis	Prolactostatin (dopamine)
Growth hormone (GH, STH)	Acidophil	Growth	GHRH (growth hormone-releasing hormone, somatoliberin)
Corticotropin (ACTH)	Basophil	Stimulation of the adrenal glands	CRH (corticoliberin)
Melanotropin (α-MSH)	Basophil	Pigmentation of the skin	CRH (corticoliberin)
β-Endorphin	Basophil	Opioid receptors	CRH (corticoliberin)
Follicle-stimulating hormone (FSH)	Basophil	Maturation of ovum/sperm	GnRH
Luteinising hormone (LH)	Basophil	Ovulation, Corpus luteum	GnRH
Thyroid-stimulating hormone (TSH)	Basophil	Stimulation of thyroid cells	TRH (thyroliberin)
Pars intermedia			
Corticotropin (ACTH)	Basophil	Stimulation of the adrenal gland	CRH (corticoliberin)
Melanotropin (MSH)	Basophil	Pigmentation of the skin	CRH (corticoliberin)
β-Endorphin	Basophil	Binding to opioid receptors	CRH (corticoliberin)
Pars tuberalis			
Specific cells of the Pars tuberalis	Chromophobe	Circadian/circa-annual rhythm	? (Melatonin)

Clinical remarks

Lesions of the Nucleus paraventricularis and particularly of the Nucleus supraopticus lead to deficiency of the **antidiuretic hormone (ADH = vasopressin),** resulting in a lack of water re-absorption in the collecting tubules of the kidney. This is called **central diabetes insipidus.** In this case, patients pass up to 20 litres of urine daily.

The adenohypophysis can be affected by various tumours. These tumours most commonly secrete prolactin, growth hormone (GH) and corticotropin (CRH). In women, prolactinomas (prolactin-secreting adenomas) suppress the menstrual cycle (amenorrhoea), induce the production of breast milk by the mammary gland (galactorrhoea), and lead to infertility with signs of masculinisation. **Acromegaly** is defined as the distinct enlargement of limbs or protruding parts (acra) of the body such as hands, feet (→ figure), chin, mandible, ears, nose, eyebrows or genitalia. The causal factor is an overproduction of growth hormone **(GH)** in the anterior lobe of the pituitary gland, mainly due to a benign, or rarely, a malignant tumour. If a GH-producing tumour develops in the anterior lobe of the pituitary gland before completion of the longitudinal growth, this results in **gigantism** (pituitary gigantism). After ossification of the epiphyses, only the extremities become enlarged. Rarely, corticotropin-producing tumours lead to **CUSHING's syndrome** (with hypertension, striae, abdominal obesity and redness of the cheeks).

Tumours of the pituitary gland can lead to compression of the Chiasma opticum (bitemporal hemianopsia; → Fig. 12.130) or nerves in the Sinus cavernosus (→ Fig. 12.53).

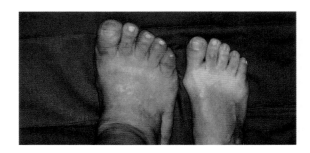

Foot of a patient with acromegaly (on the left) compared to the foot of a healthy person of the same height. The disorder is due to an overproduction of the growth hormone somatotropin (STH) in the anterior lobe of the pituitary gland. The cause is usually a benign tumour in the anterior lobe of the pituitary gland (as a part of the diencephalon). [R236]

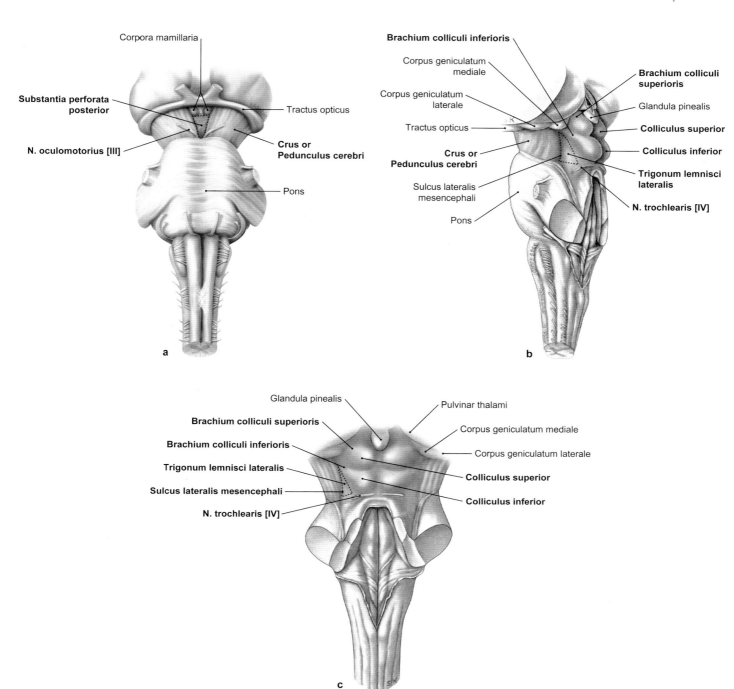

Corpora mamillaria

Substantia perforata
posterior

N. oculomotorius [III]

Tractus opticus

Crus or
Pedunculus cerebri

Pons

Brachium colliculi inferioris

Corpus geniculatum
mediale

Corpus geniculatum
laterale

Tractus opticus

Crus or
Pedunculus cerebri

Sulcus lateralis
mesencephali

Pons

Brachium colliculi
superioris

Glandula pinealis

Colliculus superior

Colliculus inferior

Trigonum lemnisci
lateralis

N. trochlearis [IV]

Glandula pinealis

Pulvinar thalami

Brachium colliculi superioris

Corpus geniculatum mediale

Brachium colliculi inferioris

Corpus geniculatum laterale

Trigonum lemnisci lateralis

Sulcus lateralis mesencephali

Colliculus superior

N. trochlearis [IV]

Colliculus inferior

a

b

c

Fig. 12.102a–c Midbrain, mesencephalon. [S702-L238]
a Anterior view.
b Lateral view.
c Posterior view.
The mesencephalon is the uppermost part of the brainstem. It is bordered from above by the diencephalon, and beneath by the pons. The Pedunculi cerebri pass along the anterior surface. The Colliculi superio-

res and inferiores of the Tectum mesencephali lie on the dorsal side; due to its characteristic form, this structure is called the quadrigeminal plate (Lamina tecti [Lamina quadrigemina]). The Glandula pinealis, as part of the diencephalon, is located above the quadrigeminal plate, and follows the fourth ventricle below the mesencephalon at the level of the pons and the Medulla oblongata.

Clinical remarks

In the case of supratentorial expanding processes (above the Tentorium cerebelli) (e.g. bleeding, tumours) medial parts of one or both temporal lobes can be compressed into the space between the mesencephalon and Tentorium cerebelli **(infratentorial herniation).** This may result in dysfunction of the ipsilateral N. oculomotorius [III] with mydriasis, compression of the pyramidal tract in the Crura cerebri combined with motor deficits, extensor spasms of the extremities and exaggerated reflexes, as well as compressions of the inner tracts and autonomic centres of the Substantia grisea centralis of the

mesencephalon. The latter can derail the circulatory regulation and the autonomic system, and lead to loss of consciousness **(midbrain syndrome).**
Endogenous endorphins deploy their effects by binding to opiate receptors – similar to opiates (e.g. morphine and its derivatives), which therefore can be used as compounds of a **central analgesic (pain) therapy.** They stimulate neurons in the Substantia grisea centralis, and thereby activate the endogenous pain-inhibiting system.

Cerebral areas

Mesencephalon

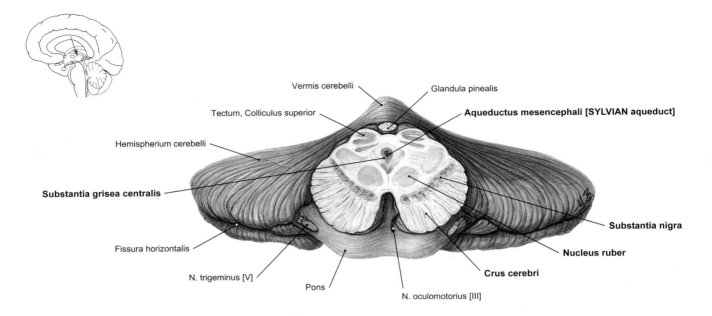

Vermis cerebelli
Glandula pinealis
Tectum, Colliculus superior
Aqueductus mesencephali [SYLVIAN aqueduct]
Hemispherium cerebelli
Substantia grisea centralis
Substantia nigra
Nucleus ruber
Fissura horizontalis
Crus cerebri
N. trigeminus [V]
Pons
N. oculomotorius [III]

Fig. 12.103   Midbrain, mesencephalon; cross-section at the level of the Colliculi superiores; anterior view. [S700]
The Aqueductus mesencephali [SYLVIAN aqueduct] passes through the mesencephalon which is divided into the Basis, Tegmentum and Tectum mesencephali. The Tegmentum and Basis mesencephali are summarised as Pedunculus cerebri.
The **Basis mesencephali** comprises the cerebral legs (Crura cerebri), traversed by different tracts (e. g. Fibrae corticonucleares).
The **Tegmentum mesencephali** comprises the Substantia grisea centralis, which surrounds the Aqueductus mesencephali [SYLVIAN aqueduct] (participates in the central suppression of pain, mediates fight or

flight reflexes, regulates autonomic processes), and the Substantia nigra, which belongs to the basal ganglia. Additional structures of the Tegmentum mesencephali include the Nucleus ruber, an important relay station of the motor system, the mesencephalic parts of the Formatio reticularis, the nuclei of the cranial nerves II and IV, as well as ascending and descending tracts.
The **Tectum mesencephali** (Lamina tecti [Lamina quadrigemina]) includes the Colliculi superiores and inferiores, which are important relay stations for visual reflexes (Colliculi superiores) and the central auditory pathway (Colliculi inferiores).

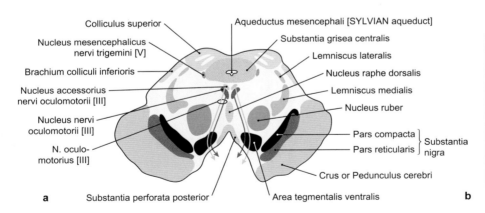

Colliculus superior
Nucleus mesencephalicus nervi trigemini [V]
Brachium colliculi inferioris
Nucleus accessorius nervi oculomotorii [III]
Nucleus nervi oculomotorii [III]
N. oculomotorius [III]
Substantia perforata posterior
Aqueductus mesencephali [SYLVIAN aqueduct]
Substantia grisea centralis
Lemniscus lateralis
Nucleus raphe dorsalis
Lemniscus medialis
Nucleus ruber
Pars compacta } Substantia nigra
Pars reticularis }
Crus or Pedunculus cerebri
Area tegmentalis ventralis

a   b

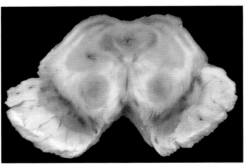

Fig. 12.104a and b   Midbrain, mesencephalon; cross-section of the rostral mesencephalon at the level of the exit of the N. oculomotorius [III].
a Schematic representation. [S700-L126]/[R247-L318]
b Anatomic specimen. [R247-L318]
The mesencephalon includes important nuclei, such as the Nucleus nervi oculomotorii, Nucleus nervi trochlearis, Nucleus accessorius nervi

oculomotorius [EDINGER-WESTPHAL], Nucleus mesencephalicus nervi trigemini, Nucleus ruber, Substantia nigra and Formatio reticularis, and several major tracts pass through it, only some of which are shown: Tractus corticospinalis, Tractus spinothalamici anterior and lateralis, Tractus tegmentalis centralis, Lemnisci mediali and lateralis, Fasciculi longitudinales mediali and dorsalis, Fibrae corticopontinae, Fibrae corticonucleares, Fibrae temporopontinae.

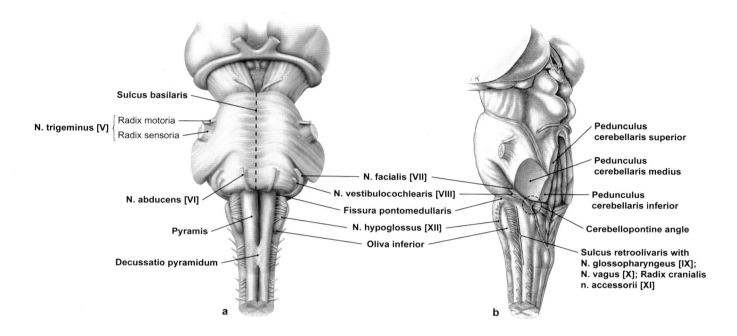

Sulcus basilaris

N. trigeminus [V] { Radix motoria
Radix sensoria

N. facialis [VII]
N. vestibulocochlearis [VIII]
Fissura pontomedullaris
N. hypoglossus [XII]
Oliva inferior

N. abducens [VI]

Pyramis

Decussatio pyramidum

a

Pedunculus cerebellaris superior

Pedunculus cerebellaris medius

Pedunculus cerebellaris inferior

Cerebellopontine angle

Sulcus retroolivaris with
N. glossopharyngeus [IX];
N. vagus [X]; Radix cranialis
n. accessorii [XI]

b

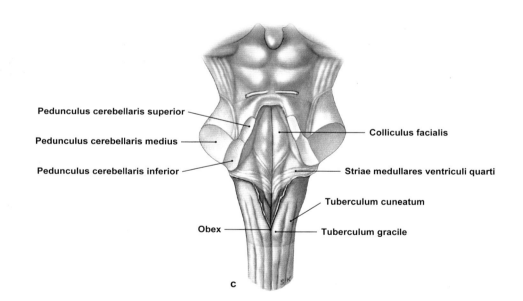

Pedunculus cerebellaris superior

Pedunculus cerebellaris medius

Pedunculus cerebellaris inferior

Obex

Colliculus facialis

Striae medullares ventriculi quarti

Tuberculum cuneatum

Tuberculum gracile

c

Fig. 12.105a–c Pons and Medulla oblongata. [S702-L238]
a Anterior view.
b Lateral view.
c Dorsal view.
Together with the cerebellum, the pons and Medulla oblongata belong to the rhombencephalon. The name is derived from the rhomboid fossa

(Fossa rhomboidea). It represents the floor of the fourth ventricle and is bordered by the cerebellar peduncles (Pedunculi cerebellares), pons and Medulla oblongata. Within the Fossa rhomboidea, the Sulcus medianus, the Colliculus facialis (fibres of the N. facialis [VII]), and the Striae medullares ventriculi quarti can be distinguished as part of the central auditory pathway.

Pons and Medulla oblongata

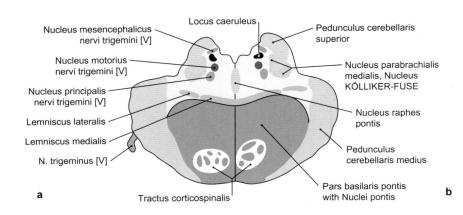

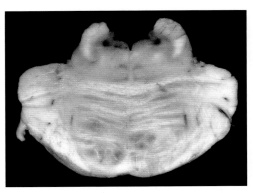

Nucleus mesencephalicus nervi trigemini [V]
Nucleus motorius nervi trigemini [V]
Nucleus principalis nervi trigemini [V]
Lemniscus lateralis
Lemniscus medialis
N. trigeminus [V]

Locus caeruleus
Pedunculus cerebellaris superior
Nucleus parabrachialis medialis, Nucleus KÖLLIKER-FUSE
Nucleus raphes pontis
Pedunculus cerebellaris medius
Pars basilaris pontis with Nuclei pontis
Tractus corticospinalis

a   **b**

Fig. 12.106a and b   **Pons;** cross-section through the rostral pons at the level of the exit of the N. trigeminus [V].
a Schematic representation. [S702-L126]/[R247-L318]
b Anatomical specimen. [R247-L318]
In the region of the Fossa rhomboidea, important nuclei responsible for the regulation of the systemic circulation, as well as the nuclei of the

cranial nerves V to X (→ Fig. 12.125, → Fig. 12.126), and partly of the cranial nerves XI and XII, are located in the pons and Medulla oblongata. The pons receives sensory information in particular from the auditory tube and the face, and sends it to the cerebellum.

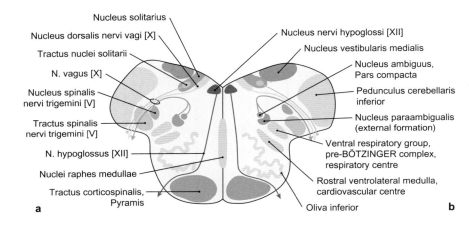

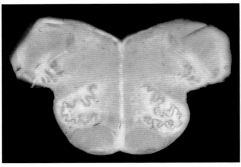

Nucleus solitarius
Nucleus dorsalis nervi vagi [X]
Tractus nuclei solitarii
N. vagus [X]
Nucleus spinalis nervi trigemini [V]
Tractus spinalis nervi trigemini [V]
N. hypoglossus [XII]
Nuclei raphes medullae
Tractus corticospinalis, Pyramis

Nucleus nervi hypoglossi [XII]
Nucleus vestibularis medialis
Nucleus ambiguus, Pars compacta
Pedunculus cerebellaris inferior
Nucleus paraambigualis (external formation)
Ventral respiratory group, pre-BÖTZINGER complex, respiratory centre
Rostral ventrolateral medulla, cardiovascular centre
Oliva inferior

a   **b**

Fig. 12.107a and b   **Medulla oblongata;** cross-section through the rostral Medulla oblongata at the level of the exit of the N. vagus [X].
a Schematic representation. [S702-L126]/[R247-L318]
b Anatomical specimen. [R247-L318]
In the Medulla oblongata, a functional distinction is made between three parts: the tegmentum, pyramids and olive. The tegmentum with

the nuclei of the cranial nerves lies dorsally, the pyramids and olive are located ventrally. The Medulla oblongata harbours important neuronal centres for the control of blood circulation, the respiratory centre, the vomiting centre and the centres for the sneezing, coughing, swallowing and sucking reflexes. In addition, the receptors for the regulation of acid-base homeostasis are found here (→ table for → Fig. 12.108).

Clinical remarks

Bulbar paralysis refers to a bilateral lesion of all motor nuclei of cranial nerves in the Medulla oblongata. This leads to paralysis of the lingual and pharyngeal muscles with subsequent atrophy, swallow-

ing and speech disorders (slurred speech). A possible cause can be a neurodegenerative disease of the motor neurons such as amyotrophic lateral sclerosis (ALS).

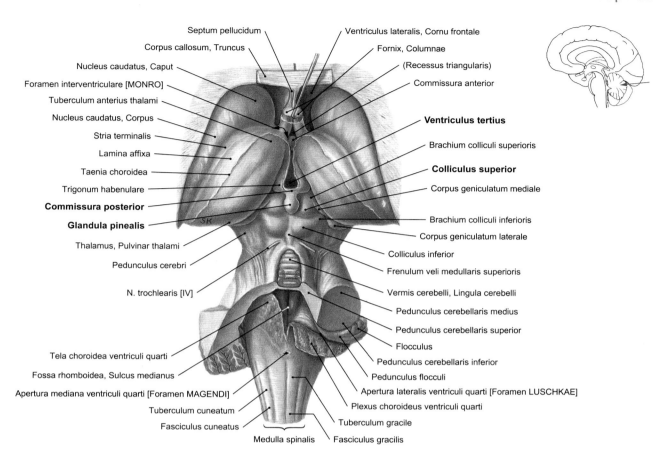

Septum pellucidum
Corpus callosum, Truncus
Nucleus caudatus, Caput
Foramen interventriculare [MONRO]
Tuberculum anterius thalami
Nucleus caudatus, Corpus
Stria terminalis
Lamina affixa
Taenia choroidea
Trigonum habenulare
Commissura posterior
Glandula pinealis
Thalamus, Pulvinar thalami
Pedunculus cerebri
N. trochlearis [IV]
Tela choroidea ventriculi quarti
Fossa rhomboidea, Sulcus medianus
Apertura mediana ventriculi quarti [Foramen MAGENDI]
Tuberculum cuneatum
Fasciculus cuneatus
Medulla spinalis

Ventriculus lateralis, Cornu frontale
Fornix, Columnae
(Recessus triangularis)
Commissura anterior
Ventriculus tertius
Brachium colliculi superioris
Colliculus superior
Corpus geniculatum mediale
Brachium colliculi inferioris
Corpus geniculatum laterale
Colliculus inferior
Frenulum veli medullaris superioris
Vermis cerebelli, Lingula cerebelli
Pedunculus cerebellaris medius
Pedunculus cerebellaris superior
Flocculus
Pedunculus cerebellaris inferior
Pedunculus flocculi
Apertura lateralis ventriculi quarti [Foramen LUSCHKAE]
Plexus choroideus ventriculi quarti
Tuberculum gracile
Fasciculus gracilis

Fig. 12.108 Brainstem, Truncus encephali; posterior view from above; after removal of the Corpus callosum and major parts of the cerebellum, the Tela choroidea of the fourth ventricle was split in the middle and folded back to the right side. [S700-L238]
Important functional **centres** (→ table) are located in the brainstem.

Overview of the functional anatomy of the brainstem

Centre/system	Function/reflex	Nuclei or brain region	Participating afferent cranial nerves	Nuclei of efferent cranial nerves or spinal cord
Eye/vision	Pupillary reflex	Area pretectalis	N. opticus [II]	Nucleus accessorius nervi oculomotorii [III]
	Oculomotor function	Preoculomotor centres, Colliculi superiores	N. opticus [II]	Nucleus nervi oculomotorii [III], Nucleus nervi trochlearis [IV], Nucleus nervi abducentis [VI]
	Corneal reflex, eyelid closure		Nucleus principalis nervi trigemini [V]	Nucleus nervi facialis [VII]
Ear/hearing	Directional hearing, head rotation to the sound source	Nucleus olivaris superior, Corpus trapezoideum, Colliculi inferiores	Nuclei cochleares [VIII]	Spinal cord (cervical anterior horn)
Balance/equilibrium	Posture, spatial orientation	Nucleus olivaris inferior, cerebellum	Nuclei vestibulares [VIII]	Spinal cord
Nose	Sneezing reflex	Respiratory centre, ventrolateral Medulla oblongata	Nucleus principalis nervi trigemini [V/2]	Nucleus ambiguus (IX, X), spinal cord (anterior horn)
Gastrointestinal tract	Taste, saliva		Rostral part of the Nucleus tractus solitarii (VII, IX, X)	Nucleus salivatorius superior [VII] and Nucleus salivatorius inferior [IX]
	Swallowing	Swallowing centre, ventrolateral Medulla oblongata	Nucleus principalis nervi trigemini (V/2, V/3), medial Nucleus tractus solitarii (IX, X)	Nucleus motorius nervi trigemini [V/3], Nucleus nervi facialis [VII], Nucleus ambiguus (IX, X), Nucleus nervi hypoglossi [XII]
	Vomiting	Area postrema	Medial Nucleus tractus solitarii [X]	Nucleus dorsalis nervi vagi [X]
	Digestion (juices and peristalsis)		Medial Nucleus tractus solitarii [X]	Nucleus dorsalis nervi vagi [X]
Breathing/respiration	Respiratory reflexes (including lung expansion reflex, cough reflex)	Respiratory centre, ventrolateral Medulla oblongata	Lateral Nucleus tractus solitarii [X]	Nucleus ambiguus (IX, X), Nucleus nervi hypoglossi [XII], spinal cord (anterior horn)
Heart/circulation	Circulatory reflexes (including baroreceptor and chemoreceptor reflexes)	Circulation centre, rostral ventrolateral Medulla oblongata (RVLM)	Dorsolateral Nucleus tractus solitarii (IX, X)	Nucleus ambiguus, external formation [X], sympathetic nervous system, spinal cord (lateral horn)

Cerebral areas

Truncus encephali and cerebellum

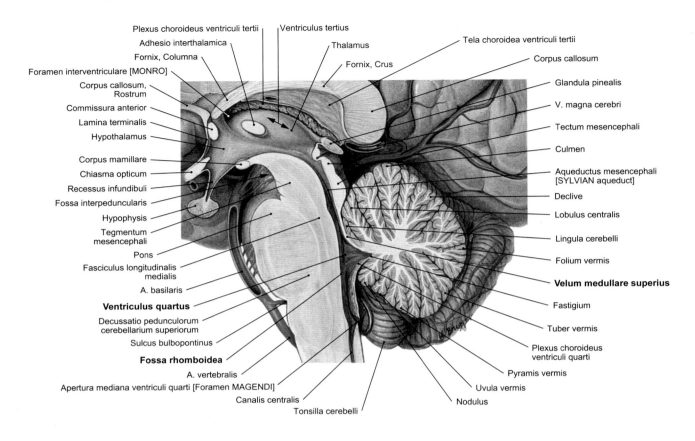

Plexus choroideus ventriculi tertii
Adhesio interthalamica
Fornix, Columna
Foramen interventriculare [MONRO]
Corpus callosum, Rostrum
Commissura anterior
Lamina terminalis
Hypothalamus
Corpus mamillare
Chiasma opticum
Recessus infundibuli
Fossa interpeduncularis
Hypophysis
Tegmentum mesencephali
Pons
Fasciculus longitudinalis medialis
A. basilaris
Ventriculus quartus
Decussatio pedunculorum cerebellarium superiorum
Sulcus bulbopontinus
Fossa rhomboidea
A. vertebralis
Apertura mediana ventriculi quarti [Foramen MAGENDI]
Canalis centralis
Tonsilla cerebelli

Ventriculus tertius
Thalamus
Fornix, Crus

Tela choroidea ventriculi tertii
Corpus callosum
Glandula pinealis
V. magna cerebri
Tectum mesencephali
Culmen
Aqueductus mesencephali [SYLVIAN aqueduct]
Declive
Lobulus centralis
Lingula cerebelli
Folium vermis
Velum medullare superius
Fastigium
Tuber vermis
Plexus choroideus ventriculi quarti
Pyramis vermis
Uvula vermis
Nodulus

Fig. 12.109 Brainstem, Truncus encephali, with the fourth ventricle, Ventriculus quartus, and the cerebellum; median section. [S700]

A few, relatively small nuclear areas located in the brainstem use the serotonergic and other aminergic (e.g. dopaminergic, histaminergic and noradrenergic) systems, to reach large portions of the brain and spinal cord via widely ramified axon fibres (→ table).

Apart from the brainstem, the median section reveals the characteristic structure of the so-called tree of life **(Arbor vitae)** of the cerebellum created by distinct grooves (surface enlargement) of the cerebellar cortex.

The Fossa rhomboidea is located in front of the cerebellum and forms the floor of the fourth ventricle. Anterior to the ventricle lies the brainstem with the mesencephalon, pons and Medulla oblongata, and even further anteriorly the A. basilaris runs along the brainstem. In the median section one can see how the posterior wall of the fourth ventricle continues as the Velum medullare superius from the cerebellum to the quadrigeminal plate (Lamina tecti [Lamina quadrigemina]). The pineal gland (Glandula pinealis) and the Corpus callosum are located on top.

Monoaminergic neurotransmitter systems in the brainstem			
Nuclei/nuclear area	**Location in the brainstem**	**Neurotransmitter used**	**Targets of projections**
Substantia nigra, Pars compacta	Border between Basis and Tegmentum mesencephali	Dopamine	Striatum
Area tegmentalis ventralis (ventral tegmental area, VTA)	Tegmentum mesencephali	Dopamine	Cerebral cortex, limbic system, Nucleus accumbens
Nucleus or Locus caeruleus	Part of the Formatio reticularis in the Tegmentum pontis	Noradrenaline	Cerebral cortex, limbic system, thalamus, hypothalamus, cerebellum
Raphe nuclei	Groups of nuclei in the area of the raphe from the mesencephalon up to the Medulla oblongata	Serotonin	CNS (whole)

Clinical remarks

Affective disorders such as depression are common psychiatric disorders. Based on current knowledge, the noradrenergic projections of the Nucleus caeruleus, as well as the serotonergic projections of the Nuclei raphe play a role in this context. It is assumed that a lack of noradrenaline and/or serotonin in the synaptic gap may be the causal factor, since in many patients a significant improvement of their symptoms could be observed if the deficiency was antagonised by continuous medication with selective noradrenaline and/or selective serotonin re-uptake inhibitors.

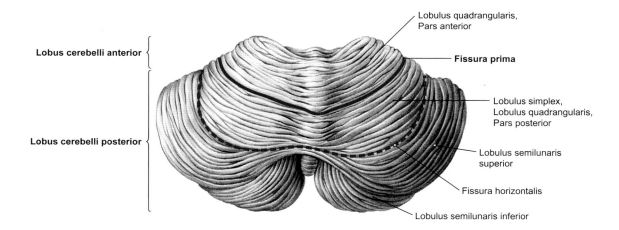

Lobulus quadrangularis,
Pars anterior

Fissura prima

Lobulus simplex,
Lobulus quadrangularis,
Pars posterior

Lobulus semilunaris
superior

Fissura horizontalis

Lobulus semilunaris inferior

Lobus cerebelli anterior

Lobus cerebelli posterior

Fig. 12.110 Cerebellum; posterior view from above (superior surface). [S700]

The cerebellum consists of the **vermis** (Vermis cerebelli) and two **hemispheres.** Of the vermis, the tuber, folium, declive and culmen are visible, as well as the Lobulus centralis and the Lingula cerebelli. The cerebellar hemispheres are divided into **three lobes,** respectively (→ Fig. 12.116):

* Lobus cerebelli anterior
* Lobus cerebelli posterior
* Lobus flocculonodularis (Nodulus + Flocculus, → Fig. 12.112).

The lobes are subdivided into **lobules** such as the Lobulus quadrangularis anterior, the Lobulus quadrangularis posterior (Lobulus simplex) as well as the Lobuli semilunares superior and inferior.

The superior surface faces the Tentorium cerebelli. The Fissura prima and the Fissura horizontalis are clearly recognisable. The Fissura horizontalis is not a functioning border, but forms a separating line between the superior and inferior surfaces.

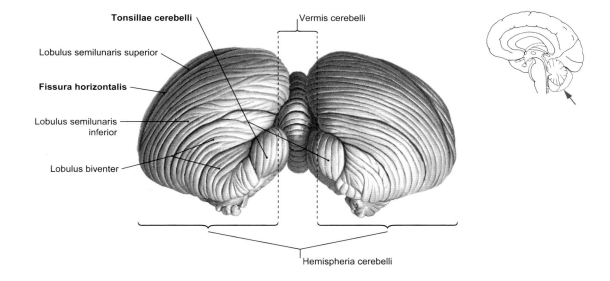

Tonsillae cerebelli

Vermis cerebelli

Lobulus semilunaris superior

Fissura horizontalis

Lobulus semilunaris inferior

Lobulus biventer

Hemispheria cerebelli

Fig. 12.111 Cerebellum; posterior view from below (inferior surface). [S700]

The inferior surface lies opposite the Os occipitale and the Cisterna cerebellomedullaris. In this view, the vermis and the two cerebellar hem-

ispheres are visible. Furthermore, one can see the paired tonsils of the cerebellum (Tonsilla cerebelli) as well as the Lobuli semilunares superior and inferior, which are separated by the Fissura horizontalis. The Lobulus biventer joins the Lobulus semilunaris inferior from below.

Clinical remarks

With increased intracranial pressure (e.g. from a tumour or bleeding), the cerebellar tonsils, as the most caudal structures of the cerebellum, can become trapped between the bone and the Medulla oblongata in the area of the Foramen magnum. The resulting compression of the Medulla oblongata can cause the failure of vital structures, such as the respiratory centre, which can be fatal. This **in-**

fratentorial herniation is juxtaposed with **supratentorial herniation** (herniation of the mesencephalon in the Incisura tentorii) with the possible consequence of midbrain syndrome (failure of the Formatio reticularis, as well as the corticobulbar and rubrospinal tracts). The latter precedes the infratentorial herniation.

Cerebellum

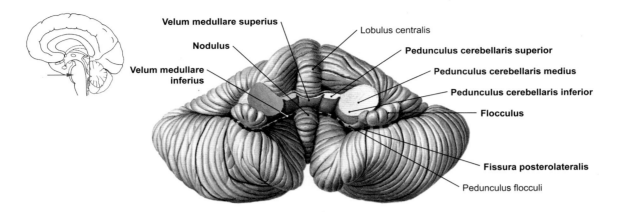

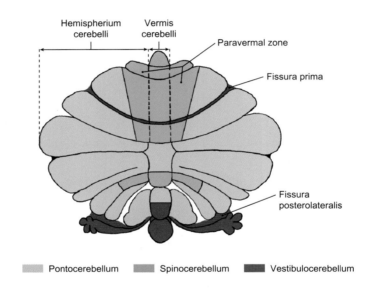

Fig. 12.112 Cerebellum; anterior view; after dissection of the cerebellar peduncles (anterior surface). [S700]
The anterior surface shows the cerebellar peduncles which connect the cerebellum to the brainstem: Pedunculi cerebellares superior, medius and inferior. The Velum medullare superius divides the vermis of the cerebellum (Vermis cerebelli) and connects both cerebellar peduncles. The paired Velum medullare inferius located on the left and the right side of the nodulus continues on both sides towards the flocculus. The cerebellar hemispheres form the outer parts.

Fig. 12.113 Cerebellum; schematic representation, functional-anatomic segmentation of the extended cerebellar cortex. [R247-L318]
Functionally, the cerebellum is divided into three parts:
- **pontocerebellum** (coordination of the precise voluntary motor activity and speech muscles)
- **spinocerebellum** (regulation of muscle tone and, together with the vestibulocerebellum, control of postural motor activity)
- **vestibulocerebellum** (control of postural motor activity = stabilisation of posture and gait, fine-tuning of eye movements, and coordination of both functions with the vestibular system = maintenance of balance).

Clinical remarks

A Typical sign of **damage to the pontocerebellum** is an intention or cerebellar tremor when executing targeted voluntary movements. This tremor in the extremities gradually increases, the closer the extremity gets to the target. The impaired muscular movement or coordination is associated with ataxia ('asynergy'), which manifests as dysmetria (also described as an inability to judge distance or scale) and dysdiadochokinesis (impaired ability to perform rapid, alternating movements).
Lesions of the spinocerebellum lead to disorders of coordinated movement sequences that are not easily corrected. The failed or severely impaired coordination of agonistic and antagonistic muscles results in ataxias of posture and gait (static and dynamic ataxias) as well as exaggerated and shortened movements (dysmetrias).
Lesions of the vestibulocerebellum are in particular associated with impaired equilibrium or balance. Only to a very limited extent are patients capable of using vestibular information to control their eye movements when moving the head, and their axial and limb muscles when standing, walking or sitting (trunk, gait and postural ataxia; disorders of movement coordination). Insufficient motor coordination of the gaze (by the eye muscles) can lead, among others, to spontaneous nystagmus and involuntary saccadic (jerky) eye movements.

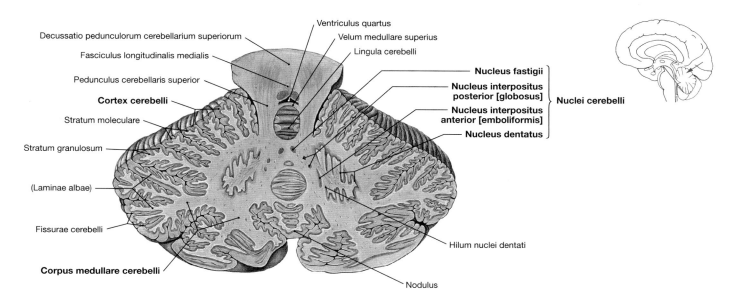

Fig. 12.114 **Cerebellum with cerebellar nuclei, Nuclei cerebelli;** flat cross-section through the upper cerebellar peduncles; posterior view. [S700]

The cerebellum consists of the **white matter** (Corpus medullare cerebelli) which surrounds the embedded cerebellar nuclei, as well as the **cerebellar cortex** (Cortex cerebelli). The flat cross-section reveals all four cerebellar nuclei in both hemispheres (pontocerebellum). The **Nucleus dentatus** ('tooth-like' nucleus) is U-shaped and jagged. The **Nucleus emboliformis** (a wedge-shaped nucleus) is located medially of the Nucleus dentatus and forms together with the further medially located **Nucleus globosus** (a ball-shaped nucleus), the **Nucleus interpositus**. Both nuclei share many functional similarities and are connected to the paravermal zone and the vermis of the cerebellum (spinocerebellum). The right and left **Nucleus fastigii**, located in the semi-oval centre of the vermis, are functionally closely related to the cortex of the Lobus flocculonodularis (vestibulocerebellum). The cerebellar nuclei contain mainly multipolar nerve cells with efferent fibres projecting into other regions of the brain.

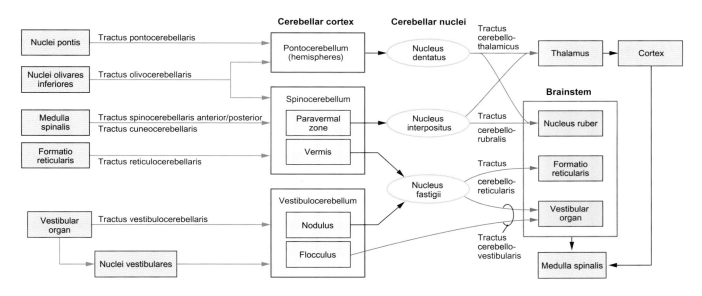

Fig. 12.115 **Schematic representation of the cerebellar compartments with corresponding afferent and efferent connections.** [R254-L141]

Clinical remarks

In the past, it was assumed that the cerebellum and its circuits had nothing to do with higher brain functions, such as social interaction and communication. Due to cerebellar malfunctions it has become evident now that this is not the case. The integrity of the PURKINJE's cells as typical cells of the cerebellum seems to play an important role. Postmortal dissections of the brains of patients with **autism** showed a reduced number of PURKINJE's cells in certain cerebellar cortical areas.

Alcoholism **(chronic alcohol abuse)** can result in irreversible damage of the cerebellum, particularly in atrophy of the Vermis cerebelli.

This pathological process leads to partial destruction of the nodulus (vestibulocerebellum), as well as of the vermis and paravermal zone (spinocerebellum). The patients can no longer coordinate their eye movements and suffer from balance disorders (stance and gait disorders with staggering and a tendency to fall).

Due to its integration into the chain 'cerebellum – Nucleus ruber – cerebellum – olive – cerebellum', **lesions of the Nucleus ruber** can cause the same symptoms as with cerebellar lesions, such as intention tremor and decreased muscle tone.

Cerebellum

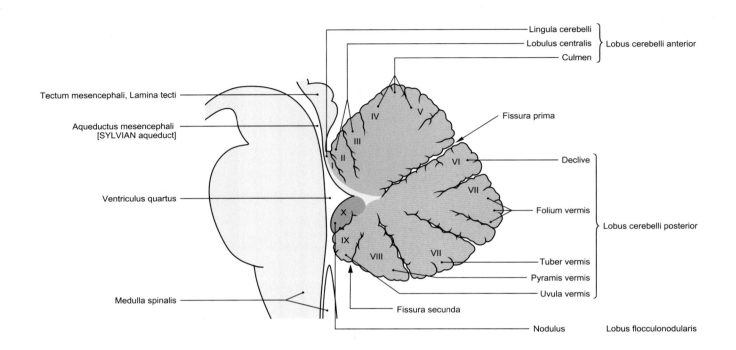

Lingula cerebelli ⎫
Lobulus centralis ⎬ Lobus cerebelli anterior
Culmen ⎭

Tectum mesencephali, Lamina tecti

Aqueductus mesencephali [SYLVIAN aqueduct]

Fissura prima

Ventriculus quartus

Declive

Folium vermis

Lobus cerebelli posterior

Tuber vermis

Pyramis vermis

Uvula vermis

Medulla spinalis

Fissura secunda

Nodulus   Lobus flocculonodularis

Fig. 12.116   Vermis of the cerebellum, Vermis cerebelli, parts I to X; median section; overview. [S700]

The Vermis cerebelli is the unpaired median part of the cerebellum, which connects the two cerebellar hemispheres (Hemispheria cerebelli).

Subdivisions of the cerebellar vermis, Vermis cerebelli (Roman numbering according to the classification of LARSELL)	
I	Lingula cerebelli
II, III	Lobus centralis
IV, V	Culmen
Fissura prima	
VI	Declive
VII A	Folium vermis
Fissura horizontalis	
VII B	Tuber vermis
VIII	Pyramis vermis
Fissura secunda	
IX	Uvula vermis
Fissura posterolateralis	
X	Nodulus

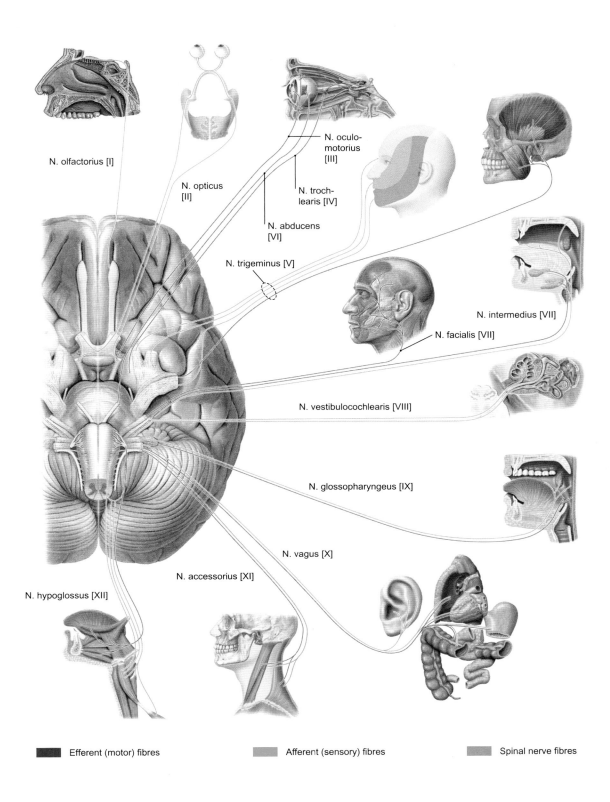

N. olfactorius [I]

N. opticus [II]

N. oculo-motorius [III]

N. troch-learis [IV]

N. abducens [VI]

N. trigeminus [V]

N. intermedius [VII]

N. facialis [VII]

N. vestibulocochlearis [VIII]

N. glossopharyngeus [IX]

N. vagus [X]

N. accessorius [XI]

N. hypoglossus [XII]

Efferent (motor) fibres   Afferent (sensory) fibres   Spinal nerve fibres

Fig. 12.117 Cranial nerves, Nn. craniales; functional overview of the cerebrum, brainstem (Truncus encephali) and cerebellum; inferior view. [S702-L127]

Twelve pairs of cranial nerves leaving the cranial base are numbered with Roman numerals (I–XII) in the order of their exit (from anterior to posterior). The first cranial nerve is formed by the Fila olfactoria, which are collectively named **N. olfactorius [I].** The bipolar olfactory neurons (the sensory ganglion in the olfactory mucosa is unnamed) project via the fila into the Bulbus olfactorius, a part of the cerebrum that was relocated cranially during development. Therefore, the olfactory bulb repre-

sents the Nucleus terminationis of the N. olfactorius [I], with the exception that it is not located in the brainstem but further advanced on the Lamina cribrosa. Thus, the first cranial nerve differs from the others because its neurons are very short, and its terminal nucleus is not located in the brainstem. Another exception applies to the **N. opticus [II],** which includes the third or even fourth neuron of the visual pathway, and in contrast to all other cranial nerves, the optic nerve is a protrusion of the diencephalon and not a peripheral nerve in the narrower sense.

→ T 58, T 60

Overview

Overview of the 12 cranial nerves and their most important innervation areas [R254]

A detailed representation of the innervation regions for each cranial nerve is shown in → Fig. 12.127 to → Fig. 12.174.
GSA: general somatic-afferent; GSE: general somatic-efferent; GVA: general visceral-afferent; GVE: general visceral-efferent; SSA: special somatic-afferent; SVA: special visceral-afferent; SVE: special visceral-efferent

Cranial nerve	Qualities	Important innervation areas
N. olfactorius [I]	SSA	Olfactory mucosa
N. opticus [II]	SSA	Retina
N. oculomotorius [III]	GSE, GVE	Eye muscles (intraocular, extraocular)
N. trochlearis [IV]	GSE	Extraocular muscles
N. trigeminus [V]	SVE, GSA	Muscles of mastication, facial skin
N. abducens [VI]	GSE	Extraocular muscles
N. facialis [VII]	GVE, SVE, SVA, GSA	Mimetic (facial) muscles, gustatory organ, glands
N. vestibulocochlearis [VIII]	SSA	Vestibular and hearing organ
N. glossopharyngeus [IX]	GVE, SVE, GSA, GVA, SVA	Pharyngeal muscles, parotid gland
N. vagus [X]	GVE, SVE, GSA, GVA, SVA	Pharyngeal muscles, larynx, internal organs
N. accessorius [XI]	SVE	M. trapezius and M. sternocleidomastoideus
N. hypoglossus [XII]	GSE	Muscles of the tongue

Overview of the cranial nerves with two or more nuclei in the brainstem [R254]

The Nn. trochlearis [IV], abducens [VI], accessorius [XI], and hypoglossus [XII] only have one eponymously named nucleus and are therefore not listed here.

Nerve	Corresponding nuclei
N. oculomotorius [III]	• Nucleus nervi oculomotorii • Nucleus accessorius nervi oculomotorii
N. trigeminus [V]	• Nucleus motorius nervi trigemini • Nucleus mesencephalicus nervi trigemini • Nucleus pontinus (sensorius principalis) nervi trigemini • Nucleus spinalis nervi trigemini
N. facialis [VII]	• Nucleus nervi facialis • Nucleus salivatorius superior • Nucleus spinalis nervi trigemini • Nuclei tractus solitarii
N. vestibulocochlearis [VIII]	• Nuclei vestibulares • Nuclei cochleares
N. glossopharyngeus [IX]	• Nucleus salivatorius inferior • Nucleus ambiguus • Nucleus spinalis nervi trigemini • Nuclei tractus solitarii
N. vagus [X]	• Nucleus dorsalis nervi vagi • Nucleus ambiguus • Nucleus spinalis nervi trigemini • Nuclei tractus solitarii

Overview of cranial nerve nuclei which serve two or more cranial nerves [R254]

All other nuclei only have one eponymously named cranial nerve.

Nucleus	Corresponding cranial nerve
Nucleus ambiguus	• N. glossopharyngeus [IX] • N. vagus [X] • N. accessorius [XI] (Radix cranialis)
Nuclei tractus solitarii	• N. facialis [VII] • N. glossopharyngeus [IX] • N. vagus [X]
Nucleus spinalis nervi trigemini	• N. trigeminus [V] • N. facialis [VII] • N. glossopharyngeus [IX] • N. vagus [X]

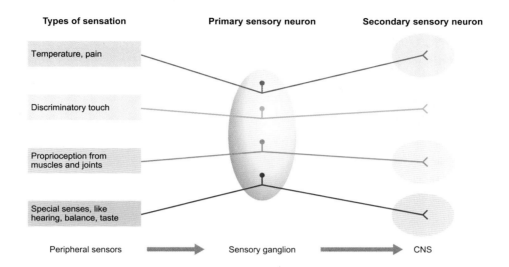

Types of sensation   Primary sensory neuron   Secondary sensory neuron

Temperature, pain

Discriminatory touch

Proprioception from muscles and joints

Special senses, like hearing, balance, taste

Peripheral sensors   →   Sensory ganglion   →   CNS

Fig. 12.118 Organisation of sensory ganglia of cranial nerves; schematic representation. [S701-L127]

Basic organisation of sensory ganglia and their role in connecting different peripheral sensory systems with defined sensory nuclei in the CNS (see individual cranial nerves for details).

Overview of cranial nerves with sensory fibre qualities			
Cranial nerves	**Sensory ganglion**	**Ganglion cell type**	**Function**
N. trigeminus [V]	Ganglion trigeminale [GASSERI]	Pseudounipolar	Sensations in face, oral cavity, nasal cavity, in the sinuses and the supratentorial meninges
N. facialis [VII]	Ganglion geniculi	Pseudounipolar	Gustatory sensation at the anterior two-thirds of the tongue, touch sensations at the outer ear canal
N. vestibulocochlearis [VIII]	Ganglion spirale	Bipolar	Hearing
		Bipolar	Balance
N. glossopharyngeus [IX]	Ganglion superius nervi glossopharyngei	Pseudounipolar	Meatus acusticus externus, middle ear, pharynx, gustatory sensations and sensory sensations of the posterior third of the tongue
	Ganglion inferius nervi glossopharyngei	Pseudounipolar	Meatus acusticus externus, middle ear, pharynx, gustatory sensations and sensory sensations of the posterior third of the tongue, Glomus caroticum
N. vagus [X]	Ganglion superius nervi vagi	Pseudounipolar	Ear, pharynx, infratentorial meninges
	Ganglion inferius nervi vagi	Pseudounipolar	Gustatory sensations in the pharynx and glottis as well as sensory sensation in the larynx, heart, aortic arch, respiratory tract, lungs, abdominal organs up to the Flexura coli sinistra [CANNON-BÖHM point; CANNON's sphinctre or point]

Structure and function

Ganglia of cranial nerves with sensory fibre qualities (GSA and SSA) contain the perikarya of the first afferent neurons. In most cases, these are pseudounipolar neurons (GSA); only the vestibulocochlear neurons are bipolar (SSA). Afferent fibres relay impulses from sensory receptors to the brain where the fibres synapse with the second neuron of the sensory path. Those cranial nerves with sensory ganglia are listed in the table given above.

Parasympathetic ganglia of the head

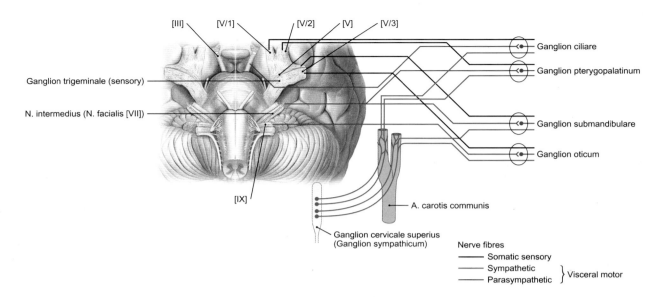

[III]   [V/1]   [V/2]   [V]   [V/3]

Ganglion ciliare

Ganglion pterygopalatinum

Ganglion trigeminale (sensory)

N. intermedius (N. facialis [VII])

Ganglion submandibulare

Ganglion oticum

[IX]

A. carotis communis

Ganglion cervicale superius
(Ganglion sympathicum)

Nerve fibres
— Somatic sensory
— Sympathetic ⎱ Visceral motor
— Parasympathetic ⎰

Fig. 12.119 Organisation of the sensory ganglia of the cranial nerves; schematic representation [S701-L127]
In the four parasympathetic ganglia of the head, pre-ganglionic parasympathetic efferent fibres of the cranial nerves [III, VII and IX] synapse with post-ganglionic parasympathetic neurons, which extend axons to

their target organs (→ table). Sensory fibres of the N. trigeminus [V] (GSA) and sympathetic post-ganglionic fibres, which synapse from sympathetic pre- to post-ganglionic fibres in the Ganglion cervicale superius, run through the parasympathetic ganglia without synapsing.

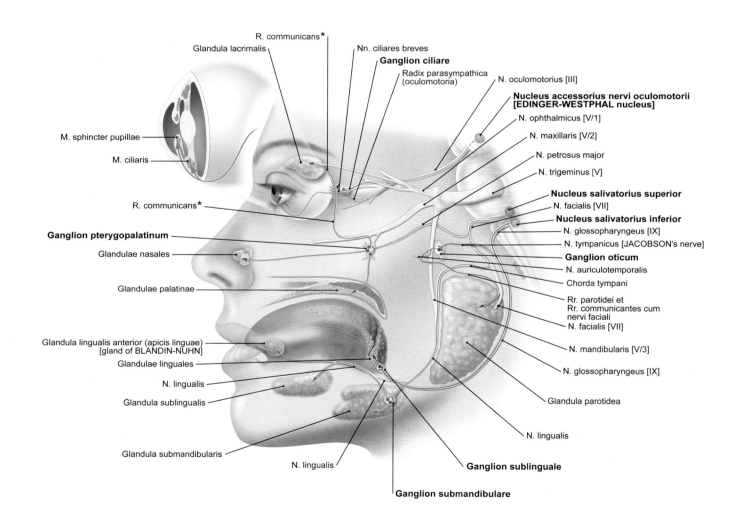

R. communicans*

Glandula lacrimalis

Nn. ciliares breves

Ganglion ciliare

Radix parasympathica
(oculomotoria)

N. oculomotorius [III]

**Nucleus accessorius nervi oculomotorii
[EDINGER-WESTPHAL nucleus]**

N. ophthalmicus [V/1]

M. sphincter pupillae

N. maxillaris [V/2]

M. ciliaris

N. petrosus major

N. trigeminus [V]

R. communicans*

Nucleus salivatorius superior
N. facialis [VII]

Nucleus salivatorius inferior
N. glossopharyngeus [IX]

Ganglion pterygopalatinum

N. tympanicus [JACOBSON's nerve]

Glandulae nasales

Ganglion oticum

N. auriculotemporalis

Chorda tympani

Glandulae palatinae

Rr. parotidei et
Rr. communicantes cum
nervi faciali

N. facialis [VII]

Glandula lingualis anterior (apicis linguae)
[gland of BLANDIN-NUHN]

N. mandibularis [V/3]

Glandulae linguales

N. glossopharyngeus [IX]

N. lingualis

Glandula sublingualis

Glandula parotidea

N. lingualis

Glandula submandibularis

Ganglion sublinguale

N. lingualis

Ganglion submandibulare

Fig. 12.120 Parasympathetic innervation to the glands of the head; schematic representation. [S700-L238]

Representation of the parasympathetic ganglia of the head with their parasympathetic fibres and corresponding nuclei of the cranial nerves (compare to → Fig. 8.192).
* lacrimal nerve anastomosis

Overview of the cranial nerves with parasympathetic ganglia

Parasympathetic nuclei in the brainstem (first neuron)	Cranial nerve with parasympathetic fibres	Parasympathetic ganglion (second neuron)	Function
Nucleus accessorius nervi oculomotorii [EDINGER-WESTPHAL nucleus]	N. oculomotorius [III]	Ganglion ciliare	Miosis (M. sphincter pupillae), accommodation (M. ciliaris)
Nucleus salivatorius superior	N. intermedius (N. facialis [VII])	Ganglion sphenopalatinum	Lacrimal gland, mucous glands of the nasal cavity, pharynx, sinuses
		Ganglion submandibulare	Glandula submandibularis, Glandula sublingualis, Glandula lingualis anterior [gland of BLANDIN-NUHN]
Nucleus salivatorius inferior	N. glossopharyngeus [IX]	Ganglion oticum	Glandula parotidea
		Ganglion sublinguale	Glandulae linguales
Nucleus ambiguus*	Plexus cardiacus	Heart	
Nucleus dorsalis nervi vagi	N. vagus [X]	• Plexus myentericus (AUERBACH's) and submucosus (MEISSNER's) • Organ-specific plexus, e.g. of the lung	Respiratory tract, lung, oesophagus, kidney, gastrointestinal tract up to the Flexura coli sinistra (CANNON-BÖHM point)

* In addition to its motor neurons for the innervation of the muscles of the soft palate, pharynx and larynx, the Nucleus ambiguus also contains cholinergic parasympathetic neurons which form the parasympathetic Plexus cardiacus.

Structure and function

There is an important difference between ganglia of the autonomic nervous system and of the sensory nervous system (GSA, SSA). In sympathetic and parasympathetic ganglia of the autonomic nervous system, pre-ganglionic axons synapse with post-ganglionic neurons. Ganglia of the sensory nervous system do not form synapses but instead contain the perikarya of the first afferent neurons.

Cranial nerves

Topography

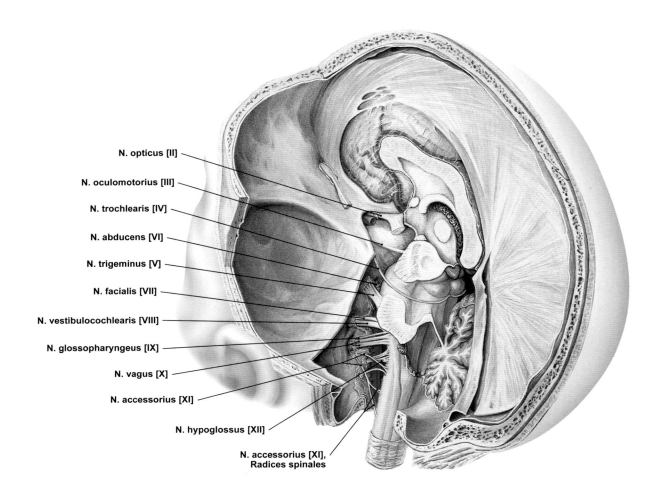

N. opticus [II]

N. oculomotorius [III]

N. trochlearis [IV]

N. abducens [VI]

N. trigeminus [V]

N. facialis [VII]

N. vestibulocochlearis [VIII]

N. glossopharyngeus [IX]

N. vagus [X]

N. accessorius [XI]

N. hypoglossus [XII]

N. accessorius [XI],
Radices spinales

Fig. 12.121 Pathway of the cranial nerves, Nn. craniales, in the subarachnoid space; posterior superior view from the left side; after removal of the left cerebral and cerebellar hemispheres as well as the Tentorium cerebelli. [S700]
The cranial nerves III to XII exit the brainstem according to their sequence in the cranial to caudal order. Some nerves exit as a bundle of nerve roots, which form the actual cranial nerve (IX–XII) later on. The N. trochlearis [IV] is the thinnest of all the cranial nerves and the only one exiting the brainstem on the posterior aspect. The N. abducens [VI] has the longest intradural passage before its exit at the cranial base.

→ T 60

A comparison of characteristic features of the cranial nerves and spinal nerves

Spinal nerves	Cranial nerves
Segmental arrangement	Without segmental arrangement
31 pairs of spinal nerves (usually)	12 pairs of cranial nerves
Exiting from the Medulla spinalis	Exiting from the Truncus encephali
Passage through segmentally arranged Foramina intervertebralia	Passage through non-segmentally arranged openings in the cranial base
Four functional fibre qualities	Seven functional fibre qualities
Target organs located primarily below the upper thoracic aperture	Target organs located primarily above the upper thoracic aperture

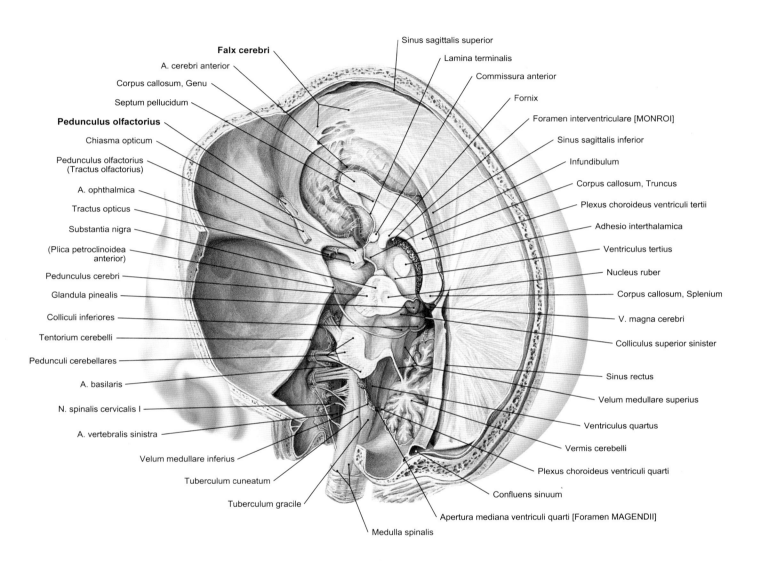

Falx cerebri
A. cerebri anterior
Corpus callosum, Genu
Septum pellucidum
Pedunculus olfactorius
Chiasma opticum
Pedunculus olfactorius (Tractus olfactorius)
A. ophthalmica
Tractus opticus
Substantia nigra
(Plica petroclinoidea anterior)
Pedunculus cerebri
Glandula pinealis
Colliculi inferiores
Tentorium cerebelli
Pedunculi cerebellares
A. basilaris
N. spinalis cervicalis I
A. vertebralis sinistra
Velum medullare inferius
Tuberculum cuneatum
Tuberculum gracile
Medulla spinalis

Sinus sagittalis superior
Lamina terminalis
Commissura anterior
Fornix
Foramen interventriculare [MONROI]
Sinus sagittalis inferior
Infundibulum
Corpus callosum, Truncus
Plexus choroideus ventriculi tertii
Adhesio interthalamica
Ventriculus tertius
Nucleus ruber
Corpus callosum, Splenium
V. magna cerebri
Colliculus superior sinister
Sinus rectus
Velum medullare superius
Ventriculus quartus
Vermis cerebelli
Plexus choroideus ventriculi quarti
Confluens sinuum
Apertura mediana ventriculi quarti [Foramen MAGENDII]

Fig. 12.122   Pathway of the cranial nerves, Nn. craniales, in the subarachnoid space; posterior superior view from the left side; after removal of the left cerebral and cerebellar hemispheres and of the Tentorium cerebelli. [S700]

In contrast with → Fig. 12.121, the names of all structures, except the cranial nerves, are shown.

→ T 60

Brain and spinal cord

Cranial nerves

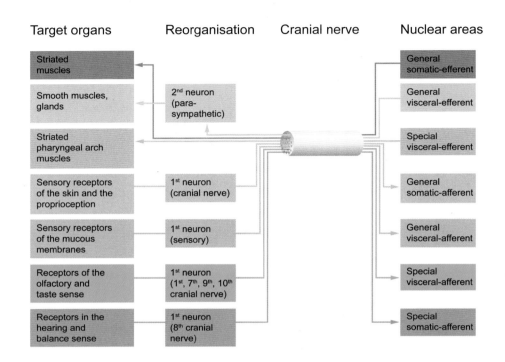

Target organs   Reorganisation   Cranial nerve   Nuclear areas

Fig. 12.123 Fibre qualities of the cranial nerves (nuclei); coloured presentation of the fibre qualities of the cranial nerves (nuclei) with possible circuits or relay stations, and the respective effector organs. [S702-L127]

Seven different fibre qualities of cranial nerves can be distinguished (→ table), but not every cranial nerve contains all of these fibre qualities.

Fibre qualities, differentiated according to efferent and afferent fibres	
Fibre quality	**Innervation**
Efferent nerve fibres	
General somatic-efferent	Motor: skeletal muscles
General visceral-efferent	Parasympathetic: glands, smooth muscles
Special visceral-efferent	Brachiomotor: pharyngeal arch muscles
Afferent nerve fibres	
General somatic-afferent	Proprioceptive (joints, muscles) and exteroceptive (sensitivity of the skin)
General visceral-afferent	Enteroceptive (sensitivity of the mucosa; blood vessels)
Special visceral-afferent	Smell and taste organ
Special somatic-afferent	Sensory: vision, hearing and vestibular organ

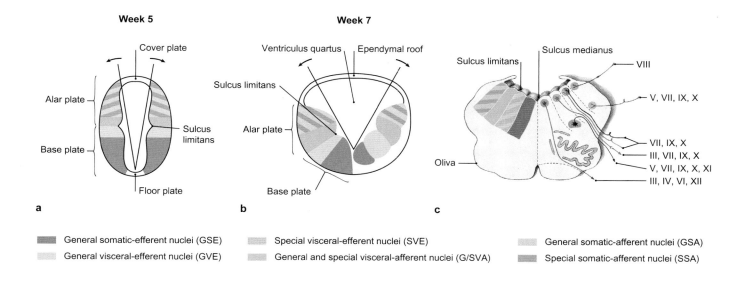

Week 5 **Week 7**

General somatic-efferent nuclei (GSE)
General visceral-efferent nuclei (GVE)

Special visceral-efferent nuclei (SVE)
General and special visceral-afferent nuclei (G/SVA)

General somatic-afferent nuclei (GSA)
Special somatic-afferent nuclei (SSA)

Fig. 12.124a–c Development of the rhombencephalon and mediolateral arrangement of the nuclei of the cranial nerves, according to their function.

a The primary arrangement in the neural tube has a dorsoventral orientation (week 5 of development). [S702-L126]/[R247-L318]
b This arrangement changes gradually with the enlargement of the Canalis centralis to the fourth ventricle (in week 7 of development), and becomes a mediolateral arrangement. [S702-L126]/[R247-L318]
c The individual fibre qualities are assigned to the respective nuclei of the cranial nerves. [S700]

In the brainstem, nuclei with similar functions are arranged one on top of the other from the top to the bottom. Due to spatial restrictions, the nuclei form four longitudinal **nuclear columns** parallel to each other. In a medial to lateral direction, this arrangement includes a somatic-efferent, a visceral-efferent, a visceral-afferent, and a somatic-afferent column of nuclei. Within the visceral-efferent, the visceral-afferent and the somatic-afferent columns, a distinction is made between general and special afferent nuclei.

Attribution of the most important cranial nerves to respective pharyngeal arches and corresponding branchiomeric muscles		
Pharyngeal arch	**Nerve of the pharyngeal arch**	**Muscles**
First pharyngeal arch (mandibular arch)	N. trigeminus [V]; N. mandibularis [V/3]	• Muscles of mastication • M. mylohyoideus • Venter anterior musculi digastrici • M. tensor tympani • M. tensor veli palatini
Second pharyngeal arch (hyoid arch)	N. facialis [VII]	• Mimetic muscles • M. stylohyoideus • Venter posterior musculi digastrici • M. stapedius
Third pharyngeal arch	N. glossopharyngeus [IX]	• Pharyngeal muscles • M. stylopharyngeus • M. levator veli palatini
Fourth pharyngeal arch (laryngeal arch)	N. vagus [X] with N. laryngeus superior	• Laryngeal muscles • Pharyngeal muscles: M. cricothyroideus
Fifth pharyngeal arch	– regresses –	– regresses –
Sixth pharyngeal arch	N. vagus [X] with N. laryngeus inferior (N. recurrens)	• Inner laryngeal muscles • Upper oesophageal muscles

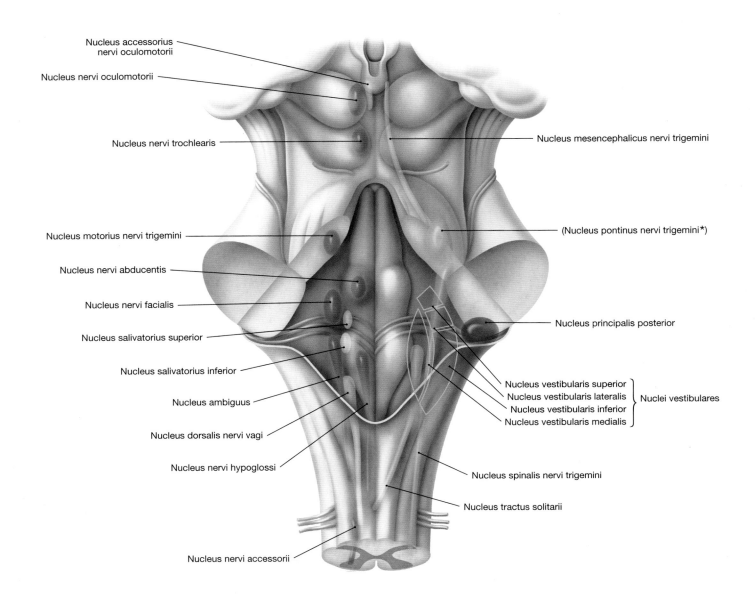

Nucleus accessorius nervi oculomotorii

Nucleus nervi oculomotorii

Nucleus nervi trochlearis

Nucleus mesencephalicus nervi trigemini

Nucleus motorius nervi trigemini

(Nucleus pontinus nervi trigemini*)

Nucleus nervi abducentis

Nucleus nervi facialis

Nucleus salivatorius superior

Nucleus principalis posterior

Nucleus salivatorius inferior

Nucleus vestibularis superior
Nucleus vestibularis lateralis
Nucleus vestibularis inferior
Nucleus vestibularis medialis

Nuclei vestibulares

Nucleus ambiguus

Nucleus dorsalis nervi vagi

Nucleus nervi hypoglossi

Nucleus spinalis nervi trigemini

Nucleus tractus solitarii

Nucleus nervi accessorii

Fig. 12.125 Cranial nerves, Nn. craniales; topographical overview of the nuclei; posterior view. [S700-L275/S700-L238]
With the exception of the cranial nerves I and II, all cranial nerves (III–XII) have nuclei located in the brainstem. The **nuclei** of the cranial nerves III and IV are located in the mesencephalon, the nuclei of the cranial nerves V to VII in the pons, and the nuclei of the cranial nerves VIII to XII in the Medulla oblongata.
It is easier to understand the arrangement of the nuclei of the cranial nerves if one keeps in mind their classification in functionally different

nuclear columns (→ Fig. 12.124). On the left, the nuclei of origin (Nuclei originis) are represented, which contain the perikarya of the efferent neurons running towards the periphery. In the terminal nuclei (Nucleus terminationis) shown on the right, the afferent fibres arriving from the periphery are synapsed onto the second neuron of the sensory tract.

* clin.: Nucleus sensorius principalis nervi trigemini

→ T 59

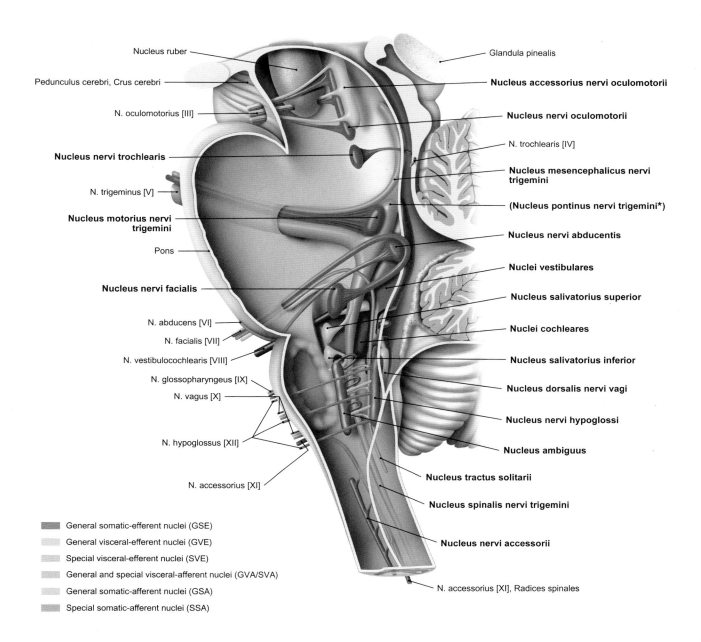

Nucleus ruber

Pedunculus cerebri, Crus cerebri

N. oculomotorius [III]

Nucleus nervi trochlearis

N. trigeminus [V]

Nucleus motorius nervi trigemini

Pons

Nucleus nervi facialis

N. abducens [VI]

N. facialis [VII]

N. vestibulocochlearis [VIII]

N. glossopharyngeus [IX]

N. vagus [X]

N. hypoglossus [XII]

N. accessorius [XI]

Glandula pinealis

Nucleus accessorius nervi oculomotorii

Nucleus nervi oculomotorii

N. trochlearis [IV]

Nucleus mesencephalicus nervi trigemini

(Nucleus pontinus nervi trigemini*)

Nucleus nervi abducentis

Nuclei vestibulares

Nucleus salivatorius superior

Nuclei cochleares

Nucleus salivatorius inferior

Nucleus dorsalis nervi vagi

Nucleus nervi hypoglossi

Nucleus ambiguus

Nucleus tractus solitarii

Nucleus spinalis nervi trigemini

Nucleus nervi accessorii

N. accessorius [XI], Radices spinales

General somatic-efferent nuclei (GSE)

General visceral-efferent nuclei (GVE)

Special visceral-efferent nuclei (SVE)

General and special visceral-afferent nuclei (GVA/SVA)

General somatic-afferent nuclei (GSA)

Special somatic-afferent nuclei (SSA)

Fig. 12.126 Cranial nerves, Nn. craniales; topographical overview of the nuclei of the cranial nerves III to XII in the median plane. [S700-L275/S700-L238]

The nuclei of origin (Nuclei originis) with the cell bodies of efferent or motor nerve fibres are divided into:

- general somatic-efferent nuclei (Nuclei nervi oculomotorii [III, extra-ocular muscles], trochlearis [IV, M. obliquus superior], abducentis [VI, M. rectus lateralis] and hypoglossi [XII, muscles of the tongue])
- general visceral-efferent nuclei (Nuclei accessorius nervi oculomoto-rii [III, Mm. sphincter pupillae and ciliaris], salivatorius superior [VII, Glandulae submandibularis, sublingualis, lacrimalis, nasales and pa-latinales], salivatorius inferior [IX, Glandula parotidea], dorsalis nervi vagi [X, viscera])
- special visceral-efferent nuclei (Nuclei motorius nervi trigemini [V, muscles of mastication and of the floor of the mouth], nervi facialis [VII, mimetic muscles], ambiguus [IX, X, Radix cranialis of XI, pharyn-geal and laryngeal muscles], and Nucleus nervi accessorii [XI, Radix spinalis, shoulder muscles]).

The terminal nuclei (Nuclei terminationis) as the targets of afferent or sensory nerve fibres, are divided into:

- general visceral-afferent nuclei (Nuclei tractus solitarii, Pars inferior [IX, X, sensory innervation of smooth muscles (viscera)])
- special visceral-afferent nuclei (Nuclei tractus solitarii, Pars superior [VII, IX, X], taste fibres)
- general somatic-afferent nuclei (Nuclei mesencephalicus nervi tri-gemini [V, proprioception in the muscles of mastication], pontinus (sensorius principalis) nervi trigemini [V, touch, vibration, position of temporomandibular joint], spinalis nervi trigemini [V, pain and tem-perature sensation in the head region])
- special somatic-afferent nuclei (Nuclei vestibulares superior, latera-lis, medialis and inferior [VIII, vestibular part, equilibrium], as well as Nuclei cochleares anterior and posterior [VIII, cochlear part, hearing]).

* clin.: Nucleus sensorius principalis nervi trigemini

→ T 59

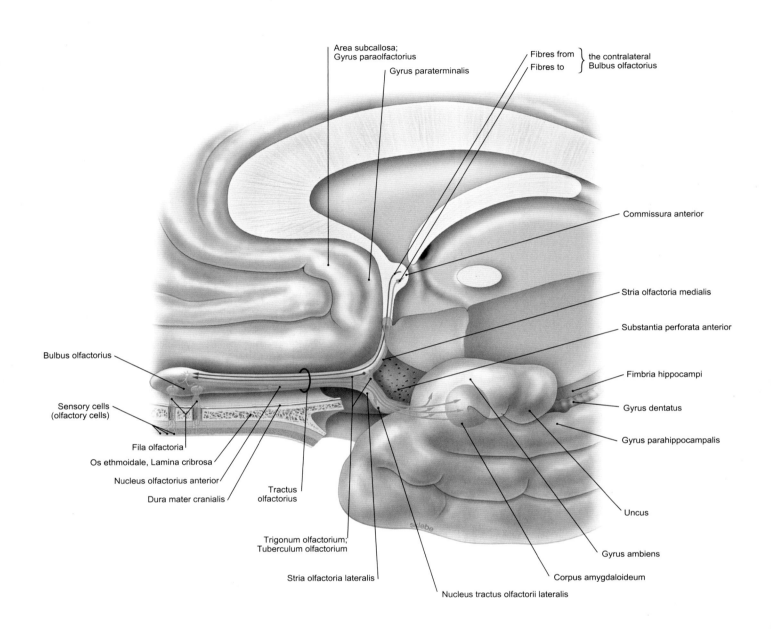

Area subcallosa;
Gyrus paraolfactorius

Gyrus paraterminalis

Fibres from ⎫ the contralateral
Fibres to ⎭ Bulbus olfactorius

Commissura anterior

Stria olfactoria medialis

Substantia perforata anterior

Bulbus olfactorius

Fimbria hippocampi

Sensory cells
(olfactory cells)

Gyrus dentatus

Gyrus parahippocampalis

Fila olfactoria

Os ethmoidale, Lamina cribrosa

Nucleus olfactorius anterior

Tractus
olfactorius

Dura mater cranialis

Uncus

Trigonum olfactorium;
Tuberculum olfactorium

Gyrus ambiens

Stria olfactoria lateralis

Corpus amygdaloideum

Nucleus tractus olfactorii lateralis

Fig. 12.127 N. olfactorius [I], with the olfactory nerves, Nn. olfactorii (Fila olfactoria), and the olfactory tract; view from the left side. [S700-L238]
An area of 3 cm² of olfactory mucosa (Regio olfactoria) is located on both sides at the roof of the nasal cavity. It contains approx. 30 million receptor cells (olfactory sensory cells) which respond to chemical signals. On the one hand, these bipolar nerve cells (olfactory neurons, first neuron, SVA) are connected to the outer environment, and on the other hand they form the **Fila olfactoria** with their axons. Olfactory neurons have a short life span of 30–60 days and are constantly throughout

one's life replaced by neuronal stem cells. The Fila olfactoria in total are referred to as the N. olfactorius [I]. In each olfactory bulb, they converge onto approx. 1,000 **glomeruli.** From there, the olfactory information is transmitted to different areas of the cranial base and the temporal lobe (primary olfactory cortical areas). From here it is transferred via direct and indirect connections to secondary olfactory cortical areas and other regions of the brain, such as the hypothalamus. Here, the conscious perception of smell takes place and becomes associated with other sensory perceptions.

→ T 60.1

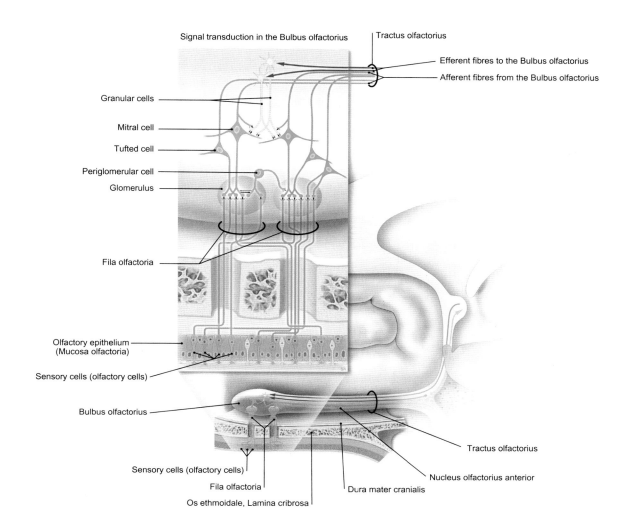

Signal transduction in the Bulbus olfactorius | Tractus olfactorius

Efferent fibres to the Bulbus olfactorius

Afferent fibres from the Bulbus olfactorius

Granular cells

Mitral cell

Tufted cell

Periglomerular cell

Glomerulus

Fila olfactoria

Olfactory epithelium (Mucosa olfactoria)

Sensory cells (olfactory cells)

Bulbus olfactorius

Sensory cells (olfactory cells)

Fila olfactoria

Os ethmoidale, Lamina cribrosa

Dura mater cranialis

Tractus olfactorius

Nucleus olfactorius anterior

Fig. 12.128 Projection and synaptic circuits schematic of the Fila olfactoria; view from the left side. [S700-L238]

In each bulbus, all Fila olfactoria converge in the olfactory bulb onto approx. 1,000 **glomeruli** (as shown in the figure for two glomeruli) which collectively form the Tractus olfactorius. Via numerous synapses in the glomeruli the signals are switched onto **mitral cells** (second neuron).

Thereby, with their axons, all neurons possessing the identical olfactory receptor reach the exact glomerulus that is specific to that particular one, out of the approx. 1,000 different olfactory receptors. Mitral cells of the olfactory bulb project to different areas at the cranial base and the temporal lobe (→ Fig. 12.127). Feedback mechanisms for better differentiation of the stimuli act upon granular cells between the mitral cells.

Clinical remarks

Viral infections, chronic sinusitis, airway obstruction due to congestion of the olfactory mucosa, e.g. allergic reaction, side effects of medication, brain tumours or head trauma with injury to the olfactory nerves along their passage through the Lamina cribrosa, can result in **hyposmia** (decreased perception of olfactory sensations) or **anosmia** (inability to perceive olfactory sensations).

N. opticus [II]

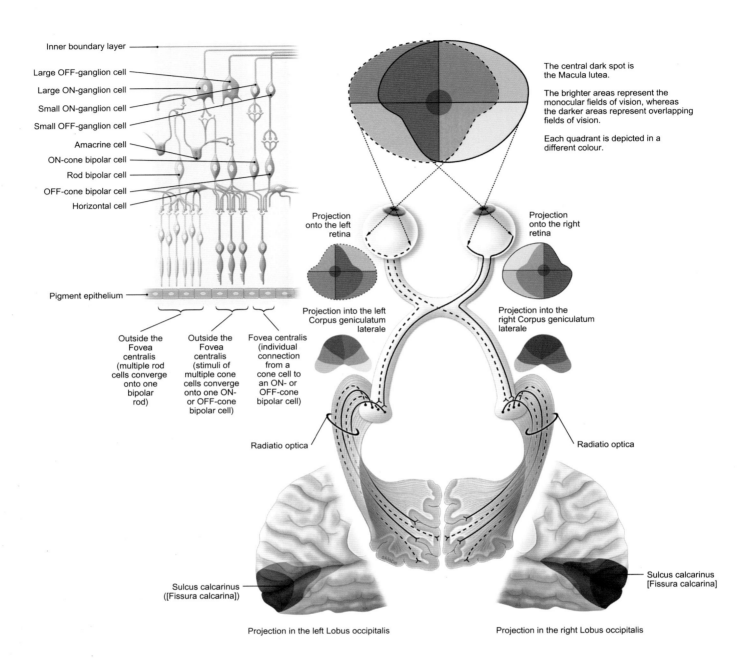

Inner boundary layer

Large OFF-ganglion cell

Large ON-ganglion cell

Small ON-ganglion cell

Small OFF-ganglion cell

Amacrine cell

ON-cone bipolar cell

Rod bipolar cell

OFF-cone bipolar cell

Horizontal cell

Pigment epithelium

Outside the Fovea centralis (multiple rod cells converge onto one bipolar rod)

Outside the Fovea centralis (stimuli of multiple cone cells converge onto one ON- or OFF-cone bipolar cell)

Fovea centralis (individual connection from a cone cell to an ON- or OFF-cone bipolar cell)

The central dark spot is the Macula lutea.

The brighter areas represent the monocular fields of vision, whereas the darker areas represent overlapping fields of vision.

Each quadrant is depicted in a different colour.

Projection onto the left retina

Projection onto the right retina

Projection into the left Corpus geniculatum laterale

Projection into the right Corpus geniculatum laterale

Radiatio optica

Radiatio optica

Sulcus calcarinus ([Fissura calcarina])

Sulcus calcarinus [Fissura calcarina]

Projection in the left Lobus occipitalis

Projection in the right Lobus occipitalis

Fig. 12.129 Neuronal circuit in the retina and central visual pathway; highly simplified schematic representation. [S700-L238] **Cone cells** (first neuron) send the information to **cone bipolar cells** (second neuron) and from here to a **ganglion cell** (third neuron). Horizontal and amacrine cells have a modifying effect on the transmission of information. The axons of the ganglionic cells join to form the N. opticus [II]. The illustrated circuitry of an **intraretinal chain** of three neurons only applies to cone cells (for rod cells → Fig. 9.79 and textbooks of histology). For the visual pathway → Fig. 9.79 and → Fig. 9.81.

→ T 60.2

Clinical remarks

A sudden, potentially reversible unilateral loss of vision can indicate an acute inflammation of the optic nerve **(neuritis of the optic nerve, retrobulbar neuritis).** The examining physician cannot see that the eye itself is hardly affected or not at all. The patient is also unable to see anything with the affected eye. In about one-third of the cases, neuritis of the optic nerve is the first symptom of multiple sclerosis (MS), a relatively frequent autoimmune disease of the central nervous system.

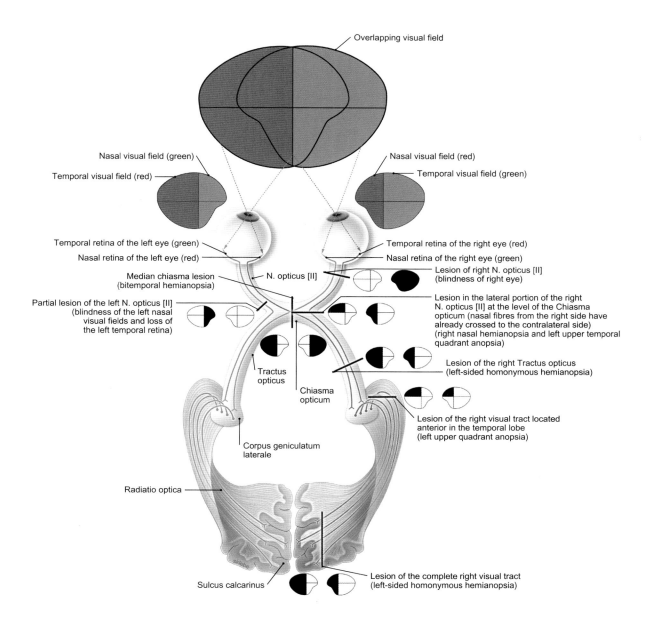

Overlapping visual field

Nasal visual field (green)

Temporal visual field (red)

Nasal visual field (red)

Temporal visual field (green)

Temporal retina of the left eye (green)

Nasal retina of the left eye (red)

Median chiasma lesion
(bitemporal hemianopsia)

N. opticus [II]

Temporal retina of the right eye (red)

Nasal retina of the right eye (green)

Lesion of right N. opticus [II]
(blindness of right eye)

Partial lesion of the left N. opticus [II]
(blindness of the left nasal
visual fields and loss of
the left temporal retina)

Lesion in the lateral portion of the right
N. opticus [II] at the level of the Chiasma
opticum (nasal fibres from the right side have
already crossed to the contralateral side)
(right nasal hemianopsia and left upper temporal
quadrant anopsia)

Tractus
opticus

Chiasma
opticum

Lesion of the right Tractus opticus
(left-sided homonymous hemianopsia)

Corpus geniculatum
laterale

Lesion of the right visual tract located
anterior in the temporal lobe
(left upper quadrant anopsia)

Radiatio optica

Sulcus calcarinus

Lesion of the complete right visual tract
(left-sided homonymous hemianopsia)

Fig. 12.130   N. opticus [II] and visual pathway. [S700-L238]/[R363]
The visual pathway starts within the retina. Here, the first three projection neurons and interneurons (horizontal and amacrine cells) of the visual pathway can be found (→ Fig. 9.81).
Up to 40 **rod cells** transmit their signals to a **bipolar rod** which sends these signals indirectly via amacrine cells (20–50 different types of these cells have now been described in the literature) to a single **ganglion cell** (thus, the first four neurons of the rod cells can be found in the retina). The axons of ganglion cells run in the N. opticus [II] to the **Chiasma opticum.** Here, the fibres from the nasal part of the retina

cross to the opposite side (red). The fibres of the temporal part do not cross (green).
The chiasma is directly followed by the Tractus opticus, which contains fibres conveying information of the opposite (contralateral) half of the visual field. The majority of these fibres (Radix lateralis) is switched in the Corpus geniculatum laterale (CGL). Some fibres (Radix medialis) already branch off before reaching the CGL, and project into the Area pretectalis, the Colliculus superior and the hypothalamus. Via the **GRATIOLET's optic radiation** (Radiatio optica), the fibres from the Corpus geniculatum laterale pass in the region of the Sulcus calcarinus to the areas 17 and 18 of the cerebral cortex (Area striata).

Clinical remarks

- Lesions of the N. opticus [II] which are located anterior to the Chiasma opticum, e.g. after a traumatic head injury, result in blindness of the affected eye (→ Fig. 12.130).
- Lateral lesions of the N. opticus [II] at the level of the Chiasma opticum (nasal fibres from the right side have already crossed to the opposite side), e.g. due to a tumour, result in a right nasal **hemianopsia** and **quadrant anopsia** of the left upper temporal quadrant (→ Fig. 12.130).
- Median lesions of the Chiasma opticum, mostly due to pituitary tumours, result in a bitemporal hemianopsia (→ Fig. 12.130).

- Lesions of the Tractus opticus (on the right side in the schematic), e.g. caused by a haemorrhage, result in a left-sided homonymous hemianopsia (→ Fig. 12.130).
- Lesions of the anterior part of the optic radiation located in the temporal lobe (on the right side in the schematic), e.g. due to ischaemia, result in anopsia of the left upper quadrant (→ Fig. 12.130).
- Lesions of the entire optic radiation (on the right side in the schematic), e.g. caused by massive bleeding, result in a left-sided homonymous hemianopsia (→ Fig. 12.130).

N. oculomotorius [III], N. trochlearis [IV], N. abducens [VI]

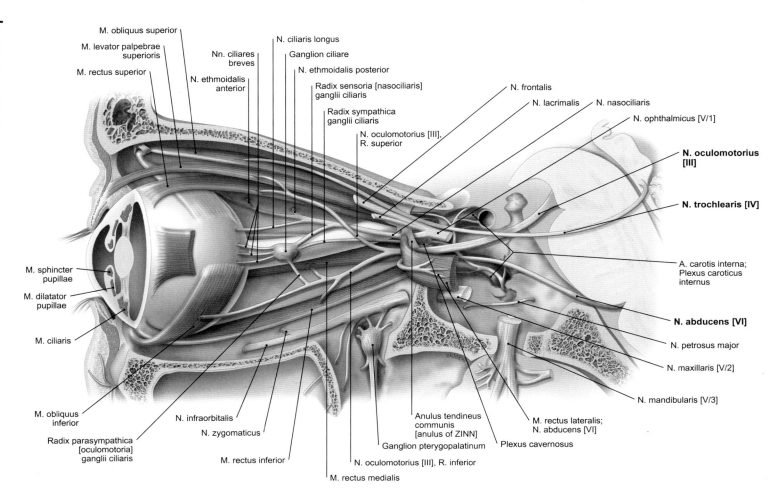

M. obliquus superior

M. levator palpebrae superioris

M. rectus superior

Nn. ciliares breves

N. ethmoidalis anterior

N. ciliaris longus

Ganglion ciliare

N. ethmoidalis posterior

Radix sensoria [nasociliaris] ganglii ciliaris

Radix sympathica ganglii ciliaris

N. oculomotorius [III], R. superior

N. frontalis

N. lacrimalis

N. nasociliaris

N. ophthalmicus [V/1]

N. oculomotorius [III]

N. trochlearis [IV]

A. carotis interna; Plexus caroticus internus

M. sphincter pupillae

M. dilatator pupillae

M. ciliaris

N. abducens [VI]

N. petrosus major

N. maxillaris [V/2]

N. mandibularis [V/3]

M. obliquus inferior

N. infraorbitalis

N. zygomaticus

Radix parasympathica [oculomotoria] ganglii ciliaris

M. rectus inferior

Anulus tendineus communis [anulus of ZINN]

Ganglion pterygopalatinum

N. oculomotorius [III], R. inferior

M. rectus medialis

M. rectus lateralis; N. abducens [VI]

Plexus cavernosus

Fig. 12.131   N. oculomotorius [III], N. trochlearis [IV] and N. abducens [VI], left side; lateral view; the orbit has been opened, the orbital fat body removed, the M. rectus lateralis has been severed near its insertion and folded back. [S700-L238]
The N. oculomotorius [III] innervates the extraocular muscles with the exception of the M. obliquus superior (N. trochlearis [IV]) and the

M. rectus lateralis (N. abducens [VI]). The third cranial nerve [CNIII] also supplies two intraocular muscles with its parasympathetic parts, the M. sphincter pupillae and M. ciliaris.

→ T 60.3, T 60.4, T 60.6

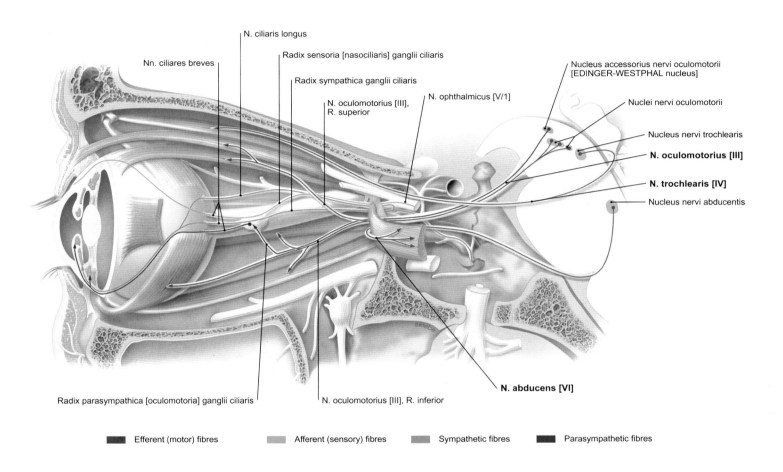

Fig. 12.132 Fibre qualities of the Nn. oculomotorius [III], trochlearis [IV] and abducens [VI], left side; lateral view. [S700-L238]

The **N. oculomotorius [III]** contains motor fibres (GSE) of the Nucleus nervi oculomotorii which supply the major part of the extraocular muscles. Within the orbit, the nerve divides into two branches: its R. superior innervates the M. rectus superior and M. levator palpebrae superioris, and its R. inferior innervates the M. rectus medialis, M. rectus inferior and M. obliquus inferior. Parasympathetic fibres (GVE) originating from the Nucleus accessorius nervi oculomotorii [EDINGER-WESTPHAL] pass via the R. inferior and Radix parasympathica (oculomotoria)

to the Ganglion ciliare. Here, the preganglionic parasympathetic fibres are switched to postganglionic fibres, which accompany the Nn. ciliares breves to the Bulbus oculi and pass via its wall to the M. ciliaris and M. sphincter pupillae.

The **N. trochlearis [IV]** contains motor fibres (GSE) of the Nucleus nervi trochlearis located in the brainstem which supply the M. obliquus superior.

The **N. abducens [VI]** contains motor fibres (GSE) of the Nucleus nervi abducentis which innervate the M. rectus lateralis.

Clinical remarks

Lesions of individual cranial nerves supplying the extraocular muscles lead to paralysis of the corresponding eye muscles with deviation of the eyeball. The direction and extent of such deviations depend on the predominant action of the muscles which are still intact (and thereby the nerves which are also still intact) against the paralysed muscles. For more details → Fig. 9.48.

Unilateral palsies of the abducent and oculomotor nerves in combination with sensory deficits of the first trigeminal branch (N. ophthalmicus [V/1]) indicate diseases of the Sinus cavernosus (**cavernous sinus syndrome:** cavernous sinus thrombosis, tumour, metastasis, aneurysm of the A. carotis interna, inflammatory infiltration). If an acute onset of the symptoms is combined with clinical signs of a drainage disorder such as venous congestion of the orbit, eyelid and conjunctival swelling, and protrusion of the eyeball, this might indicate a venous thrombosis and/or a fistula between the A. carotis interna and the Sinus cavernosus.

Cranial nerves

N. oculomotorius [III]

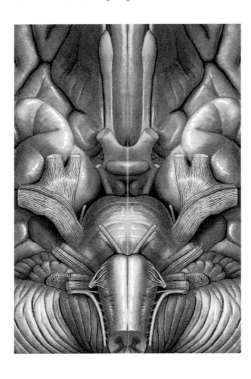

Fig. 12.133   Exit site of the N. oculomotorius [III] at the brainstem; inferior view. [S700]
The third cranial nerve [CNIII] exits directly above the pons.

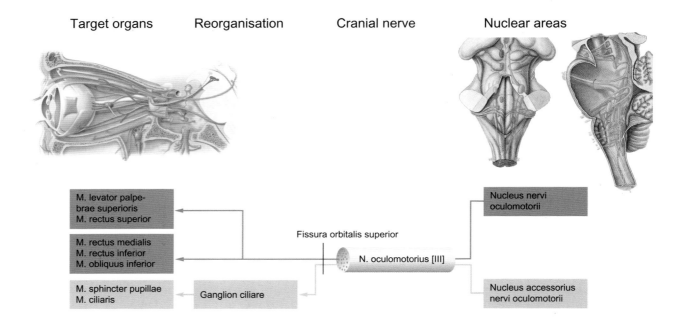

Target organs	Reorganisation	Cranial nerve	Nuclear areas

M. levator palpe-brae superioris
M. rectus superior

M. rectus medialis
M. rectus inferior
M. obliquus inferior

M. sphincter pupillae
M. ciliaris

Ganglion ciliare

Fissura orbitalis superior

N. oculomotorius [III]

Nucleus nervi oculomotorii

Nucleus accessorius nervi oculomotorii

Fig. 12.134   Pathway, branches and fibre qualities of the N. oculomotorius [III]; lateral view. [S700-L127/L238] Compare → Fig. 12.132

Clinical remarks

A complete **palsy of the oculomotor nerve** results in drooping of the eyelid **(ptosis)** across the visual axis caused by the failure of the M. levator palpebrae superioris. Paralysis of the Mm. rectus superior, rectus medialis, rectus inferior and obliquus inferior coincides with the **Bulbus oculi being directed outwards and downwards** (which depends on the contraction of the still intact Mm. rectus lateralis and obliquus superior). Because the M. sphincter pupillae is paralysed as well, the pupil is dilated **(mydriasis)** due to the outweighing action of the sympathetically innervated M. dilatator pupillae. In addition, due to the failure of the M. ciliaris, the near-point accommodation of the eye does not function, and due to the failure of the M. rectus medialis, the convergence reaction no longer works on one side. The patient complains of double images as soon as the affected eyelid is pulled up by the examiner or the patient themselves.

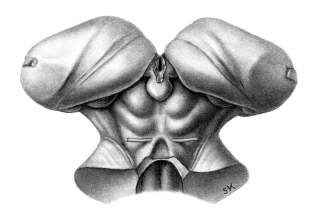

Fig. 12.135 Exit site of the N. trochlearis [IV] at the brainstem; dorsal view. [S700-L238]

The fourth cranial nerve [CNIV] exits below the Colliculi inferiores.

Target organ   Cranial nerve   Nuclear area

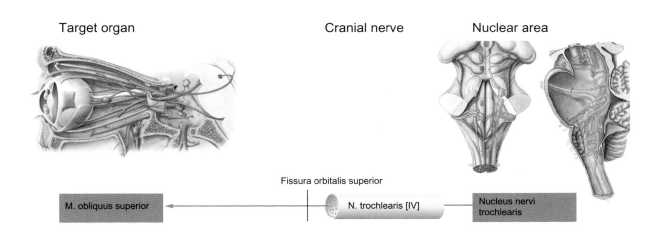

Fissura orbitalis superior

M. obliquus superior ← | → N. trochlearis [IV] ← Nucleus nervi trochlearis

Fig. 12.136 Pathway, branches and fibre qualities of the N. trochlearis [IV]; lateral view. [S700-L127/L238] Compare → Fig. 12.132

Clinical remarks

In the case of a **trochlear nerve palsy,** the failure of the M. obliquus superior and outweighing action of all other extraocular muscles result in the turning of the eyeball in a superior nasal direction. The patients report double images, especially when looking downwards nasally. They attempt to compensate for it by tilting their head to the healthy side.

Cranial nerves

N. trigeminus [V]

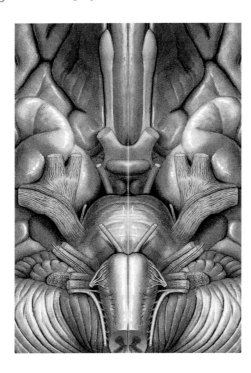

Fig. 12.137   Exit site of the N. trigeminus [V] at the brainstem; inferior view. [S700]
The fifth cranial nerve [CNV] exits on the outside of the pons.

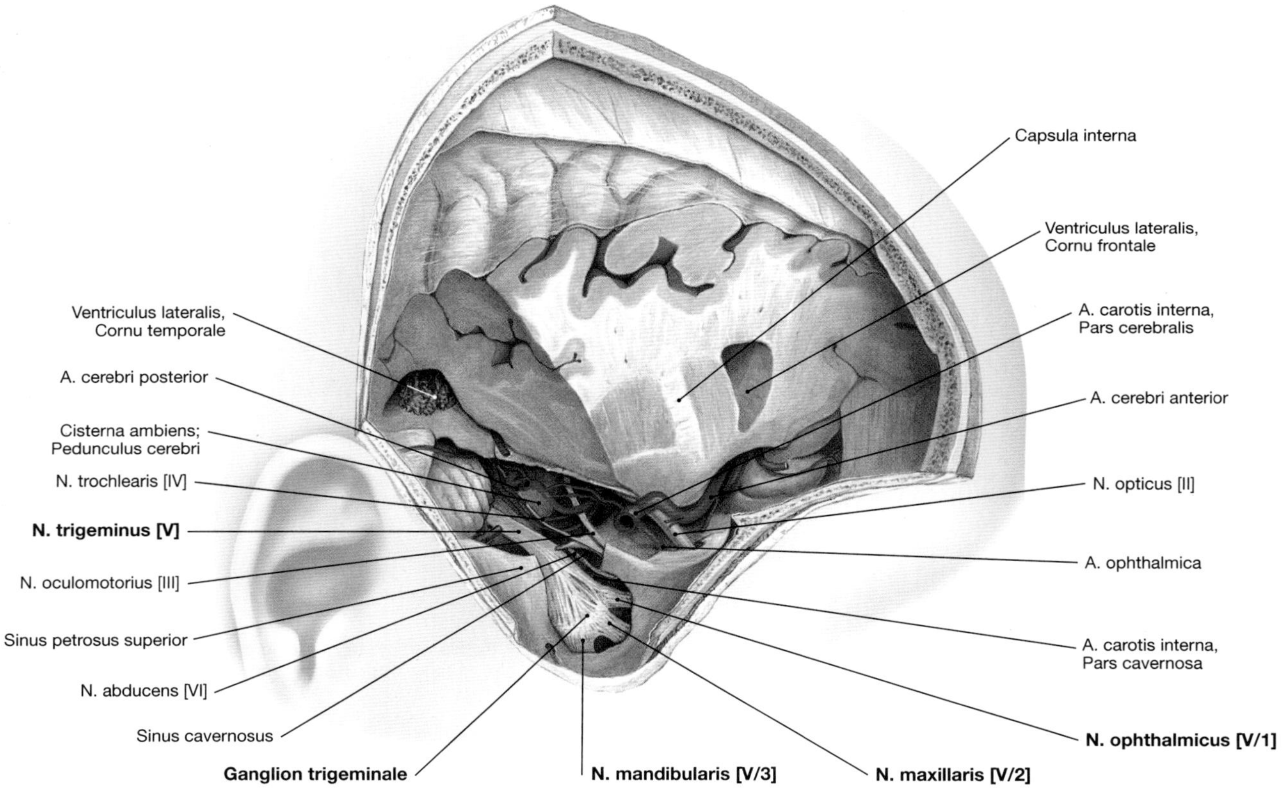

Capsula interna

Ventriculus lateralis,
Cornu frontale

A. carotis interna,
Pars cerebralis

A. cerebri anterior

N. opticus [II]

A. ophthalmica

A. carotis interna,
Pars cavernosa

N. ophthalmicus [V/1]

Ventriculus lateralis,
Cornu temporale

A. cerebri posterior

Cisterna ambiens;
Pedunculus cerebri

N. trochlearis [IV]

N. trigeminus [V]

N. oculomotorius [III]

Sinus petrosus superior

N. abducens [VI]

Sinus cavernosus

Ganglion trigeminale

N. mandibularis [V/3]

N. maxillaris [V/2]

Fig. 12.138   Pathway of the N. trigeminus [V] in the middle cranial fossa, Fossa cranii media; view from the right side. [S700]
Large parts of the frontal and temporal lobes were removed to provide a clear view onto the cranial base below. In addition, the Cavum trigeminale (MECKEL's cave) was opened. Located within is the **Ganglion trigeminale** (Ganglion semilunare, clin.: Ganglion GASSERI), from which the three main branches of the N. trigeminus originate (N. oph-thalmicus [V/1], N. maxillaris [V/2], N. mandibularis [V/3]). Besides the N. trigeminus [V], the passage of the N. opticus [II], N. oculomotorius [III] and N. trochlearis [IV] in this region of the cranial base are visible, as well as arteries branching off the Pars cerebralis of the A. carotis interna (A. ophthalmica, A. cerebri anterior).

→ T 60.5

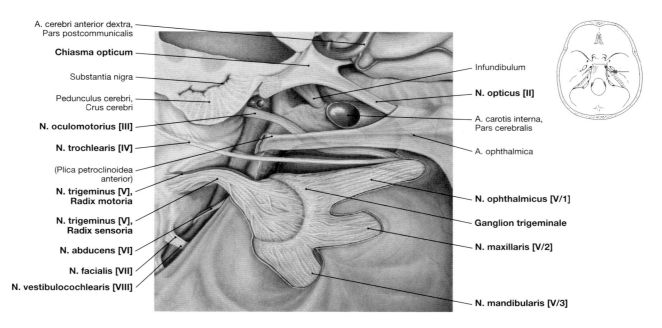

A. cerebri anterior dextra, Pars postcommunicalis
Chiasma opticum
Substantia nigra
Pedunculus cerebri, Crus cerebri
N. oculomotorius [III]
N. trochlearis [IV]
(Plica petroclinoidea anterior)
N. trigeminus [V], Radix motoria
N. trigeminus [V], Radix sensoria
N. abducens [VI]
N. facialis [VII]
N. vestibulocochlearis [VIII]

Infundibulum
N. opticus [II]
A. carotis interna, Pars cerebralis
A. ophthalmica
N. ophthalmicus [V/1]
Ganglion trigeminale
N. maxillaris [V/2]
N. mandibularis [V/3]

Fig. 12.139   Arteries and nerves in the region of the Sella turcica and Sinus cavernosus; view from the right side. [S700]
The Cavum trigeminale (MECKEL's cave) is opened after removal of the Dura mater cranialis and the Arachnoidea mater at this location. Thus, the Ganglion trigeminale (Ganglion semilunare, clin.: Ganglion GASSE-RI) is visible with the bifurcation of the three trigeminal nerve branches.

In addition, the pathway of the cranial nerves III, IV, and VI to VIII can be seen from their exit from the brainstem up to their entrance at the cranial base. The Pars cavernosa of the A. carotis interna continues as Pars cerebralis and joins the N. opticus [II]. The Chiasma opticum is located above the stalk of the pituitary gland (infundibulum).

→ T 60

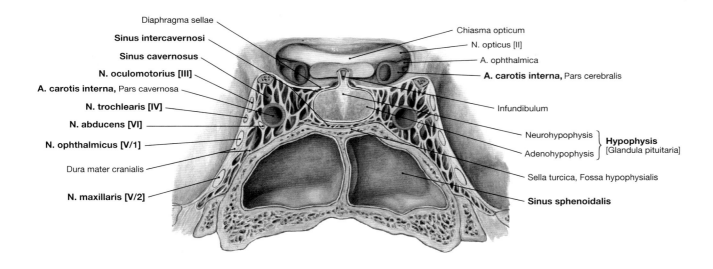

Diaphragma sellae
Sinus intercavernosi
Sinus cavernosus
N. oculomotorius [III]
A. carotis interna, Pars cavernosa
N. trochlearis [IV]
N. abducens [VI]
N. ophthalmicus [V/1]
Dura mater cranialis
N. maxillaris [V/2]

Chiasma opticum
N. opticus [II]
A. ophthalmica
A. carotis interna, Pars cerebralis
Infundibulum
Neurohypophysis
Adenohypophysis
Hypophysis [Glandula pituitaria]
Sella turcica, Fossa hypophysialis
Sinus sphenoidalis

Fig. 12.140   Arteries and nerves in the region of the Sella turcica and Sinus cavernosus; frontal section; posterior view. [S700]
The N. ophthalmicus [V/1] and N. maxillaris [V/2] run together with the N. oculomotorius [III] and N. trochlearis [IV] inside the wall of the Sinus

cavernosus; the N. abducens [VI] and the A. carotis interna pass centrally through the Sinus cavernosus on both sides; the pituitary gland lies inside the median line and is encompassed by the left and right Sinus cavernosus.

Clinical remarks

Mechanical but also visual (bright light) or acoustic stimuli trigger the **corneal reflex** (eyelid closure reflex, orbicularis oculi reflex, blink re-flex, as an eye-protecting mechanism). This is a multisynaptic reflex, which can be missing in peripheral nerve lesions but also in the context of severe brainstem lesions. It is usually tested by touching the cornea with a cotton swab. Stimulating impulses reach the complex

of the trigeminal nuclei via fibres of the N. ophthalmicus [V/1]. The polysynaptic reflex arc propagates via the Colliculi superiores, the Formatio reticularis and the nuclear complex of the N. facialis [VII], which activates the M. orbicularis oculi with motor fibres and thus triggers the eyelid closure.

N. trigeminus [V]

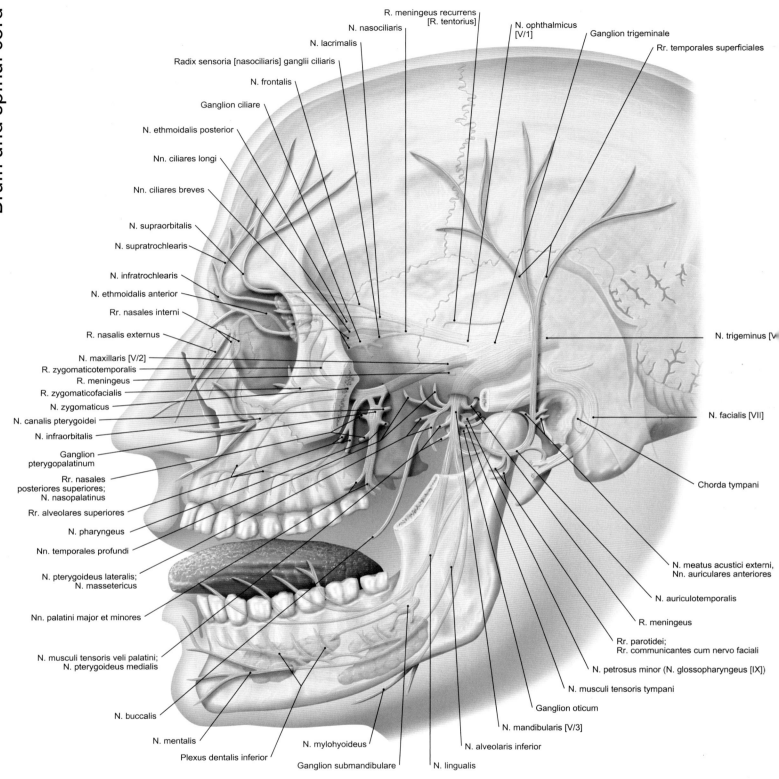

R. meningeus recurrens [R. tentorius]

N. nasociliaris

N. lacrimalis

Radix sensoria [nasociliaris] ganglii ciliaris

N. frontalis

Ganglion ciliare

N. ethmoidalis posterior

Nn. ciliares longi

Nn. ciliares breves

N. supraorbitalis

N. supratrochlearis

N. infratrochlearis

N. ethmoidalis anterior

Rr. nasales interni

R. nasalis externus

N. maxillaris [V/2]

R. zygomaticotemporalis

R. meningeus

R. zygomaticofacialis

N. zygomaticus

N. canalis pterygoidei

N. infraorbitalis

Ganglion pterygopalatinum

Rr. nasales posteriores superiores; N. nasopalatinus

Rr. alveolares superiores

N. pharyngeus

Nn. temporales profundi

N. pterygoideus lateralis; N. massetericus

Nn. palatini major et minores

N. musculi tensoris veli palatini; N. pterygoideus medialis

N. buccalis

N. mentalis

Plexus dentalis inferior

N. mylohyoideus

Ganglion submandibulare

N. lingualis

N. alveolaris inferior

N. mandibularis [V/3]

Ganglion oticum

N. musculi tensoris tympani

N. petrosus minor (N. glossopharyngeus [IX])

N. alveolaris inferior

Rr. parotidei; Rr. communicantes cum nervo faciali

R. meningeus

N. auriculotemporalis

N. meatus acustici externi, Nn. auriculares anteriores

Chorda tympani

N. facialis [VII]

N. trigeminus [V]

Rr. temporales superficiales

Ganglion trigeminale

N. ophthalmicus [V/1]

Fig. 12.141 N. trigeminus [V], left side; lateral view. [S700-L127]
The trigeminal nerve [V] is the nerve of the first pharyngeal arch and consists of three main branches: N. ophthalmicus [V/1] (light green), N. maxillaris [V/2] (orange) and N. mandibularis [V/3] (turquoise). It consists mainly of general somatic-afferent (GSA) fibres. These are completed by special visceral-efferent (SVE) fibres.

The **N. ophthalmicus [V/1]** innervates the eye (including cornea and conjunctiva), the skin of the upper eyelid, forehead, back of the nose, as well as the nasal and paranasal mucous membranes. It is accompanied by parasympathetic fibres for the innervation of the lacrimal gland on its peripheral pathway.

The **N. maxillaris [V/2]** innervates the skin of the anterior temporal region and the upper cheek as well as the skin below the eye. In addi-

tion, it provides sensory innervation to the palate, the teeth and the gingiva of the upper jaw, and the mucosa of the Sinus maxillaris.

The **N. mandibularis [V/3]** innervates the muscles of mastication, and two muscles of the floor of the mouth (M. mylohyoideus, and Venter anterior of the M. digastricus), as well as the M. tensor veli palatini and M. tensor tympani. It contributes sensory branches to the skin of the posterior temporal region, of the cheeks, and the chin, and innervates the teeth and gingiva of the lower jaw. Its branches receive parasympathetic fibres for the innervation of the large salivary glands and taste fibres for the tongue, and also provide sensory innervation to the anterior two-thirds of the tongue.

→ T 60.5

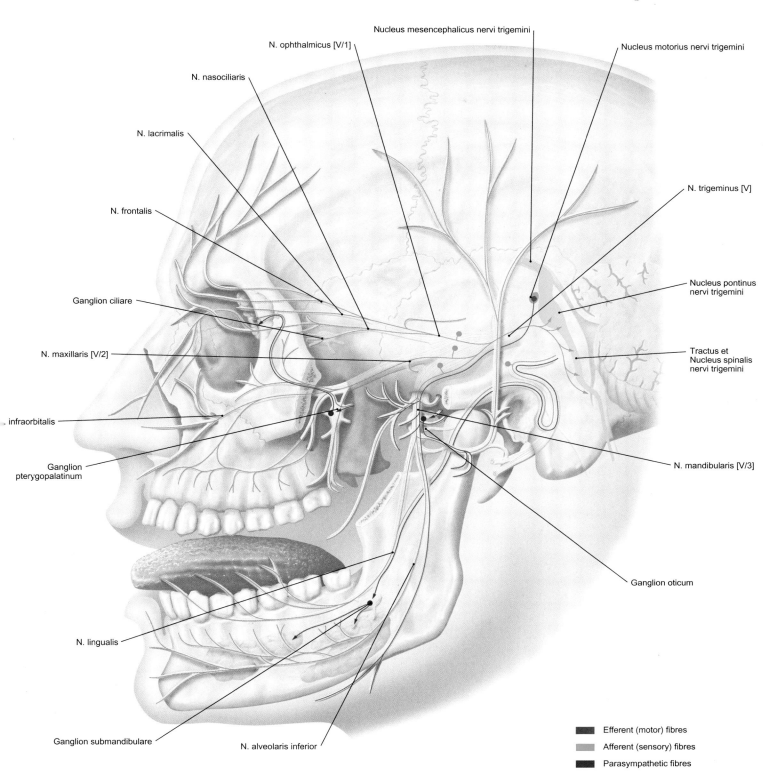

Nucleus mesencephalicus nervi trigemini

N. ophthalmicus [V/1]

N. nasociliaris

N. lacrimalis

N. frontalis

Ganglion ciliare

N. maxillaris [V/2]

. infraorbitalis

Ganglion
pterygopalatinum

N. lingualis

Ganglion submandibulare

N. alveolaris inferior

Nucleus motorius nervi trigemini

N. trigeminus [V]

Nucleus pontinus
nervi trigemini

Tractus et
Nucleus spinalis
nervi trigemini

N. mandibularis [V/3]

Ganglion oticum

Efferent (motor) fibres
Afferent (sensory) fibres
Parasympathetic fibres

Fig. 12.142 **Fibre qualities of the N. trigeminus [V], left side;** lateral view. [S700-L127]
Nuclei of origin and **terminal nuclei** of the N. trigeminus [V] are the Nucleus mesencephalicus nervi trigemini (somatosensory), the Nucleus pontinus (sensorius principalis) nervi trigemini (somatosensory), the Nucleus spinalis nervi trigemini (general somatic-afferent, GSA), and the Nucleus motorius nervi trigemini (special visceral-efferent, SVE).

The N. trigeminus [V] consists of a **Radix sensoria** (Portio major) and a **Radix motoria** (Portio minor). After exiting the pons, the nerve passes across the clivus to the Ganglion trigeminale (Ganglion semilunare, clin.: Ganglion GASSERI; contains pseudo-unipolar nerve cells for the transmission of protopathic and epicritic sensory stimuli to the Nuclei pontinus and spinalis nervi trigemini), and then divides into its three main branches, the N. ophthalmicus [V/1], N. maxillaris [V/2] and N. mandibularis [V/3].

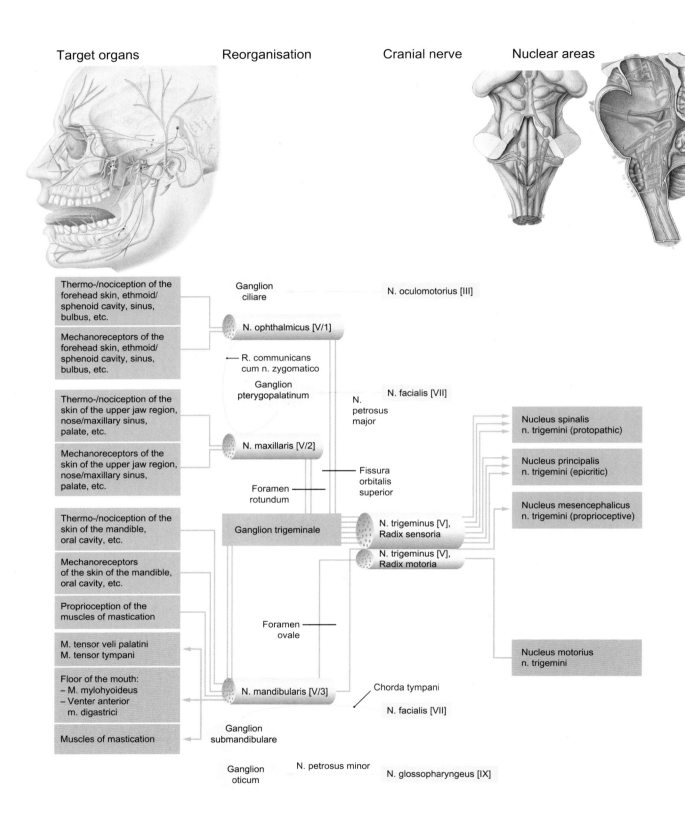

Target organs   Reorganisation   Cranial nerve   Nuclear areas

Thermo-/nociception of the forehead skin, ethmoid/sphenoid cavity, sinus, bulbus, etc.

Mechanoreceptors of the forehead skin, ethmoid/sphenoid cavity, sinus, bulbus, etc.

Thermo-/nociception of the skin of the upper jaw region, nose/maxillary sinus, palate, etc.

Mechanoreceptors of the skin of the upper jaw region, nose/maxillary sinus, palate, etc.

Thermo-/nociception of the skin of the mandible, oral cavity, etc.

Mechanoreceptors of the skin of the mandible, oral cavity, etc.

Proprioception of the muscles of mastication

M. tensor veli palatini
M. tensor tympani

Floor of the mouth:
– M. mylohyoideus
– Venter anterior
 m. digastrici

Muscles of mastication

Ganglion ciliare

N. ophthalmicus [V/1]

R. communicans cum n. zygomatico

Ganglion pterygopalatinum

N. maxillaris [V/2]

Foramen rotundum

Ganglion trigeminale

Foramen ovale

N. mandibularis [V/3]

Ganglion submandibulare

Ganglion oticum

N. oculomotorius [III]

N. facialis [VII]

N. petrosus major

Fissura orbitalis superior

N. trigeminus [V], Radix sensoria

N. trigeminus [V], Radix motoria

Chorda tympani

N. facialis [VII]

N. petrosus minor   N. glossopharyngeus [IX]

Nucleus spinalis n. trigemini (protopathic)

Nucleus principalis n. trigemini (epicritic)

Nucleus mesencephalicus n. trigemini (proprioceptive)

Nucleus motorius n. trigemini

Fig. 12.143 Fibre qualities, cranial nuclei and target organs of the N. trigeminus [V]; lateral view. [S700-L127/L238]

Branches of the N. ophthalmicus [V/1] (exclusively somatic-afferent)

Branch	Minor branches	Innervation area
R. meningeus recurrens [R. tentorius]		Parts of the meninges
N. frontalis	N. supraorbitalis	Skin of the forehead, and mucosa of the frontal sinus
	N. supratrochlearis	Skin and conjunctiva at the medial (nasal) angle of the eye
N. lacrimalis		Lacrimal gland (for the innervation of the excretory duct, it is joined by postganglionic parasympathetic fibres of the N. zygomaticus), skin and conjunctiva of the lateral (temporal) angle of the eye
N. nasociliaris	(→ table below)	Paranasal sinuses, anterior part of the nasal cavity, as well as the iris, Corpus ciliare, and cornea of the eye (→ see table below)

Branches of the N. nasociliaris [from V/1]

Branch	Pathway	Innervation area
Radix sensoria ganglii ciliaris [R. communicans cum ganglio ciliari]	Guides the sensory components to the Ganglion ciliare, from which the Nn. ciliares breves emerge	Eyeball and its conjunctiva (together with the Nn. ciliares longi)
Nn. ciliares longi	Join the N. opticus [II] and accompany the Nn. ciliares breves from the Ganglion ciliare to the Bulbus oculi; they also receive sympathetic fibres from the Plexus caroticus	Eyeball (Bulbus oculi) and its conjunctiva; the sympathetic fibres innervate the M. dilatator pupillae
N. ethmoidalis posterior	Passes through the eponymous foramen to the posterior ethmoidal cells and the sphenoidal sinus	Mucosa of the posterior ethmoidal cells and of the sphenoidal sinus
N. ethmoidalis anterior	Passes through the eponymous foramen back into the anterior cranial fossa, and then through the Lamina cribrosa into the nasal cavity; ending with Rr. nasales externi in the skin of the dorsum of the nose	Mucosa of the anterior nasal cavity and of the anterior ethmoidal cells, skin of the dorsum of the nose
N. infratrochlearis	Runs below the trochlea to the medial angle of the eye	Skin of the medial angle of the eye

Branches of the N. maxillaris [V/2] (exclusively somatic-afferent)

Branch	Minor branches	Innervation area
R. meningeus		Parts of the meninges
N. zygomaticus	R. zygomaticotemporalis	Skin in the temporal region
	R. zygomaticofacialis	Skin in the upper cheek region; for the innervation (of the excretory duct) of the lacrimal gland, its postganglionic parasympathetic fibres accompany the N. zygomaticus, which releases them to the N. lacrimalis
Rr. ganglionares ad ganglion pterygopalatinum	(→ table at the top of the next page)	Guide sensory fibres to the Ganglion pterygopalatinum; for the innervation of palate and nose (→ table at the top of the next page), they are joined by sympathetic and parasympathetic fibres of the Glandulae nasales and palatinae (special visceral-efferent) as well as by taste fibres
N. infraorbitalis	Nn. alveolares superiores with Rr. alveolares superiores posteriores, medii and anteriores	Mucosa of the maxillary sinus, teeth and gingiva of the upper jaw
		Skin and conjunctiva of the lower eyelid, lateral cutaneous region of the nasal wings, skin of the upper lip and lateral cheek region between lower eyelid and upper lip

N. trigeminus [V]

Branches of Rr. ganglionares ad ganglion pterygopalatinum [from V/2]

Branch	Pathway	Innervation area
N. palatinus major	Runs via the Canalis palatinus major via the Foramen palatinum majus	Mucosa of the hard palate, Glandulae palatinae, taste buds of the palate
Nn. palatini minores	Leave the Canalis palatinus major via the Foramina palatina minora	Mucosa of the soft palate, Tonsilla palatina, Glandulae palatinae, taste buds of the palate
Rr. nasales posteriores superiores laterales et mediales	Pass through the Foramen sphenopalatinum into the nasal cavity, and provide the N. nasopalatinus which reaches the hard palate via the Canalis incisivus	Mucosa of the nasal conchae, of the nasal septum, and of the anterior part of the hard palate, upper incisors and gingiva, Glandulae nasales

Branches of the N. mandibularis [V/3] (somatic-afferent and visceral-efferent)

Branch	Minor branches	Innervation area
R. meningeus		Parts of the meninges
N. massetericus		M. masseter
Nn. temporales profundi		M. temporalis
N. pterygoideus lateralis		M. pterygoideus lateralis
N. pterygoideus medialis		M. pterygoideus medialis
N. musculi tensoris veli palatini		M. tensor veli palatini
N. musculi tensoris tympani		M. tensor tympani
N. buccalis		Skin and mucosa of the cheek, and gingiva of the lower jaw
N. auriculotemporalis	Rr. parotidei	Postganglionic parasympathetic fibres of the Ganglion oticum conjoin and innervate the parotid gland
	Rr. communicantes cum nervo faciali	Postganglionic parasympathetic fibres of the Ganglion oticum conjoin and innervate the parotid gland
	N. meatus acustici externi	External auditory tube, tympanic membrane
	Nn. auriculares anteriores	Skin in front of the auricle
	Nn. temporales superficiales	Skin of the posterior temporal region
N. lingualis	Rr. isthmi faucium	Skin of the soft palate
	N. sublingualis	Mucosa of the floor of the mouth
		Sensory innervation of the anterior two-thirds of the tongue, taste fibres of the anterior two-thirds of the tongue in association with preganglionic parasympathetic fibres of the Chorda tympani for the innervation of the Ganglion submandibulare
N. alveolaris inferior		Teeth and gingiva of the lower jaw
	N. mylohyoideus	M. mylohyoideus and Venter anterior of the M. digastricus
	N. mentalis	Skin of the chin

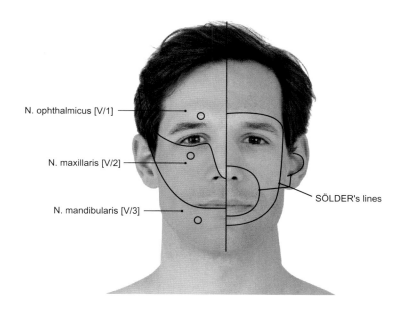

N. ophthalmicus [V/1]

N. maxillaris [V/2]

N. mandibularis [V/3]

SÖLDER's lines

Fig. 12.144 Innervation areas of the facial skin, with nerve exits and protopathic sensibility. [S700-J803]

On the right half of the face, the somatotopic segmentation of the protopathic sensibility is shown. On the left half of the face, the innervation areas and exit sites of the three trigeminal nerve branches are indicated.

Clinical remarks

Particularly in the context of circulatory disorders, **lesions of the N. trigeminus [V]** can occur. Usually only individual nuclei are affected selectively or partially, but rarely the entire N. trigeminus [V]. Such lesions may manifest, for example, as paralysis of the ipsilateral muscles of mastication or as a selective loss of epicritic sensitivity. Afferent fibres of the protopathic sensibility reach the Nucleus spinalis nervi trigemini in a somatotopic order (→ Fig. 12.144). A defined segment of the Nucleus spinalis nervi trigemini innervates a concentric area of the facial skin. To assess the extent of a nuclear lesion, one can therefore test the protopathic sensibility along the concentric **SÖLDER's lines.**

Clinical remarks

Loss of sensibility in the innervation area of a trigeminal branch generally suggests a **peripheral lesion** of the nerve. Potential causes for lesions of the N. ophthalmicus [V/1] and the N. maxillaris [V/2] are a cavernous sinus thrombosis (Clinical remarks for → Fig. 12.132), tumours and fractures of the cranial base. Sensory disturbances in the mandibular region or paralysis of the muscles of mastication often have iatrogenic causes (due to dentistry or surgical treatment).

In the common and not yet completely understood **trigeminal neuralgia** (often thought to be caused by a pathological neurovascular contact between the A. superior cerebelli and the N. trigeminus [V] at its exit site from the brainstem), hypersensitivity of the N. trigeminus [V] results repetitively in acute, strong stabbing pain in the sensory innervation area of the affected trigeminal branch. Even the slightest touch of the corresponding exit sites (→ Fig. 12.144) can trigger extremely severe and stabbing pain attacks.

Neuralgia of the N. ophthalmicus [V/1] can occur as post-zoster neuralgia (after a varicella zoster virus infection of the first trigeminal branch, so-called **zoster ophthalmicus;** or shingles → figure).

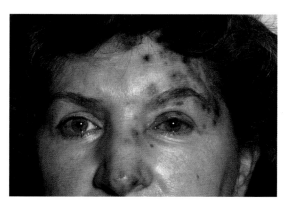

Zoster ophthalmicus. Patient with zoster ophthalmicus (viral infection of the skin in the innervation area of the first trigeminal branch with varicella zoster viruses, the so-called facial herpes zoster or shingles). The involvement of the superficial epithelium of the eye (cornea and conjunctiva) is particularly dangerous (risk of blindness) and painful. The marked redness of the conjunctiva and the narrowed lid of her left eye are clearly visible. [E943]

N. abducens [VI]

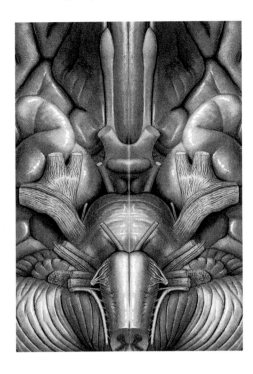

Fig. 12.145   Exit site of the N. abducens [VI] at the brainstem; inferior view. [S700]
The sixth cranial nerve [CNVI] exits below the pons.

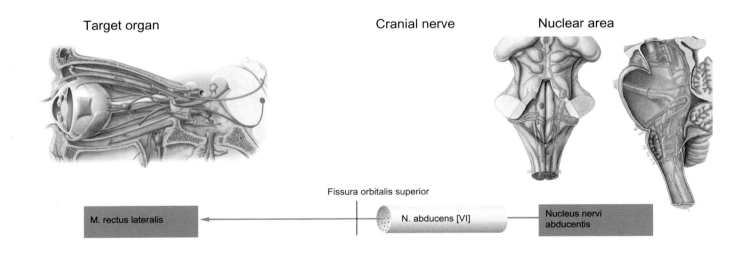

Target organ   Cranial nerve   Nuclear area

Fissura orbitalis superior

M. rectus lateralis ← N. abducens [VI] — Nucleus nervi abducentis

Fig. 12.146   Pathway, branches and fibre qualities of the N. abducens [VI]; lateral view. [S700-L127/L238] Compare → Fig. 12.132

Clinical remarks

Sixth nerve palsy or palsy of the abducent nerve is particularly frequent, due to the long extradural pathway of the N. abducens [VI] along the clivus (with cranial base fractures) and on its passage through the Sinus cavernosus (cavernous sinus thrombosis). If the patient is asked to look to the temporal side, the affected eyeball continues to look straight ahead, since the M. rectus lateralis is paralysed. The patient then has double vision.

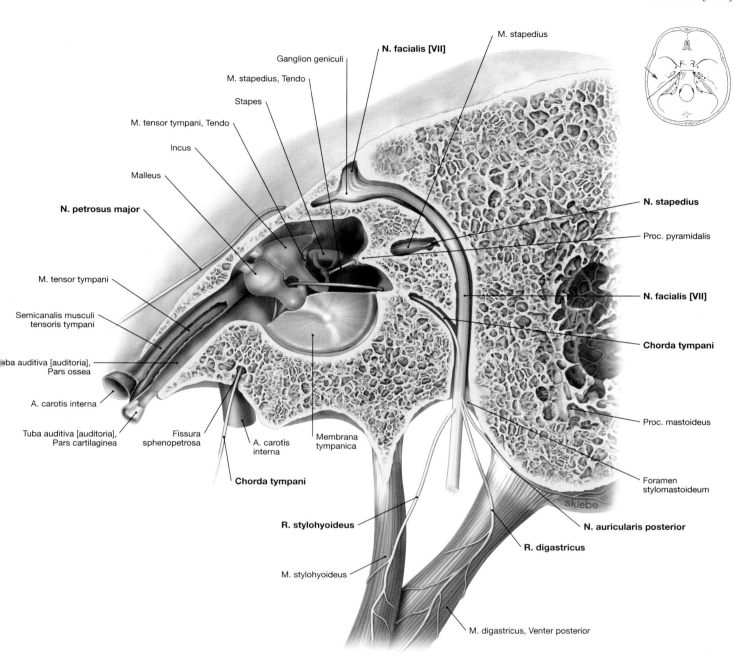

M. stapedius

N. facialis [VII]

Ganglion geniculi

M. stapedius, Tendo

Stapes

M. tensor tympani, Tendo

Incus

Malleus

N. petrosus major

M. tensor tympani

Semicanalis musculi tensoris tympani

...ba auditiva [auditoria], Pars ossea

A. carotis interna

Tuba auditiva [auditoria], Pars cartilaginea

Fissura sphenopetrosa

A. carotis interna

Membrana tympanica

Chorda tympani

R. stylohyoideus

M. stylohyoideus

M. digastricus, Venter posterior

N. stapedius

Proc. pyramidalis

N. facialis [VII]

Chorda tympani

Proc. mastoideus

Foramen stylomastoideum

N. auricularis posterior

R. digastricus

sklebe

Fig. 12.147 Pathway of the N. facialis [VII]; vertical section through the Canalis nervi facialis; view from the left side. [S700-L238]
Approx. 1 cm after entering the petrous part of the temporal bone through the Porus acusticus internus (not shown), the N. facialis [VII] forms its external genu (Ganglion geniculi). The main stem of the nerve runs within a bony canal to the Foramen stylomastoideum. Along its way through the petrous bone, the N. facialis [VII] releases the N. petrosus major, N. stapedius, and the Chorda tympani (→ table for → Fig. 12.151).

→ T 60.7

Clinical remarks

The close topographical relationship of the Canalis facialis to the tympanic cavity can lead to lesions of the N. facialis [VII] in the case of petrous bone fractures, or inflammations of the middle ear and mastoid, as well as during surgical interventions on the middle and inner ear. The symptoms depend on the location of the lesion. If the **lesion is located at or in front of the Ganglion geniculi,** it leads to paralysis of all facial (mimetic) muscles. Furthermore, this results in failure of the M. stapedius (hyperacusis), taste disorders, and impaired secretions of the lacrimal, nasal and salivary glands.
If the **lesion is located below the bifurcation of the N. stapedius,** the sense of taste and secretion functions controlled by the Chorda tympani will be impaired as well as the facial muscles. Due to its unprotected pathway between the malleus and incus, the **Chorda tympani** can also be damaged separately in the case of middle ear infections (Clinical remarks for → Fig. 10.30), or during middle ear and inner ear surgery.
The biggest problem in patients with peripheral facial palsy is a **lagophthalmos** (the eye cannot be closed properly due to paralysis of the M. orbicularis oculi; → Fig. 12.152c), causing the cornea to dry out (leading to blindness, induced by the lack of blinking and reduced production of lacrimal fluid).

N. facialis [VII]

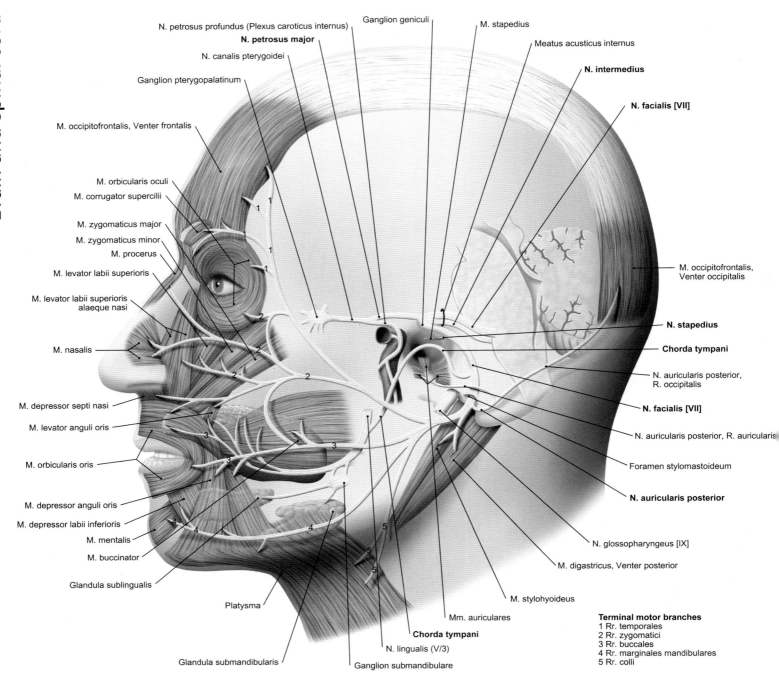

N. petrosus profundus (Plexus caroticus internus)
N. petrosus major
N. canalis pterygoidei
Ganglion pterygopalatinum
M. occipitofrontalis, Venter frontalis
M. orbicularis oculi
M. corrugator supercilii
M. zygomaticus major
M. zygomaticus minor
M. procerus
M. levator labii superioris
M. levator labii superioris alaeque nasi
M. nasalis
M. depressor septi nasi
M. levator anguli oris
M. orbicularis oris
M. depressor anguli oris
M. depressor labii inferioris
M. mentalis
M. buccinator
Glandula sublingualis
Platysma
Glandula submandibularis

Ganglion geniculi
M. stapedius
Meatus acusticus internus
N. intermedius
N. facialis [VII]
M. occipitofrontalis, Venter occipitalis
N. stapedius
Chorda tympani
N. auricularis posterior, R. occipitalis
N. facialis [VII]
N. auricularis posterior, R. auricularis
Foramen stylomastoideum
N. auricularis posterior
N. glossopharyngeus [IX]
M. digastricus, Venter posterior
M. stylohyoideus
Mm. auriculares
Chorda tympani
N. lingualis (V/3)
Ganglion submandibulare

Terminal motor branches
1 Rr. temporales
2 Rr. zygomatici
3 Rr. buccales
4 Rr. marginales mandibulares
5 Rr. colli

Fig. 12.148 N. facialis [VII], left side; lateral view. [S700-L127]
The N. facialis [VII] exits at the cerebellopontine angle together with the N. intermedius (a part of the N. facialis [VII], often viewed as a separate nerve), and the N. vestibulocochlearis [VIII]. After a short distance, the N. intermedius unites with the N. facialis [VII]. The N. facialis [VII] and N. vestibulocochlearis [VIII] run to the Pars petrosa of the Os temporale and enter the bone via the Porus and Meatus acusticus internus. After the Nn. cochlearis and vestibularis branch off, the N. facialis [VII] passes into the Canalis facialis (→ Fig. 12.147). There it turns in an almost right-angled,

posterior inferior direction (external genu of the facial nerve). The Ganglion geniculi lies just ahead of this turning point. Along its pathway in the Canalis facialis, the seventh cranial nerve [CNVII] provides several branches (→ table for → Fig. 12.151). After leaving the cranial base through the Foramen stylomastoideum, it turns rostrally, provides further branches, and then enters the Glandula parotidea, where it divides into its motor terminal branches (Plexus intraparotideus; → table for → Fig. 12.151).

→ T 60.7

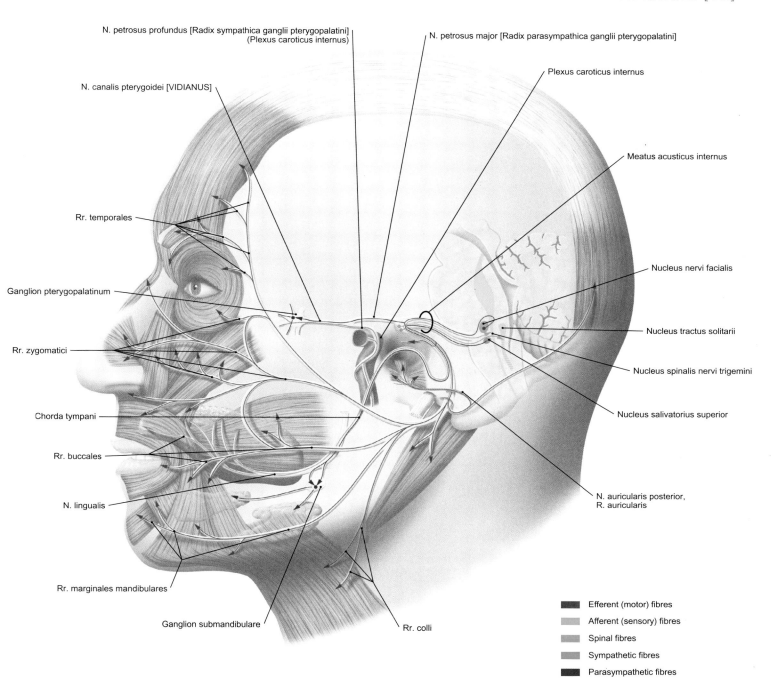

N. petrosus profundus [Radix sympathica ganglii pterygopalatini]
(Plexus caroticus internus)

N. petrosus major [Radix parasympathica ganglii pterygopalatini]

Plexus caroticus internus

N. canalis pterygoidei [VIDIANUS]

Meatus acusticus internus

Rr. temporales

Nucleus nervi facialis

Ganglion pterygopalatinum

Nucleus tractus solitarii

Rr. zygomatici

Nucleus spinalis nervi trigemini

Chorda tympani

Nucleus salivatorius superior

Rr. buccales

N. lingualis

N. auricularis posterior,
R. auricularis

Rr. marginales mandibulares

Ganglion submandibulare

Rr. colli

Efferent (motor) fibres
Afferent (sensory) fibres
Spinal fibres
Sympathetic fibres
Parasympathetic fibres

Fig. 12.149 Fibre qualities of the N. facialis [VII], left side; lateral view. [S700-L127]

The N. facialis [VII] is the second pharyngeal arch nerve. It is a complex nerve with several different fibre qualities. Its **motor fibres** (special visceral-efferent, SVE) originate from the **Nucleus nervi facialis.** They run in a posterior arch around the Nucleus nervi abducentis (internal genu of the facial nerve). The upper part of the nucleus contains the neurons for the facial (mimetic) muscles of the forehead and eye, and the lower part of the nucleus contains the neurons for the facial muscles below the eye. The upper nuclear portion has a double innervation from both hemispheres (→ Fig. 12.153). It therefore receives corticonuclear fibres from the ipsilateral and contralateral sides. The lower nuclear portion is only reached by corticonuclear fibres from the opposite (contralateral) side.

Preganglionic parasympathetic fibres originate from the **Nucleus salivatorius superior** (general visceral-efferent, GVE). They run with the intermediate nerve across the N. facialis [VII], then pass via the N. petrosus major to the Ganglion pterygopalatinum, or join the Chorda tym-

pani to continue within the N. lingualis (from V/3), and reach the Ganglion submandibulare. In these ganglia, the switching (synapsing) then takes place on the **postganglionic fibres.** These project into the lacrimal, nasal and palatine glands, as well as into the Glandulae sublingualis and submandibularis (→ table for the N. trigeminus [V], → Fig. 12.143). Special visceral-afferent (SVA) fibres of the anterior two-thirds of the tongue which mediate taste sensations, project into the upper part of the **Nucleus tractus solitarii.** The fibres join the N. lingualis and pass to the N. facialis [VII] via the Chorda tympani and from here to the brainstem.

General somatic-afferent fibres (GSA) from the posterior wall of the external acoustic meatus, and partially also from the region behind the ear, the auricle and the tympanic membrane join the N. vagus [X] (R. communicans cum nervo vago) for a short distance, leaving it in the Pars petrosa to join the N. facialis [VII]. The perikarya of these fibres as well as the perikarya of the gustatory (taste) fibres are located in the Ganglion geniculi. They reach the Nucleus spinalis nervi trigemini via the intermediate part of the N. facialis [VII].

Brain and spinal cord

N. facialis [VII]

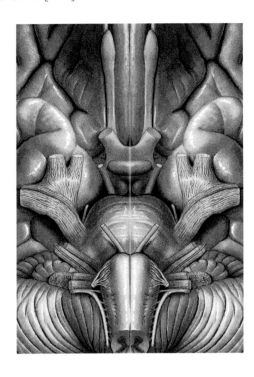

Fig. 12.150   Exit site of the N. facialis [VII] at the brainstem; inferior view. [S700]
The seventh cranial nerve [CNVII] exits at the cerebellopontine angle. Also, the N. intermedius located on the N. vestibulocochlearis [VIII] is highlighted in yellow.

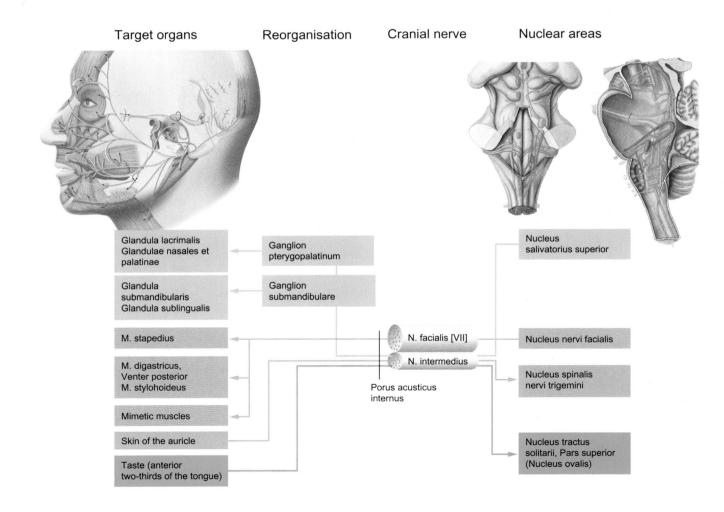

| Target organs | Reorganisation | Cranial nerve | Nuclear areas |

Glandula lacrimalis
Glandulae nasales et palatinae
← Ganglion pterygopalatinum

Nucleus salivatorius superior

Glandula submandibularis
Glandula sublingualis
← Ganglion submandibulare

M. stapedius

N. facialis [VII]

Nucleus nervi facialis

M. digastricus,
Venter posterior
M. stylohoideus

N. intermedius

Nucleus spinalis nervi trigemini

Porus acusticus internus

Mimetic muscles

Skin of the auricle

Taste (anterior two-thirds of the tongue)

Nucleus tractus solitarii, Pars superior (Nucleus ovalis)

Fig. 12.151   Pathway, branches, fibre qualities, cranial nuclei and target organs of the N. facialis [VII]; lateral view. [S700-L127/L238]

Branches of the N. facialis [VII]

Branch	Pathway	Innervation area
N. petrosus major [Radix parasympathica ganglii pterygopalatini]	Passes from the external genu of the facial nerve through the Canalis nervi petrosi majoris into the middle cranial fossa; enters the Canalis pterygoideus via the Foramen lacerum, in which it continues along with the sympathetic N. petrosus profundus as the N. canalis pterygoidei to reach the Ganglion pterygopalatinum (switching of the parasympathetic fibres)	GVE (via branches of the N. maxillaris [V/2]): Glandulae lacrimalis, nasales, palatinae and pharyngeales SVA (via branches of the N. mandibularis [V/3]): taste buds of the palate
N. stapedius	Branches off in the lower part of the Canalis facialis	SVE: M. stapedius
Chorda tympani	Shortly before the distal end of the Canalis facialis, it runs in the opposite direction within its own bony canal to the tympanic cavity, which it traverses without bony protection between the handle of the malleus and the long limb of the incus behind the tympanic membrane; joins the N. lingualis (from V/3) after passing through the Fissura petrotympanica	GVE (via the N. lingualis, switches in the Ganglion submandibulare): Glandulae submandibularis and sublingualis SVA (via N. lingualis): anterior two-thirds of the tongue
N. auricularis posterior	Branches off shortly after leaving the Canalis facialis	SVE: M. occipitofrontalis, ear muscles
Rr. digastricus and stylohyoideus	Small muscle branches	SVE: M. digastricus, Venter posterior, M. stylohyoideus
Plexus intraparotideus	The motor terminal branches to the facial (mimetic) muscles subdivide in the Glandula parotidea into a Pars temporofacialis and a Pars cervicofacialis, which in turn are fanned out into five terminal branches: Rr. temporales, Rr. zygomatici, Rr. buccales, Rr. marginales mandibulares, R. colli (or Rr. colli, → Fig. 8.95)	SVE: mimetic muscles, including M. buccinator and platysma

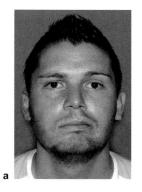
a
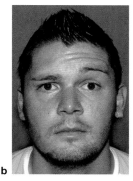
b
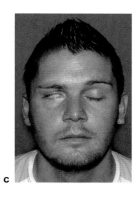
c
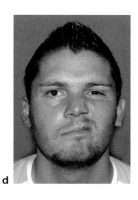
d
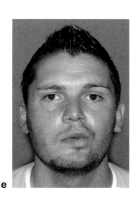
e

Fig. 12.152a–e Peripheral paralysis of the N. facialis [VII], right side.
[S700-T887]
a Admission status of the patient. The skin creases in the right half of the face have disappeared (smoothed out).
b If the patient is asked to raise his eyebrows, only the left half of the forehead displays wrinkles (loss of function of the M. occipitofrontalis indicates a peripheral facial nerve palsy).
c When the patient is asked to shut both eyes, he cannot do this on the side of the damaged facial nerve (lagophthalmos). The eyeball automatically turns upwards when closing the eyes. Because the eyelid does not close properly on the affected side, the white sclera becomes visible (BELL's palsy).
d When the patient is asked to wrinkle his nose, he cannot do this on the right side of his face.
e When the patient is asked to whistle, no tone is produced but air escapes through the lips on the paralysed side.

Clinical remarks

A **supranuclear lesion** (lesion of corticonuclear fibres, e. g. due to an infarction in the Capsula interna) results in a **central facial palsy** (so-called lower facial palsy). But in contrast to an infranuclear lesion, and due to the double innervation of the mimetic muscles of the eye and forehead, only the lower contralateral (opposite) half of the face is affected by motor deficits (→ Fig. 12.153).

An **infranuclear lesion** (lesion site below the nucleus of the facial nerve), e. g. due to a malignant tumour of the parotid gland, results in failure of all motor terminal branches of the N. facialis [VII] on the same side **(peripheral facial palsy)**.

An **acoustic neuroma** (Clinical remarks for → Fig. 12.157) is a tumour originating from the SCHWANN cells of the N. vestibulocochlearis [VIII] or the N. facialis [VII]. This slow-growing benign tumour gradually displaces and ultimately damages both nerves. This manifests as a peripheral palsy of the N. facialis [VII]. All topodiagnostic tests (see above) are negative. The diagnosis is confirmed by means of MRI or CT imaging.

N. facialis [VII]

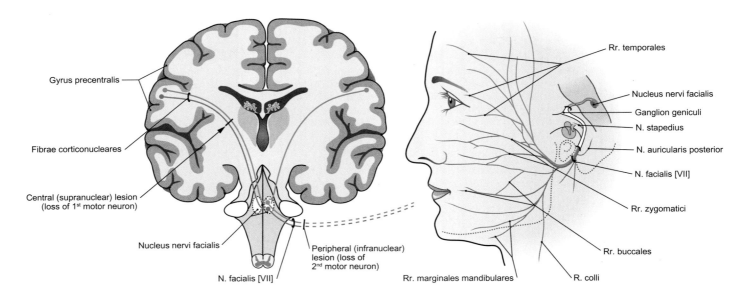

Fig. 12.153 Corticonuclear connections and peripheral pathway of the N. facialis [VII]. [S700-L126]/[B500-M282/L232]
On the left side, the central connections to the Nucleus nervi facialis are presented in simplified form. The corticonuclear tracts to the upper part of the nucleus (for Rr. temporales; green) come from both hemi-spheres. The lower nuclear portion (for Rr. zygomatici, buccales, margi-nales mandibulares and R. colli; red) is only reached from the contra-lateral (opposite) hemisphere.
On the right side, the peripheral efferent fibres (SVE) exiting the upper and lower parts of the Nucleus nervi facialis are shown.

Clinical remarks

Lesion sites of peripheral facial palsy

With the advent of modern high-resolution imaging techniques, clas-sical topodiagnostic tests have become less relevant as prognostic tools in predicting the outcome and healing time of a facial palsy. These tests are largely non-specific and lack sensitivity when com-pared to electrodiagnostic procedures. Nevertheless, several tests are clinically relevant:

- The SCHIRMER's test provides information on the amount of fluid production by the lacrimal gland (Clinical remarks for → Fig. 9.28)
- The acoustic (stapedial) reflex test determines the function of the N. stapedius
- Gustometry (test of taste perception) assesses the integrity of the Chorda tympani
- The mimetic muscles can be electrically stimulated in nerve excit-ability tests
- Electroneurography compares the nerve conduction velocity on both sides and can identify differences between the healthy and damaged sides.

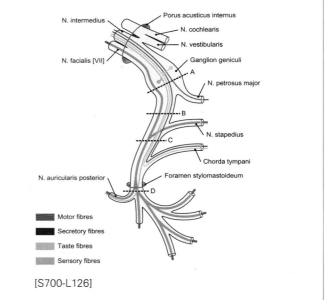

[S700-L126]

Lesion site	Topodiagnostic tests	Cause of lesion (aetiology)
Below the nucleus/nuclear area in the brainstem (A in → figure)	MRI, CT, SCHIRMER's test (testing the function of the lacrimal gland)	e.g. acoustic neuroma
After N. petrosus major has branched off (B in → figure)	Stapedial reflex test	e.g. otitis media
After Chorda tympani has branched off (C in → figure)	Gustometry (testing the perception of taste)	e.g. otitis media
After exiting the Foramen stylomastoideum (D in → figure)	Testing the motor function of facial muscles	e.g. malignant tumour of the parotid gland

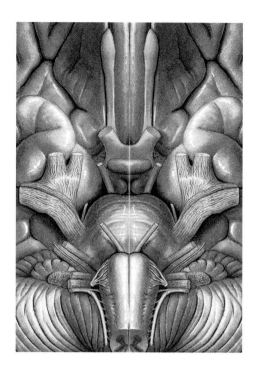

Fig. 12.154 Exit site of the N. vestibulocochlearis [VIII] at the brainstem; inferior view. [S700]
The eighth cranial nerve [CNVIII] exits at the cerebellopontine angle.

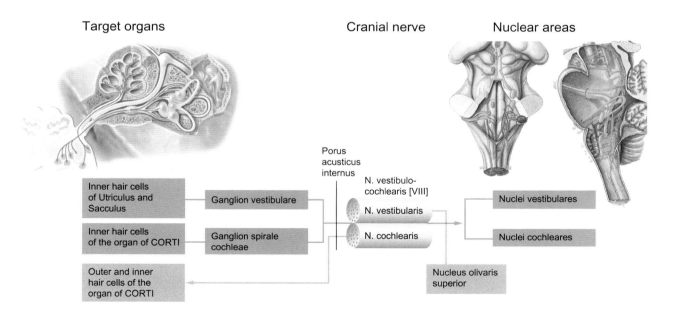

Target organs

Cranial nerve

Nuclear areas

Porus
acusticus
internus

Inner hair cells
of Utriculus and
Sacculus

Ganglion vestibulare

N. vestibulo-
cochlearis [VIII]

N. vestibularis

Nuclei vestibulares

Inner hair cells
of the organ of CORTI

Ganglion spirale
cochleae

N. cochlearis

Nuclei cochleares

Outer and inner
hair cells of the
organ of CORTI

Nucleus olivaris
superior

Fig. 12.155 Pathway, branches and fibre qualities of the N. vesti-bulocochlearis [VIII]; lateral view. [S700-L127/L238]

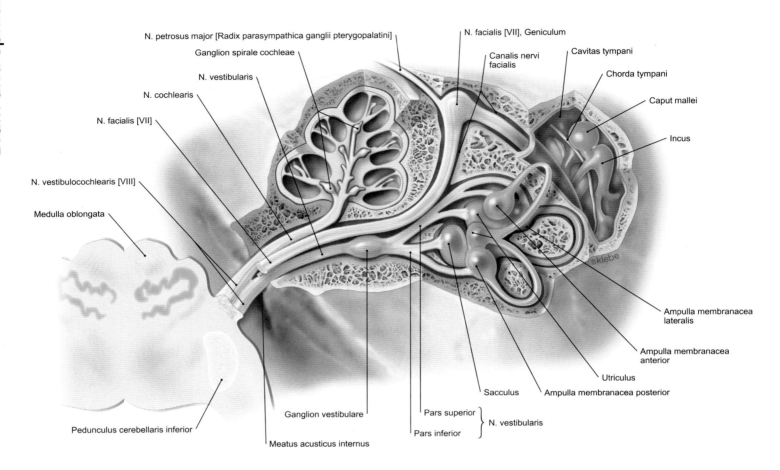

N. petrosus major [Radix parasympathica ganglii pterygopalatini]

Ganglion spirale cochleae

N. vestibularis

N. cochlearis

N. facialis [VII]

N. vestibulocochlearis [VIII]

Medulla oblongata

N. facialis [VII], Geniculum

Canalis nervi facialis

Cavitas tympani

Chorda tympani

Caput mallei

Incus

Ampulla membranacea lateralis

Ampulla membranacea anterior

Utriculus

Sacculus

Ampulla membranacea posterior

Pars superior

Pars inferior

N. vestibularis

Pedunculus cerebellaris inferior

Ganglion vestibulare

Meatus acusticus internus

Fig. 12.156 N. vestibulocochlearis [VIII], pathway in the Pars petrosa of the Os temporale; superior view; Pars petrosa opened. [S700-L238]

The nerve fibres of the **N. cochlearis** originate from the organ of CORTI in the cochlea. Their cell bodies (perikarya) are located in the Ganglion spirale cochleae within the modiolus (bipolar nerve cells). The central cell processes (axons) then form the N. cochlearis. The vestibular organ also possesses bipolar neurons. Similar to the neurons of the auditory system, they receive sensory information from the hair cells. Their cell bodies lie in the Ganglion vestibulare which is located on the floor of the Meatus acusticus internus. The central processes of the neurons form

the **N. vestibularis,** which unites with the N. cochlearis at the Meatus acusticus internus to form the N. vestibulocochlearis [VIII] (common clin.: N. statoacusticus) and enters the brainstem at the cerebellopontine angle.

The pathway of the N. facialis [VII] in the Meatus acusticus internus and subsequently in the Canalis facialis is also shown here. In addition, the Ganglion geniculi, the branching-off N. petrosus major, and the pathway of the N. facialis [VII] in the wall of the tympanic cavity are visible. The Chorda tympani runs between the malleus and the incus.

→ T 60.8

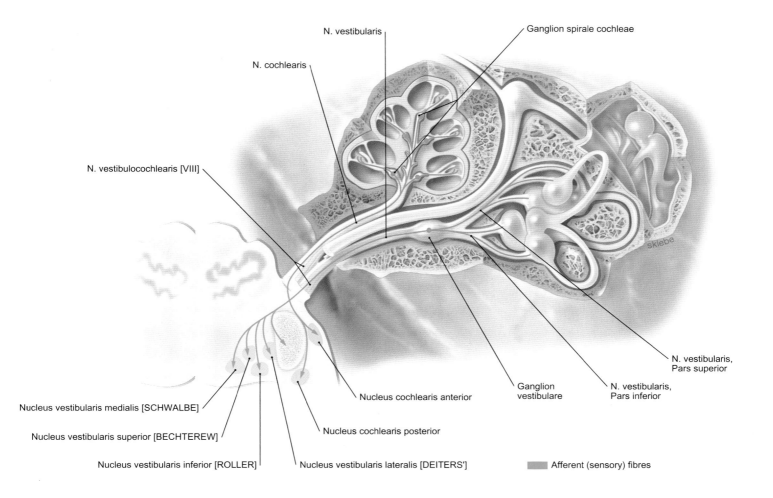

N. vestibularis

Ganglion spirale cochleae

N. cochlearis

N. vestibulocochlearis [VIII]

sklebe

N. vestibularis, Pars superior

Nucleus vestibularis medialis [SCHWALBE]

Nucleus vestibularis superior [BECHTEREW]

Nucleus vestibularis inferior [ROLLER]

Nucleus vestibularis lateralis [DEITERS']

Nucleus cochlearis posterior

Nucleus cochlearis anterior

Ganglion vestibulare

N. vestibularis, Pars inferior

Afferent (sensory) fibres

Fig. 12.157 Fibre qualities of the N. vestibulocochlearis [VIII]; superior view; Pars petrosa of the Os temporale opened. [S700-L238]
The hair cells within the organ of CORTI and the hair cells of the semicircular canals as well as the Utriculi and Sacculi of the vestibular apparatus transmit sensory information to the special somatic-afferent neuronal fibres (SSA). These fibres are the peripheral processes of bipolar neurons (first neuron of the auditory and vestibular tracts). The perikarya of these bipolar neurons lie in the Ganglion spirale cochleae or in the Ganglion vestibulare. The **central projections** of the **Ganglion spirale**

merge to form the **N. cochlearis,** and run through the Meatus acusticus internus to reach the brainstem via the cerebellopontine angle. Here they connect to the Nuclei cochleares anterior and posterior. The **central projections of the first neuron of the vestibular tract** (SSA) unite to form the **N. vestibularis,** and also reach the Medulla oblongata via the cerebellopontine angle. They project here into the Nuclei vestibulares medialis [SCHWALBE's], superior [BECHTEREW], inferior [ROLLER's] and lateralis [DEITERS'].

Clinical remarks

Sudden hearing loss, ringing in the ears, balance disorder and vertigo may be the first signs of an **acoustic neuroma.** This is a benign tumour of connective and neural tissue, which usually originates from SCHWANN cells of the vestibular part of the N. vestibulocochlearis [VIII] **(schwannoma of the vestibular nerve)** and lies in the cerebellopontine angle or in the Meatus acusticus internus. In 5 % of all cases, the acoustic neuroma occurs bilaterally. Due to the joint pathway with the N. facialis [VII], a peripheral facial palsy can occur.
a MRI, axial sectioning, 1.5 Tesla (T2-weighted).
b MRI, frontal sectioning, 3 Tesla (T1-weighted).
[S700-O534]

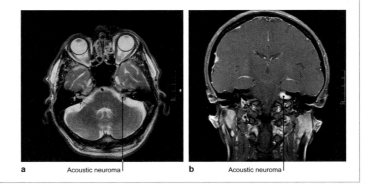

a   Acoustic neuroma

b   Acoustic neuroma

N. glossopharyngeus [IX]

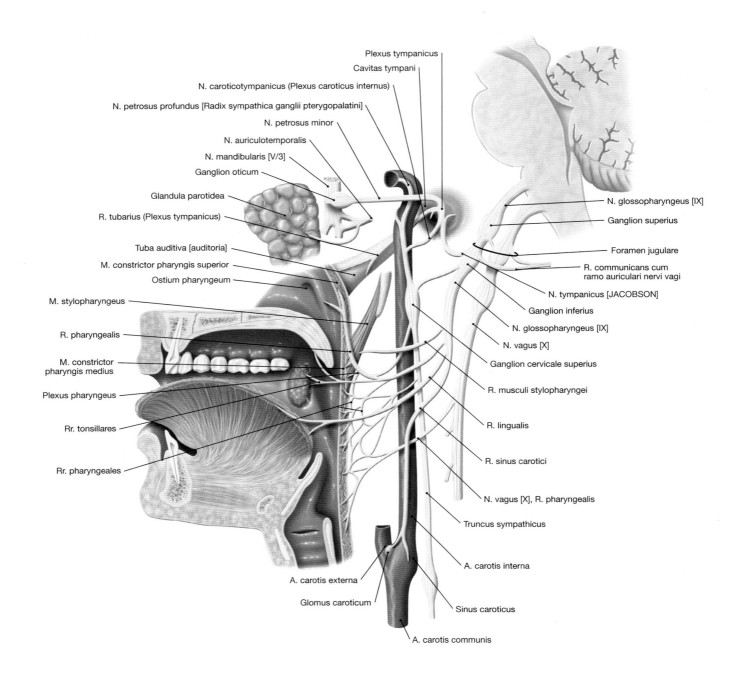

Plexus tympanicus
Cavitas tympani
N. caroticotympanicus (Plexus caroticus internus)
N. petrosus profundus [Radix sympathica ganglii pterygopalatini]
N. petrosus minor
N. auriculotemporalis
N. mandibularis [V/3]
Ganglion oticum
Glandula parotidea
R. tubarius (Plexus tympanicus)
Tuba auditiva [auditoria]
M. constrictor pharyngis superior
Ostium pharyngeum
M. stylopharyngeus
R. pharyngealis
M. constrictor pharyngis medius
Plexus pharyngeus
Rr. tonsillares
Rr. pharyngeales

N. glossopharyngeus [IX]
Ganglion superius
Foramen jugulare
R. communicans cum ramo auriculari nervi vagi
N. tympanicus [JACOBSON]
Ganglion inferius
N. glossopharyngeus [IX]
N. vagus [X]
Ganglion cervicale superius
R. musculi stylopharyngei
R. lingualis
R. sinus carotici
N. vagus [X], R. pharyngealis
Truncus sympathicus
A. carotis interna
Sinus caroticus
A. carotis communis
Glomus caroticum
A. carotis externa

Fig. 12.158 N. glossopharyngeus [IX]; schematic median section; view from the left side. [S700-L127]

The N. glossopharyngeus [IX] exits the brainstem together with the N. vagus [X], and the N. accessorius [XI] via the Sulcus retro-olivaris, and all three nerves pass through the Foramen jugulare at the cranial base. Within the foramen lies the smaller Ganglion superius of the N. glossopharyngeus, and directly below it the Ganglion inferius. Thereafter, the nerve runs between the V. jugularis interna and A. carotis interna downwards, and in an arch-like course it enters the root of the tongue from behind between the Mm. stylopharyngeus and styloglossus. Along its pathway it provides the **N. tympanicus,** which runs to the tympanic cavity, divides into the mucosa of the Plexus tympanicus, subsequently again leaving the tympanic cavity as **N. petrosus minor.** The N. petrosus minor accompanies the N. petrosus major on the anterior surface of the petrous bone, and passes through the Foramen la-

cerum to reach the Ganglion oticum. The N. glossopharyngeus [IX] innervates the parotid gland via this ganglion.

Additional **branches** are the R. musculi stylopharyngei to the M. stylopharyngeus and the Rr. pharyngeales to the Mm. constrictor pharyngis superior, palatoglossus and palatopharyngeus, as well as sensory fibres to the pharyngeal mucosa and to the Glandulae pharyngeales.

Along with the sympathetic trunk and the N. vagus [X], other fibres of the N. glossopharyngeus [IX] form the **Plexus pharyngeus,** which innervates the Mm. constrictor pharyngis inferior, levator veli palatini and uvulae.

The Rr. tonsillares supply the Tonsilla palatina and the mucosa of the Isthmus faucium, the Rr. linguales guides gustatory (taste) fibres for the posterior third of the tongue. The R. sinus carotici transmits the sensory input from mechanoreceptors and chemoreceptors of the Sinus caroticus and Glomus caroticum to the brainstem.

→ T 60.9

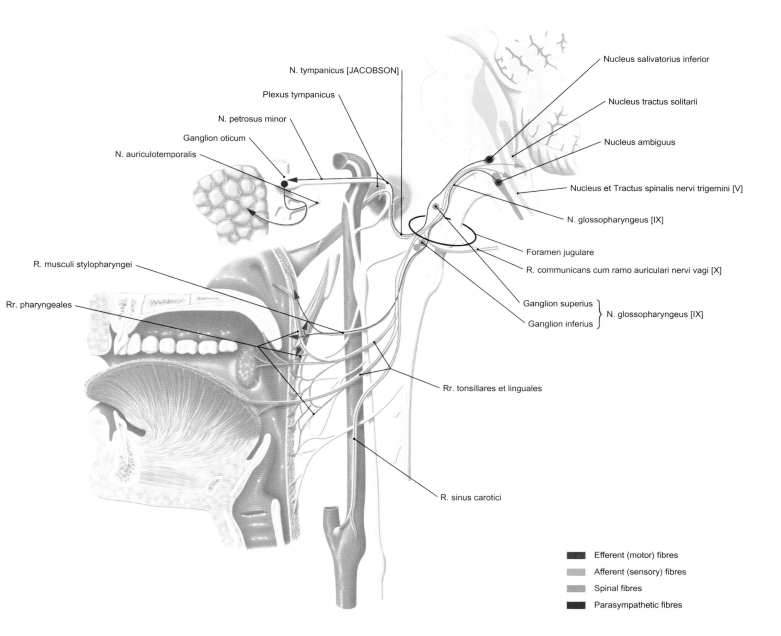

N. tympanicus [JACOBSON]

Plexus tympanicus

N. petrosus minor

Ganglion oticum

N. auriculotemporalis

R. musculi stylopharyngei

Rr. pharyngeales

Nucleus salivatorius inferior

Nucleus tractus solitarii

Nucleus ambiguus

Nucleus et Tractus spinalis nervi trigemini [V]

N. glossopharyngeus [IX]

Foramen jugulare

R. communicans cum ramo auriculari nervi vagi [X]

Ganglion superius ⎫ N. glossopharyngeus [IX]
Ganglion inferius ⎭

Rr. tonsillares et linguales

R. sinus carotici

■ Efferent (motor) fibres
▨ Afferent (sensory) fibres
▨ Spinal fibres
■ Parasympathetic fibres

Fig. 12.159 Fibre qualities of the N. glossopharyngeus [IX]; sche-matic median section; view from the left side. [S700-L127]
Motor fibres (SVE) of the N. glossopharyngeus [IX] originating from the Nucleus ambiguus innervate the pharyngeal muscles and the soft pal-ate in conjunction with motor fibres of the N. vagus [X] (also derived from the Nucleus ambiguus, SVE).
Parasympathetic fibres (GVE) originating in the Nucleus salivatorius inferior, pass via the N. tympanicus, Plexus tympanicus and N. petrosus minor to the Ganglion oticum, where they are switched from pregan-glionic to postganglionic fibres. The **postganglionic** fibres join the N. auriculotemporalis (from V/3)) and the N. facialis [VII] to reach the Glandula parotidea. Further parasympathetic fibres (GVE) pass to the pharyngeal glands.

Numerous **general somatic-afferent** fibres (GSA) that project to the Nucleus spinalis nervi trigemini come from the tympanic cavity, the pharyngeal mucosa, and from the posterior third of the tongue.
General visceral-afferent fibres (GVA) transmit the sensory input of mechanoreceptors in the Sinus caroticus (measuring blood pressure) and of chemoreceptors in the Glomus caroticum (measuring the partial pressure of O_2 and CO_2, and the pH in the blood). The impulses are transmitted to the brainstem. Here they lead to reflexive changes in the respiratory rate and blood pressure.
Special visceral-afferent fibres (SVA) conduct taste sensations from the posterior third of the tongue to the Nucleus tractus solitarius.

Clinical remarks

Lesions of the N. glossopharyngeus [IX] result in swallowing diffi-culties (paralysis of the M. constrictor pharyngis superior, lacking formation of the PASSAVANT's ridge), deviation of the uvula to the healthy side (paralysis of the Mm. levator veli palatini, palatoglossus, palatopharyngeus and uvulae), impaired sensibility of the pharyngeal region (lack of gag reflex), lack of taste sensations in the posterior

third of the tongue, as well as impaired secretion of the Glandula parotidea. In most cases, the N. glossopharyngeus [IX] is not exclu-sively affected. Frequently, the Nn. vagus [X] and accessorius [XI] can also be damaged by fractures, aneurysms, tumours and throm-bosis of cerebral blood vessels in the region of the Foramen jugulare.

Brain and spinal cord

N. glossopharyngeus [IX]

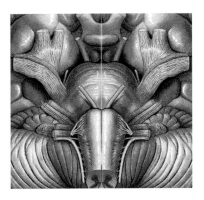

Fig. 12.160   Exit site of the N. glossopharyngeus [IX] at the brainstem; inferior view. [S700]
The ninth cranial nerve [CNIX] exits the Medulla oblongata via the Sulcus retroolivaris between the olive and the inferior cerebellar peduncle.

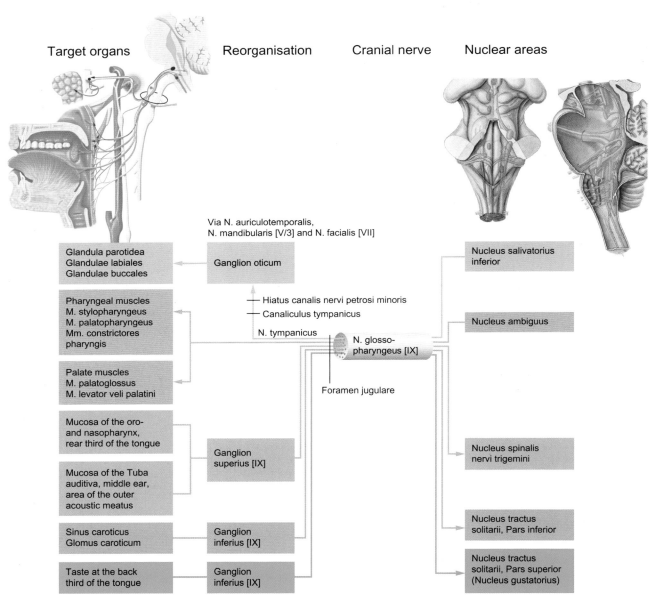

Target organs   Reorganisation   Cranial nerve   Nuclear areas

Via N. auriculotemporalis,
N. mandibularis [V/3] and N. facialis [VII]

| Glandula parotidea
Glandulae labiales
Glandulae buccales | ← | Ganglion oticum | | Nucleus salivatorius inferior |

— Hiatus canalis nervi petrosi minoris
— Canaliculus tympanicus

N. tympanicus

| Pharyngeal muscles
M. stylopharyngeus
M. palatopharyngeus
Mm. constrictores pharyngis | | | N. glosso-pharyngeus [IX] | Nucleus ambiguus |

| Palate muscles
M. palatoglossus
M. levator veli palatini | | | |

Foramen jugulare

| Mucosa of the oro-
and nasopharynx,
rear third of the tongue | | Ganglion superius [IX] | | Nucleus spinalis nervi trigemini |

| Mucosa of the Tuba auditiva, middle ear, area of the outer acoustic meatus | | | |

| Sinus caroticus
Glomus caroticum | | Ganglion inferius [IX] | | Nucleus tractus solitarii, Pars inferior |

| Taste at the back third of the tongue | | Ganglion inferius [IX] | | Nucleus tractus solitarii, Pars superior (Nucleus gustatorius) |

Fig. 12.161   Fibre qualities, cranial nuclei and target organs of the N. glossopharyngeus [IX]; lateral view. [S700-L127/L283]

Clinical remarks

In the case of an aberrant pathway of the A. inferior anterior cerebelli, e.g. between the exit points of the N. glossopharyngeus [IX] and the N. vagus [X], the arterial pulse can irritate the N. glossopharyngeus [IX]. This may cause unilateral sudden attacks of pain in the tongue, the soft palate or pharynx which result in drinking and swallowing problems **(glossopharyngeal neuralgia).** In rare cases, the N. vagus [X] can also be affected **(vagal neuralgia)** with reflex bradycardia or asystole (cardiac arrest).

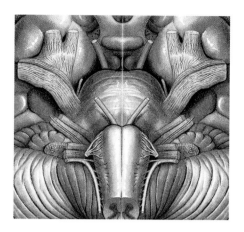

Fig. 12.162 Exit point of the N. vagus [X] at the brainstem; inferior view. [S700]
The tenth cranial nerve [CNX] exits via the Sulcus retroolivaris between the N. glossopharyngeus [IX] (cranial) and the N. accessorius [XI] (caudal).

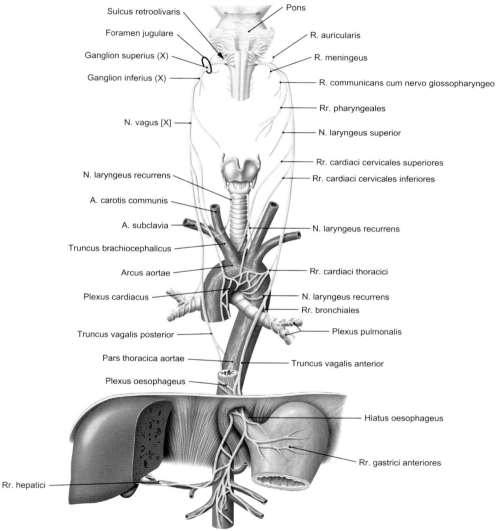

Sulcus retroolivaris
Foramen jugulare
Ganglion superius (X)
Ganglion inferius (X)
N. vagus [X]
N. laryngeus recurrens
A. carotis communis
A. subclavia
Truncus brachiocephalicus
Arcus aortae
Plexus cardiacus
Truncus vagalis posterior
Pars thoracica aortae
Plexus oesophageus
Rr. hepatici

Pons
R. auricularis
R. meningeus
R. communicans cum nervo glossopharyngeo
Rr. pharyngeales
N. laryngeus superior
Rr. cardiaci cervicales superiores
Rr. cardiaci cervicales inferiores
N. laryngeus recurrens
Rr. cardiaci thoracici
N. laryngeus recurrens
Rr. bronchiales
Plexus pulmonalis
Truncus vagalis anterior
Hiatus oesophageus
Rr. gastrici anteriores

Fig. 12.163 N. vagus [X]; both nerve branches; anterior view. [S700-L127]

The figure illustrates the slightly different pathways of the left and right Nn. vagi, as well as the pathway of the two nerve branches before the transition into the abdominal cavity.

→ T 60.10

Clinical remarks

Complete **lesions of the N. vagus [X]** occur most often near the Foramen jugulare. Frequently, the N. glossopharyngeus [IX] and the N. accessorius [XI] are also affected. Depending on the lesion site, the symptoms include swallowing difficulties and deviation of the uvula to the healthy side (damage to the Plexus pharyngeus), sensory deficits in the region of the pharynx and epiglottis (lack of gag re-

flex, gustatory impairment), hoarseness (paralysis of laryngeal muscles), tachycardia and arrhythmia (innervation of the heart). Unilateral lesions have very little effect on the autonomic functions. Bilateral lesions, however, can cause severe respiratory and circulatory problems, and can even be lethal in some patients.

N. vagus [X]

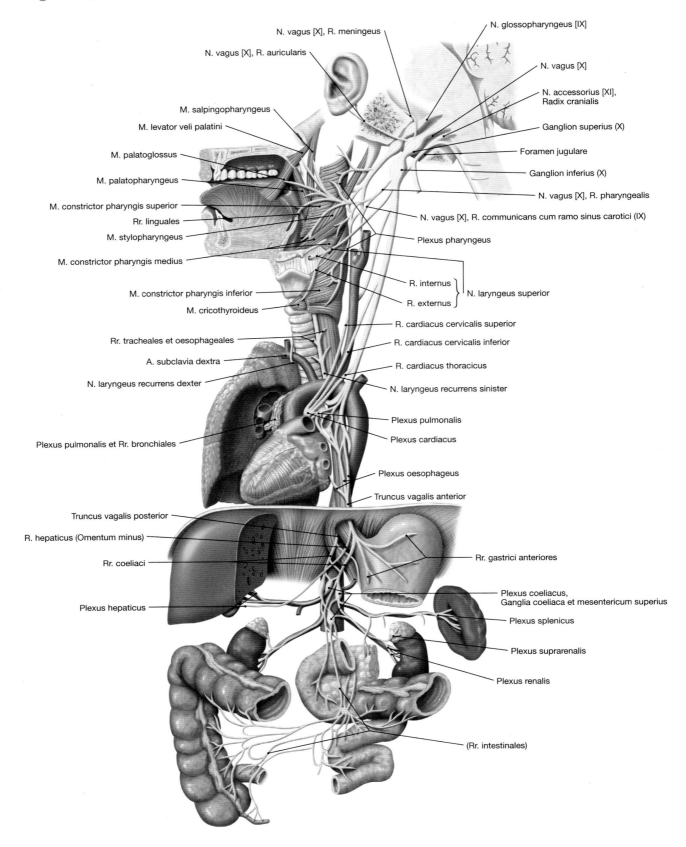

N. vagus [X], R. meningeus

N. vagus [X], R. auricularis

N. glossopharyngeus [IX]

N. vagus [X]

N. accessorius [XI], Radix cranialis

M. salpingopharyngeus

M. levator veli palatini

M. palatoglossus

Ganglion superius (X)

M. palatopharyngeus

Foramen jugulare

M. constrictor pharyngis superior

Ganglion inferius (X)

Rr. linguales

N. vagus [X], R. pharyngealis

M. stylopharyngeus

N. vagus [X], R. communicans cum ramo sinus carotici (IX)

M. constrictor pharyngis medius

Plexus pharyngeus

M. constrictor pharyngis inferior

R. internus

M. cricothyroideus

R. externus

N. laryngeus superior

Rr. tracheales et oesophageales

R. cardiacus cervicalis superior

A. subclavia dextra

R. cardiacus cervicalis inferior

N. laryngeus recurrens dexter

R. cardiacus thoracicus

N. laryngeus recurrens sinister

Plexus pulmonalis

Plexus pulmonalis et Rr. bronchiales

Plexus cardiacus

Plexus oesophageus

Truncus vagalis anterior

Truncus vagalis posterior

R. hepaticus (Omentum minus)

Rr. gastrici anteriores

Rr. coeliaci

Plexus coeliacus, Ganglia coeliaca et mesentericum superius

Plexus splenicus

Plexus hepaticus

Plexus suprarenalis

Plexus renalis

(Rr. intestinales)

Fig. 12.164   N. vagus [X]; schematic median section in the region of the head. [S700-L127]

A detailed description of the pathway of the N. vagus [X] is provided on the next page but one.

→ T 60.10

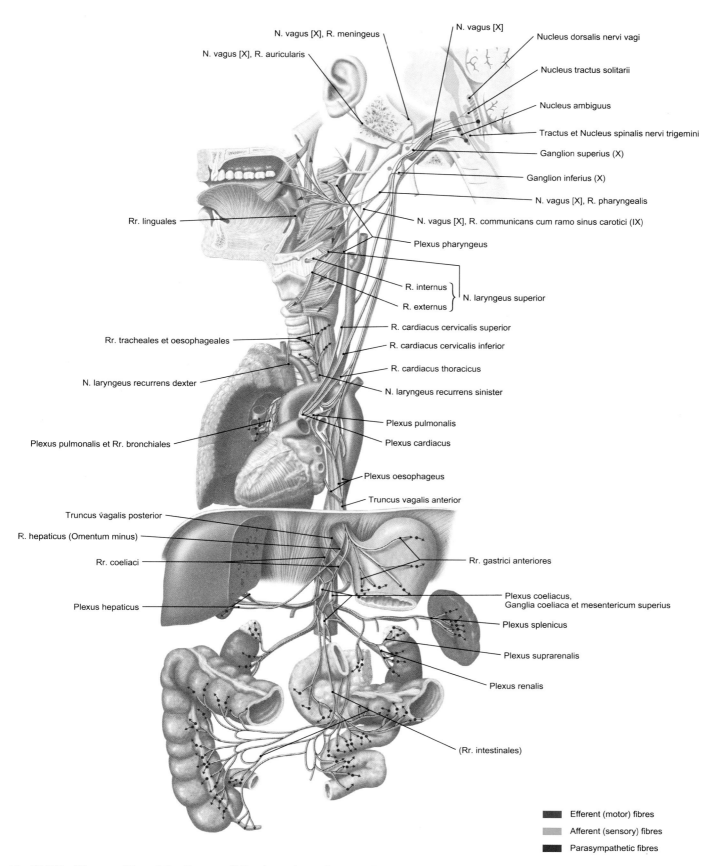

N. vagus [X], R. meningeus

N. vagus [X]

N. vagus [X], R. auricularis

Nucleus dorsalis nervi vagi

Nucleus tractus solitarii

Nucleus ambiguus

Tractus et Nucleus spinalis nervi trigemini

Ganglion superius (X)

Ganglion inferius (X)

N. vagus [X], R. pharyngealis

Rr. linguales

N. vagus [X], R. communicans cum ramo sinus carotici (IX)

Plexus pharyngeus

R. internus
R. externus } N. laryngeus superior

R. cardiacus cervicalis superior

R. cardiacus cervicalis inferior

Rr. tracheales et oesophageales

R. cardiacus thoracicus

N. laryngeus recurrens dexter

N. laryngeus recurrens sinister

Plexus pulmonalis

Plexus cardiacus

Plexus pulmonalis et Rr. bronchiales

Plexus oesophageus

Truncus vagalis anterior

Truncus vagalis posterior

R. hepaticus (Omentum minus)

Rr. gastrici anteriores

Rr. coeliaci

Plexus coeliacus,
Ganglia coeliaca et mesentericum superius

Plexus hepaticus

Plexus splenicus

Plexus suprarenalis

Plexus renalis

(Rr. intestinales)

Efferent (motor) fibres

Afferent (sensory) fibres

Parasympathetic fibres

Fig. 12.165   Fibre qualities of the N. vagus [X]; schematic median section in the region of the head. [S700-L127]

Fibre qualities of the N. vagus [X], also → Fig. 12.166 and the next page.

Cranial nerves

Brain and spinal cord

N. vagus [X]

N. vagus [X], → Fig. 12.164
Along with the N. glossopharyngeus [IX] and the N. accessorius [XI] in the Sulcus retroolivaris, the N. vagus [X] exits the brainstem and crosses the cranial base via the Foramen jugulare. The **Ganglion superius** is located in the Foramen jugulare, from which the R. meningeus branches off and returns to the posterior cranial fossa for the sensory innervation of the meninges. The R. auricularis branches off as well to innervate the outer wall of the acoustic meatus. The **Ganglion inferius** is located just below the Foramen jugulare.

The N. vagus [X] crosses the neck and the thoracic cavity, and enters the abdominal cavity. Along its pathway, the N. vagus [X] gradually loses its appearance as a coherent nerve. At the level of the oesophagus, two distinct trunks (Trunci vagales anterior and posterior) can still be discerned, but from the stomach downwards the fibres branch out more widely and reach the liver, pancreas, spleen, kidneys, adrenal glands, small intestine, and colon via multiple **plexuses.** The fibres of the N. vagus [X] terminate at the level of the left colonic flexure (CANNON-BÖHM point).

On its **cervical passage,** the N. vagus [X] provides the Rr. pharyngeales, which along with the N. glossopharyngeus [IX] and sympathetic fibres form the **Plexus pharyngeus** (motor innervation of the Mm. constrictores pharyngis medius and inferior, levator veli palatini, uvulae [SVE], parasympathetic innervation of the Glandulae pharyngeales [AVE], and sensory innervation of the pharyngeal mucosa [GVA]). Additional branches are the R. lingualis (taste fibres of the root of the tongue and epiglottis, SVA), the N. laryngeus superior (motor innervation of the Mm. cricothyroideus and constrictor pharyngis inferior with the R. externus, and the R. internus for the sensory innervation of the laryngeal mucosa above the vocal folds), and the Rr. cardiaci cervicales superiores and inferiores to the Plexus cardiacus of the heart (also responsible for the regulation of the blood pressure).

In the **thoracic part** of the N. vagus [X], the N. laryngeus recurrens branches off. On the left side, this nerve loops around the aortic arch, and on the right side around the A. subclavia, running back cranially to the larynx. There it innervates all laryngeal muscles (with the exception of the M. cricothyroideus) and the mucosa below the vocal folds. Additionally, the Rr. cardiaci thoracici of the Plexus cardiacus branch off in the thoracic part. The Rr. bronchiales join the Plexus pulmonalis and innervate the muscles and glands of the bronchial tree. The tonus of the lung tissue is continuously monitored by the N. vagus [X] and respiration will be reflexively adjusted.

On the right and left sides, the N. vagus [X] forms a wide-meshed plexus (Plexus oesophagus) around the middle part of the oesophagus, from which the two vagal trunks finally emerge, the Truncus vagalis anterior (in particular fibres of the left N. vagus [X]) and the Truncus vagalis posterior (in particular fibres of the right N. vagus [X]). Both of the trunci pass along with the oesophagus through the diaphragm into the **abdominal cavity.** From the stomach onwards, the trunci branch out progressively and form numerous plexuses before reaching the abovementioned abdominal organs.

Fibre qualities of the N. vagus [X], → Fig. 12.165 and → Fig. 12.166:
Parasympathetic fibres (GVE) of the N. vagus [X] originate from the Nucleus dorsalis nervi vagi in the Medulla oblongata, and innervate glands and smooth muscles of the viscera.
General visceral-afferent fibres (GVA) of the same organs project into the Nucleus dorsalis nervi vagi and the Nucleus tractus solitarii.
Special visceral-efferent fibres (SVE) originate from the Nucleus ambiguus and innervate the striated muscles of the palate, pharynx, larynx, and oesophagus.

General visceral-afferent fibres (GVA) from the mucosa of the same structures project into the Nucleus dorsalis nervi vagi and into the Nuclei tractus solitarii.
General somatic-afferent fibres (GSA) of the external acoustic meatus and the meninges of the posterior cranial fossa project into the Nucleus spinalis nervi trigemini.
Gustatory fibres (SVA) of the root of the tongue and the epiglottis join the Nucleus tractus solitarii.

N. vagus [X]	
Nuclei (quality)	• Nucleus ambiguus (SVE) • Nucleus tractus solitarii (SVA, GVA) • Nucleus spinalis nervi trigemini (GSA) • Nucleus dorsalis nervi vagi (GVE, GVA)
Exit point at the brain	Medulla oblongata: Sulcus retroolivaris
Location in the subarachnoid space	Cisterna basalis
Passage through the cranial base	Foramen jugulare
Areas of supply	**Motor:** • Pharyngeal muscles (caudal part), M. levator veli palatini, M. uvulae • Laryngeal muscles **Specific sensory:** Root of the tongue **Sensory:** • Dura of the Fossa cranii posterior • Meatus acusticus externus (sickle-shaped deep part) • Membrana tympanica (outer surface) **Parasympathetic:** Cervical, thoracic and abdominal organs up to the CANNON-BÖHM point

Target organs   Reorganisation   Cranial nerve   Nuclear areas

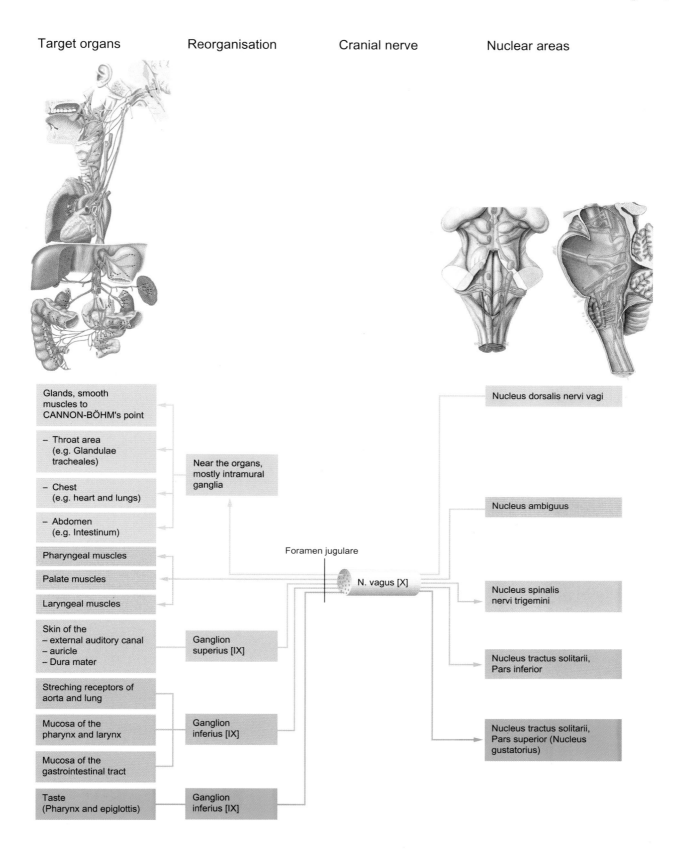

Glands, smooth
muscles to
CANNON-BÖHM's point

– Throat area
  (e.g. Glandulae
  tracheales)

– Chest
  (e.g. heart and lungs)

– Abdomen
  (e.g. Intestinum)

Pharyngeal muscles

Palate muscles

Laryngeal muscles

Skin of the
– external auditory canal
– auricle
– Dura mater

Streching receptors of
aorta and lung

Mucosa of the
pharynx and larynx

Mucosa of the
gastrointestinal tract

Taste
(Pharynx and epiglottis)

Near the organs,
mostly intramural
ganglia

Ganglion
superius [IX]

Ganglion
inferius [IX]

Ganglion
inferius [IX]

Foramen jugulare

N. vagus [X]

Nucleus dorsalis nervi vagi

Nucleus ambiguus

Nucleus spinalis
nervi trigemini

Nucleus tractus solitarii,
Pars inferior

Nucleus tractus solitarii,
Pars superior (Nucleus
gustatorius)

**Fig. 12.166   Fibre qualities, cranial nuclei and target organs of the
N. vagus [X];** lateral view. [S700-L127/L238]

N. accessorius [XI]

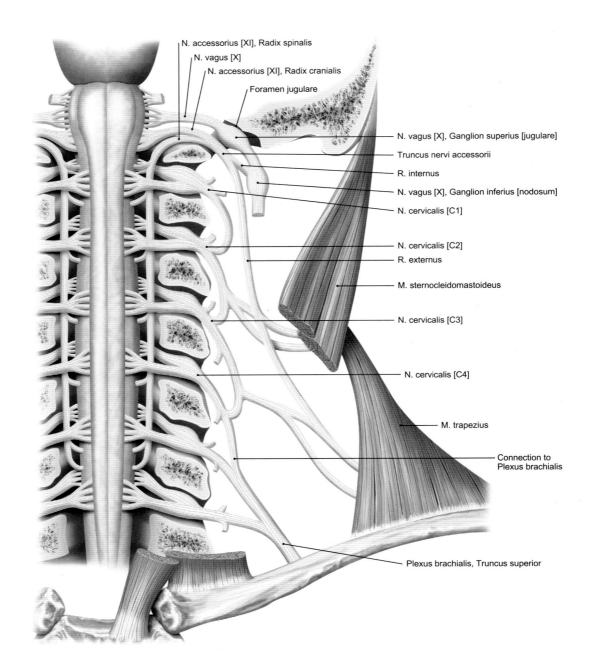

N. accessorius [XI], Radix spinalis

N. vagus [X]

N. accessorius [XI], Radix cranialis

Foramen jugulare

N. vagus [X], Ganglion superius [jugulare]

Truncus nervi accessorii

R. internus

N. vagus [X], Ganglion inferius [nodosum]

N. cervicalis [C1]

N. cervicalis [C2]

R. externus

M. sternocleidomastoideus

N. cervicalis [C3]

N. cervicalis [C4]

M. trapezius

Connection to Plexus brachialis

Plexus brachialis, Truncus superior

Fig. 12.167   N. accessorius [XI]; anterior view; the spine and skull are opened. [S700-L127]

The N. accessorius [XI] exits the brainstem in the Sulcus retroolivaris along with the N. glossopharyngeus [IX] and the N. vagus [X], and all three cranial nerves cross the cranial base via the Foramen jugulare. Its fibres originate from two roots. The **Radix cranialis** of the N. accessorius [XI] originates from the Nucleus ambiguus in the Medulla oblongata. At the level of the Foramen jugulare it joins the **Radix spinalis** of the N. accessorius [XI], of which the fibres originate segmentally from the cervical spine between the anterior and posterior roots. However, it is under discussion whether the N. accessorius [XI] is actually a true cranial nerve, because its spinal nuclear area (Nucleus nervi accessorii) lies in cells of the anterior horn of the cervical spinal cord, while the cranial nuclear area can be assigned to the basal section of the Nucleus ambi-

guus and thus to the N. vagus [X]. Accordingly, the fibres derived from C1–7 are defined as the **Radix spinalis nervi accessorii,** and the fibres originating from the Nucleus ambiguus as the **Radix cranialis nervi accessorii.** Textbooks state that the fibres of the Radix cranialis form the R. internus and converge on the N. vagus [X], inferior to the Foramen jugulare (according to newer findings which require further analysis, the N. accessorius [XI] has no cranial root and no connection to the N. vagus [X]). The Radix cranialis participates in the innervation of the pharyngeal and laryngeal muscles and is, strictly speaking, not a part of the N. accessorius [XI]. The fibres of the Radix spinalis run caudally to the M. sternocleidomastoideus which they innervate, and then pass through the lateral cervical triangle to the anterior margin of the M. trapezius, which they also innervate.

→ T 60.11

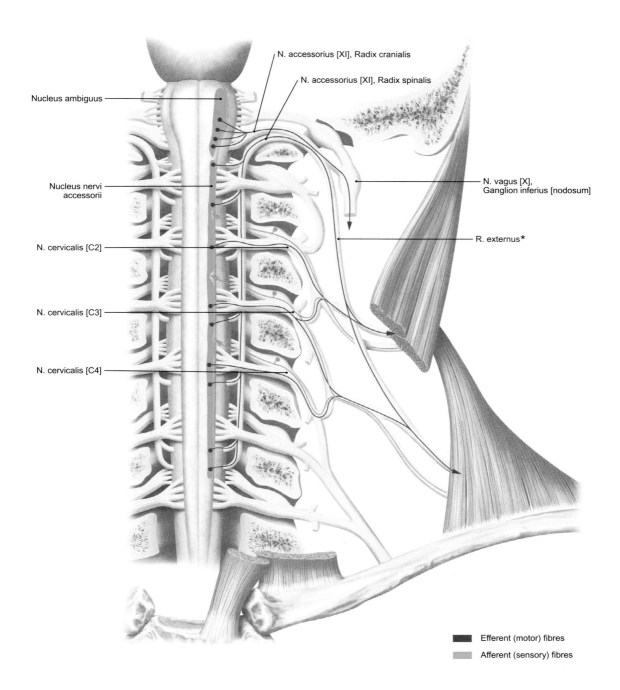

Nucleus ambiguus

N. accessorius [XI], Radix cranialis

N. accessorius [XI], Radix spinalis

Nucleus nervi accessorii

N. cervicalis [C2]

N. cervicalis [C3]

N. cervicalis [C4]

N. vagus [X], Ganglion inferius [nodosum]

R. externus*

Efferent (motor) fibres

Afferent (sensory) fibres

Fig. 12.168 Fibre qualities of the N. accessorius [XI]; anterior view, the vertebral canal and skull are opened. [S700-L127]

The N. accessorius [XI] innervates the M. sternocleidomastoideus and M. trapezius. Its nuclear area is the Nucleus nervi accessorii, from which **special visceral-efferent** fibres (SVE) emerge.

* to the M. sternocleidomastoideus and M. trapezius

Clinical remarks

Lesions of the N. accessorius [XI] occur frequently due to its relatively superficial pathway in the lateral triangle of the neck. Particularly common are iatrogenic lesions (caused by the doctor, e.g. after lymph node extirpation) or traumatic lesions following neck injuries. If the N. accessorius [XI] was damaged superior to the M. sternocleidomastoideus, patients cannot turn their heads to the healthy side (paralysis of the M. sternocleidomastoideus). In addition, they are no longer able to raise their arm above the horizontal plane (impaired arm elevation due to paralysis of the M. trapezius). But usually the lesion site is located below the outlet of the nerve branches to the M. sternocleidomastoideus in the lateral cervical triangle. The consequences are a dropped shoulder and difficulties in raising the arm above the horizontal plane.

N. accessorius [XI]

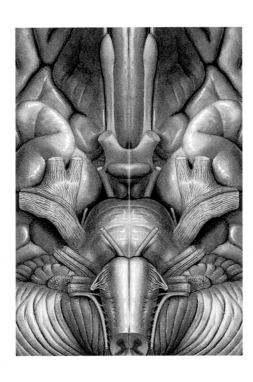

Fig. 12.169 Exit point of the N. accessorius [XI] on the brainstem; inferior view. [S700]
The 11th cranial nerve [CNXI] exits the brainstem on the ventral side, dorsally of the olive.

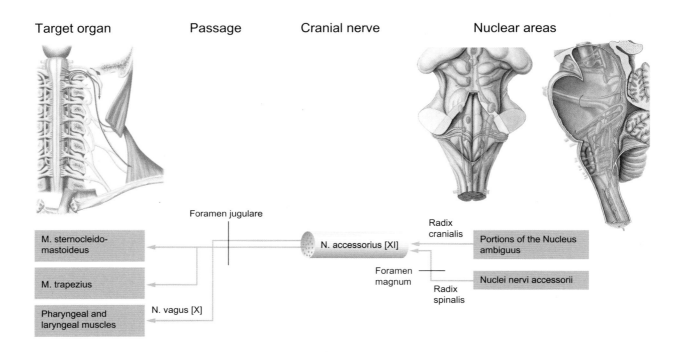

Fig. 12.170 Fibre qualities, cranial nuclei and target organs of the N. accessorius [XI]; anterior view, the spine and the skull are opened.
[S700-L127/L238]

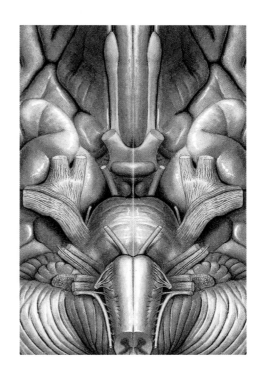

Fig. 12.171   Exit point of the N. hypoglossus [XII] on the brainstem; inferior view. [S700]
The 12th cranial nerve [CN XII] exits the brainstem on the ventral side in the Sulcus anterolateralis between the olive and the pyramid (Sulcus preolivaris).

Target organ   Passage   Cranial nerve   Nuclear area

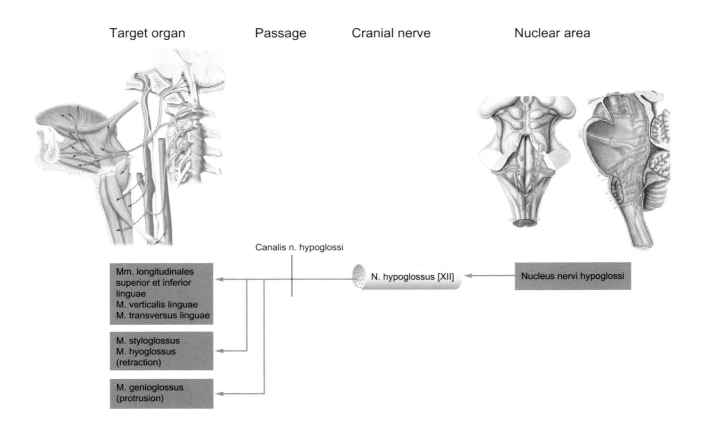

Canalis n. hypoglossi

Mm. longitudinales superior et inferior linguae
M. verticalis linguae
M. transversus linguae

M. styloglossus
M. hyoglossus
(retraction)

M. genioglossus
(protrusion)

N. hypoglossus [XII]

Nucleus nervi hypoglossi

Fig. 12.172   Fibre qualities, cranial nuclei and target organs of the N. hypoglossus [XII]; view from the left side. [S700-L127/L238]

N. hypoglossus [XII]

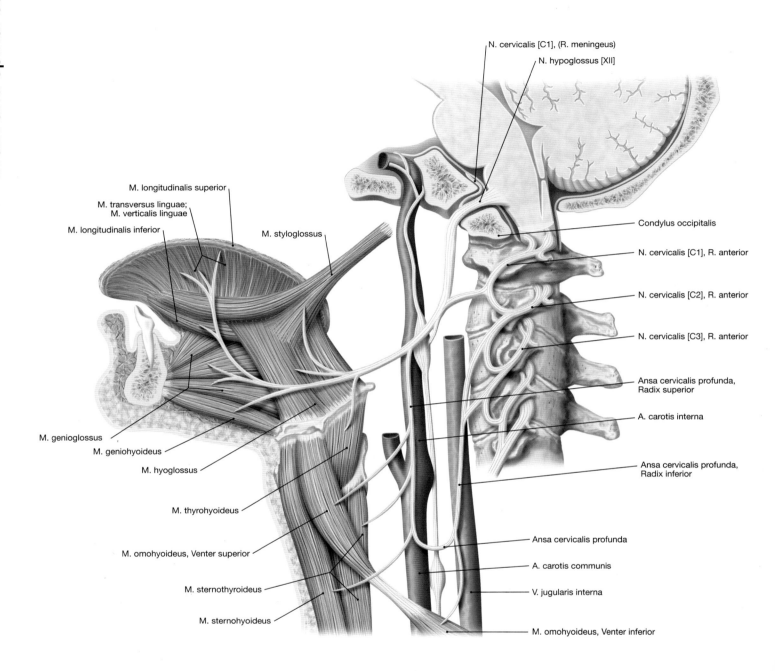

Fig. 12.173 N. hypoglossus [XII]; schematic median section; view from the left side. [S700-L127]

The fibres of the N. hypoglossus [XII] originate from the Nucleus nervi hypoglossi in the Medulla oblongata, and form several small bundles when exiting between the pyramid and the olive in the Sulcus anterolateralis. After the fibres join the N. hypoglossus [XII], the nerve passes through the **Canalis nervi hypoglossi.** Inferior to the cranial base, fibres of the spinal nerves C1 and C2 join the N. hypoglossus [XII], accompanying it over a short distance, before leaving it again. With other fibres originating from C2 and C3, they form the **Ansa cervicalis pro-** **funda** and, in addition, innervate the M. geniohyoideus. Posterior to the N. vagus [X], the N. hypoglossus [XII] passes caudally in the neurovascular bundle behind the pharynx, and then turns rostrally and medially in a right-angled arch of 90°. Passing along the upper margin of the Trigonum caroticum, it crosses the bifurcation of the A. carotis externa at the exit point of the A. lingualis, and enters between the M. hyoglossus and M. mylohyoideus to reach the tongue, of which it completely innervates the internal muscles, as well as the Mm. styloglossus, hyoglossus and genioglossus.

→ T 60.12

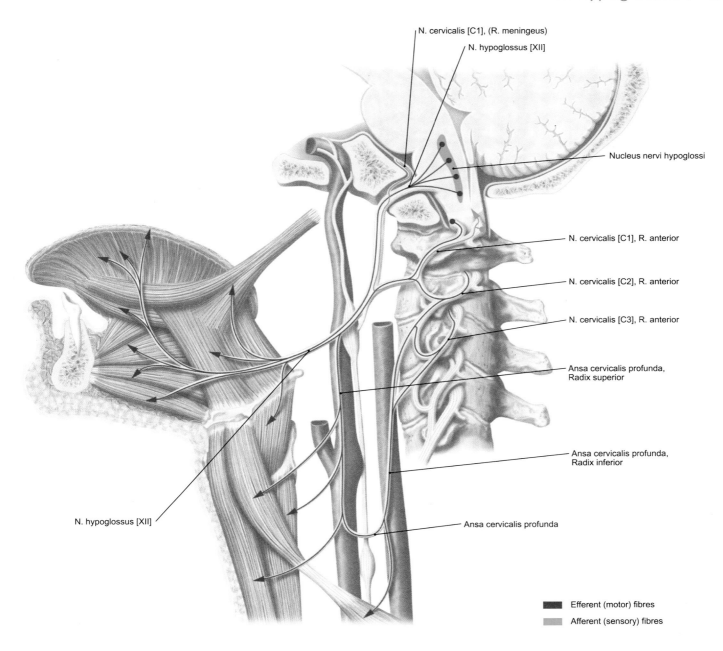

N. cervicalis [C1], (R. meningeus)

N. hypoglossus [XII]

Nucleus nervi hypoglossi

N. cervicalis [C1], R. anterior

N. cervicalis [C2], R. anterior

N. cervicalis [C3], R. anterior

Ansa cervicalis profunda,
Radix superior

Ansa cervicalis profunda,
Radix inferior

Ansa cervicalis profunda

N. hypoglossus [XII]

■ Efferent (motor) fibres

■ Afferent (sensory) fibres

Fig. 12.174 Fibre qualities of the N. hypoglossus [XII]; schematic median section; view from the left side. [S700-L127]

The N. hypoglossus [XII] consists of **general somatic-efferent** fibres (GSE) from the Nucleus nervi hypoglossi, with which it innervates the internal muscles of the tongue, as well as the Mm. styloglossus, hyoglossus and genioglossus.

Clinical remarks

Unilateral peripheral **lesions of the N. hypoglossus [XII]** or its cranial nucleus, e.g. due to a fracture of the cranial base, cause a deviation of the tongue to the affected side because the lingual muscles that are still intact on the opposite side will push the tongue to the paralysed side (→ figure). If the paralysis persists over a longer period, the signs of muscle atrophy are visible on the paretic side. In the case of a persistent paralysis of lingual muscles it leads to dysphagia (difficulty in swallowing) and dysarthria (poor articulation). In the case of a supranuclear lesion, the contralateral lingual muscles are paralysed, because the paretic site in the brain is located on the side of the tongue which is still intact. Due to the close paramedian relationship of the hypoglossal nuclei, their bilateral damage in the brainstem occurs frequently.

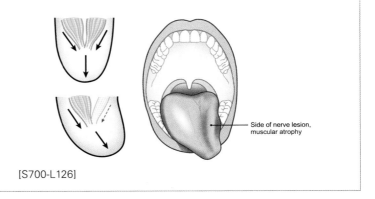

Side of nerve lesion, muscular atrophy

[S700-L126]

Spinal cord segments

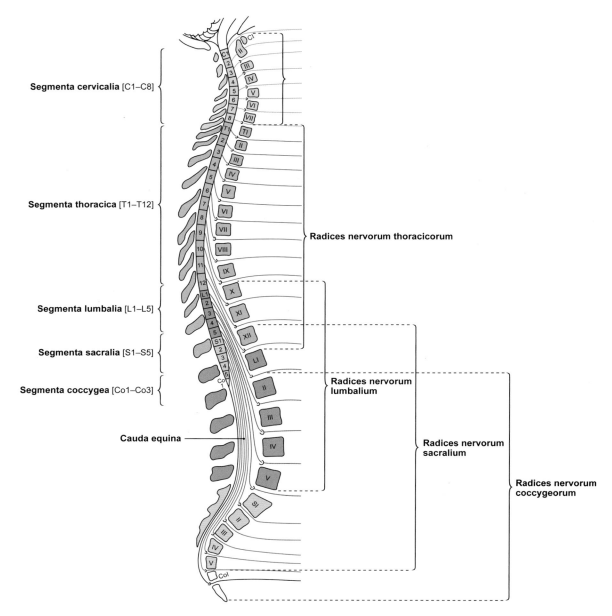

Segmenta cervicalia [C1–C8]

Segmenta thoracica [T1–T12]

Radices nervorum thoracicorum

Segmenta lumbalia [L1–L5]

Segmenta sacralia [S1–S5]

Segmenta coccygea [Co1–Co3]

Radices nervorum lumbalium

Cauda equina

Radices nervorum sacralium

Radices nervorum coccygeorum

Fig. 12.175   Spinal cord segments, Segmenta medullae spinalis; schematic median section; view from the left side; regional segments highlighted by different colours. [S700-L126]/[B500~M492/L316]/ [G1083]
The spinal cord is composed of eight cervical segments (Segmenta cervicalia [C1–C8]), 12 thoracic segments (Segmenta thoracica [T1–T12]), five lumbar segments (Segmenta lumbalia [L1–L5]), five sacral segments (Segmenta sacralia [S1–S5]) and one to three coccygeal segments (Segmenta coccygea [Co1–Co3]). In the adult, the spinal cord extends only to the level of the lumbar vertebrae LI–LII.

The segmental spinal nerve roots (Radices nervorum) pass through their corresponding Foramina intervertebralia. Due to the faster growth of the vertebral canal, the spinal cord ends much higher above the foramen belonging to the corresponding spinal nerve root in the vertebral canal, therefore the pathway of the spinal nerve roots in the vertebral canal gets increasingly longer from cranial to caudal. Below the lumbar vertebrae LI–LII, the spinal nerve roots in the vertebral canal are arranged as the so-called horse tail (Cauda equina).

Clinical remarks

Any kind of narrowing or constriction of the vertebral canal results in disorders of the corresponding segmental neurons. Tumours (→ figure) or median disc prolapses occurring below the spinal cord segment S3 can result in a **conus medullaris syndrome** (lesion of spinal cord segments S3–Co3) or a **cauda equina syndrome** (lesion of spinal nerve roots in the area of the Cauda equina). The symptoms are sensory deficits (saddle anaesthesia), flaccid paralysis, incontinence and impotence.
[R317]

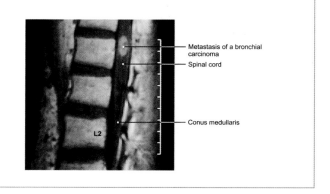

Metastasis of a bronchial carcinoma

Spinal cord

Conus medullaris

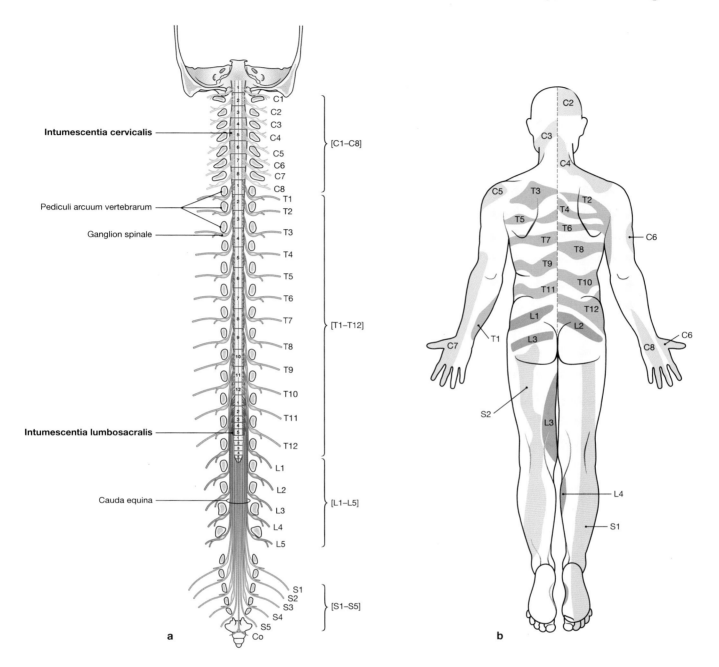

Fig. 12.176a and b   Spinal cord segments, Segmenta medullae spinalis, and corresponding dermatomes. [S700-L126]/[E402-004]
a Schematic representation of a frontal section, ventral view.
b Schematic representation of the dermatomes innervated by the corresponding spinal cord segments.
Due to its slower growth during development, the spinal cord is considerably shorter than the spine; therefore the spinal nerve roots get increasingly longer in the cranial to caudal direction and increasingly oblique in the lateral direction. In adults, the spinal cord ends approx. at the level of LI–LII (ranging from TXII to LII/LIII). Therefore, the Radices

anteriores and posteriores lie in higher segments of the spine than the exit point of the corresponding spinal nerve on the vertebral canal. Below the Conus medullaris, the Radices anteriores and posteriores of the lumbar, sacral and coccygeal nerves are bundled caudally to reach their exit points (foramina) from the vertebral canal. This collection of nerve roots is known as the Cauda equina. In the figure on the right, the skin areas (dermatomes) of the back are shown, which receive their autonomic innervation from the sensory fibres of the spinal nerves of the corresponding spinal cord segments (spinal nerve roots).

Clinical remarks

Referred pain is defined as a misinterpretation of visceral pain by the brain. The visceral pain is not perceived at the site of its origin, but projected into distant skin areas **(HEAD's zones)**. Referred pain is usually the result of nociceptive input (pain information) originating from an area such as the intestines, which only have a small number of afferent sensory fibres. Along with afferent fibres of a particular

skin area (dermatome), these fibres converge at the same spinal cord levels, which have a large number of afferent sensory fibres. Thereby the brain locates the visceral pain in the corresponding region of the skin. A typical example is the referred pain felt in the left arm with angina pectoris or a myocardial infarction.

425

Spinal cord

Spinal cord segments

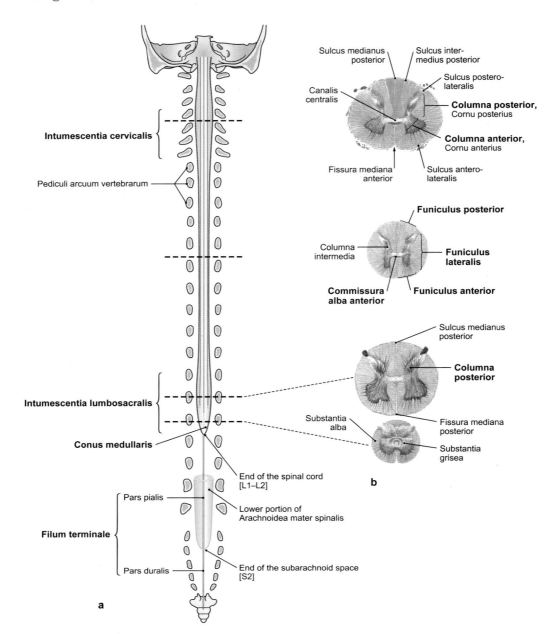

Fig. 12.177a and b   Spinal cord, Medulla spinalis, segments and cross-sections.
a Ventral view. [S700-L126]
b Cross-sections at the level of the dotted lines in the Pars cervicalis, Pars thoracica, Pars lumbalis and Pars sacralis. [S700]
The spinal cord is the part of the CNS located in the upper two-thirds of the vertebral canal. In adults, it extends from the Foramen magnum to approx. the level of LI/LII. In newborns, the spinal cord extends to the level of LIII or even LIV. The distal end is cone-shaped (Conus medullaris). Attached to the Conus medullaris is a fine network of connective tissue (Filum terminale) which comprises parts of the pia mater and

continues caudally in the vertebral canal. The spinal cord is widened in the region of the spinal nerve roots supplying the limbs. The upper (cervical) widening (Intumescentia cervicalis, C5–T1) contains neurons for the innervation of the upper limbs; the lower (lumbosacral) widening (Intumescentia lumbosacralis) lies at the level of the spinal nerve roots L1–S3 and provides the innervation of the lower limbs. The cross-sections of the Medulla spinalis show the typical distribution pattern of the grey and the white matter. In contrast to the brain, the butterfly-shaped Substantia grisea of the spinal cord lies in the centre, and is enveloped by the Substantia alba.

Most frequently clinically examined spinal cord segments, Segmenta medullae spinalis, and their corresponding key muscles		
Spinal cord segment	**Indicator muscle**	**Dermatome**
C5	M. deltoideus	Lateral upper arm; shoulder region
C6	M. biceps brachii; M. brachioradialis	Thumb; thenar region
C7	M. triceps brachii	Middle finger
C8	Mm. interossei of the hand	Digitus minimus; hypothenar region
L3	M. quadriceps femoris; M. iliopsoas	Knee, medial aspect
L4	M. tibialis anterior	Lower leg, medial aspect
L5	M. extensor hallucis longus	Big toe region
S1	M. triceps surae	Foot and leg region, lateral aspect

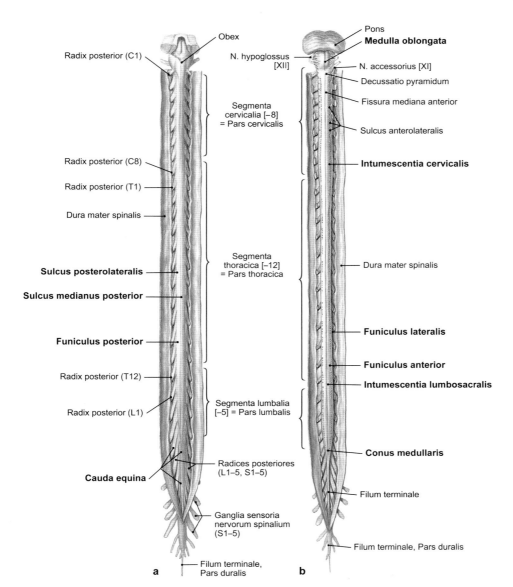

Obex

Radix posterior (C1)

Pons
Medulla oblongata

N. hypoglossus
[XII]

N. accessorius [XI]

Decussatio pyramidum

Fissura mediana anterior

Segmenta
cervicalia [–8]
= Pars cervicalis

Sulcus anterolateralis

Intumescentia cervicalis

Radix posterior (C8)

Radix posterior (T1)

Dura mater spinalis

Segmenta
thoracica [–12]
= Pars thoracica

Dura mater spinalis

Sulcus posterolateralis

Sulcus medianus posterior

Funiculus lateralis

Funiculus posterior

Funiculus anterior

Radix posterior (T12)

Intumescentia lumbosacralis

Radix posterior (L1)

Segmenta lumbalia
[–5] = Pars lumbalis

Conus medullaris

Radices posteriores
(L1–5, S1–5)

Cauda equina

Filum terminale

Ganglia sensoria
nervorum spinalium
(S1–5)

Filum terminale, Pars duralis

a

Filum terminale,
Pars duralis

b

Fig. 12.178a and b   Spinal cord, Medulla spinalis, and spinal nerves, Nn. spinales, after opening the vertebral canal and the dural sac. [S700]
a Dorsal view.
b Ventral view.
The spinal cord is shaped like a sword and has a diameter of 1–1.5 cm. It connects caudally to the Medulla oblongata of the brainstem. In the cervical and lumbar regions it is enlarged to form the Intumescentia cervicalis (C5–T1) and the Intumescentia lumbosacralis (L2–S3). Multiple neurons and nerve fibres are located here which mainly supply the

innervation of the limbs. The Conus medullaris forms the caudal tip of the spinal cord.
The surface of the spinal cord is characterised by **longitudinal grooves**. These are the Fissura mediana anterior in the midline of the ventral side and the Sulcus medianus posterior on the dorsal side. On both sides, the Funiculus anterior runs laterally of the Fissura mediana anterior. The Sulcus ventrolateralis follows, separating the Funiculus anterior from the Funiculus lateralis. The Funiculi posteriores lie dorsally on the right and left sides of the Sulcus medianus posterior, and are separated from the Funiculi laterales by the Sulci posterolaterales.

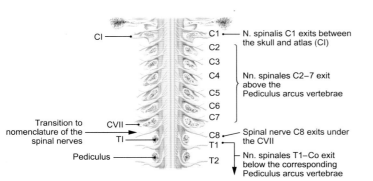

CI

C1
C2
C3
C4
C5
C6
C7

N. spinalis C1 exits between the skull and atlas (CI)

Nn. spinales C2–7 exit above the Pediculus arcus vertebrae

Transition to nomenclature of the spinal nerves

CVII

TI

C8
T1
T2

Spinal nerve C8 exits under the CVII

Nn. spinales T1–Co exit below the corresponding Pediculus arcus vertebrae

Pediculus

Fig. 12.179   Nomenclature of the spinal nerves. [S700-L284]
In contrast to the other spinal cord segments, the number of spinal cord segments in the cervical spine does not correspond with the number of the vertebrae. In the **cervical spine** there are eight cervical cord segments as opposed to only seven cervical vertebrae. The first pair of cervical nerves exits between the skull and the atlas (CI). The subsequent pairs of spinal nerves C2–C7 exit **above** the respective corresponding Pediculus arcus vertebrae. At the transition from the seventh cervical vertebra to the first thoracic vertebra, the nomenclature changes since the eighth spinal nerve exits below the seventh cervical vertebra. The subsequent pairs of spinal nerves T1–Co always exit **inferior** to the corresponding vertebral arch.

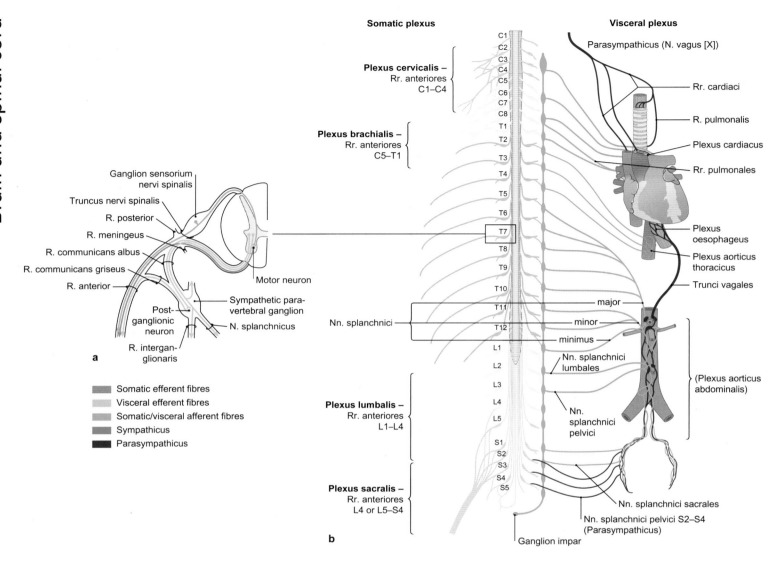

Somatic plexus

C1
C2
C3
C4
C5
C6
C7
C8

Plexus cervicalis –
Rr. anteriores
C1–C4

Plexus brachialis –
Rr. anteriores
C5–T1

T1
T2
T3
T4
T5
T6
T7
T8
T9
T10
T11
T12
L1
L2
L3
L4
L5
S1
S2
S3
S4
S5

Ganglion sensorium
nervi spinalis

Truncus nervi spinalis

R. posterior

R. meningeus

R. communicans albus

R. communicans griseus

R. anterior

Post-
ganglionic
neuron

R. intergan-
glionaris

Motor neuron

Sympathetic para-
vertebral ganglion

N. splanchnicus

a

Somatic efferent fibres
Visceral efferent fibres
Somatic/visceral afferent fibres
Sympathicus
Parasympathicus

Plexus lumbalis –
Rr. anteriores
L1–L4

Plexus sacralis –
Rr. anteriores
L4 or L5–S4

Nn. splanchnici

b

Visceral plexus

Parasympathicus (N. vagus [X])

Rr. cardiaci

R. pulmonalis

Plexus cardiacus

Rr. pulmonales

Plexus
oesophageus

Plexus aorticus
thoracicus

Trunci vagales

major
minor
minimus

Nn. splanchnici
lumbales

Nn.
splanchnici
pelvici

(Plexus aorticus
abdominalis)

Nn. splanchnici sacrales

Nn. splanchnici pelvici S2–S4
(Parasympathicus)

Ganglion impar

Fig. 12.180a and b Spinal nerve and nerve plexuses.
a Composition and bifurcation of a thoracic spinal nerve. [S700-L126]/
[B500-M492/L316]
b Illustration of the somatic (on the left) and autonomic (on the right)
nerve plexuses. [S700-L126]/[E402-004]
Spinal nerves consist of the Fila radicularia of the anterior and posterior
nerve roots, which leave the spinal cord as **Radix anterior** (Radix motoria, axons of the motor neurons) at the Sulcus anterolateralis, or enter it
dorsally as **Radix posterior** (Radix sensoria, axons of the pseudo-unipolar nerve cells of the spinal ganglion, Ganglion sensorium nervi spinalis, located in the area of the Foramen intervertebrale). The fibres of the
Radices anterior and posterior unite to form the trunk of the spinal
nerve, which therefore contains mixed fibre qualities (somatic motor,
somatic sensory, autonomic). The trunk of the spinal nerve divides
immediately into its terminal branches: **R. meningeus, R. posterior,
R. anterior,** and in the thoracolumbar region into the **R. communicans
albus** connected to the sympathetic trunk, and the **R. communicans
griseus** for the transmission of sympathetic impulses.

Nerve plexuses (b) can be somatic (shown on the left side) or visceral
(right side) and consist of fibres of different qualities and levels. Nerves
originating from the plexuses supply various target tissues and organs.
Enteric nerve plexuses can generate reflex activities independent of the
CNS.
The large **somatic plexuses** emerge from the Rr. anteriores of the spinal nerves: Plexus cervicalis (C1–C4), Plexus brachialis (C5–T1), Plexus
lumbalis (L1–L4), Plexus sacralis (L4–S4) and Plexus coccygeus (S5–
Co). With the exception of the spinal nerve T1, all thoracic spinal nerves
have Rr. anteriores, which are independent branches and do not participate in the formation of a plexus.
The **visceral nerve plexuses** develop along with the viscera, and normally contain efferent (sympathetic and parasympathetic) and afferent
parts. The visceral plexuses include the Plexus cardiacus and Plexus
pulmonalis in the thorax, as well as the Plexus aorticus abdominalis
anterior to the aorta in the abdomen, which extends caudally to the lateral pelvic walls. The Plexus aorticus abdominalis projects efferent fibres to all abdominal and pelvic organs, and receives afferents from the
same organs.

Clinical remarks

Irritation or lesions of individual nerve roots are collectively defined
as **radiculopathy.** The most common cause is a mediolateral disc
prolapse (→ Fig. 12.189). Very often, the segments C4–C7 of the cervical spine and L4/L5 and L5/S1 of the lumbosacral transition are affected. Patients typically complain of sensory dysfunctions, muscle
weakness or even paralysis. The isomuscular reflexes are weakened.

Clinically a very precise distinction has to be made between radicular
and peripheral lesions. Radicular disorders correspond to the segmental organisation of the spinal cord in their manifestation. Lesions
distal to the plexus manifest according to the innervation pattern of
the affected peripheral nerves.

Fig. 12.181 Spinal cord, Medulla spinalis; laminar organisation of the grey matter with respect to its cytoarchitecture (according to REXED, 1952) exemplified on a thoracic segment (T10). [B500-L238]
On the histological level (cytoarchitecture), the grey matter (Substantia grisea) is divided into a number of **layers** (laminae) which are numbered I to X in the dorsal to ventral order (formation and number of the layers vary in different segments of the spinal cord). In addition, various nerve **nuclei** are defined. However, these nuclei may extend onto several cytoarchitectural neuronal layers. The division into nuclei or nuclear areas is based on the functional organisation.
The **posterior horns** (Laminae I–VI: Nucleus thoracicus posterior [STILLING-CLARKE's column], Nucleus proprius, Substantia gelatinosa) contain relay neurons for the transmission of afferent sensory input (stimuli of cutaneous receptors, deep sensibility, pain perception from the periphery), which are relayed and transmitted from here. The **lateral horns** (Lamina VII) contain neurons (Nucleus intermediolateralis) for autonomic efferences. The **anterior horns** (Columna anterior, Cornu anterius; Laminae VIII, IX) contain the neurons (somatic-efferent root cells) with efferent fibres to the musculature.

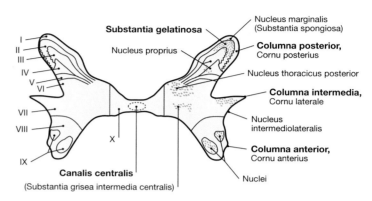

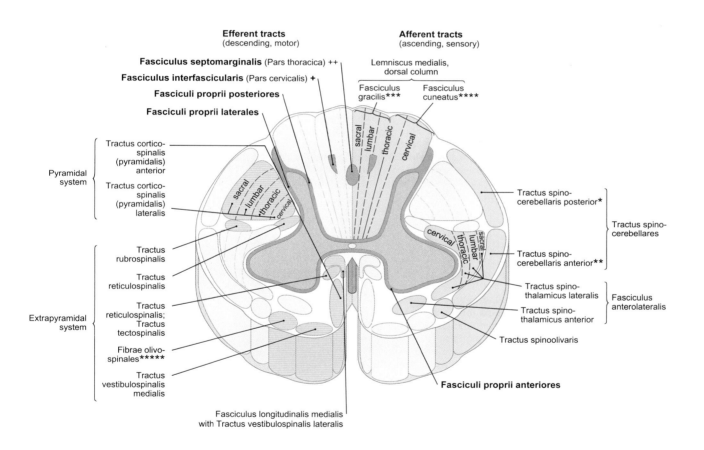

Fig. 12.182 Spinal cord, Medulla spinalis; schematic structure of the white matter exemplified by a lower cervical segment. [S700-L127]/[B500-M492/L316]
Afferent (= ascending) tracts are highlighted in blue, and efferent (= descending) tracts in red.
The regions indicated with + and ++ contain descending collateral tracts of the posterior funiculi.
*   clin.: FLECHSIG's tract
**   clin.: GOWERS' tract
***   clin.: GOLL's tract
****   clin.: BURDACH's tract
***** clin.: The existence of these fibres has not yet been evidenced conclusively.

+   SCHULTZE's comma tract (Pars cervicalis)
++   oval bundle of FLECHSIG (Pars thoracica)
The Fasciculus gracilis conducts fibres for the epicritic sensibility of the lower extremities up to spinal cord segment T6. Upwards of T6, epicritic sensibility, including the upper extremities, is conducted via the Fasciculus cuneatus. Fibres for protopathic sensibility are conducted via the Tractus spinothalamici anterior and lateralis. The unconscious proprioception is conducted via the Tractus spinocerebellares anterior and posterior to the cerebellum. Motor efferences (descending) regulate the muscle contractions in the body. The innermost layer of efferent fibres in the pyramidal tract associate with the cervical region. These are the first fibres that synapse with α-motor neurons in the neck region and innervate the neck muscles. The pyramidal fibre tracts for the thoracic, lumbar and sacral regions are layered outwards on top of the cervical fibres.

Tracts of the spinal cord

Efferent and afferent tract systems of the Substantia alba of the spinal cord		
Type	**Tracts/systems**	**Tractus/fasciculi**
Descending (efferent) tract systems		
Autonomic fibres		
Motor nerve fibres	Pyramidal tracts	• Tractus corticospinalis lateralis • Tractus corticospinalis anterior

	Extrapyramidal tracts	• Lateral tract: Tractus rubrospinalis
		• Medial tracts:
		  – Tractus tectospinalis
		  – Tractus reticulospinalis
		  – Tractus vestibulospinales medialis and lateralis

Ascending (afferent) tract systems		
Proprioceptive fibres	Posterior funiculus	• Fasciculus gracilis • Fasciculus cuneatus
Pain-conducting fibres	Spinothalamic system	• Tractus spinothalamicus lateralis • Tractus spinothalamicus anterior • Tractus spinoreticularis • Tractus spinotectalis
	Spinocerebellar system	• Tractus spinocerebellaris posterior • Tractus spinocerebellaris anterior • Tractus spinocerebellaris superior • Tractus spinoolivaris

---

Clinical remarks

Due to a consistent immunisation/vaccination programme (initially with the vaccine of living micro-organisms and since 1998 with dead vaccine), the infectious disease of **poliomyelitis** (infantile paralysis) is now considered largely eradicated in Western industrialised nations. Infection with the polio virus leads to an isolated destruction of α-motor neurons (second neuron of the motor tract system). This results in flaccid muscle paralysis and loss of isomuscular reflexes with preserved sensitivity. The first motor neuron in the Gyrus precentralis is intact, but the motor neurons of the spinal cord and the motor nuclei of the cranial nerves are damaged by the endemically occurring polio virus. In 95 % of all cases, the infection is asymptomatic, but in 5 % it results in poliomyelitis.

Clinical remarks

Damage or compression of the spinal cord can be caused by intramedullary (Clinical remarks for → Fig. 12.175) or extramedullary tumours, medial disc prolapses (→ figure), dorsal spondylophytes, or due to an accident. A complete **paraplegia** results in the loss of all qualities of sensory, motor and autonomic functions below the lesion site. Initially a flaccid paralysis develops below the lesion site (spinal shock), which converts into a spastic paralysis over time.
BROWN-SÉQUARD syndrome is defined as a spinal hemiplegia with spastic paresis below the lesion site, and dissociative sensory dysfunctions combined with a loss of proprioception (deep sensibility, dorsal tracts) on the affected side and a loss of pain and temperature sensation on the contralateral side (lateral spinothalamic tract system; Clinical remarks for → Fig. 12.203).

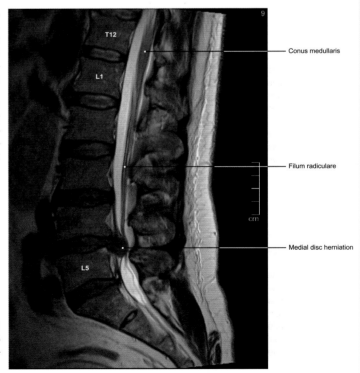

Conus medullaris

Filum radiculare

Medial disc herniation

MRI of the lumbar spine at the thoracolumbar and lumbosacral transition (T2-weighted). Median prolapse of the vertebral disc at L5 with typical clinical symptoms of a weak dorsal extension of the hallux and back pain on the left side. [S700-O534]

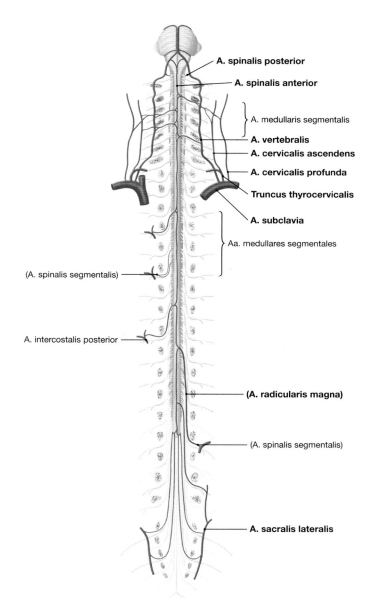

A. spinalis posterior

A. spinalis anterior

A. medullaris segmentalis

A. vertebralis

A. cervicalis ascendens

A. cervicalis profunda

Truncus thyrocervicalis

A. subclavia

Aa. medullares segmentales

(A. spinalis segmentalis)

A. intercostalis posterior

(A. radicularis magna)

(A. spinalis segmentalis)

A. sacralis lateralis

Fig. 12.183 Arteries of the spinal cord, Medulla spinalis; ventral view; not all segmental spinal arteries are shown. [S700-L284]
The arterial blood supply of the spinal cord is fed by three sources:
* through the **A. subclavia** (cervical segment) via the A. spinalis anterior and Rr. radiculares anteriores and posteriores from the Aa. vertebralis, cervicalis ascendens and cervicalis profunda
* through the **Aorta thoracica** (thoracic segment) via the A. intercostalis suprema and Aa. intercostales posteriores

* through the **Aorta abdominalis** (lumbosacral segment) via the Aa. lumbales.

The A. iliaca interna supplies the Cauda equina via the A. iliolumbalis and A. sacralis lateralis. All of these arteries provide the Rr. spinales. The largest R. spinalis is the **A. radicularis magna** [ADAMKIEWICZ], which emerges between T8 and L3: in 50 % of all cases at the level of T9/T10, and in 75 % of all cases on the left side. Additional radiculomedullary arteries occur in 43 % of all cases.

Clinical remarks

Occlusions of the A. spinalis anterior (supply area → Fig. 12.184) can be caused by thrombosis, tumours, etc., and can lead to an **anterior spinal artery syndrome** in the artery's supply area. At the level of the arterial occlusion, lesions to both anterior horns lead to flaccid paralysis of the muscles and muscular parts innervated by the affected segment of the spinal cord. Simultaneously, the tracts in the Funiculus anterolateralis become dysfunctional. In regions of the body which are innervated by spinal cord segments below the arterial occlusion, spas-

tic paraparesis, loss of pain and temperature perception (but preservation of touch perception) will occur, as well as micturition and defecation disorders and sexual dysfunctions (→ Fig. 12.207).
Blockage of blood supply by the largest anterior radicular vessel results in a **A. radicularis magna syndrome.** Depending on the level of the blockage, this results in symptoms of paraplegia in the lower thoracic or upper lumbar regions with complete loss of function of spinal cord segments below the lesion.

Arteries and meninges of the spinal cord

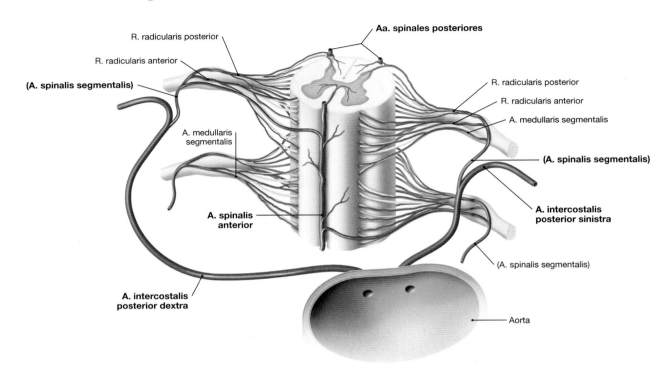

Fig. 12.184 **Segmental arterial blood supply of the spinal cord;** oblique ventral view. [S700-L275]

The blood supply of the spinal cord is provided by the **A. spinalis anterior** and the **Aa. spinales posteriores,** which originate in the cervical region and are arranged longitudinally along the spinal cord. Additional contributors are feeder arteries (spinal segmental arteries from the Aa. vertebrales, the deep cervical arteries, the Aa. intercostales and

Aa. lumbales), which enter the vertebral canal via the Foramina intervertebralia and divide into **Rr. radiculares anteriores and posteriores** at the level of each spinal cord plane. The Rr. radiculares anteriores and posteriores follow the spinal nerves and supply them with blood. On different planes, segmental **Aa. medullares** branch off the spinal segmental arteries, which project directly to the longitudinal arteries and anastomose with them.

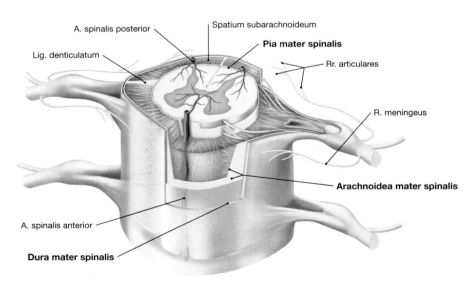

Fig. 12.185 **Meninges of the spinal cord;** oblique ventral view. [S700-L275]

Like the brain, the spinal cord is also surrounded by the three meninges, which protect and suspend it within the vertebral canal.

The **Dura mater spinalis** is the strongest and most external membrane. The laterally exiting spinal nerves and their roots are surrounded by tubular dural sheaths which radiate into and fuse with the neural sheath (epineurium) of the spinal nerves. The spinal arachnoid follows on the inside of the dura. It is separated from the Pia mater spinalis by the subarachnoid space which is filled with cerebrospinal fluid (CSF, Liquor cerebrospinalis). Delicate trabeculations (Trabeculae arachnoideae, not shown) connect the arachnoid mater of one side with the Pia

mater spinalis on the other side. This connective tissue also surrounds the blood vessels located within the subarachnoid space.

The **Pia mater spinalis** is a highly vascularised membrane and tightly attached to the surface of the spinal cord, which it surrounds. It extends deeply into the Fissura mediana anterior, envelops the Radices posteriores and anteriores of the spinal nerves like a sheath, and accompanies them on their way through the subarachnoid space. At the exit or entry sites of the radices, the Pia mater spinalis transitions into the **Arachnoidea mater spinalis.** Extensions of the Pia mater spinalis continue laterally on both sides of the spinal cord as Ligg. denticulata to the spinal arachnoid and dura mater. They serve to attach the spinal cord in the centre of the subarachnoid space.

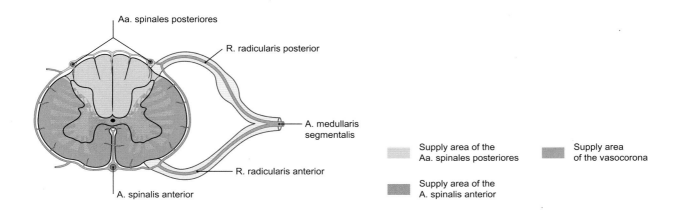

Fig. 12.186 Blood supply of the spinal cord; cross-section. [S700-L126]/[R247-L318]

The blood supply of the spinal cord is divided into the areas of the A. spinalis anterior, the Aa. spinales posteriores and the vasocorona.

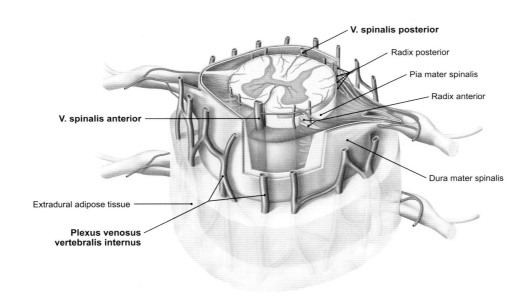

Fig. 12.187 Veins of the vertebral canal, Canalis vertebralis; oblique ventral view. [S700-L275]

The veins draining the spinal cord form for the most part longitudinally arranged vascular trunks. On both sides, two pairs of longitudinal veins are located around the exit or entry sites of the Radix anterior and Radix posterior out of or into the spinal cord, respectively. In addition, the **V. spinalis anterior** runs along the Fissura mediana anterior, and the **V. spinalis posterior** along the Sulcus medianus posterior. These veins drain blood into the **Plexus venosus vertebralis internus** in the epidural space of the vertebral canal. This venous plexus communicates via segmentally arranged veins with the large venous trunks of the body, such as the azygos system, and also with the intracranial veins.

433

Reflexes of the spinal cord

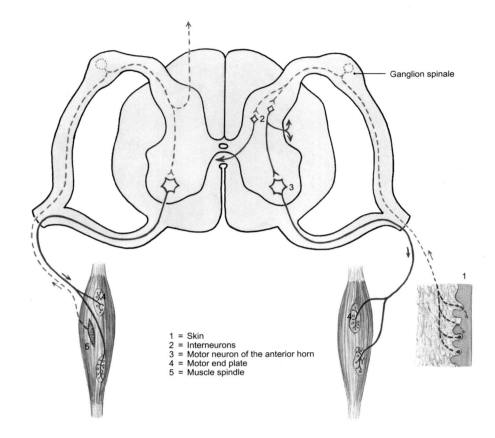

Ganglion spinale

1 = Skin
2 = Interneurons
3 = Motor neuron of the anterior horn
4 = Motor end plate
5 = Muscle spindle

Fig. 12.188   Reflexes of the spinal cord, Medulla spinalis. [S700]
The spinal cord is linked to supraspinal centres via a **connection mechanism,** and has an **intrinsic neuronal network** enabling autonomous spinal reflex loops, which bypass the brain. Spinal reflexes are needed, for example, to maintain a constant muscle tone when at rest or when moving, or to protect against harmful stimuli (e.g. the withdrawal reflex when an extremity is exposed to extreme heat).
Due to the connectivity and complexity, two different **types of reflex circuitry** can be differentiated: monosynaptic (proprioceptive) and poly-

synaptic reflexes. In particular, the polysynaptic reflexes can be modified by supraspinal centres.
Left side of the illustration: local reflex circuitry (monosynaptic, bineuronal, proprioceptive reflex; e.g. a typical stretch reflex such as knee-jerk or patellar, ACHILLES tendon or ankle jerk reflexes, etc.).
Right side of the illustration: complex reflex circuitry (polysynaptic, polyneuronal; e.g. abdominal, cremaster, plantar reflexes, etc.).

Somatic monosynaptic and polysynaptic reflexes with corresponding spinal cord segments for clinical neurological diagnostics			
Reflex	**Triggering stimulus**	**Reflex response**	**Spinal cord segments**
Monosynaptic reflexes			
Biceps tendon reflex	Tapping the biceps tendon	Contraction of the M. biceps brachii (flexion in the elbow joint, supination)	C6 (C5–C6)
Triceps tendon reflex	Tapping the triceps tendon	Contraction of the M. triceps brachii (extension in the elbow joint)	C7 (C6–C8)
Patellar tendon/knee jerk reflex	Tapping the Lig. patellae	Contraction of the M. quadriceps femoris (extension in the knee joint)	L3 (L2–L4)
ACHILLES tendon/ankle jerk reflex	Tapping the ACHILLES tendon	Contraction of the M. triceps surae (plantar flexion of the foot)	S1 (L5–S2)
Polysynaptic reflexes			
Cremaster reflex	Stroking the skin of the medial thigh	Contraction of the M. cremaster (pulls the testicle towards the body)	L1–L2
Abdominal (wall/skin) reflex	Stroking the skin of the lateral abdominal wall	Contraction of ipsilateral abdominal musculature (e.g. M. obliquus externus abdominis)	T6–T12
Anal reflex	Stroking the anal skin	Contraction of the M. sphincter ani externus	S3–S5

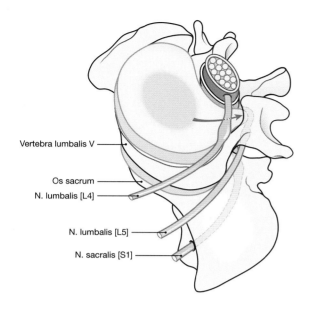

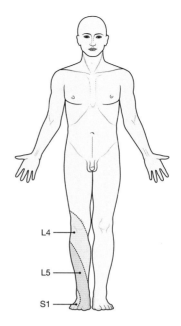

**Fig. 12.189   Mediolateral herniation of the intervertebral disc be-
tween the fourth and fifth lumbar vertebrae** (schematic representation); lateroventral superior view. [S700-L126]/[R363]
This disc prolapse ('slipped disc') results in compression of the spinal
nerve root L5 exiting in the segment below; the more medially located
spinal nerve root L4 exiting in the same segment, however, remains
unaffected.

**Fig. 12.190   Dysfunctional cutaneous innervation due to lesions
(paraesthesia or anaesthesia) of some frequently affected spinal
nerves.** [S700-L126]
The spinal nerves L4, L5, and S1 are particularly affected by disc prolapses.

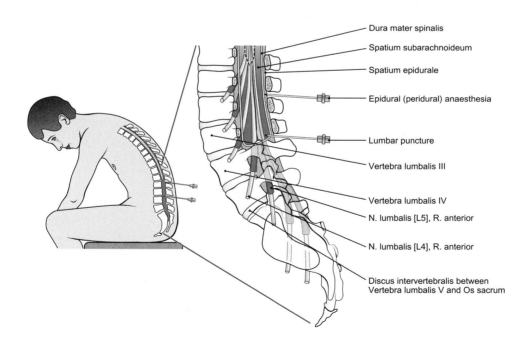

Fig. 12.191   Epidural anaesthesia and spinal anaesthesia. [S700-
L126]/[R363]
Anaesthetics are injected into the epidural space (epidural anaesthesia)
to selectively anaesthetise individual spinal nerves. The local adipose
tissue restricts the anaesthetic from spreading into other spinal cord
segments.
In contrast to epidural anaesthesia, in **spinal anaesthesia** the anaesthetics are applied into the subarachnoid space. The drug mixes with
the cerebrospinal fluid (CSF), but with gravity this is restricted to below

the injection site (in a patient sitting upright), so that only the nerve
branches passing below the injection site are anaesthetised.
For a **lumbar puncture** (with the knees drawn up to the chest) the
needle is usually inserted between the spinous processes of the lumbar vertebrae III and IV or IV and V. Then the needle is carefully pushed
forward until it has penetrated the Dura mater spinalis, and the tip of
the needle lies within the subarachnoid space. Now CSF can be taken
for diagnostic purposes or an anaesthetic can be applied.

Spinal cord and vertebral canal, imaging

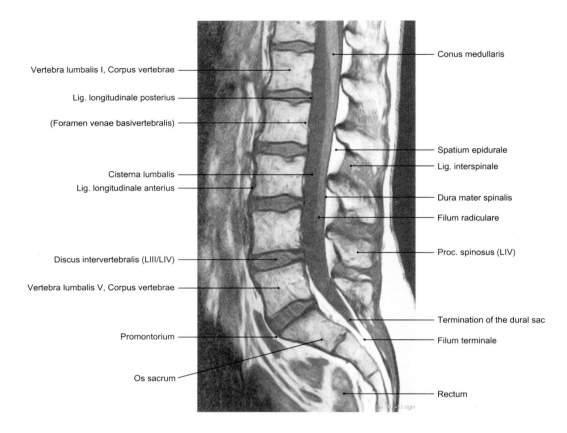

Vertebra lumbalis I, Corpus vertebrae

Lig. longitudinale posterius

(Foramen venae basivertebralis)

Cisterna lumbalis
Lig. longitudinale anterius

Discus intervertebralis (LIII/LIV)

Vertebra lumbalis V, Corpus vertebrae

Promontorium

Os sacrum

Conus medullaris

Spatium epidurale
Lig. interspinale

Dura mater spinalis
Filum radiculare

Proc. spinosus (LIV)

Termination of the dural sac
Filum terminale

Rectum

Fig. 12.192 Lumbar spine; magnetic resonance imaging (MRI) scan of the lumbar and lower thoracic parts of the spinal column, median section, T1-weighted. [R316-007]

It is clearly visible that the spinal cord ends at the level of LI/LII, and that the Cauda equina only partially fills the vertebral canal.

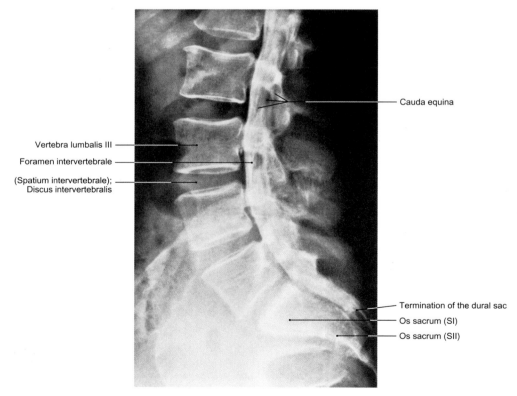

Vertebra lumbalis III
Foramen intervertebrale
(Spatium intervertebrale);
Discus intervertebralis

Cauda equina

Termination of the dural sac
Os sacrum (SI)
Os sacrum (SII)

Fig. 12.193 Myelography of the lumbosacral transition zone; X-ray image in lateral projection. [R316-007]

The contrast medium was distributed in the subarachnoid space. The distal end of the dural sac (CSF space, subarachnoid space) is at the level of the second sacral vertebra (SII).

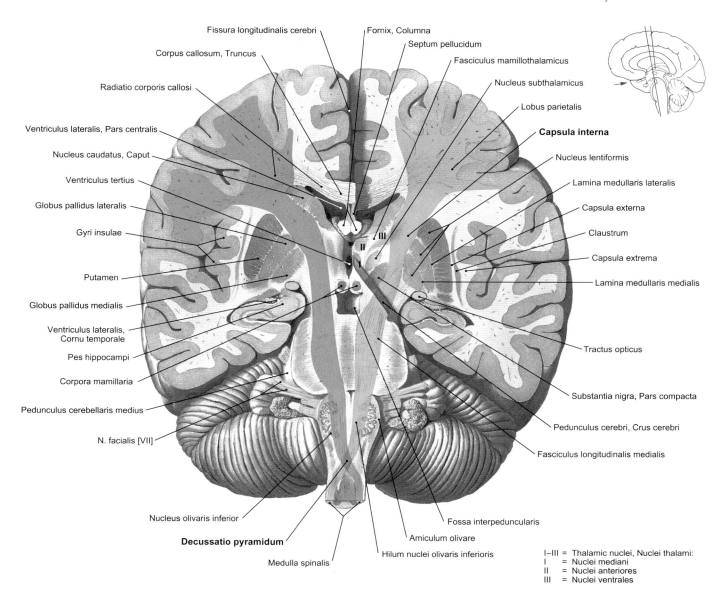

Fissura longitudinalis cerebri

Corpus callosum, Truncus

Radiatio corporis callosi

Ventriculus lateralis, Pars centralis

Nucleus caudatus, Caput

Ventriculus tertius

Globus pallidus lateralis

Gyri insulae

Putamen

Globus pallidus medialis

Ventriculus lateralis, Cornu temporale

Pes hippocampi

Corpora mamillaria

Pedunculus cerebellaris medius

N. facialis [VII]

Nucleus olivaris inferior

Decussatio pyramidum

Medulla spinalis

Fornix, Columna

Septum pellucidum

Fasciculus mamillothalamicus

Nucleus subthalamicus

Lobus parietalis

Capsula interna

Nucleus lentiformis

Lamina medullaris lateralis

Capsula externa

Claustrum

Capsula extrema

Lamina medullaris medialis

Tractus opticus

Substantia nigra, Pars compacta

Pedunculus cerebri, Crus cerebri

Fasciculus longitudinalis medialis

Fossa interpeduncularis

Amiculum olivare

Hilum nuclei olivaris inferioris

I–III = Thalamic nuclei, Nuclei thalami:
I   = Nuclei mediani
II   = Nuclei anteriores
III   = Nuclei ventrales

Fig. 12.194 Pyramidal tract, Tractus pyramidalis, and basal ganglia, Nuclei basales; oblique staggered section through the posterior limb of the internal capsule, the cerebral peduncles, and the Medulla oblongata; anterior view; pyramidal tracts highlighted, right tract: pink, left tract: green. [S700]

The pyramidal tract transmits motor impulses from the motor cortex to the motor corticonuclear fibres (Fibrae corticonucleares) and to the motor neurons in the anterior horn of the spinal cord (Fibrae corticospinales). The fibres **originate** in the Gyrus precentralis, in secondary motor fields, and in somatosensory cortical areas. They **converge** in the Coro-

na radiata, and in a somatotopic arrangement they pass through the genu and Crus posterius of the Capsula interna (→ Fig. 12.196). Along their way they pass through the **Crura cerebri** in the mesencephalon. In the area of the brainstem, the Fibrae corticonucleares leave the pyramidal tract at different levels. In the decussation (crossing over) of the pyramids **(Decussatio pyramidum),** the major part of the remaining fibres (Fibrae corticospinales) cross to the opposite side, whereas a smaller part continues on the ipsilateral side downwards and crosses to the opposite side only within the spinal cord.

Clinical remarks

Lesions of the pyramidal tract initially result in a flaccid paralysis of the muscles on the contralateral side, although the potential for conduction of excitation in the peripheral nervous system and in the muscles is still intact. In particular, the fine motor skills of the hand and foot are affected. Gross movements of the proximal limbs and of the torso are usually still quite intact. In the context of the lesion, primitive reflexes, which are normally blocked by the pyramidal tract, return. These reflexes can be triggered in healthy children up to the age of two years, as the nerve fibres of the pyramidal tract are not yet

completely myelinated. For example, the **BABINSKI reflex** can be triggered again (stroking the lateral sole of the foot leads to dorsiflexion of the big toe).

With time, patients with a lesion of the pyramidal tract develop increased muscular tone and monosynaptic reflexes, but weakened or absent polysynaptic reflexes. This syndrome of spastic paralysis is however caused by an additional lesion of the reticulospinal (extrapyramidal) tracts.

Pyramidal tract

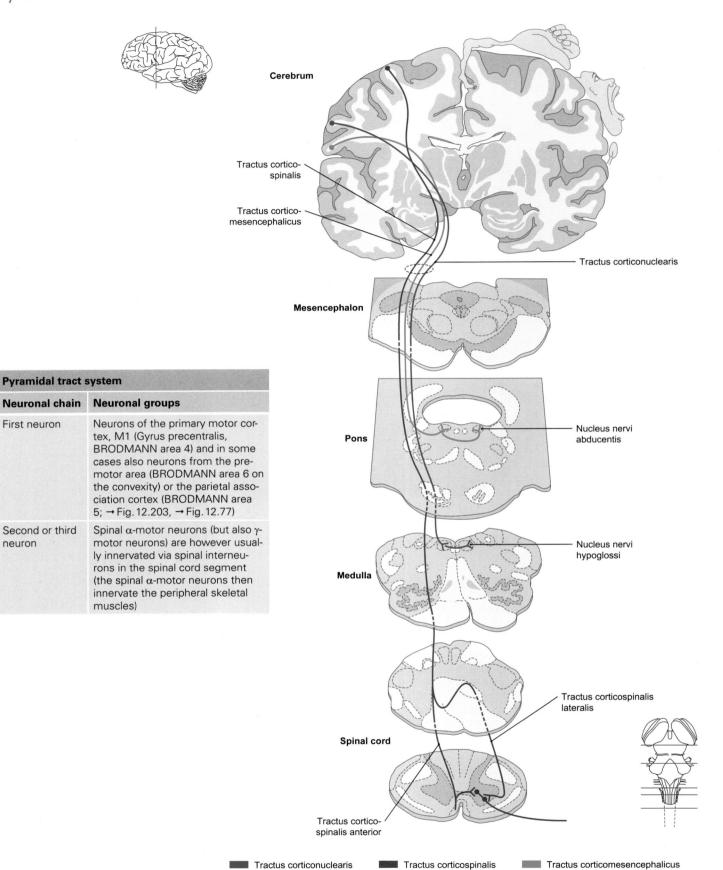

Cerebrum

Tractus cortico-
spinalis

Tractus cortico-
mesencephalicus

Tractus corticonuclearis

Mesencephalon

Pyramidal tract system	
Neuronal chain	**Neuronal groups**
First neuron	Neurons of the primary motor cortex, M1 (Gyrus precentralis, BRODMANN area 4) and in some cases also neurons from the premotor area (BRODMANN area 6 on the convexity) or the parietal association cortex (BRODMANN area 5; → Fig. 12.203, → Fig. 12.77)
Second or third neuron	Spinal α-motor neurons (but also γ-motor neurons) are however usually innervated via spinal interneurons in the spinal cord segment (the spinal α-motor neurons then innervate the peripheral skeletal muscles)

Pons

Nucleus nervi
abducentis

Nucleus nervi
hypoglossi

Medulla

Tractus corticospinalis
lateralis

Spinal cord

Tractus cortico-
spinalis anterior

■ Tractus corticonuclearis   ■ Tractus corticospinalis   ■ Tractus corticomesencephalicus

Fig. 12.195   Parts and pathway of the pyramidal tract; schematic representation. [S702-L127]/[G1081]
The Tractus corticospinalis (red) passes through the Capsula interna and forms the Tractus corticospinales anterior and lateralis at the level of the pyramids. The Tractus corticonuclearis ends crossed and uncrossed at the motor nuclei of the cranial nerves. The Tractus corticomesencephalicus (green) includes fibres from the central visual field, which end at the motor nuclei of the cranial nerves III, IV and VI (e.g. the Nucleus nervi abducentis, as shown here).

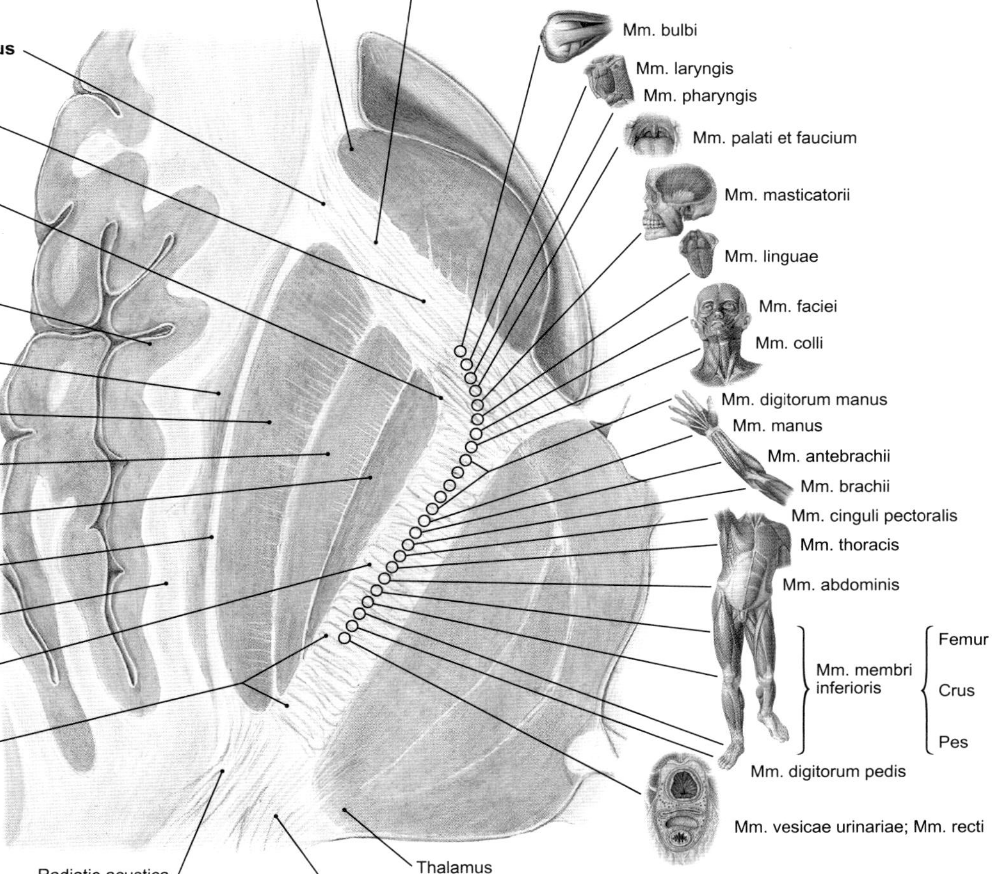
Nucleus caudatus, Caput
Radiationes thalami anteriores
Capsula interna, Crus anterius
Tractus frontopontinus
Capsula interna, Genu
Insula [Lobus insularis]
Claustrum
Putamen
Globus pallidus lateralis
Globus pallidus medialis
Capsula externa
Capsula extrema
Capsula interna, Crus posterius
Crus posterius; Fibrae corticospinales; Fibrae corticorubrales; Fibrae corticoreticulares; Fibrae corticothalamicae; Fibrae thalamoparietales; Radiationes thalami centrales
Radiatio acustica
Radiatio optica
Thalamus
Mm. bulbi
Mm. laryngis
Mm. pharyngis
Mm. palati et faucium
Mm. masticatorii
Mm. linguae
Mm. faciei
Mm. colli
Mm. digitorum manus
Mm. manus
Mm. antebrachii
Mm. brachii
Mm. cinguli pectoralis
Mm. thoracis
Mm. abdominis
Mm. membri inferioris
Femur
Crus
Pes
Mm. digitorum pedis
Mm. vesicae urinariae; Mm. recti

Fig. 12.196 Internal capsule, Capsula interna; functional organisation. [S700]

The Capsula interna is clinically particularly relevant because almost all **cortical projection tracts** are concentrated here in a small space. The Capsula interna is confined by the Nucleus caudatus medially anterior, by the thalamus medially posterior, and by the Globus pallidus and the putamen laterally. In the horizontal section, the Capsula interna appears angled. A distinction is made between the anterior limb (Crus anterius), the 'knee-like' genu and the posterior limb (Crus posterius) of the Capsula interna. Within the Capsula interna, the descending tracts are arranged somatotopically**.** The corticonuclear fibres run in the genu, and the corticospinal fibres passing in the Crus posterius towards the upper limb, torso and lower limb have a somatotopic arrangement (from anterior to posterior).

Tracts and arterial blood supply of the Capsula interna

Localisation	Tracts*	Blood supply
Anterior limb (Crus anterius)	• Tractus frontopontinus (from the frontal lobe to the pons) • Radiatio thalami anterior (from the thalamus to the frontal cortex)	Aa. centrales anteromediales (from the A. cerebri anterior)
Genu	Tractus corticonuclearis (part of the pyramidal tract)	Aa. centrales anterolaterales (from the A. cerebri media) = Aa. lenticulostriatae
Posterior limb (Crus posterius)	• Tractus corticospinalis • Tractus corticorubralis and Tractus corticoreticularis • Radiatio centralis thalami (from the rostral thalamic nuclei to the motor cortex) • Radiatio thalami posterior (from the Corpus geniculatum laterale and further thalamic nuclei to the Lobus parietalis and Lobus occipitalis) • Tractus parietotemporopontinae and Tractus occipitopontinus (from the Lobus temporalis or Lobus occipitalis to the pons) • Radiatio optica (optic/visual radiation; from the Corpus geniculatum laterale to the Lobus occipitalis) • Radiatio acustica (acoustic radiation; from the Corpus geniculatum mediale to the Lobus temporalis)	Rr. capsulae internae (from the A. choroidea anterior)

* Analogous to the clinical usage of the terms, fibrae and tractus are synonyms here.

Clinical remarks

The blood vessels supplying the Capsula interna are terminal arteries. **Vascular occlusions** and **massive bleeding** after rupture of a blood vessel (especially Aa. centrales anterolaterales) with capsular haemorrhage are not rare. Because of the destruction of the tracts, a **stroke** (apoplexy) can occur. Its severity depends on the localisation (lesion site) in the Capsula interna. Common symptoms are a contralateral paralysis (hemiplegia), sensory deficits, and loss of the contralateral half of the visual field (hemianopsia).

Extrapyramidal motor system

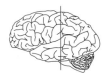

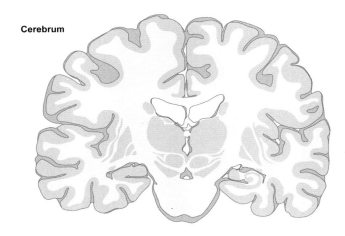

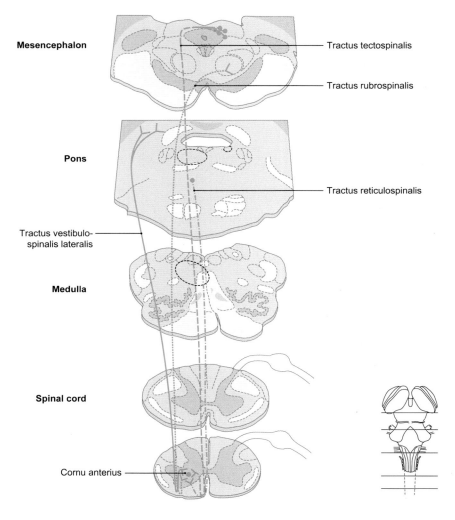

Cerebrum

Mesencephalon — Tractus tectospinalis

— Tractus rubrospinalis

Pons

— Tractus reticulospinalis

Tractus vestibulo-
spinalis lateralis

Medulla

Spinal cord

Cornu anterius

Fig. 12.197 Extrapyramidal motor system (EPMS); schematic representation. [S700-L127]

Phylogenetically, the extrapyramidal motor system (EPMS) is older than the pyramidal system; it consists of descending fibre systems which originate in different nuclear areas of the brainstem. They run crossed or uncrossed in the anterolateral column of the spinal cord. Nuclei or nuclear areas are the Formatio reticularis (Tractus reticulospinalis), Nucleus ruber (Tractus rubrospinalis), tectum (Colliculi superiores, Tractus tectospinalis) and the Nuclei vestibulares lateralis and medialis (Tractus vestibulospinalis). The nuclei or nuclear areas receive primary afferent impulses from the cerebellum and the cortex, and are closely connect-

ed to the basal ganglia (especially to the striatum). They play a role in the control of conscious and unconscious movements by coordinating the processes ('fluency') of the movements, guiding the mostly involuntary movements, and maintaining the muscle tone and balance. The Tractus reticulospinalis, Tractus vestibulospinalis and Tractus tectospinalis are functional-anatomical components of the medial system for the innervation of the axial-skeletal and leg musculature (including stance or postural motility); in contrast, the Tractus rubrospinalis belongs to the lateral system that mainly mediates the movement patterns of arms and hands via the innervation of the upper limbs.

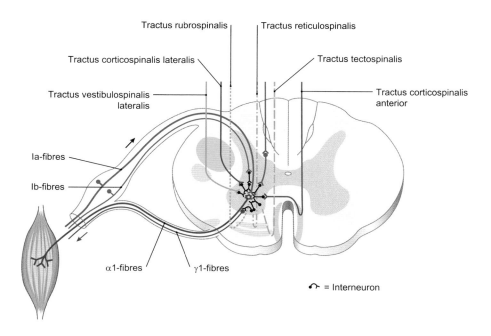

Tractus rubrospinalis

Tractus reticulospinalis

Tractus corticospinalis lateralis

Tractus tectospinalis

Tractus vestibulospinalis
lateralis

Tractus corticospinalis
anterior

Ia-fibres

Ib-fibres

α1-fibres   γ1-fibres

↶ = Interneuron

Fig. 12.198   Final motor pathway and motor unit; schematic representation. [S702-L127]
The α- and γ-motor neurons in the spinal cord are innervated (mostly via interneurons) by various tracts of the pyramidal and extrapyramidal systems. Individual motor neurons (nerve cells of the anterior horn) with their axons and the muscle fibres innervated by them are referred to as a **motor unit.** Via afferent fibres, the motor neurons also receive information from the corresponding muscle fibres (e.g. via stretch receptors).

Clinical remarks

Lesions of the motor unit lead to a **flaccid paralysis.** This is associated with decreased gross motor skills, muscular hypotonia or atonia, hyporeflexia or areflexia, and muscle atrophy.
Damage to the central motor tracts results in **spastic paralysis.** This includes a reduction in muscle strength and fine motor skills, increased spastic tone and stretch reflexes, attenuated multisynaptic reflexes, and the appearance of **pathological reflexes** (e.g. the BABINSKI reflex, OPPENHEIM's sign), while muscle mass remains initially unchanged. In the early stages of a lesion of the central tracts a flaccid paralysis occurs because stretch reflexes are suppressed. However, this quickly transitions into a spastic paralysis.
Positive **BABINSKI reflex:** stroking the lateral sole of the foot triggers a dorsal movement of the big toe with simultaneous plantar movement of the other toes (this is a physiological reflex in newborns, which disappears in the course of early neuronal maturation).
Positive **OPPENHEIM's sign:** identical movements of the toes as in the BABINSKI reflex test, but after stroking the anterior tibia.

In the case of neurodegenerative diseases (affecting the motor neurons), a distinction is made in English-speaking countries between **upper motor neuron disease** and **lower motor neuron disease.** As stated above, lesions of the first motor neuron result in a spastic paralysis (e.g. due to a stroke, multiple sclerosis, traumatic brain injury). Exceptions are isolated lesions of the first motor neuron causing a flaccid paralysis. Lesions of the second motor neuron result in a flaccid paralysis (e.g. associated with **poliomyelitis, GUILLAIN-BARRÉ syndrome,** nerve plexus or peripheral nerve lesions). Sometimes with this disease, both motor neurons are damaged (e.g. **amyotrophic lateral sclerosis** which manifests with a mixed picture of spastic and flaccid paralysis). Diseases of central areas which play a decisive role in the motor pathways can also lead to striking pathologies (e.g. **PARKINSON's disease, HUNTINGTON's disease, hemiballism**).

Voluntary movements

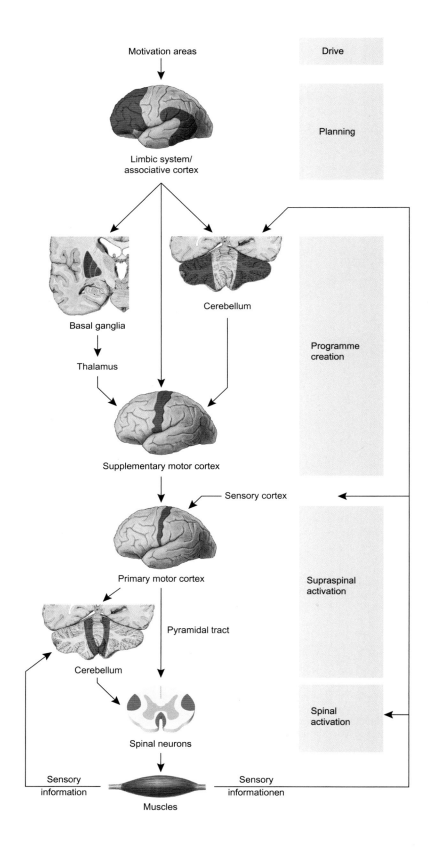

Fig. 12.199 Planning and realisation of voluntary movements; schematic representation. [S702-L127]
The structures shown in the diagram work closely together when carrying out controlled, voluntary movements. This is a sequence of tightly coupled processes in a given time, so that they are perceived as a single process.

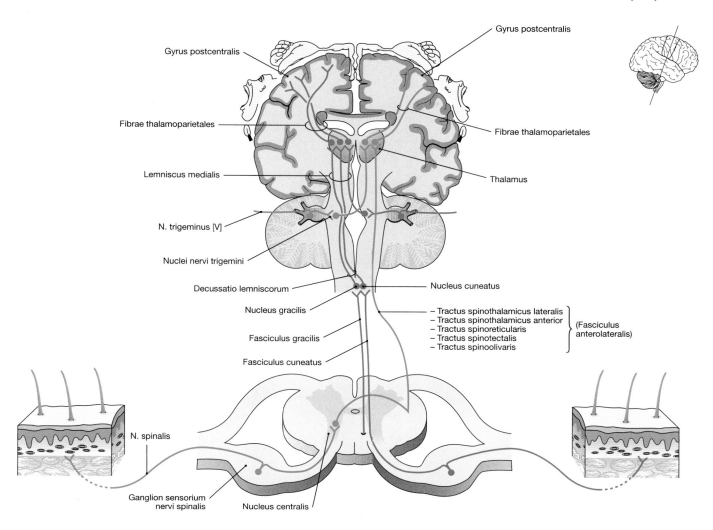

Fig. 12.200   Conduction of epicritic sensibility and pathway of the **Funiculus posterior (blue), and of the spinal afferent and the trigeminal afferent tracts;** conduction of pain/temperature and pathway of neospinothalamic tracts (green). [S700]

Circuitry of epicritic sensibility (somatosensory system; → table), and circuitry of **protopathic sensibility** (nociceptive pathway, for the perception of pain, temperature and pressure sensations):

- **first neuron** (uncrossed): from receptors (exteroceptors) in the skin and mucosa, etc. to the posterior horn, Laminae I to V (root cells, perikarya in the spinal ganglia)

- **second neuron** (crossed, some fibres possibly uncrossed): from the posterior horn to the thalamus, into the Formatio reticularis and to the Tectum mesencephali (Tractus spinothalamici anterior and lateralis, Tractus spinoreticularis, Tractus spinotectalis; perikarya in the dorsal column)

- **third neuron** (uncrossed): from the thalamus among others to the cerebral cortex, particularly to the Gyrus postcentralis (thalamocortical fibres, perikarya in the thalamus).

Somatosensory system	
Neuronal chain	**Localisation**
First neuron	Perikarya of pseudo-unipolar ganglion cells in the Ganglion spinale or Ganglion trigeminale
Second neuron	• in the Cornu posterius • in the Nucleus cuneatus or Nucleus gracilis of the Medulla oblongata • in the Nucleus dorsalis thalami • in the Nucleus spinalis nervi trigemini
Third neuron	Perikarya in the contralateral Nucleus ventralis posterolateralis of the thalamus
Fourth neuron	Primary somatosensory cortex: Gyrus postcentralis and Lobulus paracentralis
Fifth neuron	Secondary somatosensory cortex: Operculum parietale

Spinal cord

Somatosensory system

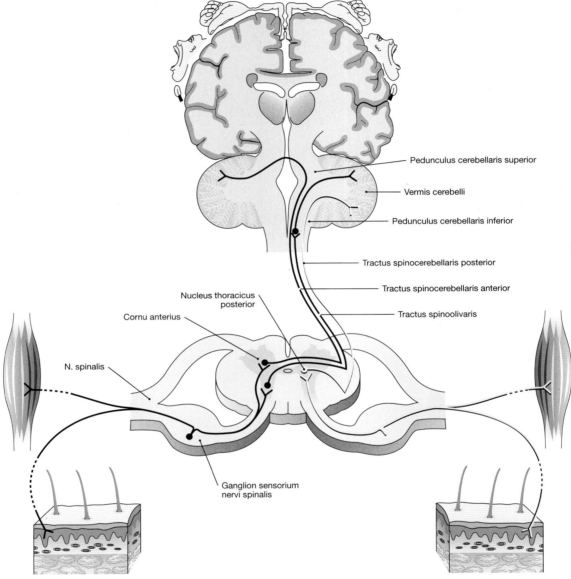

Pedunculus cerebellaris superior

Vermis cerebelli

Pedunculus cerebellaris inferior

Tractus spinocerebellaris posterior

Tractus spinocerebellaris anterior

Tractus spinoolivaris

Nucleus thoracicus posterior

Cornu anterius

N. spinalis

Ganglion sensorium nervi spinalis

Fig. 12.201 Pathway of unconscious deep sensibility (afferent tract). Anterior spinocerebellar tract (Tractus spinocerebellaris anterior, black) and posterior spinocerebellar tract (Tractus spinocerebellaris posterior, yellow). [S700]

The body's sense of position, movement and strength are perceived by proprioception (deep sensibility). The pathway of the unconscious deep sensibility (unconscious, but with precise spatial differentiation as a prerequisite for the coordination of movement by the cerebellum) is conducted via the **anterior spinocerebellar tract** (Tractus spinocerebellaris anterior, black):

- **first neuron** (uncrossed): from proprioceptive receptors in muscles, tendons and connective tissue to the nuclei in the Zona intermedia and to the anterior (ventral) column (root cells, perikarya in the spinal ganglia)
- **second neuron** (double-crossed): from the anterior horn as the Tractus spinocerebellaris anterior within the anterolateral tract, and via

the Pedunculus cerebellaris superior to the cerebellum (cells of the tract, perikarya in the Zona intermedia and the anterior horn).

Another pathway of the unconscious deep sensibility or proprioception is the **posterior spinocerebellar tract** (Tractus spinocerebellaris posterior, yellow):

- **first neuron** (uncrossed): from the end organs (proprioceptive receptors) in muscles, tendons and connective tissue to the nuclei of the posterior (dorsal) column and to the Nucleus thoracicus (root cells, perikarya in the spinal ganglia)
- **second neuron** (uncrossed): from the posterior horn and the Nucleus thoracicus as Tractus spinocerebellaris posterior within the lateral tract, and via the Pedunculus cerebellaris inferior to the cerebellum (cells of the tract, perikarya in the Nucleus thoracicus and at the base of the posterior column).

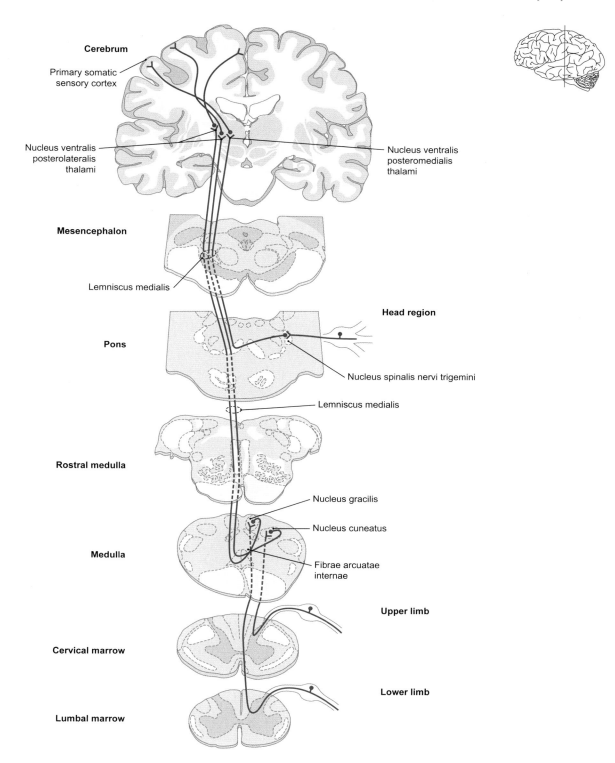

Cerebrum

Primary somatic
sensory cortex

Nucleus ventralis
posterolateralis
thalami

Nucleus ventralis
posteromedialis
thalami

Mesencephalon

Lemniscus medialis

Head region

Pons

Nucleus spinalis nervi trigemini

Lemniscus medialis

Rostral medulla

Nucleus gracilis

Nucleus cuneatus

Medulla

Fibrae arcuatae
internae

Upper limb

Cervical marrow

Lower limb

Lumbal marrow

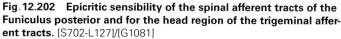

Fig. 12.202 Epicritic sensibility of the spinal afferent tracts of the Funiculus posterior and for the head region of the trigeminal afferent tracts. [S702-L127]/[G1081]

The system of the posterior tracts is characterised by the fact that the fibres run in the ipsilateral Funiculus posterior to the cranial Nuclei cuneatus and gracilis without switching or crossing over to the opposite side. Only after being relayed within the two nuclear areas of the Medulla oblongata, the axons (of the second neuron) cross over to the opposite side as **Fibrae arcuatae internae** in the Decussatio lemnisci medialis. The somatotopic arrangement (somatotopy) remains unchanged along the rest of its pathway as the Tractus bulbothalamicus within the **Lemniscus medialis** to the Nucleus ventralis posterolateralis in the thalamus, during the re-switching and along the pathway as thalamocortical fibres (Fibrae thalamoparietales) through the Crus posterius of the Capsula interna and up to the primary somatosensory cortical areas (Gyrus postcentralis of the parietal lobe). The first relay station of the N. trigeminus [V] lies in the Nucleus spinalis nervi trigemini in the pons. The fibres join the Tractus bulbothalamicus within the Lemniscus medialis and are switched in the Nucleus ventralis posteromedialis of the thalamus before they reach their respective cortical areas as thalamocortical fibres. Here too, the somatotopy remains unchanged along the length of its pathway.

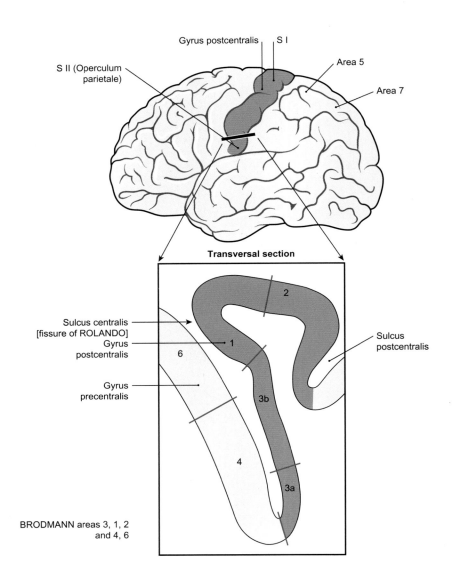

Fig. 12.203   Primary somatosensory cortical area (S I: BROD-MANN areas 3, 1, 2), secondary somatosensory cortical area in the Operculum parietale (S II), and somatosensory association cortex (BRODMANN areas 5 and 7) of the Lobus parietalis. [S700-L126]/[B500~M492/L316]/[G1077]

In the primary somatosensory cortex, apart from the primary perception of sensations, an initial subjective perception also takes place. However, the essential interpretation of the somatosensory information only succeeds in the secondary somatosensory cortex. This small area

is the Operculum parietale located in the Sulcus lateralis [SYLVIAN aqueduct]. Here, stimuli from both body halves (via the Corpus callosum) are united. From the secondary somatosensory cortical areas, the fibres continue to the somatosensory association areas (postparietal cortex, BRODMANN areas 5 and 7), as well as to the insular region and to the limbic system. In the association areas, the afferent somatosensory stimuli are processed along with visual stimuli, and influence motor control via efferent fibres to the precentral region.

Clinical remarks

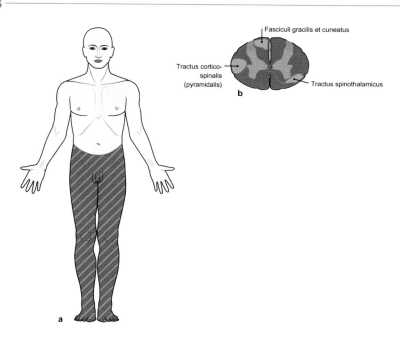

Complete paraplegia at the level of the 11ᵗʰ thoracic segment. [S700-L126]

a This leads to a loss of all the motor and sensory functions in the marked (cross-hatched) area.
b Cross-section of the spinal cord, lesion highlighted.

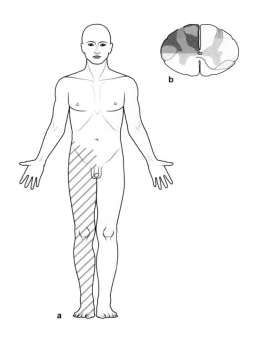

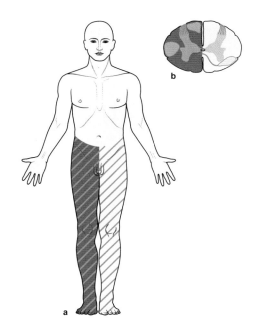

Hemiplegia (BROWN-SÉQUARD) due to a right-sided (hemilateral) disruption of the spinal cord at the level of the 11ᵗʰ thoracic segment. [S700-L126]
a On the right side (homolateral), this results in a loss of motor function, initially of a flaccid type, and later in a spastic paralysis. Furthermore, this is combined with a loss of fine touch sensation, and the sense of position and vibration. The crude touch sensation, however, remains intact. On the left side (contralateral), the result is a loss of pain and temperature sensation (→ Fig. 12.200).
b Cross-section of the spinal cord, lesion highlighted.

Lesion of the tracts of the right Funiculus posterior at the level of the 11ᵗʰ thoracic segment. [S700-L126]
a The fine touch sensation and sense of position and vibration are lost. The crude touch sensation, however, remains intact.
b Cross-section of the spinal cord, lesion highlighted.

Clinical remarks

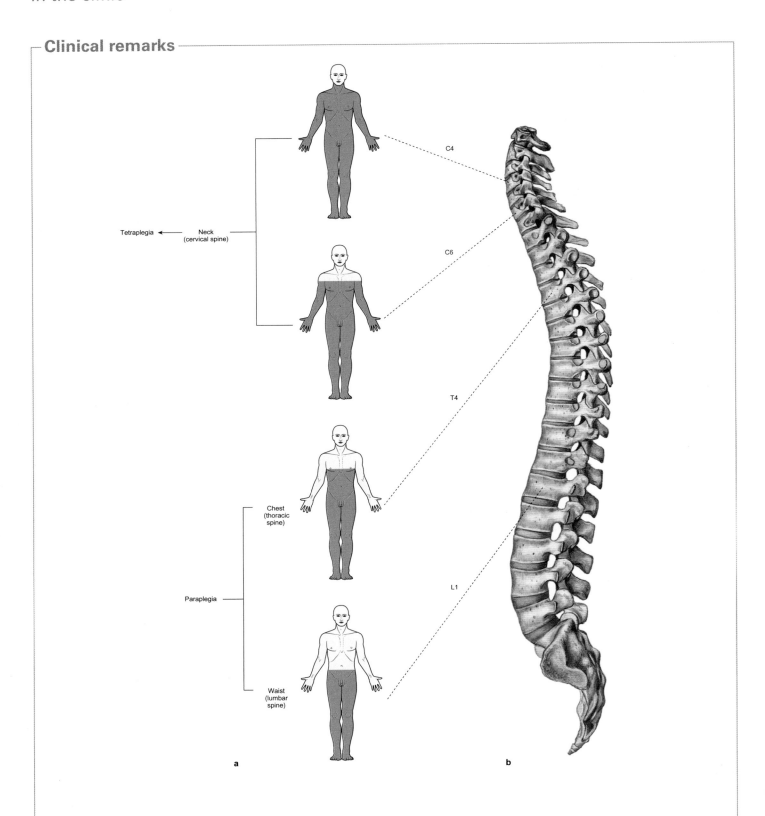

Relationship between the extent of the paralysis and the location of the lesion in the spinal cord.
a Extent of the paralysis. Areas labelled in red represent the paralysed body regions [S701-L126].
b Corresponding location of the spinal cord lesion. [S700]
Tetraplegia or quadriplegia describe the complete paralysis (plegia) of all extremities, e.g. a lesion in the spinal cord segments C1–C7.
Paraplegia refers to the complete plegia of both legs, e.g. lesions from thoracic T4 to lumbar L1 spinal cord segments. Tetraplegia and paraplegia may be complete loss (of all motor and sensory functions)

or incomplete loss (only partial loss of predominantly motor or sensory functions).
Tetraparesis (quadriparesis) is distinct from tetraplegia and refers to a spastic or flaccid muscle weakness in all four extremities, e.g. that occurs as a result of a stroke or GUILLAIN-BARRÉ syndrome.
Hemiplegia is the loss of motor and/or sensory functions on one side of the body.
Monoplegia refers to a complete paralysis of a group of muscles or a body part, mostly the paralysis of one arm or leg.

Clinical remarks

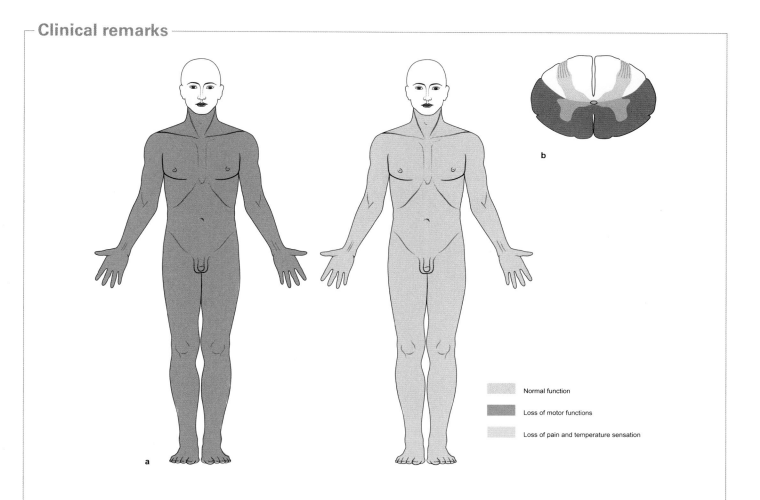

Normal function

Loss of motor functions

Loss of pain and temperature sensation

Spinalis anterior syndrome. [S701-L126]
a Lesion at the level of C4.
b Cross-section of the spinal cord, lesion highlighted.
The **Spinalis anterior syndrome** comprises a range of symptoms as a consequence of reduced arterial blood supply via the A. spinalis anterior to the spinal cord, which can have several causes, e.g. athe- rosclerosis, thrombosis, embolism or trauma. Motor functions are lost below the spinal cord lesion (paraparesis (= partial paralysis) with im- paired micturition and defecation functions). Additionally, a dissociated sensitivity disorder caudal to the lesion results in the loss of pain and temperature sensations (protopathic sensations), while epicritic sen- sations remain intact (sense of position, vibration and touch).

Brain and spinal cord

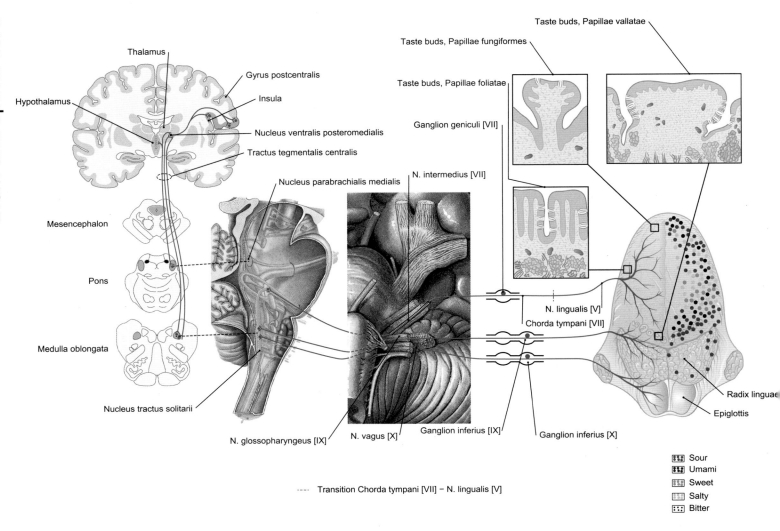

Thalamus
Gyrus postcentralis
Insula
Hypothalamus
Nucleus ventralis posteromedialis
Tractus tegmentalis centralis
Nucleus parabrachialis medialis
Mesencephalon
Pons
Medulla oblongata
Nucleus tractus solitarii
N. glossopharyngeus [IX]
N. vagus [X]
Ganglion inferius [IX]
Ganglion inferius [X]

Taste buds, Papillae vallatae
Taste buds, Papillae fungiformes
Taste buds, Papillae foliatae
Ganglion geniculi [VII]
N. intermedius [VII]
N. lingualis [V]
Chorda tympani [VII]
Radix linguae
Epiglottis

Sour
Umami
Sweet
Salty
Bitter

---- Transition Chorda tympani [VII] – N. lingualis [V]

Fig. 12.204 Human tongue with epiglottis and gustatory (taste) system. [S700-L126/L238]

Approximately 2,000 **taste buds (Caliculi gustatorii)** can be found on the human tongue (in the **Papillae vallatae, fungiformes and foliatae**), the soft palate and the epiglottis. Each taste bud consists of different cell types. The actual receptor cells are epithelial cells, which perceive the five primary taste categories (→ Fig. 8.172) – sweet, sour, salty, bitter, umami. (The sixth could possibly also be oily.) The sensory cells of taste form synapses with axonal plexuses located on the basal side of the taste buds. These are sometimes referred to as **secondary sensory cells,** since the sensory cells do not depolarise, but their action potential arises only when they synapse with the first afferent neuron. Corresponding to their location, the information is transmitted to the **Nucleus tractus solitarii** in the Medulla oblongata:
- from the anterior two-thirds of the tongue via the N. facialis [VII] (Pars intermedia)
- from the posterior third of the tongue and the soft palate via the N. glossopharyngeus [IX]
- from the epiglottis and the soft palate via the N. vagus [X].

Corresponding to the respective nerves, the perikarya of the first neuron are located in the **Ganglion geniculi [VII],** in the **Ganglion inferius [IX]** (Ganglion petrosum) or in the Ganglion inferius [X] (Ganglion nodosum).

In the **Pars gustatoria (Nucleus gustatorius)** of the brainstem, the fibres are relayed onto the second neuron. The axons of the second neuron pass within the ipsilateral **Tractus tegmentalis centralis** (accompanying the Lemniscus medialis) to the **Nucleus ventralis posteromedialis of the thalamus,** where they are switched onto the third neuron. As thalamocortical fibres, they pass to the strictly somatotopically arranged (corresponding to the position of the homunculus, → Fig. 12.79) inferior parts of the Gyrus postcentralis, as well as to **anterior regions of the insular cortex** of the temporal lobe and the operculum of the frontal lobe. These are the areas of conscious taste perception. Some axons pass directly from the thalamus or indirectly from the Nucleus tractus solitarii via the **Nucleus parabrachialis medialis** to the hypothalamus and the amygdala as well (which influences autonomic body functions, such as appetite, satiation, emotional connection).

Clinical remarks

Since the excitation threshold for the action potential of taste receptors increases with age, the perception of the sense of taste is age-dependent. Deficiency or complete loss of the sense of taste is referred to as **hypogeusia** or **ageusia,** respectively. Because of the common secondary cortical area of the gustatory and olfactory pathways in the orbital-frontal cortex, there is a close functional relationship between taste and smell.

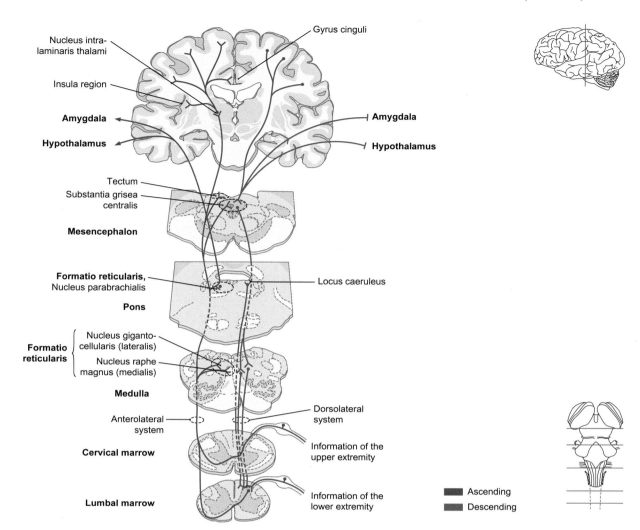

Nucleus intra-laminaris thalami

Insula region

Amygdala

Hypothalamus

Gyrus cinguli

Amygdala

Hypothalamus

Tectum
Substantia grisea centralis

Mesencephalon

Formatio reticularis,
Nucleus parabrachialis

Locus caeruleus

Pons

Formatio reticularis
Nucleus giganto-cellularis (lateralis)
Nucleus raphe magnus (medialis)

Medulla

Anterolateral system

Cervical marrow

Dorsolateral system

Information of the upper extremity

Lumbal marrow

Information of the lower extremity

Ascending
Descending

Fig. 12.205   Ascending tracts of pain conduction in the Tractus paleospinothalamicus (shown on the left side) and descending tracts of pain-modulating fibres (on the right); simplified illustration. [S702-L127]

The perception of pain is highly subjective and is determined by a complex neuronal and modulation process. A distinction is made between **acute and chronic pain, peripherally induced pain** (superficial somatic pain via nociceptive receptors in the skin and muscles; deep somatic pain from joints and tendons; visceral pain due to chemical stimuli, stretching or distension of hollow organs or spasms of smooth visceral muscles), and **centrally mediated pain** (thalamic pain, psychosomatic pain, referred spinal pain).

Pain is essential for the survival and integrity of the human body. A distinction is made between the three ascending pain tracts:

- archispinothalamic tract (→ table): runs mainly in the Fasciculi proprii of the spinal cord, conveys visceral, emotional and autonomic pain reactions via collateral fibre tracts to the hypothalamus and limbic system

- paleospinothalamic tract: dull, slow, somatic and deep pain sensations, often associated with autonomic (vegetative) reactions
- neospinothalamic tract: classic somatic pain sensations perceived as quick and sharp, from the skin and muscles of the upper and lower limbs.

The central neurons end in the Cornu posterius (Lamina I) (→ Fig. 12.181 and → Fig. 12.182) and, after the switching and crossing of the fibres in the Commissura anterior, the Tractus spinothalamicus lateralis continues to the thalamus. With a maintained somatotopic arrangement, the input is transmitted via thalamocortical fibres to the sensory cortex (Gyrus postcentralis), where pain is consciously located. From the head and neck, the transmission continues via the Ganglion trigeminale to the Nucleus spinalis nervi trigemini in the Medulla oblongata, and via the contralateral Tractus trigeminothalamicus within the Lemniscus medialis to the Nucleus ventralis posteromedialis of the thalamus. From here the fibres pass to the corresponding brain regions of the Gyrus postcentralis.

Stations of the nociceptive system	
Neuronal chain	**Neuronal groups**
First neuron	Perikarya of pseudo-unipolar ganglion cells in the Ganglion spinale or Ganglion trigeminale
Second neuron	Within the Cornu posterius (Laminae II, IV–VIII) or Nucleus spinalis nervi trigemini
Third neuron	Perikarya of the thalamus: • ipsilateral Nucleus ventralis posterolateralis (for the Tractus spinothalamicus) • contralateral Nucleus ventralis posteromedialis (for the Tractus trigeminothalamicus) • Perikarya of intralaminar nuclei
Fourth neuron	• Primary somatosensory cortex: Gyrus postcentralis • Hypothalamus, limbic system • Brainstem (Substantia grisea centralis, tectum, Formatio reticularis)

Spinal cord

Autonomic nervous system

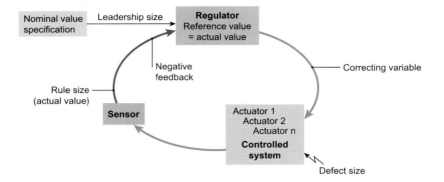

Fig. 12.206 **Homeostasis via feedback loops;** schematic representation. [S701-L127]/[E984]
Within the human body, a constant (steady) state of the internal milieu **(homeostasis)** must be maintained. For this purpose, the actual value is measured by a **sensor** (e.g. chemoreceptor), and this information is transmitted to a **regulator** (e.g. the respiratory centre in the brain-stem). The regulator compares the actual value with the physiological nominal value, and, if needed, counteracts the measured difference by using appropriate **actuators** (e.g. respiratory drive), to align actual and nominal values. This type of regulation is referred to as **feedback loop**. There are negative and positive feedback loops.

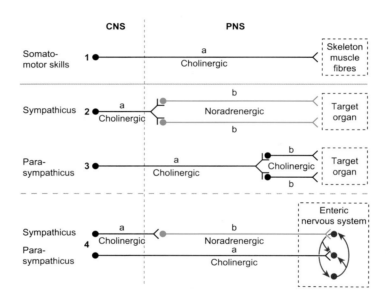

Fig. 12.207 **Circuitry of the peripheral motor innervation in the somatic and autonomic nervous system.** 1 = somatic motor neuron, 2 = visceral motor neuron of the sympathetic nervous system, 3 = visceral motor neuron of the parasympathetic nervous system, 4 = visceral motor neurons and their impact on the enteric nervous system; a = first neuron, b = second neuron. [S701-L141]
The somatic motor innervation of skeletal muscle fibres is provided directly (without further circuitry) via the axons of α-motor neurons of the spinal cord. In contrast, the visceral motor axons are switched at least once in an autonomic ganglion (exception: medulla of the suprarenal gland). In the case of the sympathicus and parasympathicus, the first neuron **(preganglionic neuron)** lies in the central nervous system (brainstem or spinal cord). The corresponding axon **(preganglionic axon)** passes to an autonomic ganglion. There it is relayed onto the second neuron (postganglionic neuron). The latter continues to the target organ.

Clinical remarks

The body's response to **negative stress (distress)** is a reinforced activation of the sympathetic nervous system and increased tension. Long-lasting stress situations may cause a persistent hyperactivity of the sympathetic nervous system. This is associated with an increased release of 'stress hormones', such as glucocorticoids (e.g. cortisol) and catecholamines (e.g. adrenaline). This is accompanied by dys- functional autonomic symptoms, such as increased heart rate and blood pressure (hypertension), cardiac dysrhythmias, irritability and restlessness, all of which is felt and perceived as additional stress by the patient. If the distress continues (sympathetic hyperactivity and excessive secretion of stress hormones over a long period of time), this can cause a **physical and mental fatigue (burn-out).**

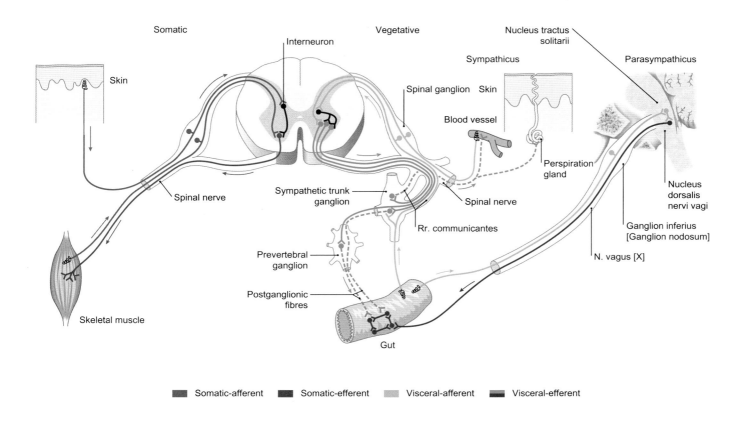

Fig. 12.208 Organisation of the somatic nervous system as compared to the autonomic nervous system (spinal cord and PNS); schematic representation. [S702-L127]/[G1076]

In the **somatic nervous system** (left side), afferent information is transmitted directly via the processes of the spinal ganglionic cells (monosynaptic reflex arc) or indirectly to the α-motor neurons of the anterior horn.

In the case of the **sympathicus** (right side), visceral-afferent information is passed in a first step via spinal ganglionic cells to interneurons of the spinal cord. Via one or more relay stations, the information finally arrives in visceral-efferent neurons of the lateral horn. From here, pre-

ganglionic visceral-efferent axons (green, solid line) continue to the paravertebral ganglia of the sympathetic trunk or the prevertebral ganglia near the aorta. After switching in the ganglia, the postganglionic axons (green, dotted line) reach their target organ. In the case of the **parasympathicus** (N. vagus [X] is given in the example), visceral-afferent information is transmitted via the Ganglion inferius [Ganglion nodosum] of the N. vagus [X] to the Nucleus tractus solitarii in the brainstem, and then relayed onto the Nucleus dorsalis nervi vagi. The visceral motor fibres pass back into the body's periphery (vasovagal reflex arc) via the N. vagus [X].

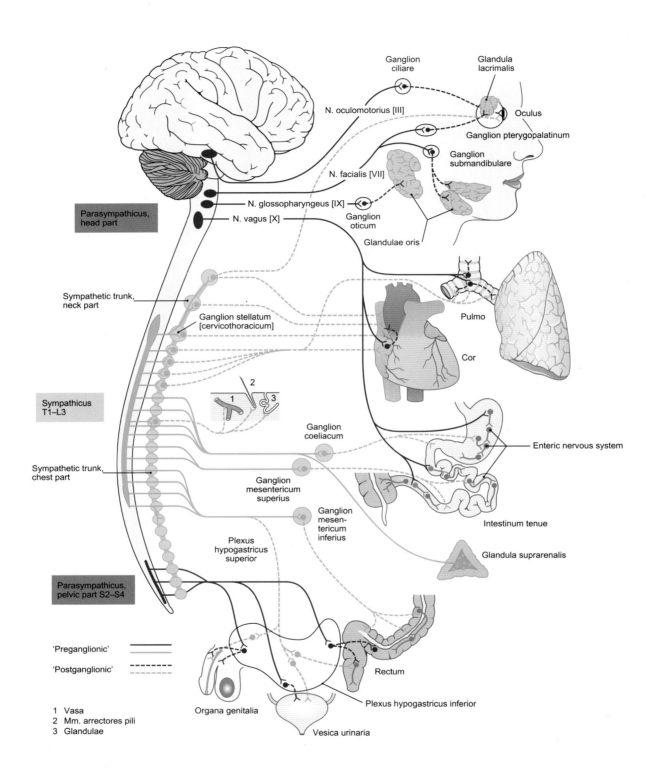

Ganglion ciliare

Glandula lacrimalis

N. oculomotorius [III]

Oculus

Ganglion pterygopalatinum

N. facialis [VII]

Ganglion submandibulare

N. glossopharyngeus [IX]

N. vagus [X]

Ganglion oticum

Parasympathicus, head part

Glandulae oris

Sympathetic trunk, neck part

Pulmo

Ganglion stellatum [cervicothoracicum]

Cor

Sympathicus T1–L3

Ganglion coeliacum

Enteric nervous system

Sympathetic trunk, chest part

Ganglion mesentericum superius

Ganglion mesentericum inferius

Intestinum tenue

Plexus hypogastricus superior

Glandula suprarenalis

Parasympathicus, pelvic part S2–S4

Rectum

'Preganglionic'

'Postganglionic'

Plexus hypogastricus inferior

1 Vasa
2 Mm. arrectores pili
3 Glandulae

Organa genitalia

Vesica urinaria

Fig. 12.209 Autonomic nervous system (sympathicus and parasympathicus). [S700-L106]~[S130-6-L126]
The autonomic nervous system comprises the sympathetic (green), the parasympathetic (purple), and the enteric nervous system.
The neurons of the **sympathicus** are located in the lateral horn of the thoracolumbar segment of the spinal cord. Their axons project to the ganglia of the sympathetic trunk and of the digestive tract. Here they are switched onto postganglionic neurons which project to the target organs. The sympathetic excitation serves to mobilise the body for activity, and in emergency situations. The sympathetic nervous system also comprises the medulla of the adrenal gland, which can release adrenaline and noradrenaline.

The nuclear areas of the **parasympathicus** are located in the brainstem and the sacral spinal cord. The axons project onto ganglia adjacent to the target organs, which are found in the head, thorax and abdominal cavity. Here they are switched onto postganglionic neurons, which reach the target organs via short axons. The parasympathetic nervous system plays an important role in the intake and processing (digestion) of food, as well as in sexual arousal, and forms the counterpart of the sympathicus.

The **enteric nervous system** regulates the intestines (intestinal activity), and is modulated by sympathetic and parasympathetic influences.

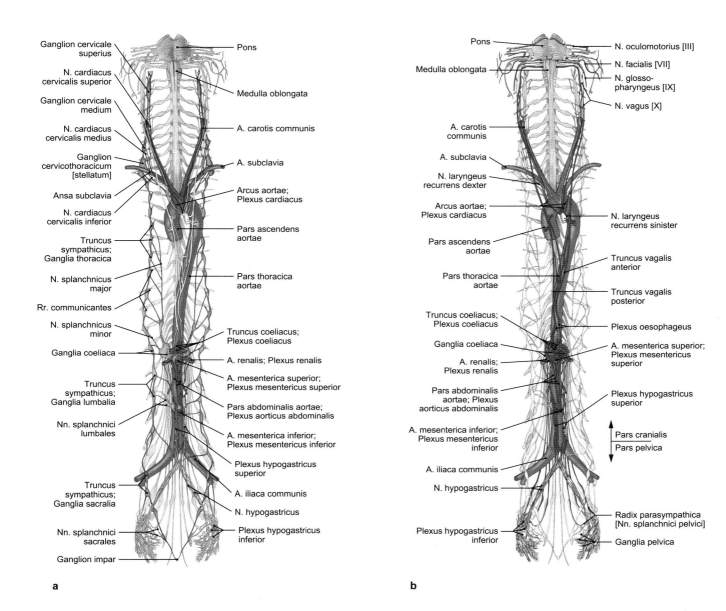

Ganglion cervicale superius
Pons
N. cardiacus cervicalis superior
Medulla oblongata
Ganglion cervicale medium
A. carotis communis
N. cardiacus cervicalis medius
A. subclavia
Ganglion cervicothoracicum [stellatum]
Arcus aortae; Plexus cardiacus
Ansa subclavia
N. cardiacus cervicalis inferior
Pars ascendens aortae
Truncus sympathicus; Ganglia thoracica
Pars thoracica aortae
N. splanchnicus major
Rr. communicantes
N. splanchnicus minor
Truncus coeliacus; Plexus coeliacus
Ganglia coeliaca
A. renalis; Plexus renalis
A. mesenterica superior; Plexus mesentericus superior
Truncus sympathicus; Ganglia lumbalia
Pars abdominalis aortae; Plexus aorticus abdominalis
Nn. splanchnici lumbales
A. mesenterica inferior; Plexus mesentericus inferior
Plexus hypogastricus superior
Truncus sympathicus; Ganglia sacralia
A. iliaca communis
N. hypogastricus
Nn. splanchnici sacrales
Plexus hypogastricus inferior
Ganglion impar

a

Pons
N. oculomotorius [III]
N. facialis [VII]
Medulla oblongata
N. glosso-pharyngeus [IX]
N. vagus [X]
A. carotis communis
A. subclavia
N. laryngeus recurrens dexter
Arcus aortae; Plexus cardiacus
N. laryngeus recurrens sinister
Pars ascendens aortae
Truncus vagalis anterior
Pars thoracica aortae
Truncus vagalis posterior
Truncus coeliacus; Plexus coeliacus
Plexus oesophageus
Ganglia coeliaca
A. mesenterica superior; Plexus mesentericus superior
A. renalis; Plexus renalis
Pars abdominalis aortae; Plexus aorticus abdominalis
Plexus hypogastricus superior
A. mesenterica inferior; Plexus mesentericus inferior
Pars cranialis
Pars pelvica
A. iliaca communis
N. hypogastricus
Radix parasympathica [Nn. splanchnici pelvici]
Plexus hypogastricus inferior
Ganglia pelvica

b

Fig. 12.210a and b Sympathicus and parasympathicus. Semi-schematic representations in a topographic-anatomical context. [S700]
a Sympathicus. Sympathetic axons exit the spinal cord with the Nn. spinales, pass to ganglia in the sympathetic trunk, and finally accompany blood vessels or nerves to their target organs.

b Parasympathicus. Parasympathetic axons in the head region pass with cranial nerves to the parasympathetic ganglia and from there to their target organs in the head. The thoracic and abdominal organs are mainly innervated by the N. vagus [X]. Only the last section of the intestines and the pelvic organs receive their parasympathetic innervation from the sacral spinal cord.

Autonomic nervous system, topography

Cranial parasympathicus (cranial nerves III, VII, IX)

Cranial nerve	First neuron	Second neuron	Target organs
N. oculomotorius [III]	Nucleus accessorius nervi oculomotorii [EDINGER-WESTPHAL]	Ganglion ciliare	• M. ciliaris • M. sphincter pupillae
N. facialis [VII]	Nucleus salivatorius superior	Ganglion pterygopalatinum	• Glandula lacrimalis • Mucous membranes
		Ganglion submandibulare	• Glandula submandibularis • Glandula sublingualis • Mucous membranes
N. glossopharyngeus [IX]	Nucleus salivatorius inferior	Ganglion oticum	• Glandula parotidea • Mucous membranes

Parasympathicus

Cranial nerve	First neuron	Second neuron	Target organs
Cranial parasympathicus			
N. vagus [X]	Nucleus ambiguus (external formation)	Intramural ganglia	Cervical viscera, heart and lungs
	Nucleus dorsalis nervi vagi	Intramural ganglia	Intra-abdominal glands
		Ganglia of the enteric nervous system	Intestines
Sacral parasympathicus			
Sacral parasympathicus		Ganglia pelvica	Genitalia
		Intramural ganglia	Distal colon, rectum, urinary bladder, parts of the ureter

Visceral sensory afferent fibres/impulses to the brainstem

Nerve	Ganglion	Central nucleus	Origin (in organs)
N. glossopharyngeus [IX]	Ganglion inferius	Nucleus tractus solitarii	• Glomus caroticum • Sinus caroticus
N. vagus [X]	Ganglion inferius [Ganglion nodosum]	Nucleus tractus solitarii	• Glomera in the neck and thoracic region • Thoracic viscera • Gastrointestinal tract

Nuclear areas of the hypothalamus and their function in homeostasis

Area	Nuclear area	Function
Area hypothalamica anterior	Nucleus suprachiasmaticus	Circadian rhythm
	Nuclei preoptici	Regulation of the gonadotropin release in the anterior pituitary gland (adenohypophysis)
	Nucleus supraopticus	ADH, oxytocin secretion
	Nucleus paraventricularis	ADH, oxytocin secretion, food intake; regulation of stress hormone secretion via CRH
Area hypothalamica intermedia	Nucleus infundibularis [arcuatus], periventricular nerve cells	Control of the anterior pituitary gland (adenohypophysis); food intake (nutritional) behaviour
	Nucleus ventromedialis hypothalami, Nucleus dorsomedialis hypothalami	Regulation of food and fluid intake behaviour
Area hypothalamica posterior	Nucleus hypothalamicus posterior, Corpora mamillaria	Thermal regulation, autonomic control
Area hypothalamica lateralis		Food intake behaviour

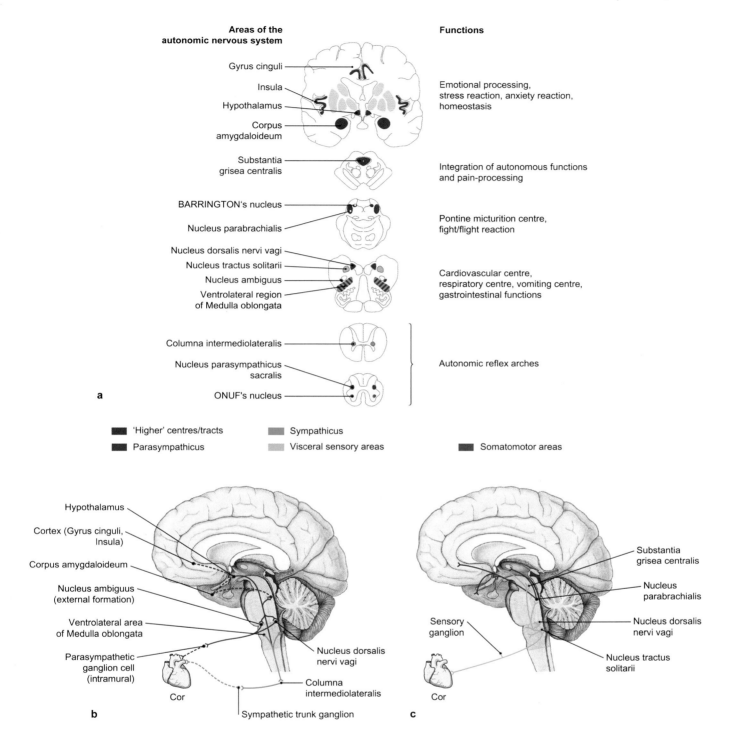

Fig. 12.211a–c Central autonomic brain regions and nuclear areas.
[S702-L127]/[G1091]
Nuclei and neuronal groups, which are involved in the central control of the autonomic nervous system and are closely interconnected, are located on different levels of the CNS.

a Autonomic nerve cells are located in the spinal cord, as well as in the brainstem, the diencephalon and the frontal lobe. Up to the level of the lower brainstem, it is possible to track the differences between sympathetic and parasympathetic neurons; but the two parts can no longer be clearly differentiated in the levels above.

b Example of the interaction between visceral motor neurons in the control of internal organs. Neurons in the hypothalamus, as the most significant autonomic relay station in the central nervous system, and neurons in the nuclear areas of the brainstem reach the autonomic cen-

tres in the Medulla oblongata or in the spinal cord directly with their axons or via an intermediary neuronal chain. From here, the preganglionic parasympathetic axons pass via the cranial nerves (N. vagus [X] is given in the example) to their target organs. Via descending fibres, the same centres can also influence sympathetic neurons in the lateral horn of the spinal cord. In this way, the autonomic nervous system is controlled in two directions.

c Example of visceral sensory afferent fibres/impulses to the central nuclear areas. Visceral sensory information is transmitted to the brain via the Nucleus tractus solitarii. In the Nucleus tractus solitarii, the fibres are switched and pass either directly to centres in the lower brainstem (autonomic reflex arches at the level of the brainstem) or via ascending neuronal chains to more centrally located regions of the brain.

In the clinic

Clinical remarks

Sympathetic trunk lesions result in **HORNER's syndrome** (HORNER's triad, CLAUDE BERNARD-HORNER syndrome) on the affected side. It is characterised by the following symptoms (→ Fig. b):
- Drooping of the upper eyelid (ptosis; loss of function of the M. tarsalis)
- Miosis (constricted pupils due to loss of function of M. dilatator pupillae) and
- (Pseudo-)enophthalmus (loss of function of the M. orbitalis).

Depending on the location of the lesion, there are (→ Fig. a):
- Central lesions (lesion of the first neuron which extends from the hypothalamus through the brainstem, the cervical and upper thoracic spinal cord to the ciliospinal centre [Centrum ciliospinale]) can occur as a result of strokes in the brainstem, as with WALLENBERG's syndrome, or traumatic cervical spinal cord lesions. Additional neurological deficits include anhydrosis of the face and arm.
- Preganglionic lesions (lesions located along the Centrum ciliospinale via the Ganglion stellatum to the Ganglion cervicale superius), e.g. due to bronchial cell carcinoma, breast cancer or PANCOAST tumours. Preganglionic lesions frequently associate with anhydrosis of the face and arms.

- Postganglionic lesions (lesion located between the Ganglion cervicale superius and M. dilatator pupillae), e.g. resulting from surgical dissection of the A. carotis interna and tumours. Anhydrosis of the face can also occur.

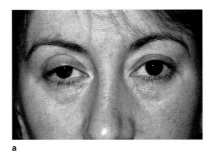

HORNER's syndrome

Sympathetic pathway injury
Miosis (constricted pupil)
Ptosis (droopy eyelid)

a

a Clinical image.
[F276-007]

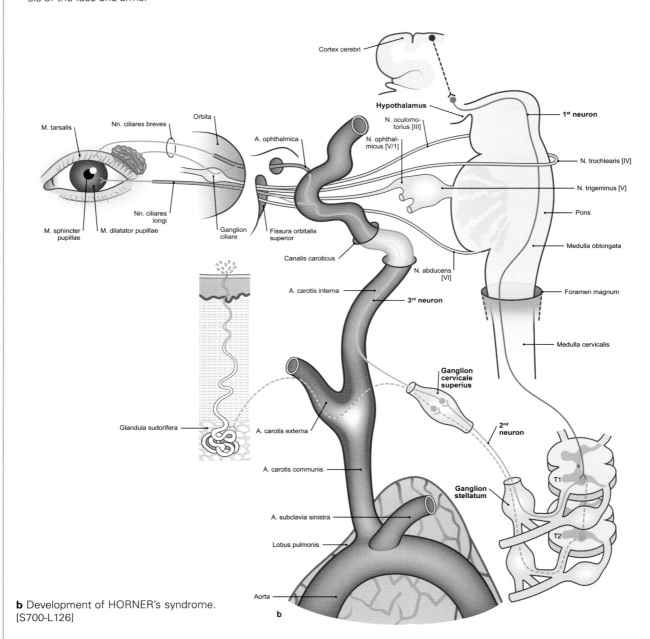

b Development of HORNER's syndrome.
[S700-L126]

b

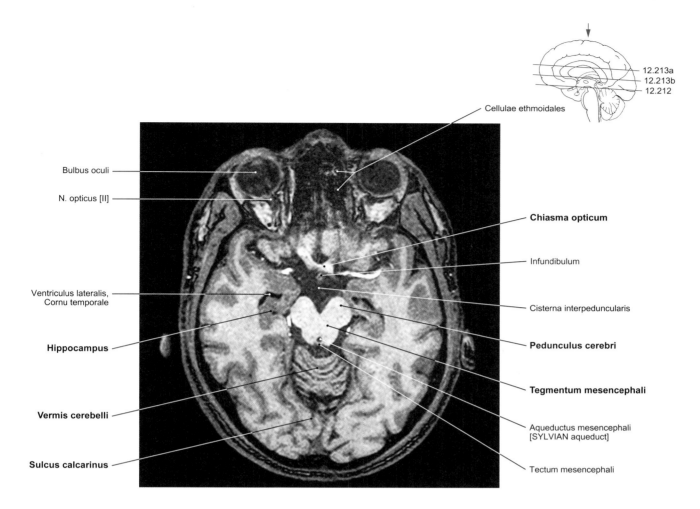

12.213a
12.213b
12.212

Cellulae ethmoidales

Bulbus oculi

N. opticus [II]

Chiasma opticum

Infundibulum

Ventriculus lateralis,
Cornu temporale

Cisterna interpeduncularis

Hippocampus

Pedunculus cerebri

Tegmentum mesencephali

Vermis cerebelli

Aqueductus mesencephali
[SYLVIAN aqueduct]

Sulcus calcarinus

Tectum mesencephali

Fig. 12.212   Brain, encephalon; magnetic resonance imaging (MRI) scan, horizontal section at the level of the mesencephalon and the temporal horns of the lateral ventricles; superior view. [S700]

The Chiasma opticum and Pedunculi cerebri of the mesencephalon are visible. The cerebellar vermis (Vermis cerebelli) also lies in this sectional plane. In the occipital lobe, the Sulcus calcarinus can be seen.

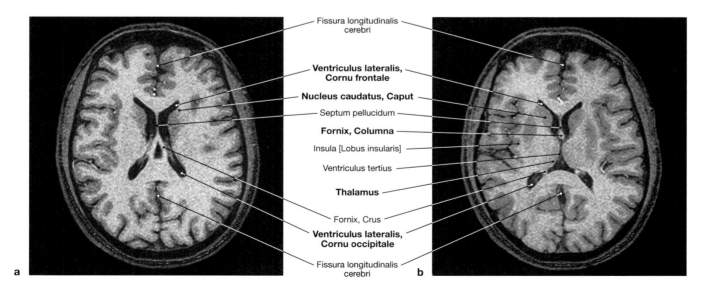

Fissura longitudinalis
cerebri

**Ventriculus lateralis,
Cornu frontale**

Nucleus caudatus, Caput

Septum pellucidum

Fornix, Columna

Insula [Lobus insularis]

Ventriculus tertius

Thalamus

Fornix, Crus

**Ventriculus lateralis,
Cornu occipitale**

Fissura longitudinalis
cerebri

a   b

Fig. 12.213a and b   Brain, encephalon. [S700]
a Magnetic resonance imaging (MRI) scan, horizontal section at the level of the floor of the central parts of the lateral ventricles; superior view. The Cornua frontale and occipitale, the Septum pellucidum and the crus of the fornix are visible here. On the left side, the Lobus insularis can also be identified.

b Magnetic resonance imaging (MRI) scan, horizontal section at the level of the third ventricle and the temporal horns of the lateral ventricles; superior view. In addition to the Lobi insulares and the structures mentioned in **a,** the thalamus and the columns of the fornix are visible.

Brain and spinal cord

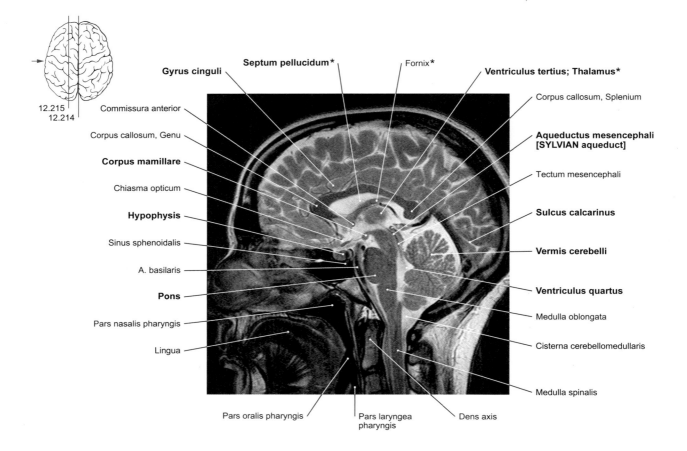

12.215
12.214

Septum pellucidum*   Fornix*   Ventriculus tertius; Thalamus*

Gyrus cinguli   Corpus callosum, Splenium

Commissura anterior   Aqueductus mesencephali [SYLVIAN aqueduct]

Corpus callosum, Genu   Tectum mesencephali

Corpus mamillare   Sulcus calcarinus

Chiasma opticum   Vermis cerebelli

Hypophysis   Ventriculus quartus

Sinus sphenoidalis   Medulla oblongata

A. basilaris   Cisterna cerebellomedullaris

Pons

Pars nasalis pharyngis   Medulla spinalis

Lingua

Pars oralis pharyngis   Pars laryngea pharyngis   Dens axis

Fig. 12.214 Brain, encephalon; magnetic resonance imaging (MRI) scan, median section. [S700]
This MRI scan shows all the clearly delineated brain structures, such as the Gyrus cinguli, Septum pellucidum, third ventricle, thalamus, Aque-ductus mesencephali [SYLVIAN aqueduct], Corpus mamillare, hypotha-lamus, hypophysis (pituitary gland), mesencephalon, pons, cerebellum and Medulla oblongata. The structures marked with a star (*) appear partly distorted due to the 'partial volume effect'.

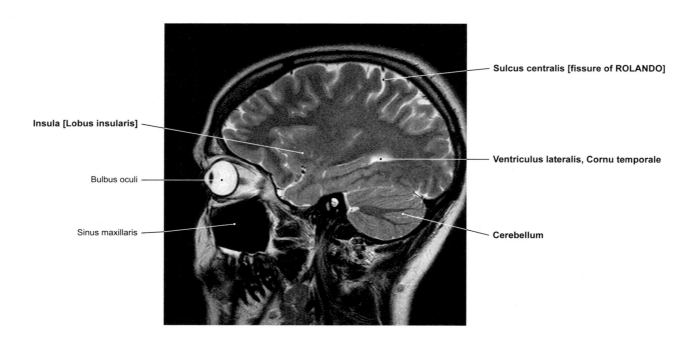

Insula [Lobus insularis]   Sulcus centralis [fissure of ROLANDO]

Bulbus oculi   Ventriculus lateralis, Cornu temporale

Sinus maxillaris   Cerebellum

Fig. 12.215 Brain, encephalon; magnetic resonance imaging (MRI) scan, sagittal section at the level of the mesencephalon and the tem-poral horns of the lateral ventricles; view from the left side. [S700]
The sagittal section displays the cerebellum and the Sulcus centralis. Also a small part of the Cornu temporale of the lateral ventricle lies in this sectional plane.

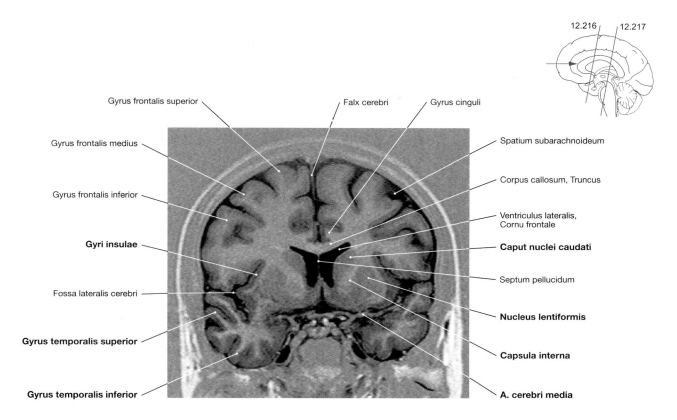

Gyrus frontalis superior
Falx cerebri
Gyrus cinguli

Gyrus frontalis medius
Spatium subarachnoideum

Gyrus frontalis inferior
Corpus callosum, Truncus

Gyri insulae
Ventriculus lateralis, Cornu frontale

Caput nuclei caudati

Fossa lateralis cerebri
Septum pellucidum

Gyrus temporalis superior
Nucleus lentiformis

Gyrus temporalis inferior
Capsula interna

A. cerebri media

Fig. 12.216 Brain, encephalon; magnetic resonance imaging (MRI) scan, frontal section at the level of the anterior part of the third ventricle; anterior view. [S700]
On the right side, the pathway of the A. cerebri media towards the Sulcus lateralis can be recognised. On both sides, the large gyri of the Lobus frontalis and Lobus temporalis are visible. With this imaging technique, the Nucleus caudatus, the Capsula interna and the Nucleus lentiformis can be delineated in the region of the nuclei of the cerebrum.

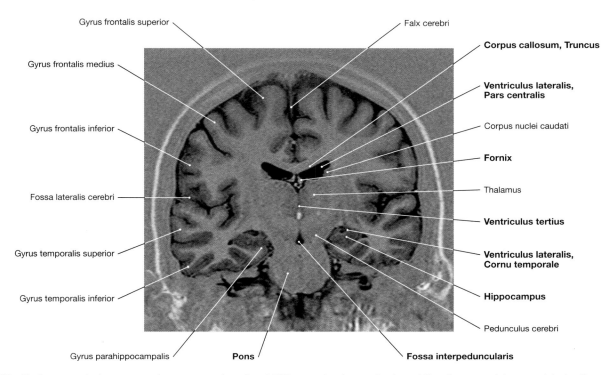

Gyrus frontalis superior
Falx cerebri

Corpus callosum, Truncus

Gyrus frontalis medius
Ventriculus lateralis, Pars centralis

Gyrus frontalis inferior
Corpus nuclei caudati

Fornix

Thalamus

Fossa lateralis cerebri
Ventriculus tertius

Gyrus temporalis superior
Ventriculus lateralis, Cornu temporale

Gyrus temporalis inferior
Hippocampus

Pedunculus cerebri

Gyrus parahippocampalis
Pons
Fossa interpeduncularis

Fig. 12.217 Brain, encephalon; magnetic resonance imaging (MRI) scan, frontal section at the level of the thalamus; anterior view. [S700]
This scan shows the Cornu temporale of the lateral ventricles and the hippocampus. Further cranially, the Pars centralis of the lateral ventricles is cut. In the midline from cranial to caudal, the Truncus corporis callosi, the fornix, the third ventricle, the Fossa interpeduncularis of the brainstem and the pons can be delineated.

Brain, frontal sections

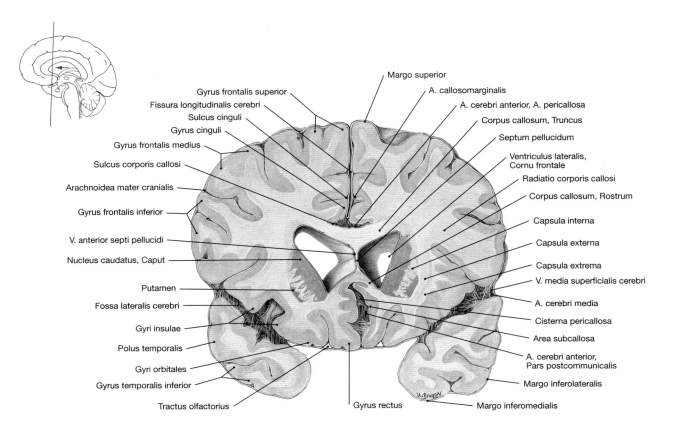

Gyrus frontalis superior
Fissura longitudinalis cerebri
Sulcus cinguli
Gyrus cinguli
Gyrus frontalis medius
Sulcus corporis callosi
Arachnoidea mater cranialis
Gyrus frontalis inferior
V. anterior septi pellucidi
Nucleus caudatus, Caput
Putamen
Fossa lateralis cerebri
Gyri insulae
Polus temporalis
Gyri orbitales
Gyrus temporalis inferior
Tractus olfactorius

Margo superior
A. callosomarginalis
A. cerebri anterior, A. pericallosa
Corpus callosum, Truncus
Septum pellucidum
Ventriculus lateralis, Cornu frontale
Radiatio corporis callosi
Corpus callosum, Rostrum
Capsula interna
Capsula externa
Capsula extrema
V. media superficialis cerebri
A. cerebri media
Cisterna pericallosa
Area subcallosa
A. cerebri anterior, Pars postcommunicalis
Margo inferolateralis
Margo inferomedialis
Gyrus rectus

Fig. 12.218 Brain, encephalon; frontal section at the level of the anterior parts of the frontal horns of the Ventriculi laterales; posterior view. [S700]

The two Ventriculi laterales are visible with the Corpus callosum above them, as well as the caput of the Nucleus caudatus and the putamen, which are located laterally of the Ventriculi laterales.

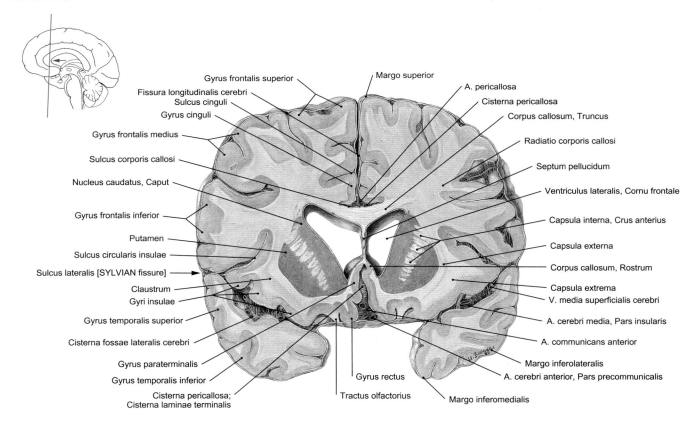

Gyrus frontalis superior
Fissura longitudinalis cerebri
Sulcus cinguli
Gyrus cinguli
Gyrus frontalis medius
Sulcus corporis callosi
Nucleus caudatus, Caput
Gyrus frontalis inferior
Putamen
Sulcus circularis insulae
Sulcus lateralis [SYLVIAN fissure]
Claustrum
Gyri insulae
Gyrus temporalis superior
Cisterna fossae lateralis cerebri
Gyrus paraterminalis
Gyrus temporalis inferior
Cisterna pericallosa; Cisterna laminae terminalis

Margo superior
A. pericallosa
Cisterna pericallosa
Corpus callosum, Truncus
Radiatio corporis callosi
Septum pellucidum
Ventriculus lateralis, Cornu frontale
Capsula interna, Crus anterius
Capsula externa
Corpus callosum, Rostrum
Capsula extrema
V. media superficialis cerebri
A. cerebri media, Pars insularis
A. communicans anterior
Margo inferolateralis
A. cerebri anterior, Pars precommunicalis
Margo inferomedialis
Gyrus rectus
Tractus olfactorius

Fig. 12.219 Brain, encephalon; frontal section at the level of the posterior part of the frontal horns of the Ventriculi laterales; posterior view. [S700]

The truncus of the Corpus callosum can be seen above the Ventriculi laterales, whereas the caput of the Nucleus caudatus, the putamen and the Crus anterius of the Capsula interna in between are visible laterally of the Ventriculi laterales.

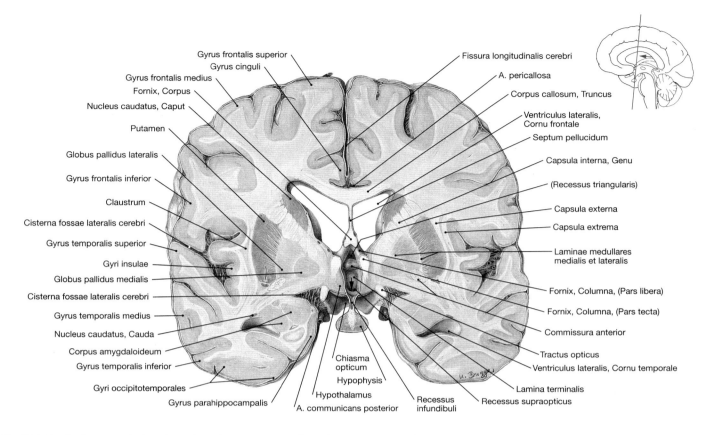

Fig. 12.220 Brain, encephalon; frontal section at the level of the Foramina interventricularia; posterior view. [S700]
The sectional plane cuts directly through the pituitary gland. Below the Ventriculi laterales, the caput of the Nucleus caudatus, the Capsula interna, the Globus pallidus, the putamen, the claustrum and several Gyri insulae are visible.

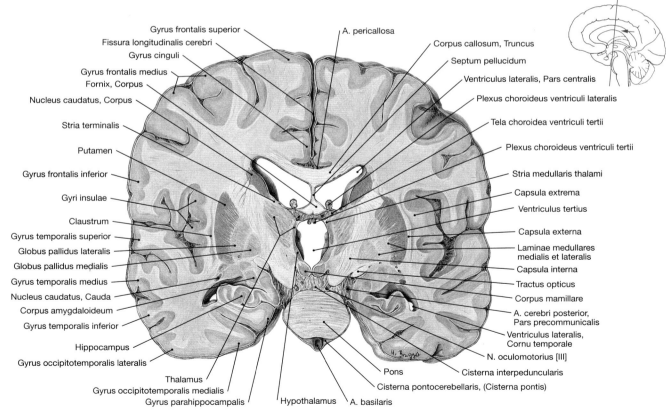

Fig. 12.221 Brain, encephalon; frontal section at the level of the Corpora mamillaria; posterior view. [S700]
At the level of the Corpora mamillaria, the lumen of the Ventriculus tertius is visible below the Ventriculi laterales. Lateral thereof from inside to outside are the thalamus, Capsula interna, Globus pallidus, putamen, Capsula externa, claustrum, Capsula extrema and Gyri insulae.

Brain, frontal sections

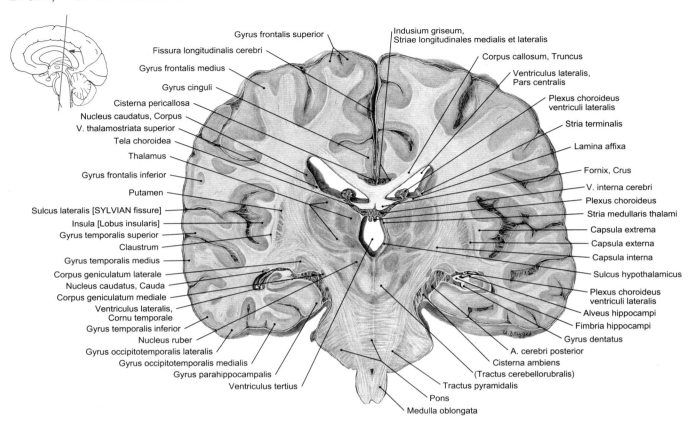

Fig. 12.222 **Brain, encephalon;** frontal section through the centre of the third ventricle; posterior view. [S700]
At this level, the left and right thalami are often cross-connected by the Adhesio interthalamica. Below the thalamus, the Nucleus ruber is clear-

ly discernible. In the brainstem, the Tractus pyramidalis appears as a prominent structure of the pons.

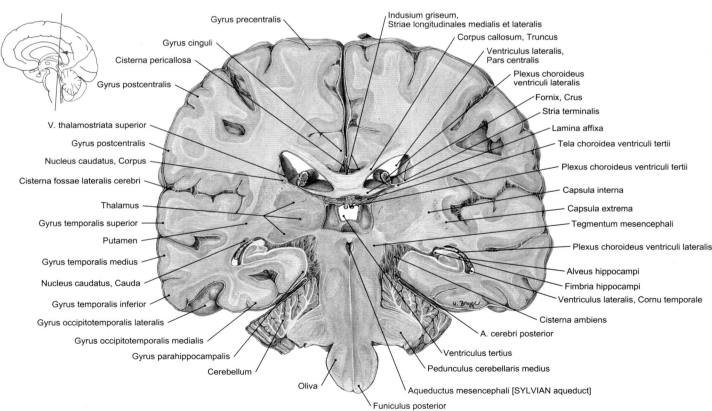

Fig. 12.223 **Brain, encephalon;** frontal section at the level of the posterior wall of the third ventricle; posterior view. [S700]
Inferior to the Ventriculi laterales, a number of thalamic nuclei can be recognised, and further caudally the occipital part of the hippocampus

is visible. In this sectional plane, the brainstem is cut at the level of the Aqueductus mesencephali [SYLVIAN aqueduct].

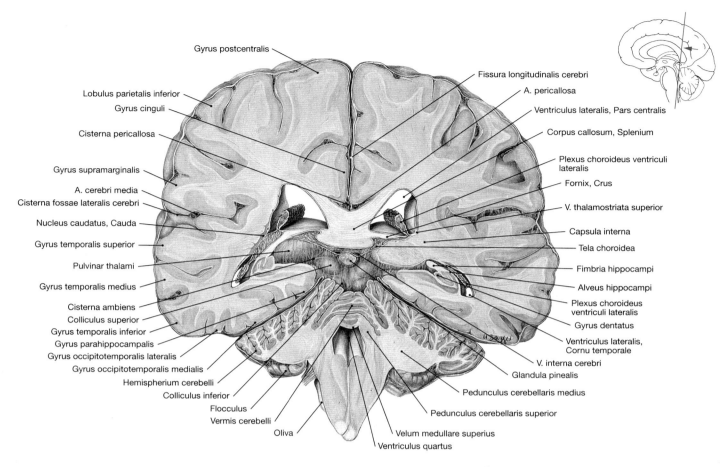

Gyrus postcentralis
Lobulus parietalis inferior
Gyrus cinguli
Cisterna pericallosa
Gyrus supramarginalis
A. cerebri media
Cisterna fossae lateralis cerebri
Nucleus caudatus, Cauda
Gyrus temporalis superior
Pulvinar thalami
Gyrus temporalis medius
Cisterna ambiens
Colliculus superior
Gyrus temporalis inferior
Gyrus parahippocampalis
Gyrus occipitotemporalis lateralis
Gyrus occipitotemporalis medialis
Hemispherium cerebelli
Colliculus inferior
Flocculus
Vermis cerebelli
Oliva

Fissura longitudinalis cerebri
A. pericallosa
Ventriculus lateralis, Pars centralis
Corpus callosum, Splenium
Plexus choroideus ventriculi lateralis
Fornix, Crus
V. thalamostriata superior
Capsula interna
Tela choroidea
Fimbria hippocampi
Alveus hippocampi
Plexus choroideus ventriculi lateralis
Gyrus dentatus
Ventriculus lateralis, Cornu temporale
V. interna cerebri
Glandula pinealis
Pedunculus cerebellaris medius
Pedunculus cerebellaris superior
Velum medullare superius
Ventriculus quartus

Fig. 12.224 Brain, encephalon; frontal section at the level of the pineal gland and of the fourth ventricle; posterior view. [S700]
The splenium of the Corpus callosum and the Glandula pinealis are displayed in the centre of the image, with the laterally located Colliculi superiores and the Pulvinar thalami. Laterally and slightly above the Ventriculus quartus, the Pedunculi cerebellares superiores are visible in the brainstem.

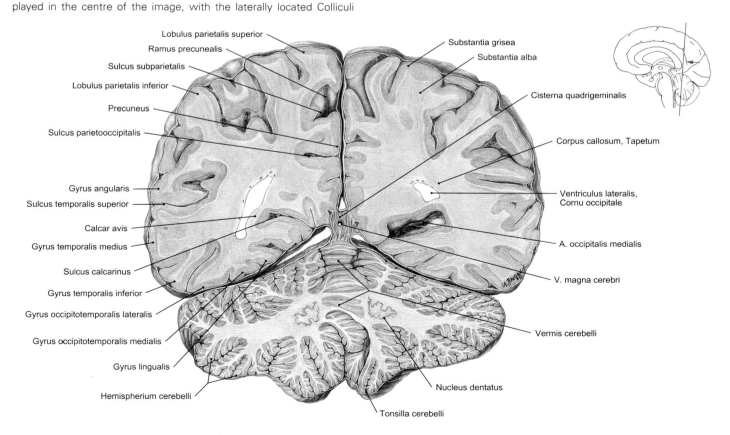

Lobulus parietalis superior
Ramus precunealis
Sulcus subparietalis
Lobulus parietalis inferior
Precuneus
Sulcus parietooccipitalis
Gyrus angularis
Sulcus temporalis superior
Calcar avis
Gyrus temporalis medius
Sulcus calcarinus
Gyrus temporalis inferior
Gyrus occipitotemporalis lateralis
Gyrus occipitotemporalis medialis
Gyrus lingualis
Hemispherium cerebelli

Substantia grisea
Substantia alba
Cisterna quadrigeminalis
Corpus callosum, Tapetum
Ventriculus lateralis, Cornu occipitale
A. occipitalis medialis
V. magna cerebri
Vermis cerebelli
Nucleus dentatus
Tonsilla cerebelli

Fig. 12.225 Brain, encephalon; frontal section at the level of the posterior horns of the Ventriculi laterales; posterior view. [S700]
The Nucleus dentatus and large parts of the Vermis cerebelli are visible in the cerebellum.

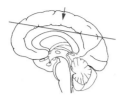

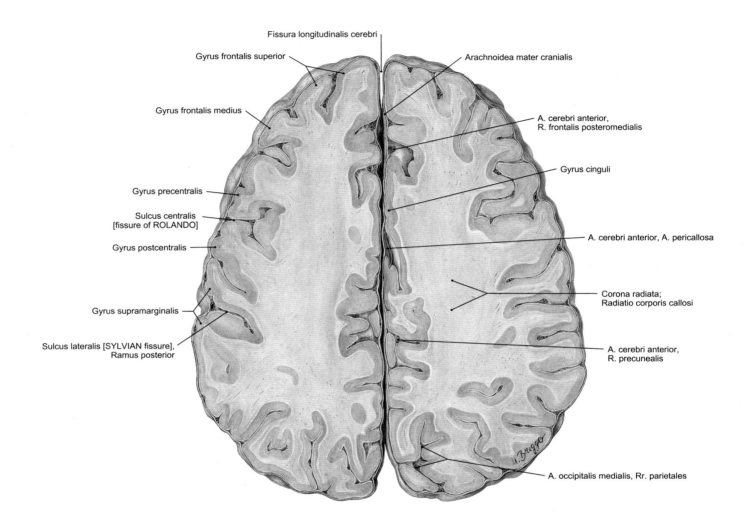

Fissura longitudinalis cerebri

Gyrus frontalis superior

Gyrus frontalis medius

Gyrus precentralis

Sulcus centralis
[fissure of ROLANDO]

Gyrus postcentralis

Gyrus supramarginalis

Sulcus lateralis [SYLVIAN fissure],
Ramus posterior

Arachnoidea mater cranialis

A. cerebri anterior,
R. frontalis posteromedialis

Gyrus cinguli

A. cerebri anterior, A. pericallosa

Corona radiata;
Radiatio corporis callosi

A. cerebri anterior,
R. precunealis

A. occipitalis medialis, Rr. parietales

Fig. 12.226   Brain, encephalon; horizontal section just above the Corpus callosum; superior view. [S700]
The sectional plane lies directly above the Corpus callosum. At this level, the nuclei are not yet visible. In the broad band of white matter, fibre tracts projecting from the thalamus to the cortex (Corona radiata) mix with commissural fibres of the Corpus callosum, connecting the two hemispheres (Radiatio corporis callosi). In addition, there are tracts converging downwards onto the Capsula interna (not shown here; → Fig. 12.28 and → Fig. 12.29). Due to the age-related atrophy of the brain, the subarachnoid space appears enlarged or wider (→ Fig. 12.227 to → Fig. 12.236).

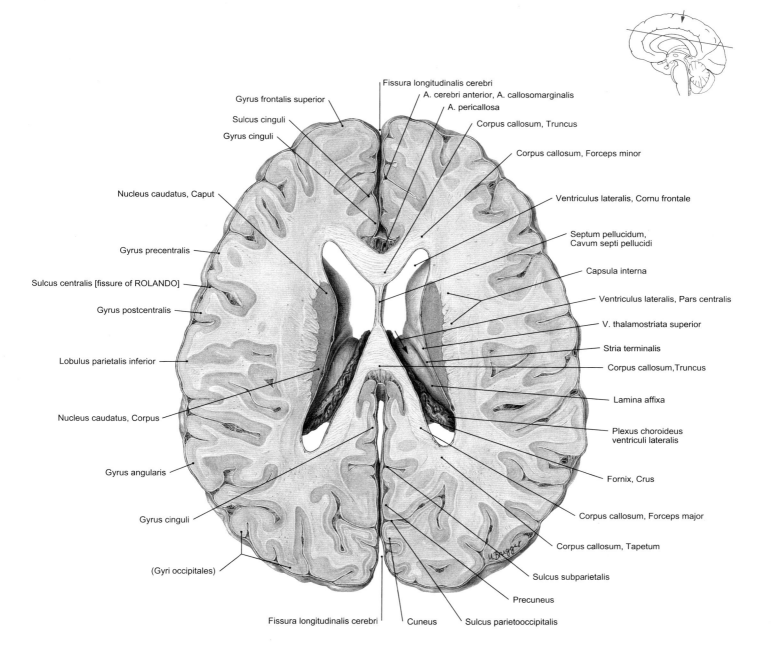

Fissura longitudinalis cerebri
A. cerebri anterior, A. callosomarginalis
A. pericallosa
Corpus callosum, Truncus
Corpus callosum, Forceps minor
Ventriculus lateralis, Cornu frontale
Septum pellucidum, Cavum septi pellucidi
Capsula interna
Ventriculus lateralis, Pars centralis
V. thalamostriata superior
Stria terminalis
Corpus callosum, Truncus
Lamina affixa
Plexus choroideus ventriculi lateralis
Fornix, Crus
Corpus callosum, Forceps major
Corpus callosum, Tapetum
Sulcus subparietalis
Precuneus
Sulcus parietooccipitalis
Cuneus
Fissura longitudinalis cerebri
(Gyri occipitales)
Gyrus cinguli
Gyrus angularis
Nucleus caudatus, Corpus
Lobulus parietalis inferior
Gyrus postcentralis
Sulcus centralis [fissure of ROLANDO]
Gyrus precentralis
Nucleus caudatus, Caput
Gyrus cinguli
Sulcus cinguli
Gyrus frontalis superior

Fig. 12.227 Brain, encephalon; horizontal section through the central part of the lateral ventricles; superior view. [S700]
The Septum pellucidum extends between the truncus and the fornix (not visible here) of the Corpus callosum and separates the Ventriculi laterales. The caput and corpus of the Nucleus caudatus are sectioned laterally of the Ventriculi laterales and the Capsula interna is located even further laterally.

467

Brain, horizontal section

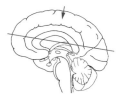

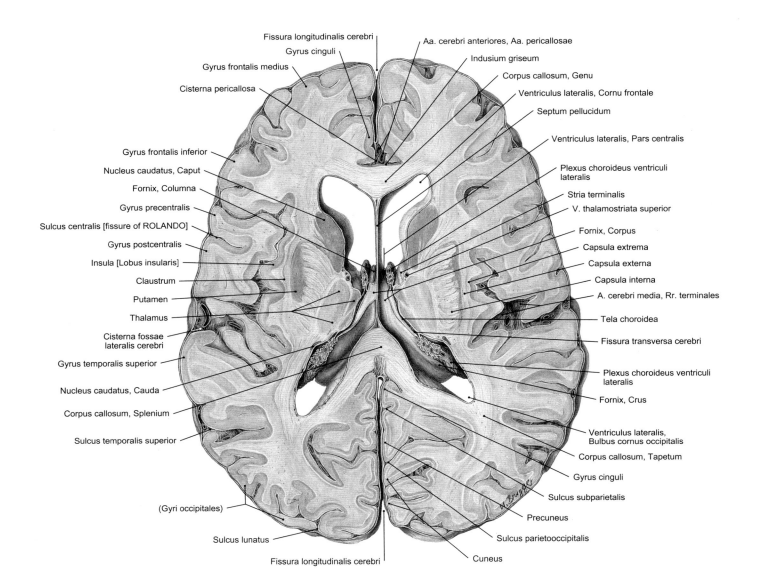

Fissura longitudinalis cerebri

Gyrus cinguli

Gyrus frontalis medius

Cisterna pericallosa

Gyrus frontalis inferior

Nucleus caudatus, Caput

Fornix, Columna

Gyrus precentralis

Sulcus centralis [fissure of ROLANDO]

Gyrus postcentralis

Insula [Lobus insularis]

Claustrum

Putamen

Thalamus

Cisterna fossae
lateralis cerebri

Gyrus temporalis superior

Nucleus caudatus, Cauda

Corpus callosum, Splenium

Sulcus temporalis superior

(Gyri occipitales)

Sulcus lunatus

Fissura longitudinalis cerebri

Aa. cerebri anteriores, Aa. pericallosae

Indusium griseum

Corpus callosum, Genu

Ventriculus lateralis, Cornu frontale

Septum pellucidum

Ventriculus lateralis, Pars centralis

Plexus choroideus ventriculi
lateralis

Stria terminalis

V. thalamostriata superior

Fornix, Corpus

Capsula extrema

Capsula externa

Capsula interna

A. cerebri media, Rr. terminales

Tela choroidea

Fissura transversa cerebri

Plexus choroideus ventriculi
lateralis

Fornix, Crus

Ventriculus lateralis,
Bulbus cornus occipitalis

Corpus callosum, Tapetum

Gyrus cinguli

Sulcus subparietalis

Precuneus

Sulcus parietooccipitalis

Cuneus

Fig. 12.228 Brain, encephalon; horizontal section at the level of the floor of the central part of the lateral ventricles; superior view. [S700] This central section shows thalamic sections located lateral of the lateral ventricles. Anterior to the thalamus the caput is visible and posteriorly a small area of the cauda of the Nucleus caudatus is visible. Located lateral of the thalamus from medial to lateral lie the Capsula interna, putamen, Capsula externa, claustrum, Capsula extrema and Gyri insulae. The genu and the splenium of the Corpus callosum are both visible in the anterior and posterior section of the midline, respectively.

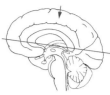

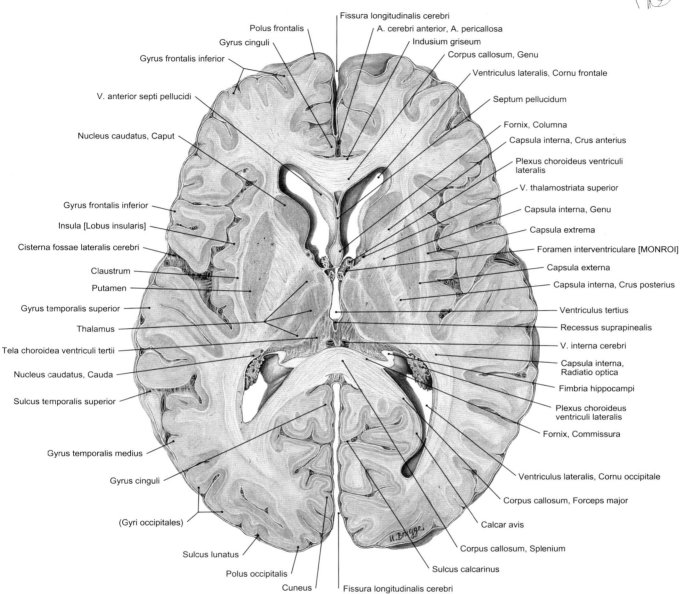

Fissura longitudinalis cerebri
Polus frontalis
A. cerebri anterior, A. pericallosa
Gyrus cinguli
Indusium griseum
Gyrus frontalis inferior
Corpus callosum, Genu
Ventriculus lateralis, Cornu frontale
V. anterior septi pellucidi
Septum pellucidum
Fornix, Columna
Nucleus caudatus, Caput
Capsula interna, Crus anterius
Plexus choroideus ventriculi lateralis
V. thalamostriata superior
Gyrus frontalis inferior
Capsula interna, Genu
Insula [Lobus insularis]
Capsula extrema
Cisterna fossae lateralis cerebri
Foramen interventriculare [MONROI]
Claustrum
Capsula externa
Putamen
Capsula interna, Crus posterius
Gyrus temporalis superior
Ventriculus tertius
Thalamus
Recessus suprapinealis
Tela choroidea ventriculi tertii
V. interna cerebri
Nucleus caudatus, Cauda
Capsula interna, Radiatio optica
Sulcus temporalis superior
Fimbria hippocampi
Plexus choroideus ventriculi lateralis
Gyrus temporalis medius
Fornix, Commissura
Gyrus cinguli
Ventriculus lateralis, Cornu occipitale
(Gyri occipitales)
Corpus callosum, Forceps major
Calcar avis
Sulcus lunatus
Corpus callosum, Splenium
Polus occipitalis
Sulcus calcarinus
Cuneus
Fissura longitudinalis cerebri

Fig. 12.229 Brain, encephalon; horizontal section through the upper part of the third ventricle; superior view. [S700]
The third ventricle (Ventriculus tertius) lies in the central part of the image, and the Ventriculi laterales, as well as the genu and splenium of the Corpus callosum are visible anterior and posterior to the third ven-tricle. The caput and cauda of the Nucleus caudatus, thalamus, puta-men, and claustrum constitute the **cerebral nuclei.** The Capsula interna with its characteristic genu is located between the large nuclei. In ad-dition, the Radiatio optica of the Capsula interna can be seen.

Sections

Brain, horizontal section

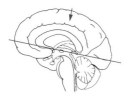

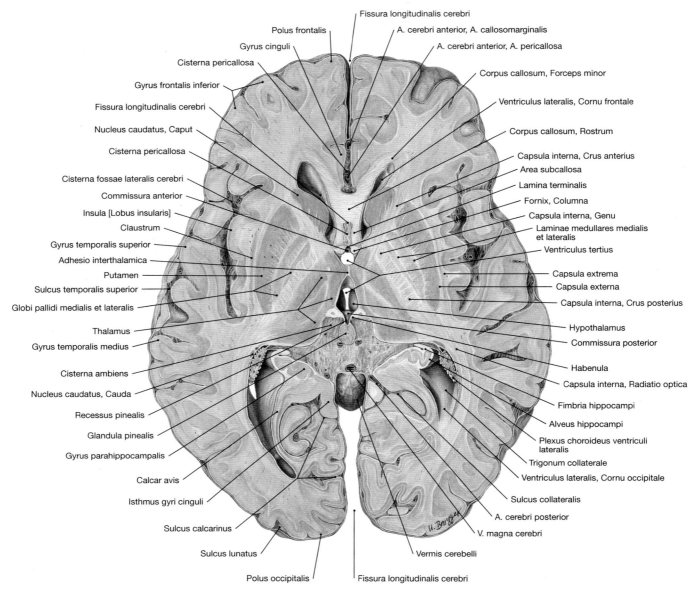

Fissura longitudinalis cerebri
Polus frontalis
Gyrus cinguli
Cisterna pericallosa
Gyrus frontalis inferior
Fissura longitudinalis cerebri
Nucleus caudatus, Caput
Cisterna pericallosa
Cisterna fossae lateralis cerebri
Commissura anterior
Insula [Lobus insularis]
Claustrum
Gyrus temporalis superior
Adhesio interthalamica
Putamen
Sulcus temporalis superior
Globi pallidi medialis et lateralis
Thalamus
Gyrus temporalis medius
Cisterna ambiens
Nucleus caudatus, Cauda
Recessus pinealis
Glandula pinealis
Gyrus parahippocampalis
Calcar avis
Isthmus gyri cinguli
Sulcus calcarinus
Sulcus lunatus
Polus occipitalis

A. cerebri anterior, A. callosomarginalis
A. cerebri anterior, A. pericallosa
Corpus callosum, Forceps minor
Ventriculus lateralis, Cornu frontale
Corpus callosum, Rostrum
Capsula interna, Crus anterius
Area subcallosa
Lamina terminalis
Fornix, Columna
Capsula interna, Genu
Laminae medullares medialis et lateralis
Ventriculus tertius
Capsula extrema
Capsula externa
Capsula interna, Crus posterius
Hypothalamus
Commissura posterior
Habenula
Capsula interna, Radiatio optica
Fimbria hippocampi
Alveus hippocampi
Plexus choroideus ventriculi lateralis
Trigonum collaterale
Ventriculus lateralis, Cornu occipitale
Sulcus collateralis
A. cerebri posterior
V. magna cerebri
Vermis cerebelli
Fissura longitudinalis cerebri

Fig. 12.230 Brain, encephalon; horizontal section through the centre of the third ventricle at the level of the Adhesio interthalamica; superior view. [S700]
The sectional plane cuts directly through the Glandula pinealis and the Adhesio interthalamica. Lateral thereof lie the thalamus, Capsula inter-
na, Globus pallidus, putamen, Capsula externa, claustrum, Capsula extrema and Lobus insularis. The Fimbria hippocampi, the Alveus hippocampi and the Gyrus parahippocampalis are also discernible.

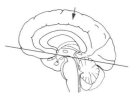

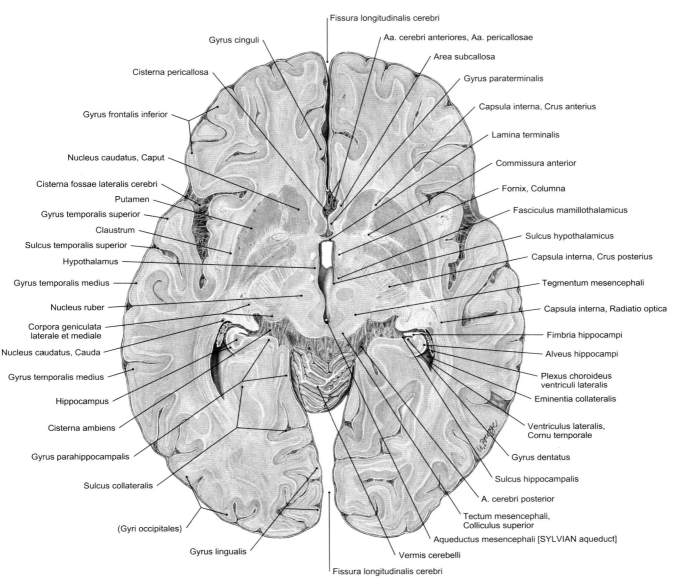

Fissura longitudinalis cerebri

Gyrus cinguli

Aa. cerebri anteriores, Aa. pericallosae

Cisterna pericallosa

Area subcallosa

Gyrus frontalis inferior

Gyrus paraterminalis

Nucleus caudatus, Caput

Capsula interna, Crus anterius

Cisterna fossae lateralis cerebri

Lamina terminalis

Putamen

Commissura anterior

Gyrus temporalis superior

Fornix, Columna

Claustrum

Fasciculus mamillothalamicus

Sulcus temporalis superior

Sulcus hypothalamicus

Hypothalamus

Capsula interna, Crus posterius

Gyrus temporalis medius

Tegmentum mesencephali

Nucleus ruber

Capsula interna, Radiatio optica

Corpora geniculata laterale et mediale

Fimbria hippocampi

Nucleus caudatus, Cauda

Alveus hippocampi

Gyrus temporalis medius

Plexus choroideus ventriculi lateralis

Hippocampus

Eminentia collateralis

Cisterna ambiens

Ventriculus lateralis, Cornu temporale

Gyrus parahippocampalis

Gyrus dentatus

Sulcus collateralis

Sulcus hippocampalis

A. cerebri posterior

(Gyri occipitales)

Tectum mesencephali, Colliculus superior

Gyrus lingualis

Aqueductus mesencephali [SYLVIAN aqueduct]

Vermis cerebelli

Fissura longitudinalis cerebri

Fig. 12.231 Brain, encephalon; horizontal section through the Ventriculus tertius, at the level of the opening of the Aqueductus mesencephali; superior view. [S700]
Due to its reddish colour, the Nucleus ruber is a prominent structure in this sectional plane. The close relationship between the Nucleus caudatus and putamen also becomes obvious. The Crus anterius of the Capsula interna runs between the two structures. The sectional plane is located at the level of the transition from the Ventriculus tertius in the Aqueductus mesencephali [SYLVIAN aqueduct]. Both structures are displayed. The upper rim of the Vermis cerebelli is also shown on this sectional plane.

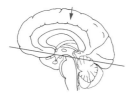

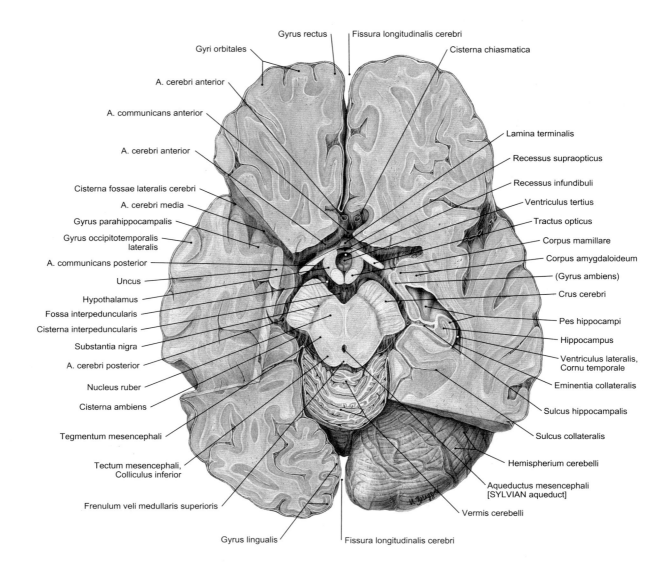

Gyrus rectus — Fissura longitudinalis cerebri

Gyri orbitales — Cisterna chiasmatica

A. cerebri anterior

A. communicans anterior — Lamina terminalis

A. cerebri anterior — Recessus supraopticus

Cisterna fossae lateralis cerebri — Recessus infundibuli

A. cerebri media — Ventriculus tertius

Gyrus parahippocampalis — Tractus opticus

Gyrus occipitotemporalis lateralis — Corpus mamillare

A. communicans posterior — Corpus amygdaloideum

Uncus — (Gyrus ambiens)

Hypothalamus — Crus cerebri

Fossa interpeduncularis

Cisterna interpeduncularis — Pes hippocampi

Substantia nigra — Hippocampus

A. cerebri posterior — Ventriculus lateralis, Cornu temporale

Nucleus ruber — Eminentia collateralis

Cisterna ambiens — Sulcus hippocampalis

Tegmentum mesencephali — Sulcus collateralis

Tectum mesencephali, Colliculus inferior — Hemispherium cerebelli

Frenulum veli medullaris superioris — Aqueductus mesencephali [SYLVIAN aqueduct]

Gyrus lingualis — Vermis cerebelli

Fissura longitudinalis cerebri

Fig. 12.232   Brain, encephalon; staggered horizontal section through the floor of the third ventricle at the level of the Corpora mamillaria; superior view. [S700]
The sectional plane is made through the Tractus optici, the hypothalami, the Corpora mamillaria, the Crura cerebri, the Nuclei rubri and the Colliculi inferiores of the Tectum mesencephali. On the right side, the hippocampus is visible, on the left side sectioned parts of the grey and white matter of the temporal and occipital lobes are shown. After removal of the occipital pole on the right side, the Hemispherium cerebelli is exposed.

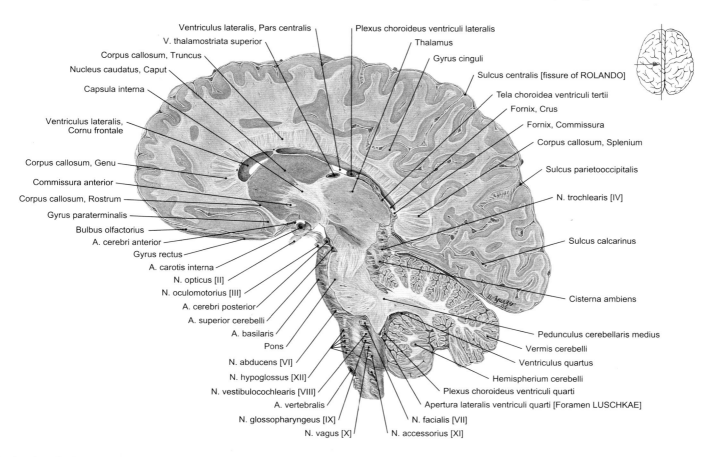

Ventriculus lateralis, Pars centralis
V. thalamostriata superior
Corpus callosum, Truncus
Nucleus caudatus, Caput
Capsula interna
Ventriculus lateralis, Cornu frontale
Corpus callosum, Genu
Commissura anterior
Corpus callosum, Rostrum
Gyrus paraterminalis
Bulbus olfactorius
A. cerebri anterior
Gyrus rectus
A. carotis interna
N. opticus [II]
N. oculomotorius [III]
A. cerebri posterior
A. superior cerebelli
A. basilaris
Pons
N. abducens [VI]
N. hypoglossus [XII]
N. vestibulocochlearis [VIII]
A. vertebralis
N. glossopharyngeus [IX]
N. vagus [X]

Plexus choroideus ventriculi lateralis
Thalamus
Gyrus cinguli
Sulcus centralis [fissure of ROLANDO]
Tela choroidea ventriculi tertii
Fornix, Crus
Fornix, Commissura
Corpus callosum, Splenium
Sulcus parietooccipitalis
N. trochlearis [IV]
Sulcus calcarinus
Cisterna ambiens
Pedunculus cerebellaris medius
Vermis cerebelli
Ventriculus quartus
Hemispherium cerebelli
Plexus choroideus ventriculi quarti
Apertura lateralis ventriculi quarti [Foramen LUSCHKAE]
N. facialis [VII]
N. accessorius [XI]

Fig. 12.233 Brain, encephalon; sagittal section through the left hemisphere at the level of the caput of the Nucleus caudatus; view from the left side. [S700]
The paramedian section shows the entire rostro-occipital dimension of the Corpus callosum. The Ventriculus lateralis is located beneath it, and further below, the Nucleus caudatus, thalamus, Capsula interna and N. opticus [II] follow. The A. basilaris runs in front of the brainstem. The Pedunculus cerebellaris medius marks the transition from the pons to the cerebellum.

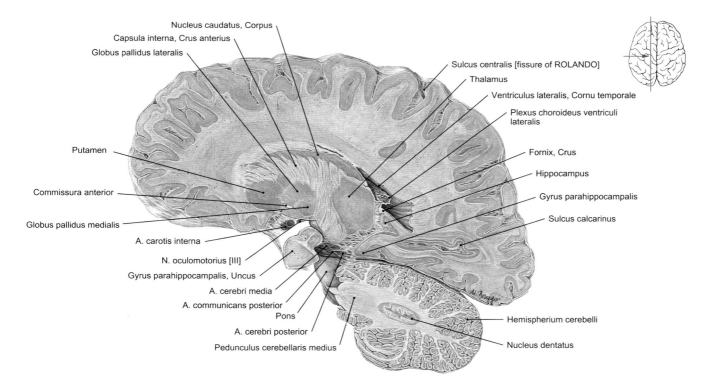

Nucleus caudatus, Corpus
Capsula interna, Crus anterius
Globus pallidus lateralis
Putamen
Commissura anterior
Globus pallidus medialis
A. carotis interna
N. oculomotorius [III]
Gyrus parahippocampalis, Uncus
A. cerebri media
A. communicans posterior
Pons
A. cerebri posterior
Pedunculus cerebellaris medius

Sulcus centralis [fissure of ROLANDO]
Thalamus
Ventriculus lateralis, Cornu temporale
Plexus choroideus ventriculi lateralis
Fornix, Crus
Hippocampus
Gyrus parahippocampalis
Sulcus calcarinus
Hemispherium cerebelli
Nucleus dentatus

Fig. 12.234 Brain, encephalon; sagittal section through the left hemisphere at the level of the corpus of the Nucleus caudatus; view from the left side. [S700]
Apart from the corpus of the Nucleus caudatus, the Crus anterius of the Capsula interna, the thalamus, the putamen, the Globus pallidus and the uncus of the Gyrus parahippocampalis are sectioned in this plane. In the cerebellum, the sectional plane cuts through the Nucleus dentatus.

Brain, sagittal sections

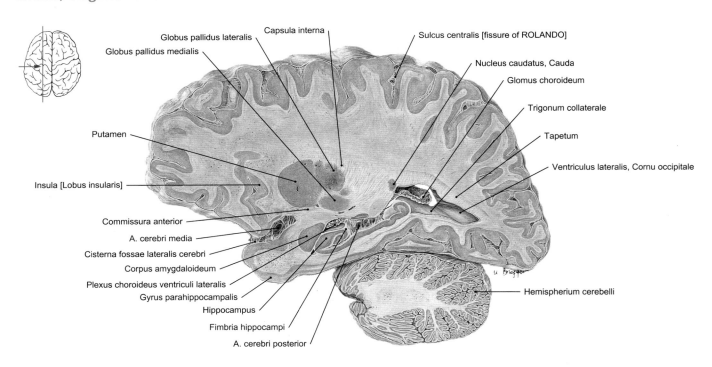

Globus pallidus lateralis
Globus pallidus medialis
Capsula interna
Sulcus centralis [fissure of ROLANDO]
Nucleus caudatus, Cauda
Glomus choroideum
Trigonum collaterale
Tapetum
Ventriculus lateralis, Cornu occipitale

Putamen

Insula [Lobus insularis]

Commissura anterior
A. cerebri media
Cisterna fossae lateralis cerebri
Corpus amygdaloideum
Plexus choroideus ventriculi lateralis
Gyrus parahippocampalis
Hippocampus
Fimbria hippocampi
A. cerebri posterior

Hemispherium cerebelli

Fig. 12.235 Brain, encephalon; sagittal section through the left hemisphere at the level of the Corpus amygdaloideum; view from the left side. [S700]
In this section, the hippocampus, the Fimbria hippocampi, and the cauda of the Nucleus caudatus are located behind the Corpus amygdaloideum. In addition, the putamen, the Globus pallidus and the Capsula interna are visible. The inferior part of this section shows the Hemispherium cerebelli.

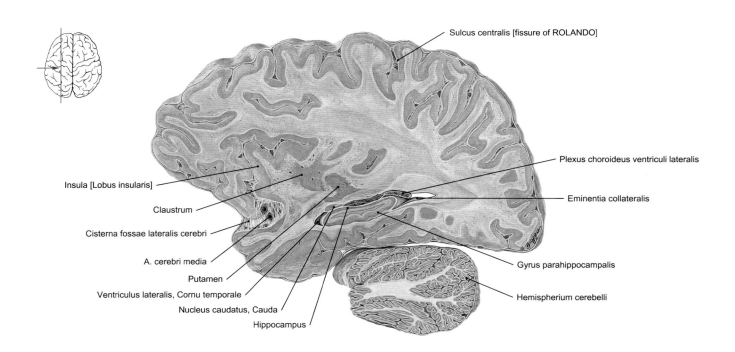

Sulcus centralis [fissure of ROLANDO]

Plexus choroideus ventriculi lateralis

Insula [Lobus insularis]

Eminentia collateralis

Claustrum

Cisterna fossae lateralis cerebri

A. cerebri media

Putamen

Ventriculus lateralis, Cornu temporale

Nucleus caudatus, Cauda

Hippocampus

Gyrus parahippocampalis

Hemispherium cerebelli

Fig. 12.236 Brain, encephalon; sagittal section through the left hemisphere at the level of the apex of the Cornu temporale of the lateral ventricle; view from the left side. [S700]
The lateral section shows the Lobus insularis. In addition, the hippocampus is visible along with the Gyrus parahippocampalis, the claustrum and the putamen.

Sample exam questions

To check that you are completely familiar with the content of this chapter, sample questions from an oral anatomy exam are listed here.

Explain the development of the nervous system:

- From which embryonic layer do the CNS and PNS develop?
- From which tissue/structure does the CNS develop?
- From which tissue/structure does the PNS develop?
- Describe the development of the mesencephalon.
- How does the pituitary gland develop?
- What originates from the prosencephalon?
- From which tissue/structure do the internal cerebrospinal fluid (CSF) spaces develop?
- Explain the development of the spinal cord.

Describe the organisation of the nervous system:

- Which parts form the brain?
- How are the respective morphological and the functional structures of the nervous system organised?
- Which lobes does the cerebrum have? Please show them.
- Describe the boundaries of the diencephalon; which parts are assigned to it?
- Describe the function of the thalamus.
- How is the grey matter respectively distributed in the brain and in the spinal cord?
- What are the functions of the hypothalamus?
- Which parts belong to the Truncus encephali?
- Name the most important fibre systems of the CNS.

Describe the structure of the meninges:

- Where is the dura mater attached to the skull? What are the Tentorium cerebelli and the Falx cerebri?
- How are the meninges supplied with blood?
- What is the Spatium subarachnoideum?
- Which nerves are involved in the innervation of the meninges?
- What is meant by bridging veins?
- How do epidural, subdural and subarachnoid haemorrhages differ from each other?

Explain the structure of the ventricular system:

- What are the internal cerebrospinal fluid (CSF) spaces?
- Describe the flow of cerebrospinal fluid.
- Where is the CSF produced?
- What is BOCHDALEK's flower basket?
- Which structures form the walls of the lateral ventricles?
- Where are physiological constrictions in the cerebrospinal fluid (CSF) system?
- Where does the cerebrospinal fluid resorption take place?
- How much cerebrospinal fluid is produced and reabsorbed each day?
- Where are enlargements of the external cerebrospinal fluid spaces?
- Where is a cerebrospinal fluid puncture typically made? Why there?
- What are the circumventricular organs?
- What are tanycytes and where do they occur?

Explain the pathway of the cerebral blood vessels:

- Make a sketch of the typical Circulus arteriosus cerebri [circle of WILLIS].

- Describe the pathway of the Aa. cerebri anterior, media and posterior.
- Name the terminal arteries provided by the A. basilaris or its branches.
- Which segments does the A. carotis interna have?
- A patient presents with a hemiparesis of the leg. Which cerebral artery can cause the blood flow/circulatory disorder?
- Which segments does the A. vertebralis have?
- What is an aneurysm? Where do aneurysms most frequently occur?
- Describe the blood supply of the cerebellum.
- Which cerebral artery is responsible, along with its branches, for the blood supply to the Capsula interna? What are the supplying blood vessels called?
- Which blood vessels supply the spinal cord?
- What signifies the A. radicularis magna, and where is it typically located? Why is it of major clinical importance to know this artery?
- Show the supply areas of the Aa. cerebri posterior, media and anterior.
- How is the venous blood drained from the surface of the brain?
- Where do intracranial veins connect with extracranial veins? Where are these venous connections located on the head?
- What are the names of the deep cerebral veins? Point them out.

Describe the structure of the cerebrum:

- What are the different parts of the cerebrum?
- Which fibre systems are found in the cerebrum?
- Show and name functional cortical areas of the cerebral hemispheres.
- Where is the primary auditory cortex located, and where is the secondary?
- What is the insula? Point it out.
- What is the hippocampal formation? Where is it?
- Which structures are connected to the hippocampus? Name connections of the hippocampal formation.
- What is called the PAPEZ circuit?
- What is meant by the cortical olfactory centre?
- To what structure do the Gyrus ambiens and the Gyrus semilunaris belong?
- Where is the Area prepiriformis?
- What are the basal ganglia? Show the corresponding nuclear areas.
- How do the basal ganglia communicate with each other?
- What is the cause of PARKINSON's disease? How does the disease manifest itself? What is its anatomic-pathological correlation?

Explain the structure of the diencephalon:

- What levels does the diencephalon have?
- Which structures are part of the epithalamus? Point them out.
- Describe afferent and efferent connections of the thalamus.
- Explain a thalamic nucleus and its associated cortical projection.
- Which regions belong to the hypothalamus?
- Which important hypothalamic nuclei and neuronal connections do you know?
- Name the hormones of the anterior pituitary gland (adenohypophysis) and of the posterior pituitary gland (neurohypophysis).
- What is described as acromegaly? What can be the cause?

Explain the structure of the mesencephalon, pons and Medulla oblongata:

- Where is the mesencephalon located? What structures are part of the mesencephalon? Point them out.
- Label horizontal sections through the mesencephalon, pons and Medulla oblongata.
- Which nuclei of cranial nerves are located in the mesencephalon, which in the pons and which in the Medulla oblongata?
- Which functional systems does the brainstem contain?
- Where is the rhomboid fossa? Point it out.
- What is meant by brainstem reflexes?

Explain the structure of the cerebellum:

- Describe the structure of the cerebellum.
- Which cerebellar nuclei do you know? Point them out.
- Which afferent and efferent connections does the cerebellum have?
- What is the main function of the cerebellum?
- Explain the blood supply of the cerebellum.

Explain the nuclear areas, pathway, fibre qualities, target organs and functions of the 12 cranial nerve pairs:

- Where do the individual cranial nerves or their branches pass through the cranial base?
- Where does/do the nuclear area(s) of the individual cranial nerves lie?
- Describe the deficits of the individual cranial nerves.
- Which cranial nerves have parasympathetic fibres?

Explain the structure of the spinal cord:

- What is an intumescentia?
- At which level does the spinal cord end?
- How is the spinal cord held in the vertebral canal?
- Which segments of the spinal cord contain parts of the sympathetic chain, and which spinal cord segments contain parts of the parasympathetic system?
- How is the grey matter arranged in the spinal cord, and how is the white matter arranged?
- How is the unconscious proprioception interconnected?
- What is the epidural space? What is inside it?
- Which reflexes are interconnected at the level of the spinal cord?

- What is the difference between a monosynaptic and a polysynaptic reflex?

Explain the somatic motor system:

- Name and point out the cortical areas that are involved in the coordination of motor functions.
- Describe the pathway of the pyramidal tract. Which fibres/tracts form the pyramidal tract?
- Explain the functional structure of the Capsula interna.
- What is the extrapyramidal motor system (EPMS)?
- What is meant by the motor end plate and the motor unit?
- How is a voluntary movement planned and executed?

Explain the somatosensory system:

- Describe the pathway of conduction of the epicritic sensibility of the spinal afferent system of the posterior funiculus and of the trigeminal afferent system for the head region.
- Describe the pathway of the unconscious proprioception (deep sensibility).
- Describe the BROWN-SÉQUARD's syndrome in the hemisection of the spinal cord at the level of, for example, T11.

Explain the olfactory, gustatory and nociceptive systems:

- Describe the stations of the olfactory tract.
- Explain the gustatory (taste) pathway and its interconnections.
- Explain the neuronal chain of the nociceptive system.
- Which ascending and descending tracts belong to the nociceptive system?

Explain the autonomic nervous system:

- Where are the sympathicus and parasympathicus located?
- How is the autonomic nervous system organised?
- Describe the interconnections, including the respective neurotransmitters.
- Explain the cranial parasympathetic system.
- Explain the sacral parasympathetic system.
- What is the sympathetic trunk?
- Name the central autonomic regions and nuclear areas in the brain.

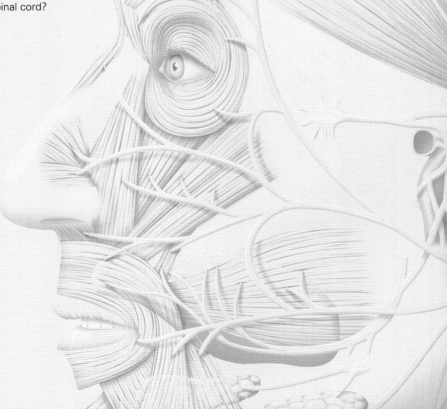

Appendix

Page numbers are in **bold** when the corresponding entries on that page are also in bold.

Index

Appendix

Index

Index

Index

Appendix

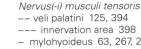

Appendix

Appendix

Appendix

Appendix

All you need for anatomy:
compatible with the 17th edition of Sobotta Atlas

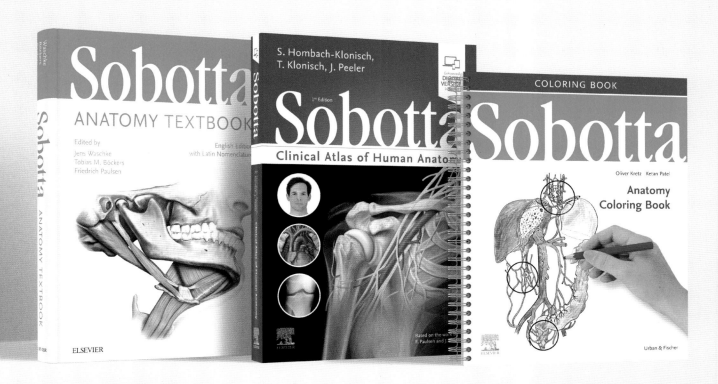
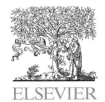